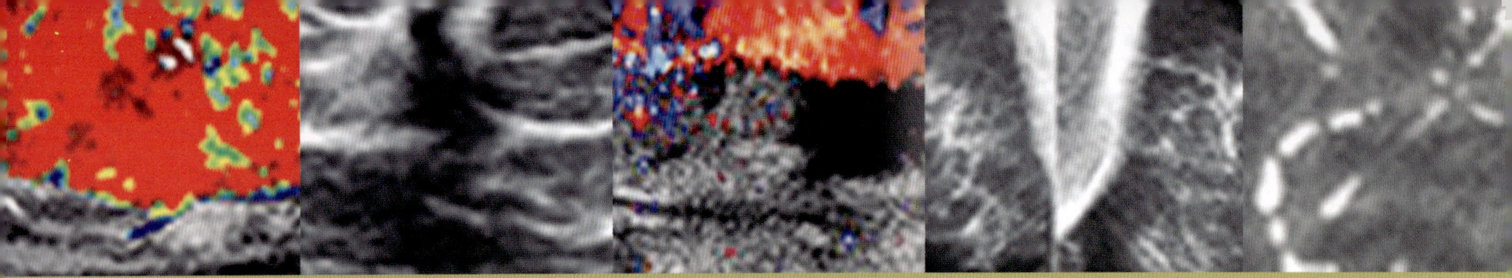

# Gastrointestinal Imaging

## THE ESSENTIALS

**Ajay K. Singh, MD**

Associate Professor of Radiology
Harvard Medical School
Associate Director of Emergency Radiology
Department of Radiology
Massachusetts General Hospital
Boston, Massachusetts

Wolters Kluwer

Philadelphia • Baltimore • New York • London
Buenos Aires • Hong Kong • Sydney • Tokyo

*Acquisitions Editor*: Ryan Shaw
*Product Development Editor*: Lauren Pecarich
*Production Project Manager*: Marian Bellus
*Senior Manufacturing Coordinator*: Beth Welsh
*Marketing Manager*: Dan Dressler
*Design Coordinator*: Joan Wendt
*Prepress Vendor*: SPi Global



9 8 7 6 5 4 3 2 1

Printed in China

---

**Library of Congress Cataloging-in-Publication Data**
Names: Singh, Ajay, 1971- , editor.
Title: Gastrointestinal imaging : the essentials / [edited by] Ajay Singh.
Other titles: Gastrointestinal imaging (Singh) | Essentials series (Philadelphia, Pa.)
Description: Philadelphia : Wolters Kluwer, [2016] | Series: Essentials series | Includes bibliographical references and index.
Identifiers: LCCN 2015040534 | ISBN 9781496307194
Subjects: | MESH: Diagnostic Imaging—methods. | Digestive System Diseases—diagnosis. | Diagnostic Techniques, Digestive System.
Classification: LCC RC78.7.D53 | NLM WI 141 | DDC 616.07/54—dc23 LC record available at http://lccn.loc.gov/2015040534

---



LWW.com

RRS1602

*I dedicate this book to my children, Avani and Ashvin Singh. Thank you for your love and support every step of the way. I also want to thank my parents for their unconditional support for my pursuits.*

# CONTRIBUTORS


**Kamran Ali, MD**
Associate Clinical Professor
Department of Radiology
University of Kansas—Wichita
Wichita, Kansas

**Shweta Bhatt, MD**
Associate Professor of Radiology
Department of Imaging Sciences
University of Rochester Medical Center
Rochester, New York

**Akshya Gupta, MD**
Department of Imaging Sciences
University of Rochester Medical Center
Rochester, New York

**Rathachai Kaewlai, MD**
Department of Diagnostic and Therapeutic Radiology
Ramathibodi Hospital, Mahidol University
Bangkok, Thailand

**Alexander Kessler, MD**
Radiology Resident
University of Rochester Medical Center
Rochester, New York

**Amisha Khicha, MD**
Assistant Clinical Professor
Department of Radiology
University of Kansas—Wichita
Wichita, Kansas

**Vijetha Vinod Maller, MD**
Department of Radiology
University of Tennessee Health Science Center
Memphis, Tennessee

**Travis McKenzie, DO**
Department of Radiology
University of Kansas—Wichita
Wichita, Kansas

**Caterina Missiroli, MD**
Department of Radiology
Azienda Ospedaliera della Provincia di Lecco
Lecco, Italy
Azienda Ospedaliera ASST Nord, Ospedale Bassini
Milano, Italy

**Refky Nicola, MS, DO**
Assistant Professor of Imaging Sciences and Emergency Medicine
Department of Radiology
University of Rochester Medical Center
Rochester, New York

**J. Paul Nielsen, MD, MPH**
Clinical Fellow (Body Imaging)
Department of Radiology
University of Colorado Anschutz Medical Campus
Golden, Colorado

**Randall L. Scott, MD**
Department of Radiology
University of Tennessee Health Science Center
Memphis, Tennessee

**Sridhar Shankar, MD, MBA**
Professor of Radiology
Department of Radiology
University of Tennessee Health Science Center
Memphis, Tennessee

**Ajay K. Singh, MD**
Associate Director of Emergency Radiology
Department of Radiology
Massachusetts General Hospital
Harvard Medical School
Boston, Massachusetts

**Sirote Wongwaisayawan, MD**
Department of Diagnostic and Therapeutic Radiology
Ramathibodi Hospital, Mahidol University
Bangkok, Thailand

# SERIES FOREWORD

The *Essentials* series is a collection of radiology textbooks following a standardized format. Each book in the *Essentials* series is a practical tool for those wanting to quickly acquire a broad base of knowledge in a specialty area. The content is limited to the essentials of that specialty so as not to overwhelm the novice, yet provides enough detail that it can serve as a quick review for residents or practicing radiologists, a guide for those who teach the specialty, and a reference for specialty physicians and other health care professionals whose patients are referred for imaging in that specialty area. What sets *Essentials* texts apart from other similar texts is that they (a) are compact and of practical size for a resident to read during an initial 4-week rotational experience, (b) include learning objectives at the beginning of each chapter, and (c) provide an exercise for self-assessment. Each book includes citations from the most recent literature that are called out in the text.

Self-assessment is a key component of the *Essentials* texts. Multiple-choice items are included at the end of every chapter, and a self-assessment examination is included at the end of each text. This should be of particular benefit to those who are preparing for the new image-rich computer-based examinations that are a component of professional certification and maintenance of certification.

The series not only includes texts related to clinical specialties that are rich with radiologic images and illustrations but also texts related to noninterpretive subjects such as radiologic physics and quality and safety in medical imaging. The goal of the *Essentials* series is to provide a collection of practical references to accompany a well-rounded education in diagnostic imaging and imaging-guided therapy.

JANNETTE COLLINS, MD, MED, FCCP, FACR

# PREFACE

Because of the rapid advances in imaging technology, it has become necessary for the radiologist to be familiar not only with the conventional fluoroscopy imaging techniques but also with the contemporary cross-sectional imaging modalities. Imaging plays a pivotal role in the early detection as well as treatment of a number of gastrointestinal pathologies, including appendicitis and diverticulitis. The rapid advances in the field of radiology have significantly improved our ability to diagnose a gastrointestinal pathology as well as triage the patient.

The chapters in this book are divided into a didactic section, followed by multiple choice questions, most of which involve careful assessment of conventional or advanced imaging. We have compiled a group of well-known experts in the field of gastrointestinal radiology to author the 11 chapters in this book. Barium studies and MR imaging have been given extra emphasis in the chapters and subsequent multiple choice questions.

**Ajay K. Singh, MD**

# ACKNOWLEDGMENTS

First, I am grateful to hundreds of my residents who helped me in collecting the clinical material needed to embark on the first addition of this book. I am also indebted to them for providing honest feedbacks to make this book effective in terms of its content and multiple choice questions.

I must thank my colleagues, especially Dr. Michael Lev, Robert Novelline, Laura Avery, Parul Penkar, Efren Flores, and Stephanie Geohagen, for their help in providing relevant suggestions.

Finally, I want to thank my son Ashvin Singh and daughter Avani Singh, who have always facilitated this project.

# CONTENTS

# Barium Studies: The Basics 1

*Ajay K. Singh*

## LEARNING OBJECTIVES

1. Describe various barium studies used to diagnose gastrointestinal pathologies.
2. Study the imaging features of bowel wall masses, ulcers, polyps, strictures, and diverticula.

## BARIUM SWALLOW AND UPPER GASTROINTESTINAL SERIES

- At the beginning of the examination, 0.1 mg of glucagon is injected intravenously (hypotonic agent to relax the duodenum and stomach).
- Use of thick barium along with effervescent crystals to produce double-contrast effect (best to evaluate mucosal abnormalities).
- Effervescent crystals are ingested with 10 mL of water (releases 300 to 400 mL of carbon dioxide).
- As a general rule, one should back up verbal command to the patient with tactile command while performing barium studies.
- Palpation of a specific organ is best performed in supine position with a gloved hand.
- Keep the image intensifier as close to the patient as possible. The spot images for upper GI series are typically taken at 100 kVp.

## EVALUATION OF THE ESOPHAGUS

- With the patient upright in *left posterior oblique* position (to prevent the spine from obscuring the esophagus), high-density barium (250% w/v) is given and multiple spot views of the esophagus are obtained (Figs. 1.1 and 1.2).
- With the patient lying prone *right anterior oblique* on the table, thin barium is given to get single-contrast images of the thoracic esophagus.
- Gastroesophageal reflux can be tested with Valsalva maneuver and water siphon test. Water siphon test: With the patient in supine position, 50 mL of water is given through a straw. If no gastroesophageal reflux is demonstrated, the patient lies in the *right posterior oblique* position and again drinks water. In this position, the GE junction is in dependent position. The sensitivity of barium study in detecting spontaneous gastroesophageal reflux is 20% to 35%. The sensitivity increases to 70% with the use of water siphon test, when compared with pH monitoring. The sensitivity for detection of reflux esophagitis is up to 90% on double-contrast study.
- If there is a sensation of food getting stuck in the esophagus, a 13-mm tablet is given with a mouthful of water.

## EVALUATION OF THE STOMACH AND DUODENUM

- The patient is laid supine, following which the patient is made to roll 360 degrees so as to coat all walls of the stomach. Multiple views of the stomach and duodenum are obtained, including *supine*, *right posterior oblique*, and *left posterior oblique*.
- The patient rests with the *right side down*, and views of the gastroesophageal junction and cardia are taken.
- With the table positioned at 45 degrees, additional views of the stomach are taken in *oblique positions*.
- Double-contrast view of the duodenal bulb is taken in *left posterior oblique* position (Fig. 1.3). Single-contrast view of the duodenal bulb is obtained with the patient *prone and left side up*.

## SMALL BOWEL FOLLOW-THROUGH

- Small bowel follow-through study is a single-contrast study of the small bowel, which uses a minimum of 16 ounces (500 to 1,000 mL) of 30% to 50% w/v low-density barium. A combination of fluoroscopy and spot images of the small bowel is obtained every 15 to 45 minutes in the *prone* position (Fig. 1.4).
- The duration of the small bowel follow-through can be shortened by giving 20 mg of metoclopramide orally 30 minutes before the start of the study.
- The ileocecal junction visualization is best obtained using spot films, often in the *left posterior oblique* position.

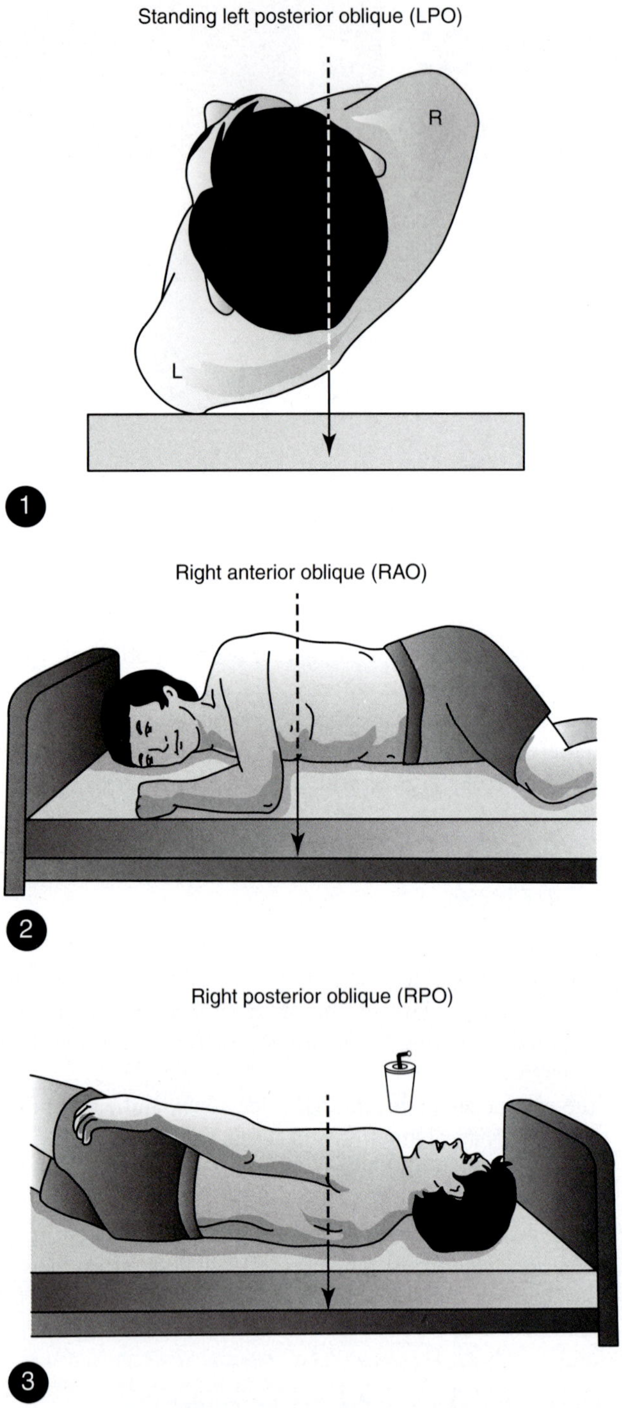


**FIG. 1.1 • Patient positioning during barium swallow study.** The schematic diagram depicts the three most important positions of the patient during barium swallow study. The standing left posterior oblique and prone right anterior oblique positions allow double- and single-contrast assessment of the esophagus, respectively. The supine right posterior oblique position is for the evaluation of gastroesophageal reflux during the siphon test.

- *Peroral pneumocolon* involves inflation of the colon with air injected through a rectal tube. It is performed at the end of the small bowel follow-through study to provide a double-contrast evaluation of the terminal ileum. The rectal tube is introduced in *lateral decubitus* position, following which the patient is placed *prone* to allow air to reflux into the terminal ileum. This is most often used in patients with Crohn disease with terminal ileitis.
- The normal transit time ranges from 30 to 120 minutes.
- Limitation of the small bowel follow-through study is incomplete distention of the small bowel loops because of which strictures and filling defects may not be well evaluated.

## ENTEROCLYSIS

- The patient's small bowel and colon are cleared using clear liquid diet and bisacodyl on the day prior to the examination.
- Metoclopramide is given IV (10 mg; just before the test) or orally (20 mg; 30 minutes before test) before the examination.
- A 10-French enteroclysis catheter is passed just beyond the duodenojejunal junction for double-contrast enteroclysis study. The balloon is inflated so as to prevent reflux of contrast into the stomach.
- For single-contrast enteroclysis, approximately 1 L of low-density barium is injected at the rate of 75 mL/m.
- For double-contrast enteroclysis, 50% w/v barium is injected at the rate of 75 mL/m, following which either air or methylcellulose is injected to produce a double-contrast effect (Fig. 1.5).[1]

## BARIUM ENEMA

- Single-contrast barium enema examination is performed using 20% w/v barium preparation, while double-contrast barium enema is performed using 80% to 100% w/v barium preparation.
- The patient is on clear liquid diet for 24 hours and also takes a laxative (bisacodyl tablets + suppository) for 24 hours.
- One milligram of glucagon can be given IV to induce colonic hypotonia. This is contraindicated in patients with insulinoma and pheochromocytoma.
- During double-contrast examination, the barium is injected through a rectal tube with the patient in prone or left lateral position until the barium reaches the mid–transverse colon. Following this, air is injected via the rectal tube to produce a double-contrast effect and push the barium into the proximal colon.
- The patient is rolled on his or her right side so as to help move the barium into the hepatic flexure, following which he or she is placed supine to move the contrast into the ascending colon. To help move the contrast into the cecum, the patient can be turned left side down or semierect.
- Spot fluoroscopic images are obtained after injection of air, starting from the rectum to the cecum. Spot images of the sigmoid colon should be obtained before the barium reaches the cecum as reflux of contrast into the ileum can obscure visualization of the sigmoid colon.[2]

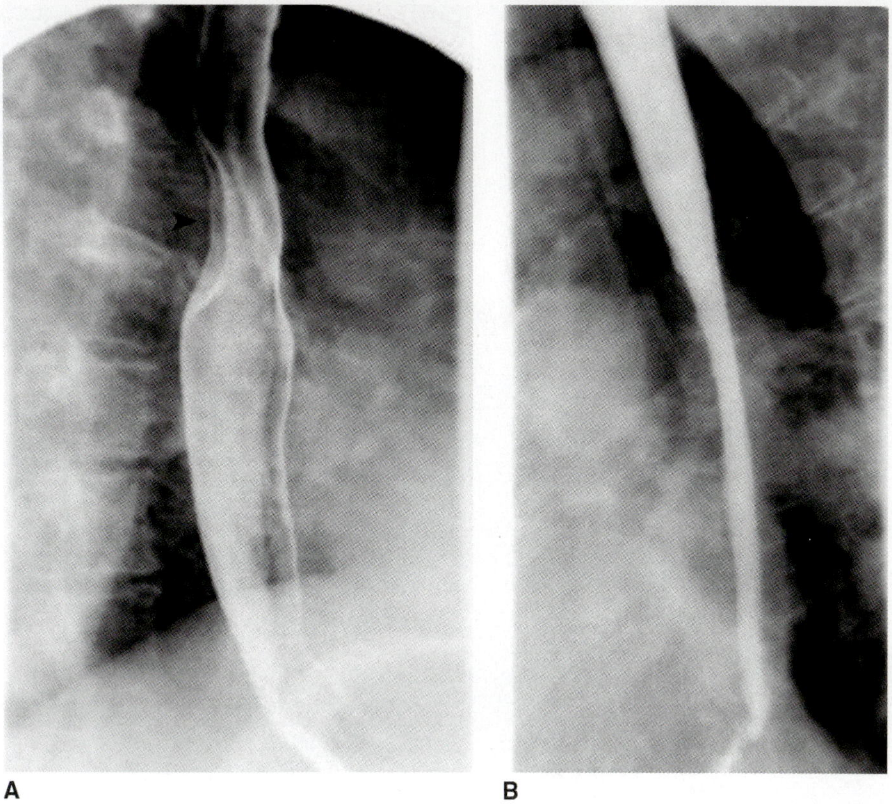

**FIG. 1.2 • Barium swallow study views.** **A:** The left posterior oblique view of the esophagus demonstrates double-contrast assessment of the esophagus. Note that the esophagus does not overlap the spine on this view. The patient has a submucosal leiomyoma in the posterior esophageal wall. **B:** The prone right anterior oblique view of the esophagus demonstrates a single-contrast assessment of the esophagus with long smooth narrowing of the lower thoracic esophagus in a patient with reflux esophagitis.

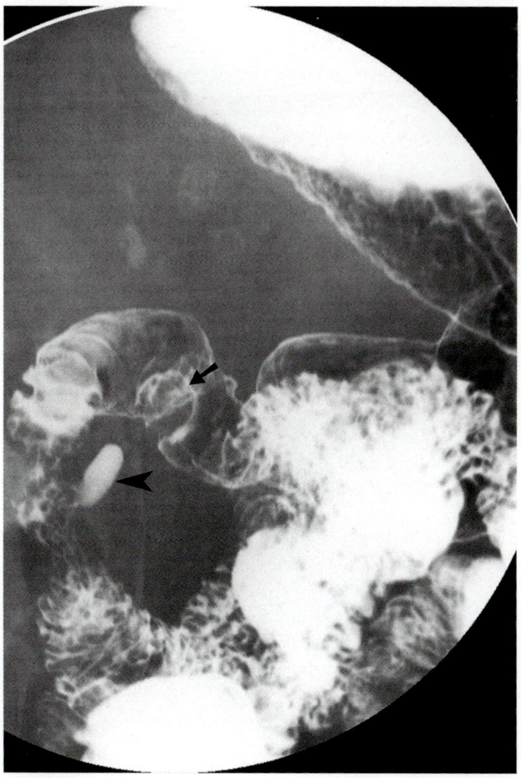

**FIG. 1.3 • Duodenal assessment on UGI series.** Left posterior oblique view of the duodenum demonstrates double-contrast assessment of the duodenum bulb. The patient has an incidental duodenal diverticulum (*arrowhead*) and antral polyp (*arrow*).

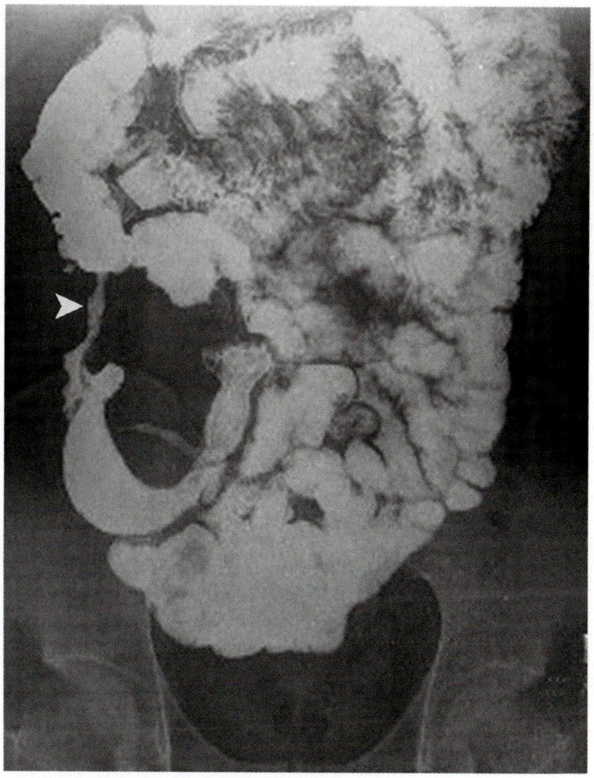

**FIG. 1.4 • Small bowel follow-through.** Prone film of the abdomen demonstrates opacification of the small bowel loops at 30 minutes. There is a terminal ileal stricture (*arrowhead*) secondary to chronic Crohn disease.

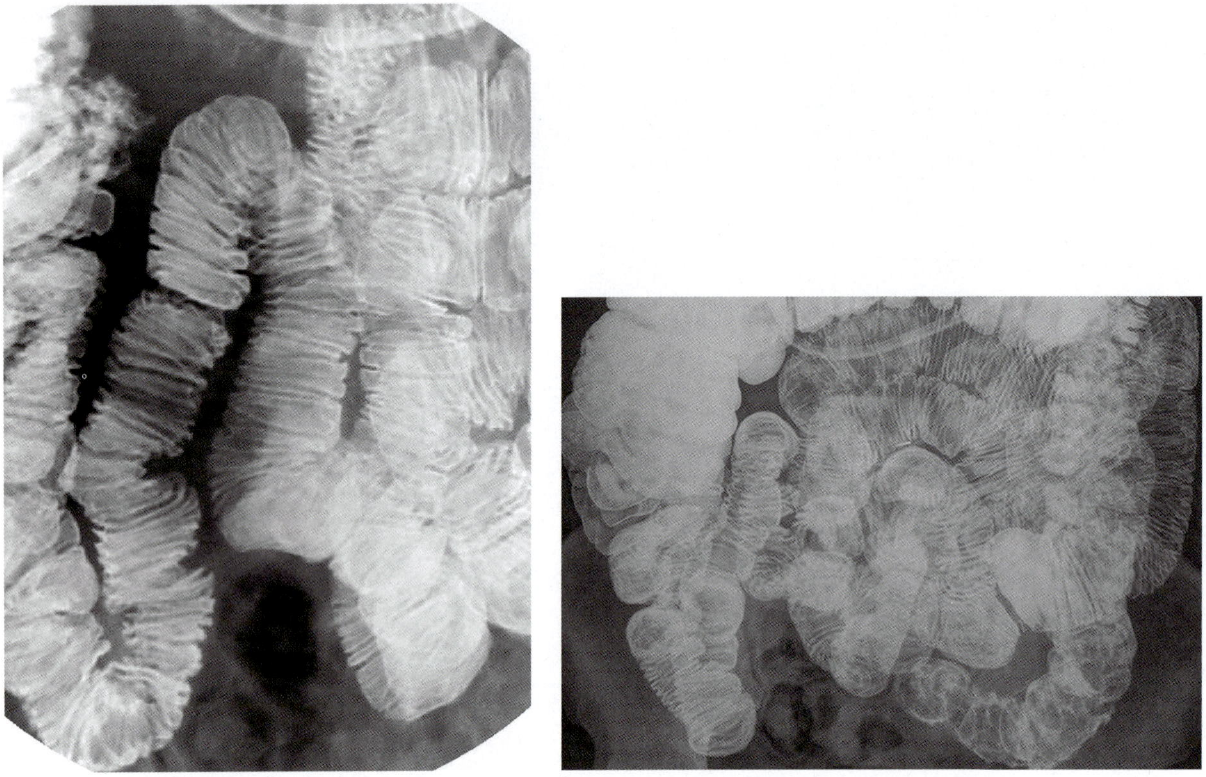

A B

**FIG. 1.5 • Double-contrast enteroclysis.** Spot film **(A)** and prone film **(B)** of the abdomen demonstrates excellent double-contrast evaluation of the valvulae conniventes in the small bowel loops. The overhead film also demonstrates opacification of the colonic loop, which can sometimes obscure the adjacent small bowel loops.

- The spot images obtained during barium enema include the following:
  1. *Lateral and PA views* of the rectum
  2. *Lateral view* of the rectosigmoid junction
  3. Sigmoid colon views in the *left posterior oblique position*
  4. Distal sigmoid colon, often best seen in the *supine or right posterior oblique position*
  5. *Upright views* of the hepatic flexure, transverse colon, and splenic flexure
  6. Splenic flexure, best imaged upright, in the *right posterior oblique position*
  7. Hepatic flexure, best imaged upright, in the *left posterior oblique position*
  8. The cecum, viewed in the *left posterior oblique and right posterior oblique* positions
- To remove excess of barium from the cecum, the patient can be placed in Trendelenburg position so as to remove the contrast into the ascending colon, following which the patient can be turned to the left.
- Overhead abdominal radiographs are obtained after spot images (prone-angled and right and left lateral decubitus views). Rectosigmoid junction can be well evaluated on the prone overhead film with the tube angled 30 degrees caudally (Fig. 1.6).
- Single-contrast barium enema examination involves rectal infusion of low-density barium contrast with the patient in the left lateral position. After examination of the rectum, the patient is still into the supine position, and graded manual compression is applied to evaluate different parts of the colon.

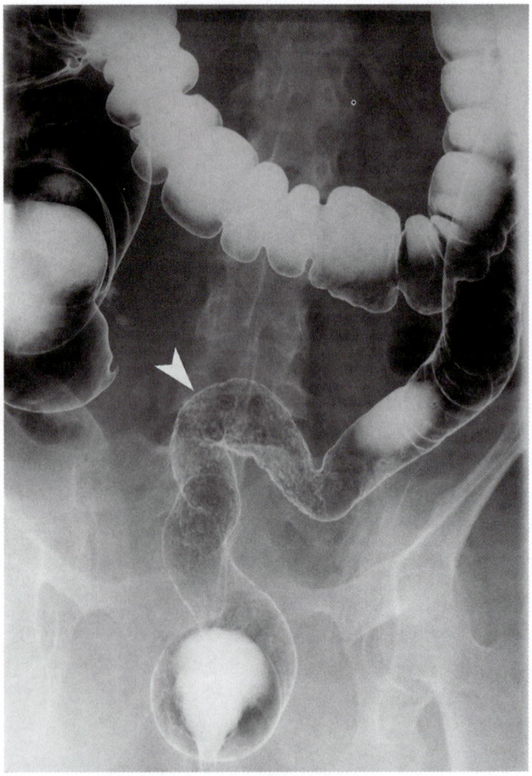

**FIG. 1.6 • Barium enema.** Overhead prone film of the abdomen with 30-degree caudal angulation of the tube allows clear assessment of the granular mucosa (*arrowhead*) of the sigmoid colon in a patient with Crohn colitis.

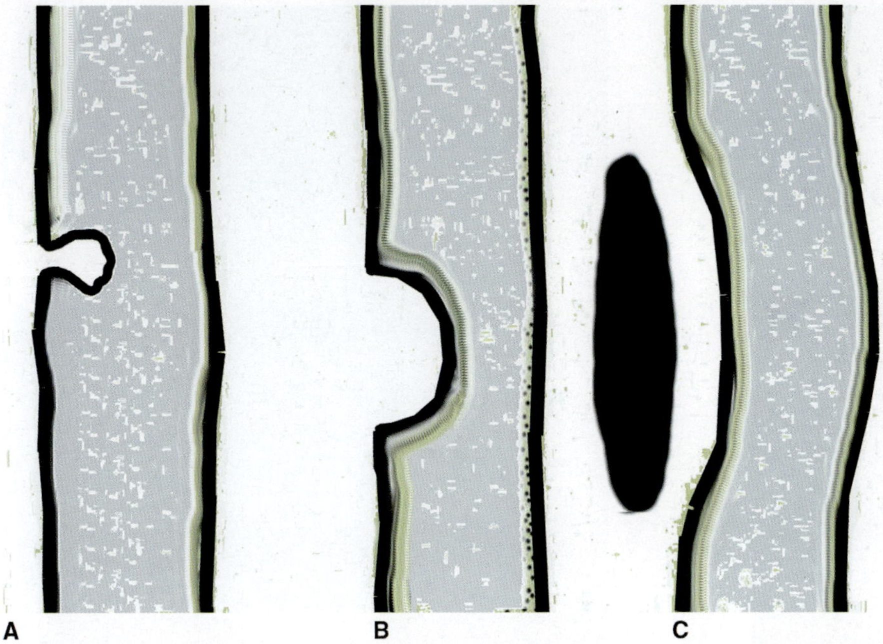


**FIG. 1.7 • Bowel mass assessment in relation to the bowel wall.** Schematic diagram depicts mucosal **(A)**, submucosal **(B)**, and extrinsic lesions **(C)**. The mucosal lesion forms an acute angle, while the submucosal lesion forms a right angle or slightly obtuse angle with the bowel wall. Extrinsic impression by a mass causes an obtuse angle with the bowel wall and often displaces the bowel wall away from its normal location.

## LOCALIZING A MASS IN THE BOWEL WALL

- Mucosal mass: Mucosal polyps can be sessile or pedunculated. Mucosal polyps that are pedunculated form an acute angle with the adjacent bowel wall (Figs. 1.7 and 1.8). These polyps are most commonly hyperplastic in the stomach and adenomatous or hamartomatous in the small bowel. Multiple mucosal polyps indicate the presence of a polyposis syndrome such as familial adenomatous polyposis and Peutz-Jeghers syndrome.

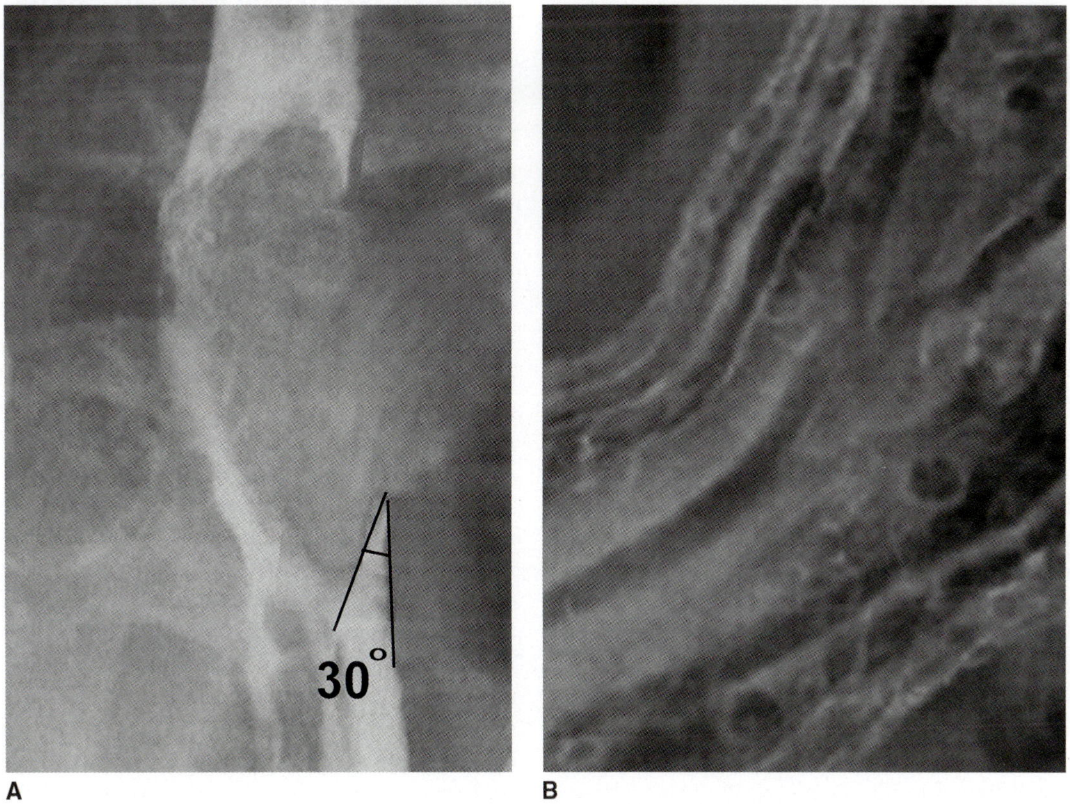


**FIG. 1.8 • Mucosal mass (squamous cell carcinoma and hyperplastic polyps). A:** Barium swallow study demonstrates an irregular marginated, large filling defect in the upper thoracic esophagus, forming an acute angle with the esophageal wall. **B:** Double-contrast upper GI series demonstrates multiple polyps in the stomach, seen as round or oval filling defects, etched in white.

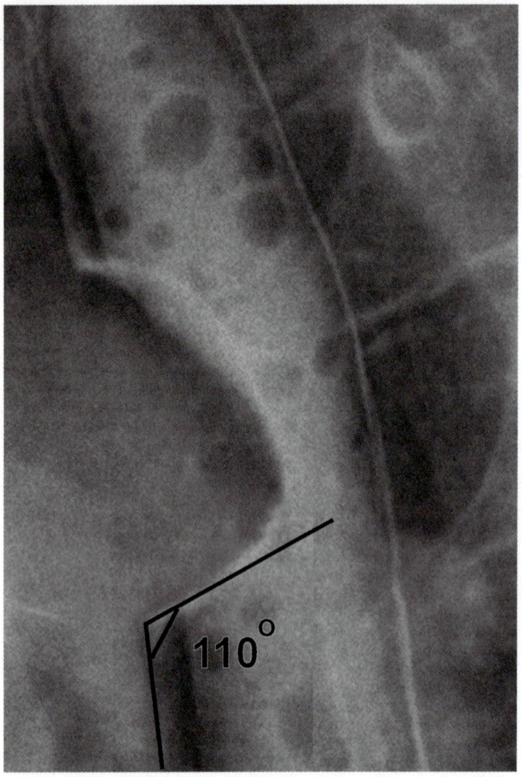


**FIG. 1.9 • Submucosal mass (leiomyoma).** Barium swallow study demonstrates a smooth hemispherical filling defect in the upper thoracic esophagus, forming a slightly obtuse angle with the esophageal wall.

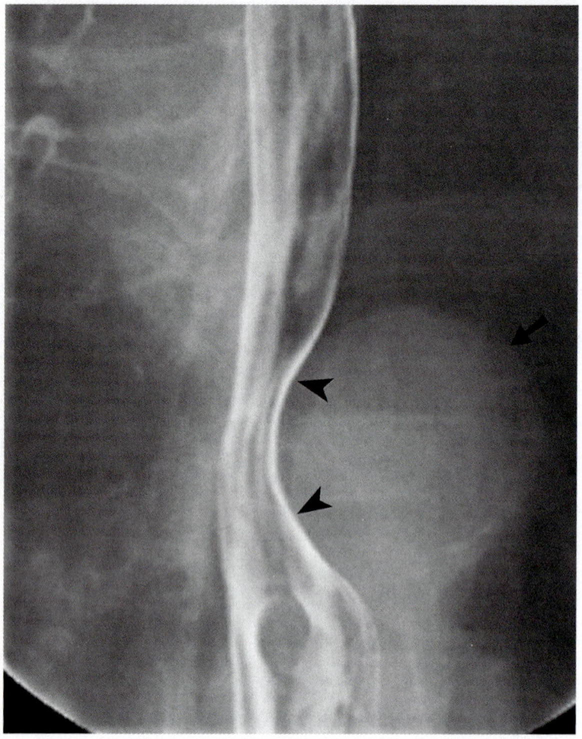

**FIG. 1.10 • Extrinsic impression by aortic aneurysm.** Double-contrast barium swallow study demonstrates an extrinsic impression (*arrowheads*) on the anterior aspect of the upper thoracic esophagus, caused by aneurysm (*arrow*) of the aortic arch.

The Mexican hat sign is seen on en face view of a pedunculated polyp, where the outer ring is produced by the head of the polyp and the inner ring is produced by the stalk of the polyp. The bowler hat sign can be seen with a polyp or a diverticulum. If the bowler hat points toward the bowel lumen, it represents a polyp. If it points away from the bowel lumen, it represents a diverticulum.

- Submucosal mass: On double-contrast barium swallow study, a submucosal mass is typically seen as a smooth hemispherical filling defect, which forms a right angle or slightly obtuse angle with the adjacent bowel wall (Fig. 1.9). The differential diagnosis of submucosal bowel mass includes leiomyoma, gastrointestinal stromal tumor, lipoma, hamartoma, hemangioma, neurofibroma, granular cell tumor, and duplication cyst. Multiple submucosal masses could be from granular cell tumor, hemangioma, Kaposi sarcoma, and lymphoma. Approximately 50% of these submucosal masses develop central necrosis resulting in an ulcerated submucosal mass, known as bull's-eye or target lesion. The differential diagnosis of multiple submucosal masses in the small bowel includes metastasis (melanoma—breast and lung carcinoma), lymphoma, carcinoid, neurofibroma, and Kaposi sarcoma.[3]
- Extrinsic mass: Extrinsic impression results in an obtuse angle with the bowel wall. The epicenter of the apparent filling defect is outside the bowel wall (Fig. 1.10).

## DIFFERENTIATING A BENIGN FROM MALIGNANT STRICTURE

Benign strictures are often smooth, symmetric, long-segment, tapered, concentric narrowing without associated ulcerations or nodular defects (Figs. 1.11 and 1.12).[4] Malignant structures are often short-segment, asymmetric narrowing with mucosal ulcerations, nodularity, and shouldering (Fig. 1.13).

## DIFFERENTIATING A BENIGN FROM MALIGNANT ULCER

Erosion refers to mucosal or lamina propria necrosis, not extending into the muscularis mucosa. Unlike ulcer, erosion does not extend into submucosa. They are 1 to 2 mm deep collections of barium, surrounded by rims of edematous mucosa and often located on antral rugal folds (Fig. 1.14).[5]

Ninety-five percent of the ulcers in the United States are benign ulcers. The imaging features of a benign gastric ulcer includes ulcer crater that extends beyond the expected outline of the bowel contour (on profile view) (Fig. 1.15). A benign ulcer has a smooth ulcer mound caused by edema with gastric folds extending to the edge of the ulcer crater. Hampton line is considered diagnostic of benign gastric ulcer and is seen as a thin lucent line across the neck of the gastric ulcer, produced by undermining of the gastric mucosa. Small ulcers along the lesser curvature and antrum are most often benign.

Malignant gastric ulcers do not protrude beyond the expected outline of the bowel. They often demonstrate an irregular ulcer

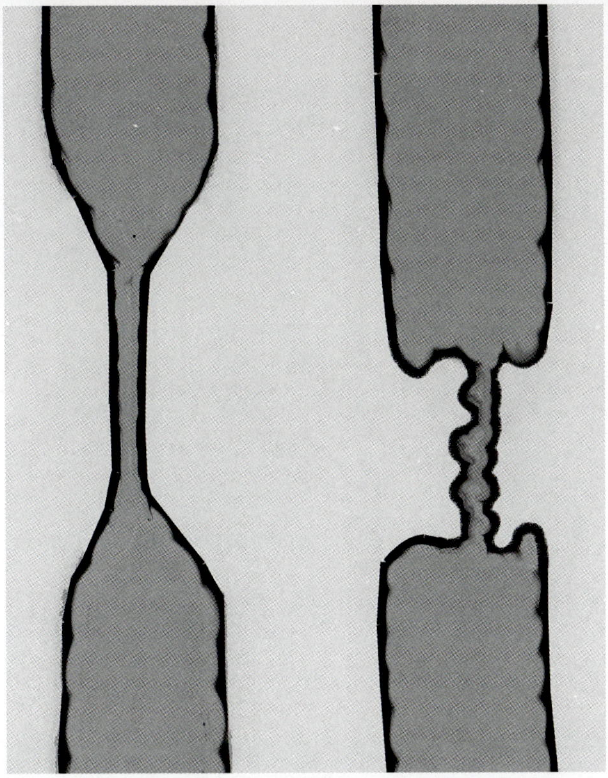

**A** **B**

**FIG. 1.11 • Benign and malignant strictures of bowel.** The schematic diagram depicts the configuration of benign and malignant strictures of the bowel. A benign stricture **(A)** shows long, symmetrical, smooth, and concentric narrowing, while a malignant stricture **(B)** shows more focal, asymmetric narrowing with nodular filling defects, ulcerations, and proximal as well as distal shouldering.

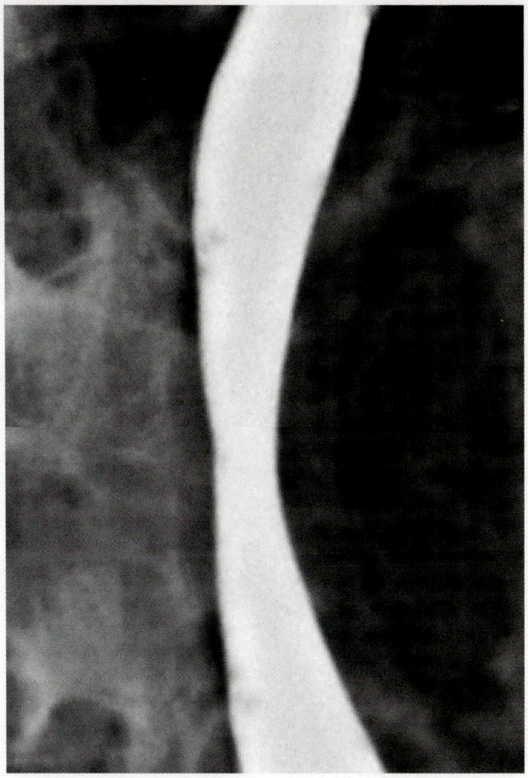

**FIG. 1.12 • Benign stricture of the esophagus.** Single-contrast barium swallow study demonstrates a long tapered narrowing of the thoracic esophagus in a patient with reflux esophagitis.

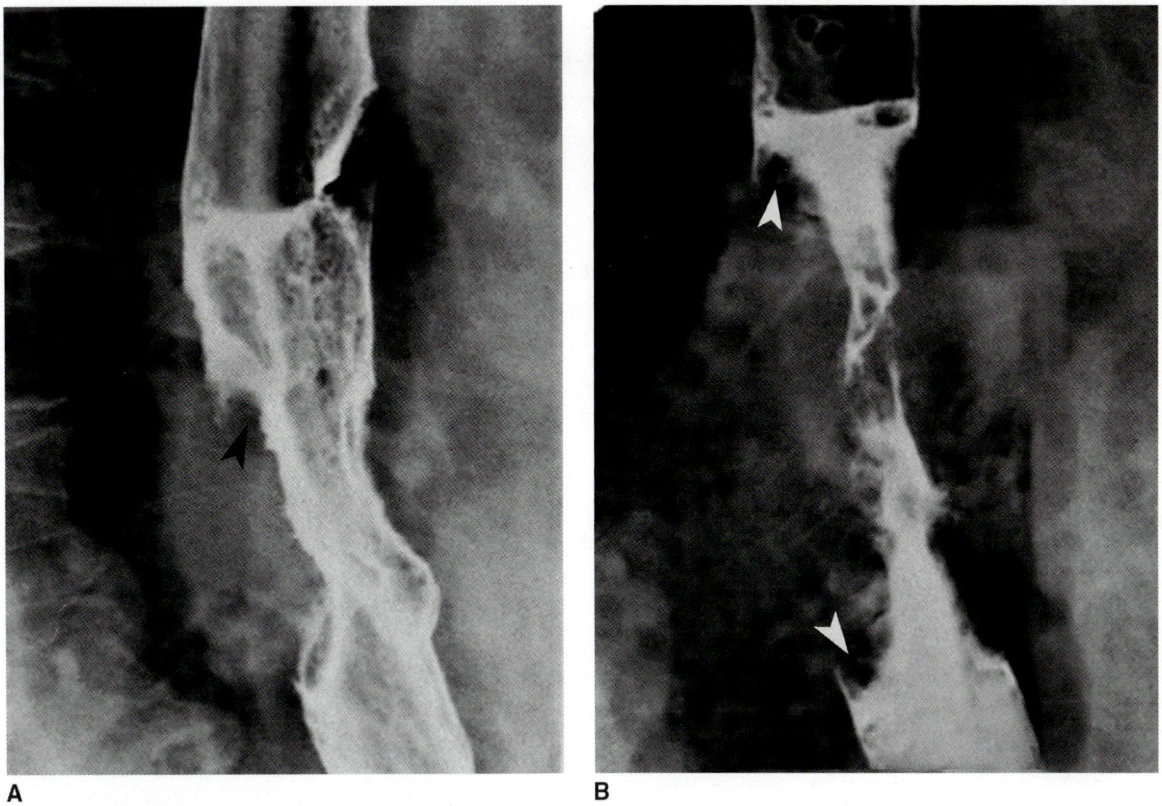

**A** **B**

**FIG. 1.13 • Malignant stricture from squamous cell carcinoma. A, B:** Double-contrast barium swallow examination demonstrates malignant strictures of the esophagus with shouldering (*arrowheads*), ulcerations, and nodular filling defects.

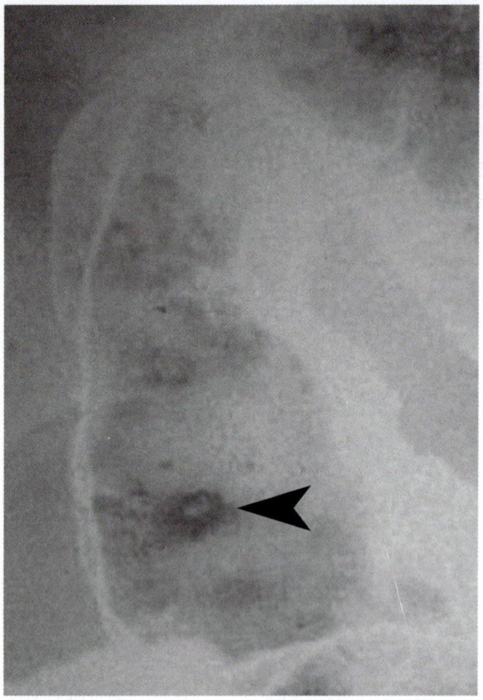

**FIG. 1.14 • Aphthoid ulcer in Crohn disease.** Double-contrast barium enema examination demonstrates an aphthoid ulcer (*arrowhead*) in the colonic wall.

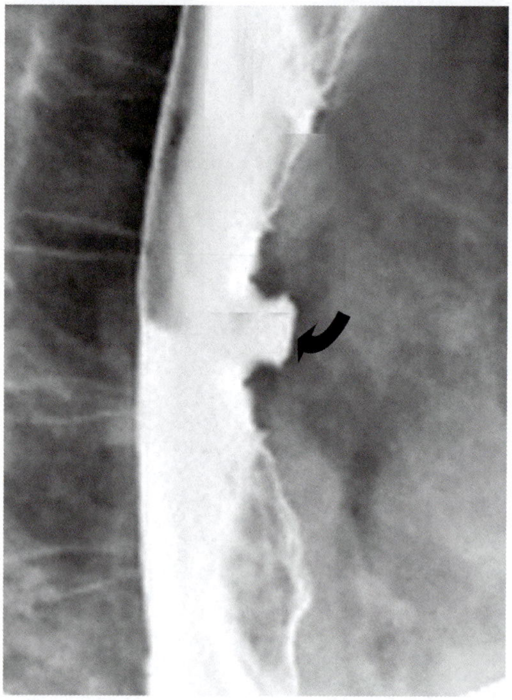

**FIG. 1.16 • Malignant ulcer in esophageal cancer.** Barium swallow study demonstrates an ulcer crater (*curved arrow*) present within an esophageal mass with an irregular ulcer mound.

crater with nodularity in the margin and surrounding mucosal folds, which do not extend to the edge of the ulcer crater (Fig. 1.16). The majority of the ulcers in the gastric fundus are malignant.

## DIVERTICULUM

A diverticulum is a smoothly marginated outpouching from the bowel, most commonly arising from the colon (Fig. 1.17). True diverticula are congenital and contain all layers of the bowel wall. False diverticula constitute the majority of the gastrointestinal tract diverticula and consist only of the mucosal layer herniating out through a defect in the muscular layer. True diverticula of the small bowel arise on the antimesenteric border, while false diverticula arise on the mesenteric border of the small bowel. The bowler hat sign points away from the bowel lumen in a diverticulum.[6] A traction diverticulum has a muscular layer in the wall and is caused by inflammatory process, such as tubercular lymphadenitis. A pulsion diverticulum does not have a muscle layer in the wall and is caused by bowel wall dysmotility. It often has a rounded configuration with a wide neck, while a traction diverticulum often has a tented or triangular configuration.

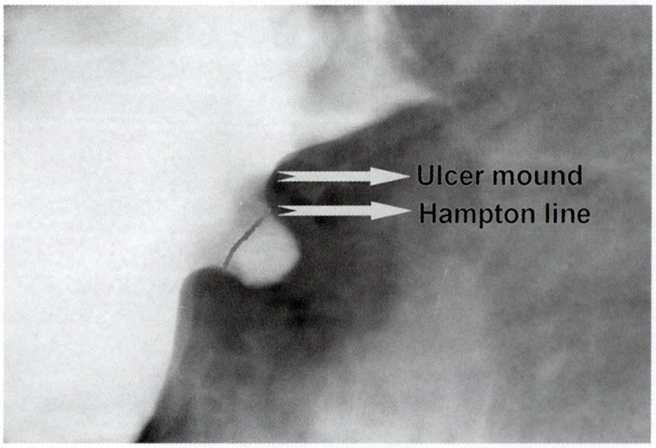


**FIG. 1.15 • Benign gastric benign ulcer.** In profile view demonstrates a benign gastric ulcer with symmetrical ulcer mound caused by edema. A thin Hampton line is drawn across the neck of the ulcer crater and is due to undermining of the mucosa.

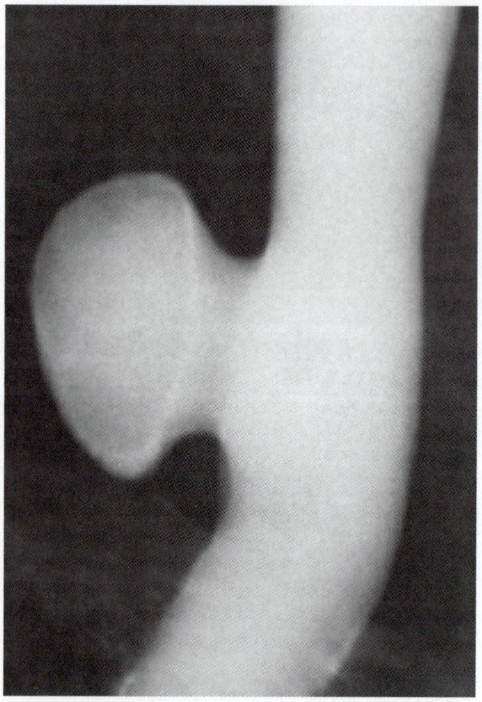

**FIG. 1.17 • Pulsion diverticulum of the esophagus.** Single-contrast esophagram study demonstrates a smooth mushroom-shaped outpouching with no mucosal irregularity or ulceration.

## ANATOMICAL MEASUREMENTS

- Schatzki ring: less than 12 mm (symptomatic)
- Esophageal longitudinal fold thickness: 1 to 3 mm
- Areae gastricae size: Antrum 2 to 3 mm, and body/fundus 3 to 5 mm (seen in 70%)
- Gastric rugal fold thickness: 3 to 5 mm[5]
- Valvulae conniventes thickness: Jejunum 2 to 3 mm, and ileum 1 to 2 mm (less than 3 mm thickness in jejunum and less than 2 mm thickness in ileum is considered abnormal)
- Bowel wall thickness: Stomach 2 to 5 mm, and small bowel 1 to 1.5 mm
- Small bowel caliber: Jejunum less than 3 cm, ileum less than 2.5 cm, and colon less than 6 cm
- Small bowel caliber (enteroclysis) Jejunum less than 4 cm, and ileum less than 3 cm
- Air–fluid levels: Up to two are normal on upright abdominal radiograph[7]

### References

1. Richard M, Gore RM, Levine MS. *Textbook of Gastrointestinal Radiology*. 3rd ed. Philadelphia, PA: Saunders; 2007.
2. Rubesin SE, Levine MS, Laufer I, et al. Double-contrast barium enema examination technique. *Radiology*. 2000;215:642–650.
3. Levine MS, Rubesin SE, Laufer I. Pattern approach for diseases of mesenteric small bowel on barium studies. *Radiology*. 2008;249:445–460.
4. Gupta S, Levine MS, Rubesin SE, et al. Usefulness of barium studies for differentiating benign and malignant strictures of the esophagus. *AJR Am J Roentgenol*. 2003;180(3):737–744.
5. Rubesin SE, Levine MS, Laufer I. Double-contrast, upper gastrointestinal radiography: a pattern approach for diseases of the stomach. *Radiology*. 2008;246(1):33–48.
6. Miller WT Jr, Levine MS, Rubesin SE, et al. Bowler-hat sign: a simple principle for differentiating polyps from diverticula. *Radiology*. 1989 Dec;173(3):615–617.
7. Silva AC, Pimenta M, Guimarães LS. Small bowel obstruction: what to look for. *Radiographics*. 2009;29(2):423–439. http://www.ncbi.nlm.nih.gov/pubmed/19325057

## SELF-ASSESSMENT QUESTIONS

1. A barium enema depicted an abnormality (arrowhead) on the spot film. What is the likely cause of the abnormality?

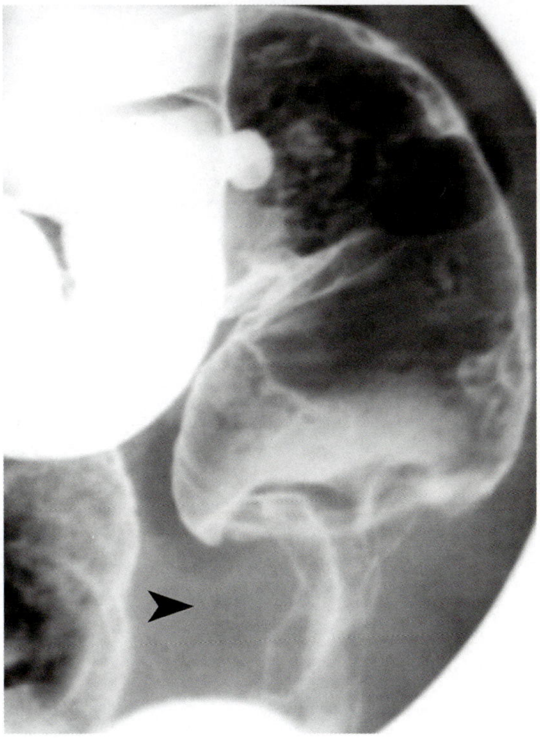

A. Crohn disease
B. Adenocarcinoma
C. Tuberculosis
D. Villous polyp

2. What is the best view to evaluate the splenic flexure during barium enema?

A. Upright right posterior oblique position
B. Upright left posterior oblique position
C. Left lateral position
D. Supine left posterior oblique position

3. What is the abnormality depicted on the barium swallow of a patient with dysphagia?

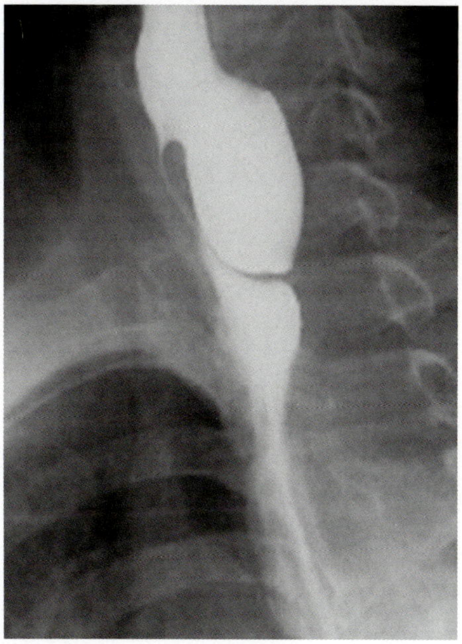

A. Diverticulum
B. Ulcer
C. Neoplasm
D. Perforation

4. What is the abnormality depicted on a single-contrast barium enema of a patient with chronic recurrent abdominal pain?

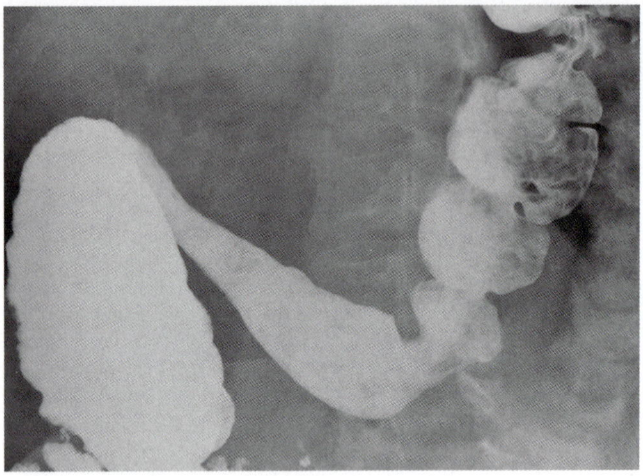

   A. Malignant stricture
   B. Benign stricture
   C. Extrinsic impression
   D. Colonic spasm

5. What is the dose of glucagon used intravenously before barium enema examination?
   A. 0.1 mg
   B. 0.2 mg
   C. 1.0 mg
   D. 5 mg

## *Answers to Self-Assessment Questions*

**1. B.** The double-contrast barium enema demonstrates an apple core lesion (arrowhead), which is diagnostic of a malignant stricture.

**2. A.** The upright right posterior oblique view demonstrates the splenic flexure, while the upright left posterior oblique view demonstrates the hepatic flexure.

**3. A.** Diverticulum. The barium swallow study demonstrates a Zenker diverticulum arising posteriorly. It is a pulsion pharyngeal diverticulum arising at the Killian dehiscence (between circular and oblique fibers of the cricopharyngeus).

**4. B.** Benign stricture. The barium enema demonstrates a long symmetric stricture in the proximal transverse colon, in a patient with Crohn colitis.

**5. C.** The dose of glucagon is 1.0 mg IV for barium enema and 0.1 mg IV for hypotonic duodenography.

# Esophagus 2

*Vijetha Vinod Maller and Sridhar Shankar*

## LEARNING OBJECTIVE

**1.** Review the imaging features of the benign and malignant pathologies of the esophagus.

Contrast studies of the esophagus play a very important role in the evaluation of causes of esophageal obstruction, tumors, inflammation, and leaks and for the radiologic evaluation of motility disorders. Both single- and double-contrast studies continue to be useful despite advances in cross-sectional imaging studies. The probable reason that CT and MRI are not the primary imaging modalities is the small caliber and location of the esophagus. Barium studies also demonstrate lesions involving the valleculae, tongue base, lower hypopharynx, and pharyngoesophageal segment that are difficult to visualize at endoscopy. The role of CT or MRI is to further clarify the findings on other studies and particularly to assess the areas surrounding the esophagus such as would be required in the staging of esophageal cancers.

## NORMAL ANATOMY

The upper esophageal sphincter, formed by the cricopharyngeal muscle, is located at the C5–C6 level, which relaxes with the ingested bolus. Abnormalities of this region like delayed closure, early closure, and nonrelaxation also known as cricopharyngeal achalasia (Fig. 2.1) can be detected on esophagram.

Lower esophageal sphincter (LOS): The distal 2 to 4 cm of the esophageal is a high-pressure zone defined by manometry, which corresponds to the bulbous distention of the distal esophagus, also known as the vestibule or phrenic ampulla (Fig. 2.2) on esophagram.

## ESOPHAGEAL RINGS

*A ring*: The A ring represents the LOS and is caused by the muscular contraction at the junction of the tubular and vestibular esophagus (Fig. 2.2). It represents the upper boundary of the phrenic ampulla and is located 2 to 4 cm above the B ring.

*B ring*: The B ring is the mucosal ring at the squamocolumnar junction or the Z line (Fig. 2.2). It represents the lower boundary of the phrenic ampulla and corresponds to the Z line, which represents the squamocolumnar junction. The B ring is seen normally with the esophageal distension but is not identified in 15% cases, where the diagnosis of hiatus hernia is difficult to make. However, this may cause episodic dysphagia, which is then termed as the Schatzki ring (Fig. 2.3). The B ring with a maximum luminal diameter of more than 20 mm rarely causes dysphagia, whereas rings with a maximum diameter of less than 13 mm almost always cause dysphagia.[1,2]

## VASCULAR IMPRESSIONS

*Aberrant right subclavian artery* is an arterial anomaly, which produces a dorsal diagonal impression on the esophagus and rarely causes symptoms (Fig. 2.4).

*Right aortic arch with aberrant left subclavian artery* produces a dorsal indentation on the esophagus as the left subclavian artery arises low from the right-sided arch and extends from right to left, dorsal to the esophagus (Fig. 2.5).

*The double aortic arch* most often presents with airway obstruction, dysphagia, and aspiration in children. The arches indent the esophagus at different levels on the right and left.

*Aberrant left pulmonary artery* indents the trachea dorsally and the esophagus ventrally as it extends between them. Narrowing of the right bronchus can cause air trapping or atelectasis.

*Tortuous aorta* or aortic aneurysm can also produce extrinsic impression on the esophagus (Fig. 2.6).

*Coarctation of the aorta* will produce reverse 3 figure indentation of the esophagus caused by pre- and post-stenotic aortic dilatation.

*Intrinsic vascular impressions*: Uphill varices and downhill varices occur in portal hypertension and superior vena cava obstruction, respectively, with reversal of flow and dilated esophageal and periesophageal veins. Barium esophagram produces linear filling defects, which change in appearance during examination with breath-holding maneuver.[3] CT scan can further confirm the diagnosis by demonstration of the varices (Fig. 2.7).

## HIATUS HERNIA

Hiatus hernia may be asymptomatic and an incidental finding in many patients. However, patients may present with epigastric or chest pain, postprandial fullness, nausea, and vomiting

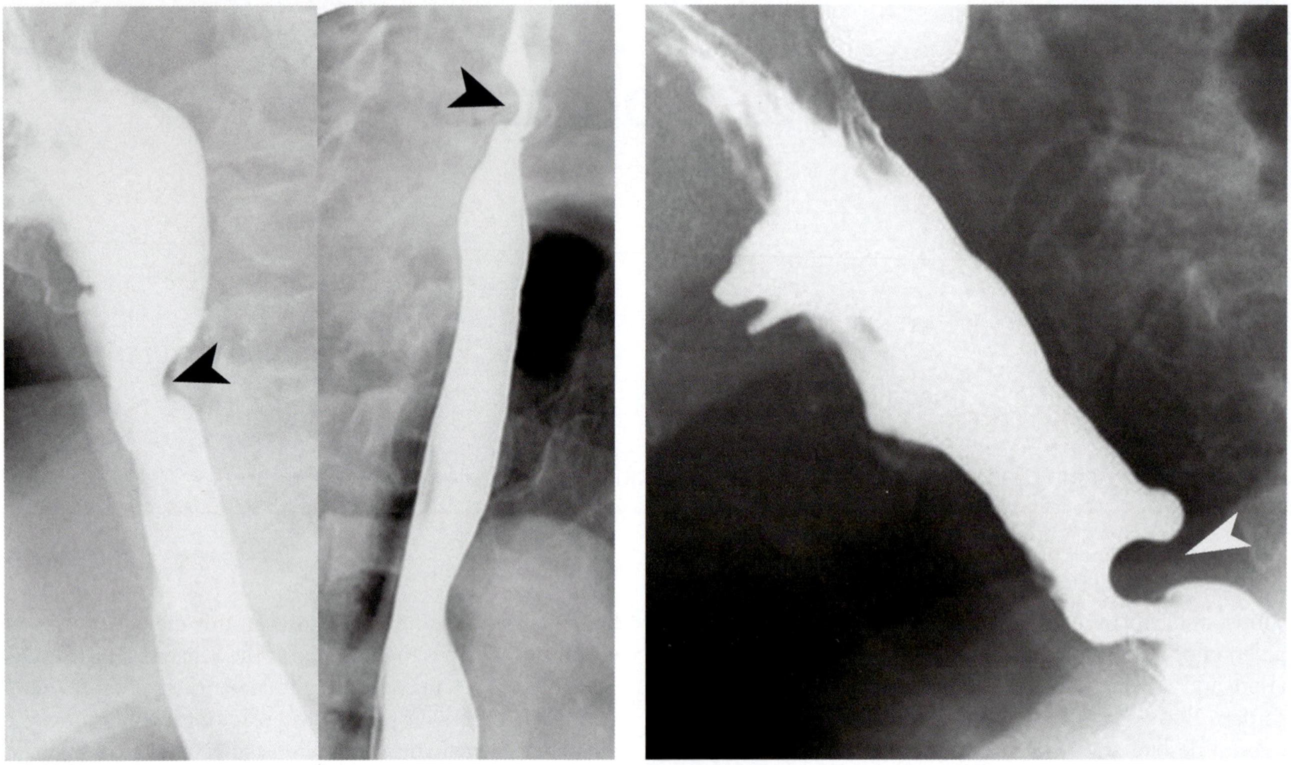

A B

**FIG. 2.1 • Cricopharyngeal achalasia. A,B:** Spot images from barium esophagram show persistent indentation by the cricopharyngeus muscle (*arrowheads*). An incidental esophageal web is seen anteriorly on Figure A.

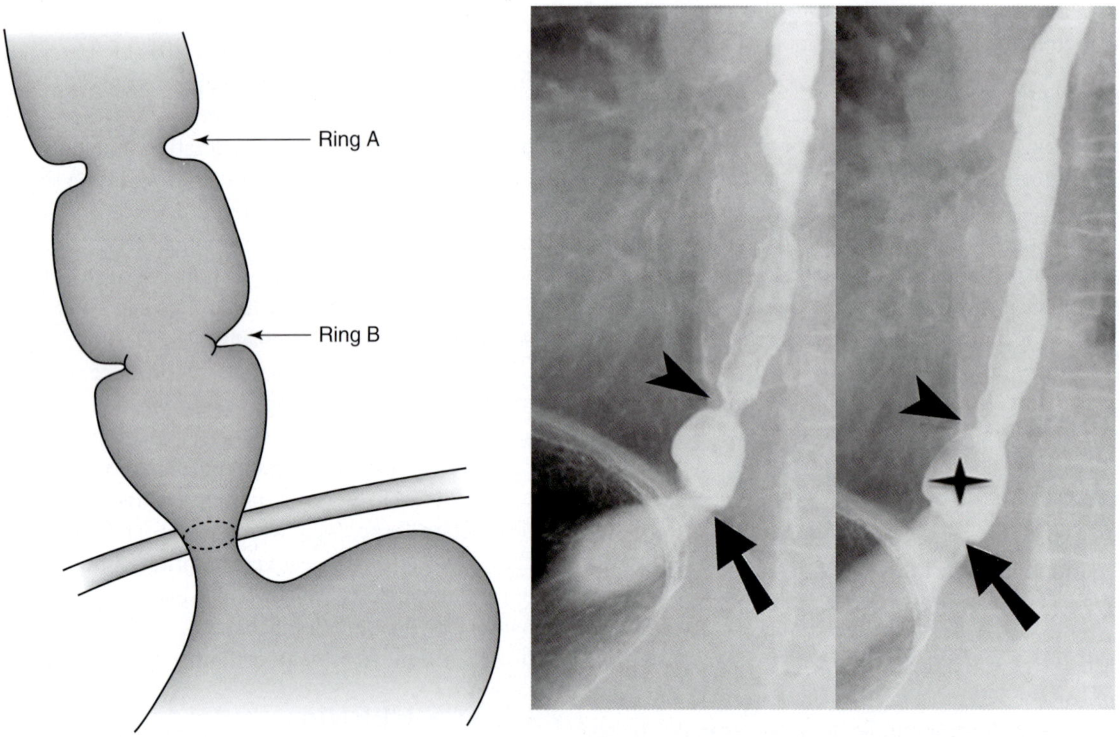


**FIG. 2.2 • A ring and B ring.** Spot images of barium esophagram demonstrate the A ring (*arrowheads*), which is due to muscular contraction and varies during examination. The B ring (*arrow*) corresponds to the squamocolumnar junction and does not change during examination. The bulbous distended part of the lower esophagus (*black star*) between A and B rings is the vestibule and corresponds to the anatomical LOS.

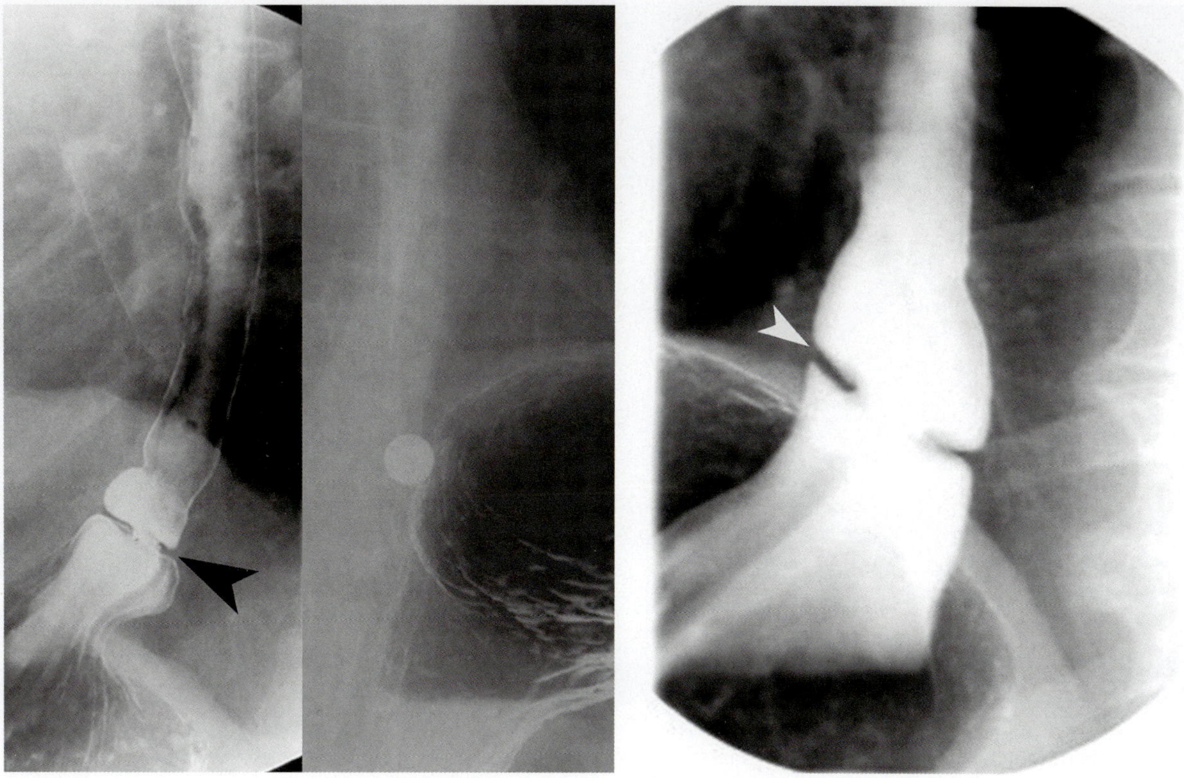

A B

**FIG. 2.3 • Schatzki ring. A,B:** Spot image from double-contrast barium esophagram in two patients presenting with dysphagia demonstrates the Schatzki ring at the anatomical squamocolumnar junction at the apex of the hiatus hernia (*arrowheads*). Spot image (A) shows hold up of the barium tablet at this level.

due to associated reflux.[4] On plain radiographs, retrocardiac opacity may be seen with air-fluid level. On esophagram, the diagnosis of hiatus hernia is made when the B ring is more than 2 cm above the diaphragmatic indentation.

- *Sliding hiatus hernia* is the most common type of hiatus hernia (95% cases).[4] The gastroesophageal (GE) junction is displaced by more than 2 cm above the hiatus due to the widening of the esophageal hiatus (Fig. 2.8). Small sliding hiatus hernias may reduce in the upright position.

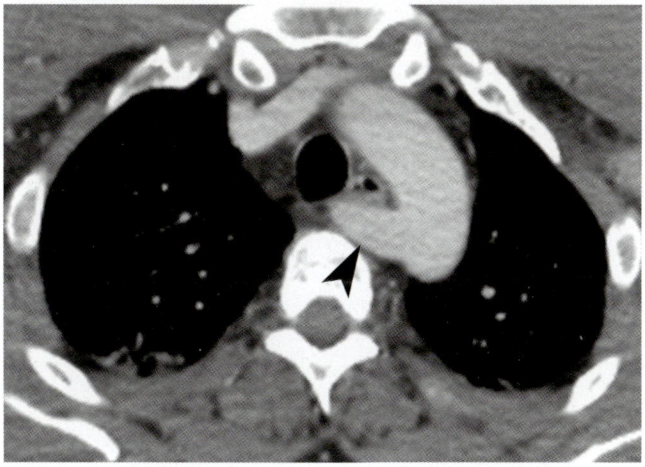

**FIG. 2.4 • Aberrant right subclavian artery.** The aberrant right subclavian artery (*arrowhead*) arises from the aortic arch, on the left side, and crosses toward the right, dorsal to the esophagus.

- *Rolling (paraesophageal) hiatus hernia* is less common (5% cases) than the sliding type. The GE junction remains in its normal location, while the gastric fundus herniates above the diaphragm (Fig. 2.9). Large hernias can be progressive with rotation of the stomach leading to gastric volvulus, obstruction, strangulation, and perforation.[4]
- *Mixed or compound hiatal hernia*: The GE junction is displaced into the thorax along with the fundus of the stomach (Fig. 2.10).

## ESOPHAGEAL WEB

*Esophageal web* can be congenital or acquired. The web is usually seen in the hypopharynx and cervical esophagus with the majority protruding from the anterior esophageal wall (Fig. 2.11). Symptoms occur when the lumen is more than 50% compromised.[5] Plummer-Vinson syndrome is esophageal web with dysphagia caused by iron deficiency anemia. There is increased incidence of carcinoma in Plummer-Vinson syndrome.[6]

## ESOPHAGEAL DIVERTICULA

Pulsion diverticula are caused due to increased intraluminal pressure. Traction diverticulum occurs due to hilar granulomatous disease.[3,7]

A *Zenker diverticulum* is a pulsion hypopharyngeal diverticulum due to the mucosal and submucosal protrusion through the triangular weak site between horizontal and oblique

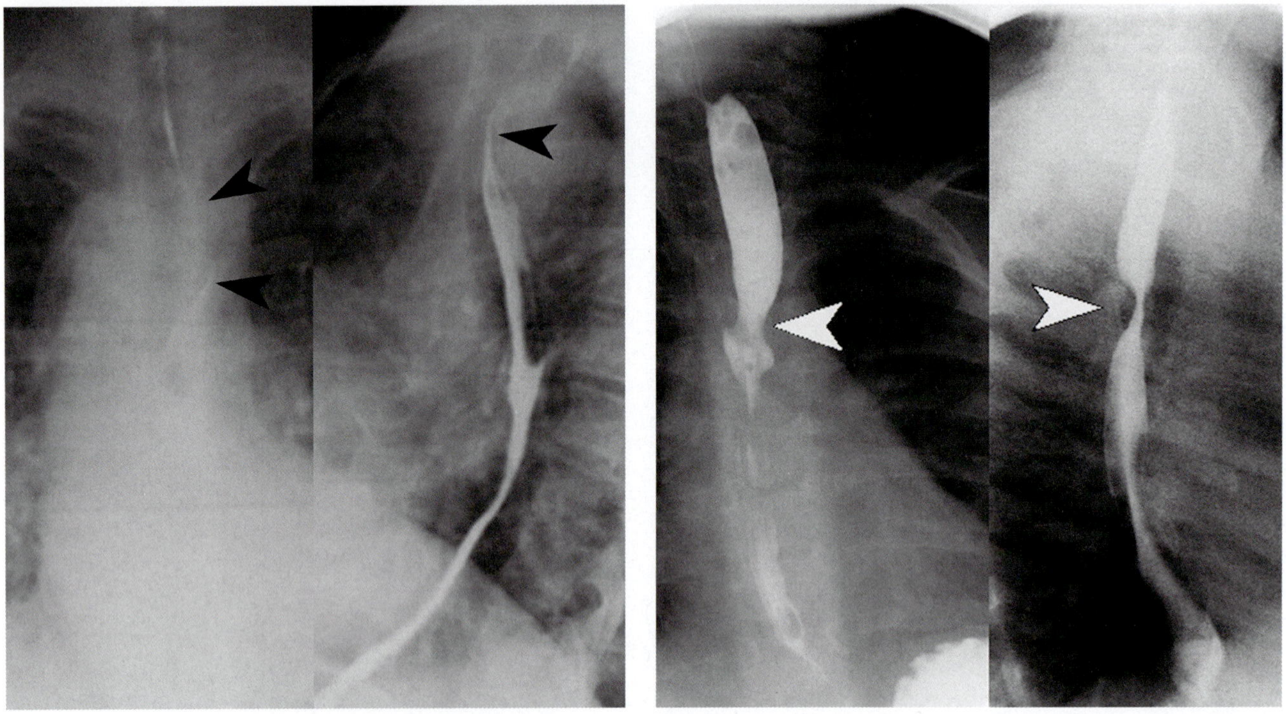

A B

**FIG. 2.5 • Aberrant subclavian artery. A:** Aberrant left subclavian artery: Barium esophagram demonstrates right-sided aortic arch with aberrant left subclavian artery, causing right-sided and dorsal indentation (*arrowheads*) on the esophagus. **B:** Aberrant right subclavian artery: Barium esophagram demonstrates dorsal indentation (*arrowheads*) on the esophagus as the right subclavian artery passes dorsal to the esophagus.

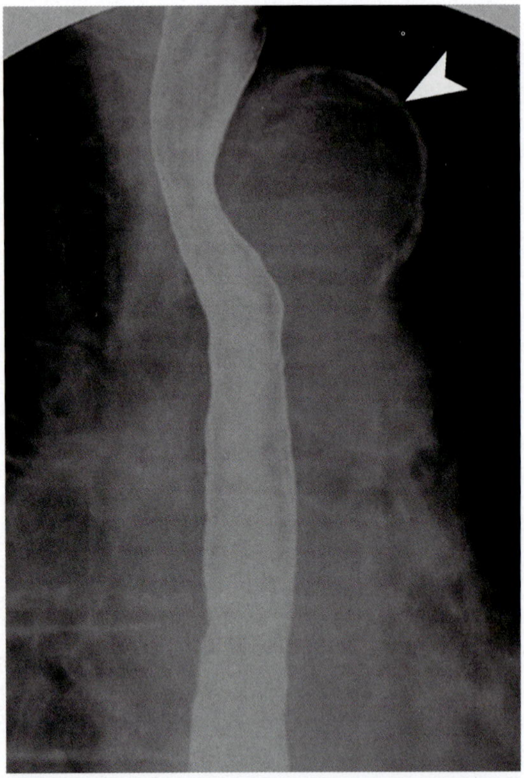

**FIG. 2.6 • Vascular impression.** Spot image from barium esophagram shows the esophageal impression from the aortic arch, which is exaggerated by tortuous and ectatic aortic arch (*arrowhead*).

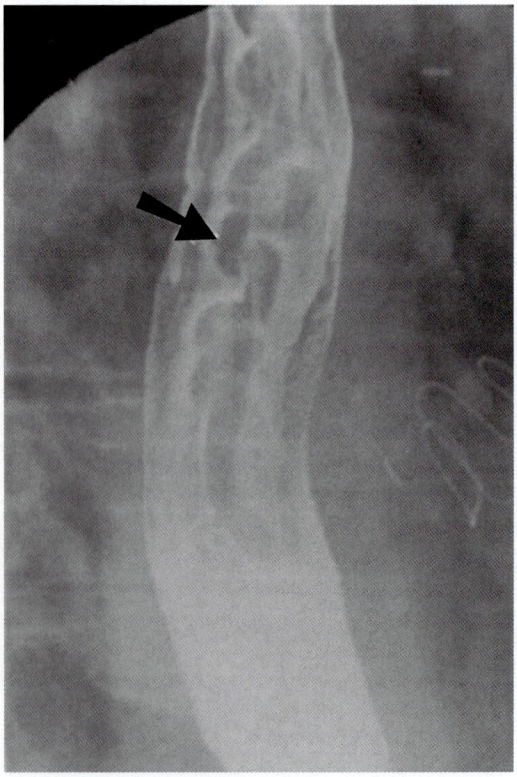

**FIG. 2.7 • Esophageal varices.** Barium esophagram shows serpiginous filling defects (*arrow*) due to varices, which were confirmed on contrast-enhanced CT.

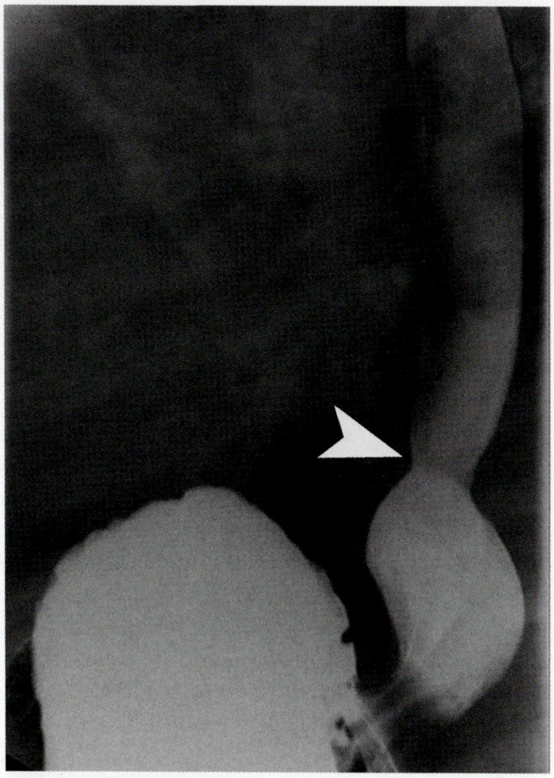

**FIG. 2.8 • Sliding hiatus hernia.** Spot image from barium esophagram shows GE junction (*arrowhead*), which is displaced by more than 2 cm above the hiatus.

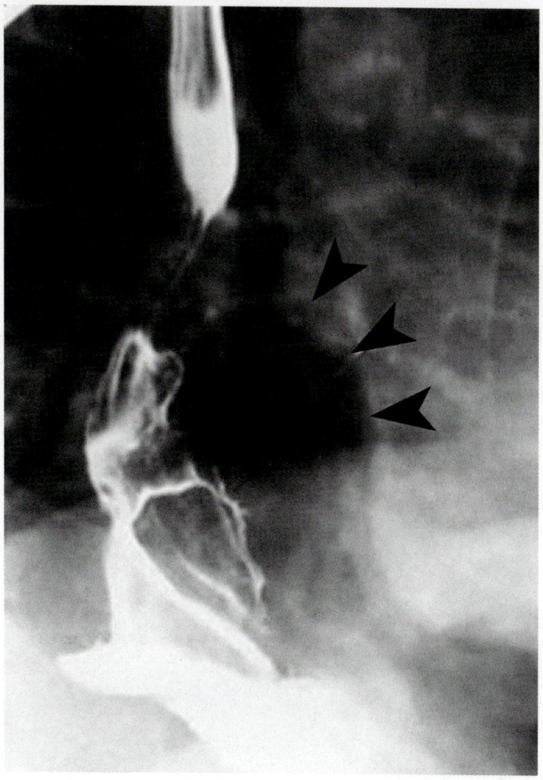

**FIG. 2.9 • Paraesophageal hernia.** Spot image from barium esophagram shows fundus (*arrowheads*) of the stomach above the diaphragmatic hiatus.

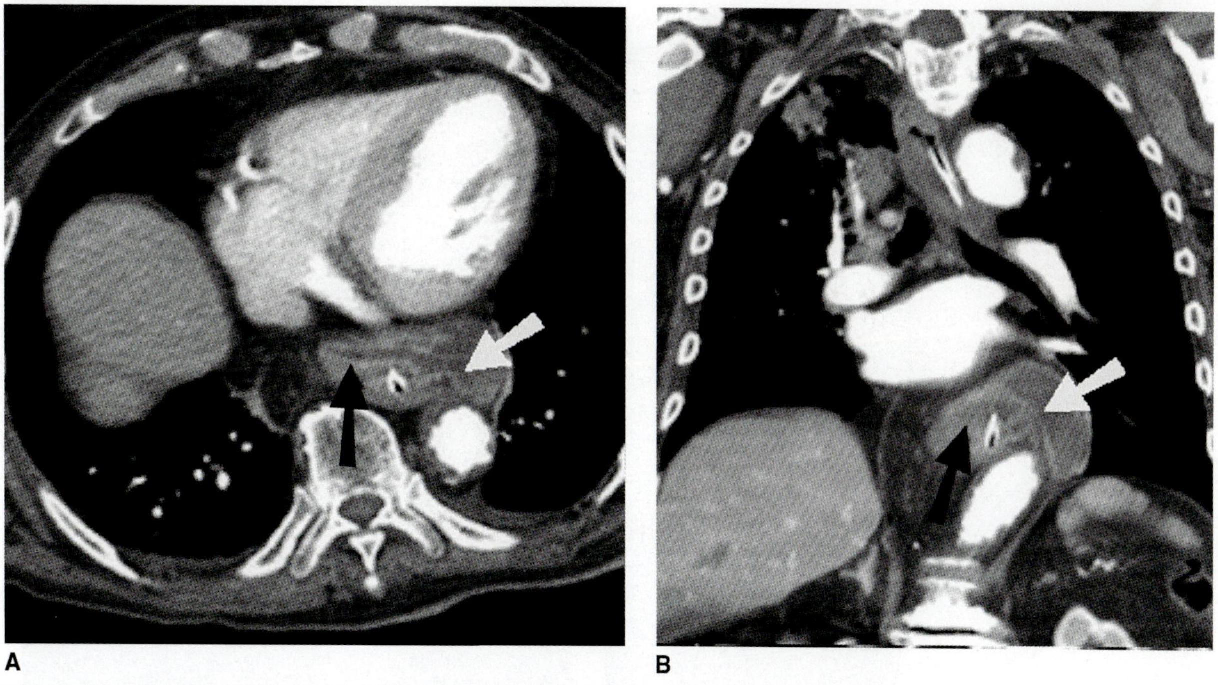

**FIG. 2.10 • Mixed hiatus hernia.** Axial and coronal contrast-enhanced CT images **(A, B)** show the fundus of the stomach (*white arrow*) protruding through the hiatus and lying adjacent to the esophagus. The GE junction is above the hiatus (*black arrow*).

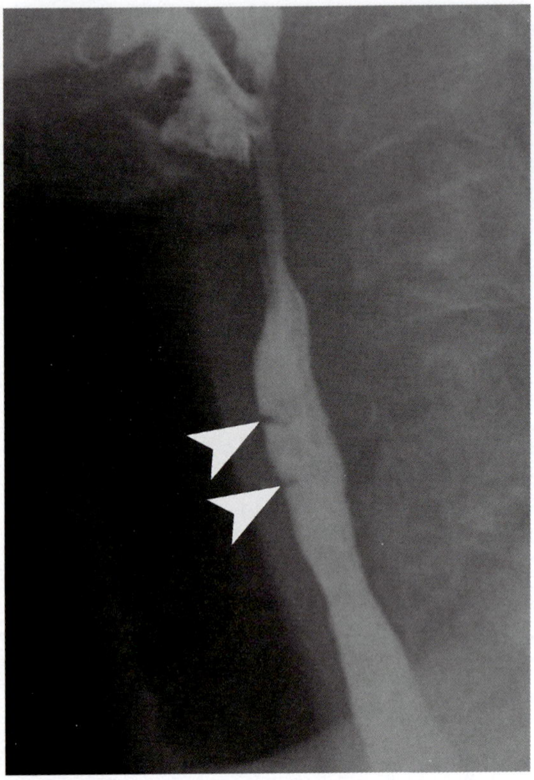

**FIG. 2.11 • Esophageal web.** Spot image of barium esophagram shows two short thin webs (*arrowheads*) arising from the anterior wall of the esophagus.

components of the cricopharyngeus muscle called the Killian' dehiscence. The likely etiology is the elevated upper esophageal pressure with cricopharyngeus dysfunction.[7] The patient presents with dysphagia, regurgitation, or aspiration. On plain radiographs, a mass or air-fluid level may be seen in the neck. The esophagram shows outpouching arising from the midline posterior wall just above the cricopharyngeus projecting caudally and is best demonstrated on lateral view (Fig. 2.12A).

*Killian-Jamieson diverticulum* is a pulsion diverticulum, which protrudes through the lateral anatomic weak site of the cervical esophagus below the cricopharyngeus muscle. This type of diverticulum originates laterally and is best demonstrated on the AP view (Fig. 2.12B).[7]

*Midesophageal diverticula* develop at the middle third of the esophagus at the level of bifurcation of the trachea. Traction-type midesophageal diverticulum is formed when periesophageal inflammation causes adhesions between inflammatory foci and esophagus. Midesophageal diverticula have been associated with nutcracker esophagus, diffuse esophageal spasm, achalasia, hypertensive LOS, and nonspecific esophageal motility disorder.[7] Classic midesophageal diverticula are small in size with a large neck, and they rarely become symptomatic or require surgical intervention (Fig. 2.13).

*Epiphrenic diverticulum* is a pulsion diverticulum from the esophagus adjacent to the diaphragm (Fig. 2.14). The persistently increased tone in the distal esophagus usually produces epiphrenic diverticula. Epiphrenic diverticula have

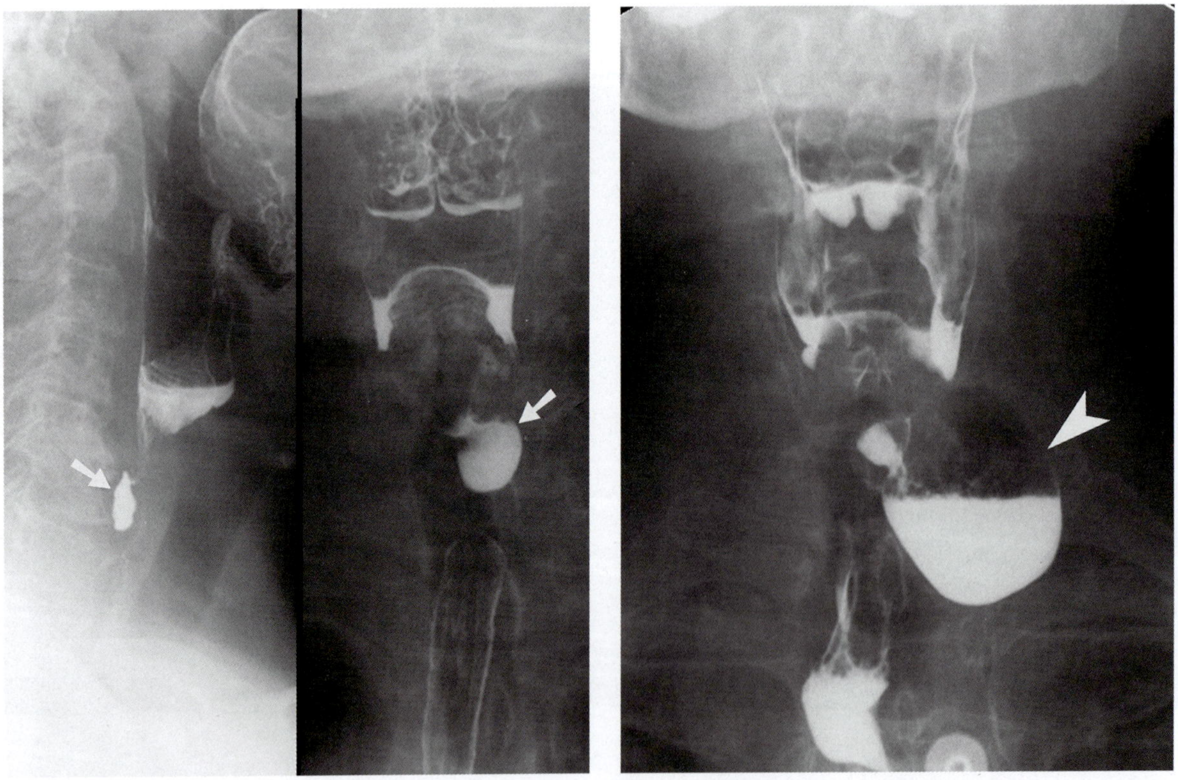

A B

**FIG. 2.12 • Zenker and Killian-Jamieson diverticulum. A: Zenker diverticulum**—spot images from barium esophagram show a diverticulum (*arrows*) projecting posteriorly from the pharyngoesophageal junction. **B: Killian-Jamieson diverticulum**—spot images from barium esophagram show a diverticulum (*arrowhead*) projecting to the left side from the pharyngoesophageal junction.

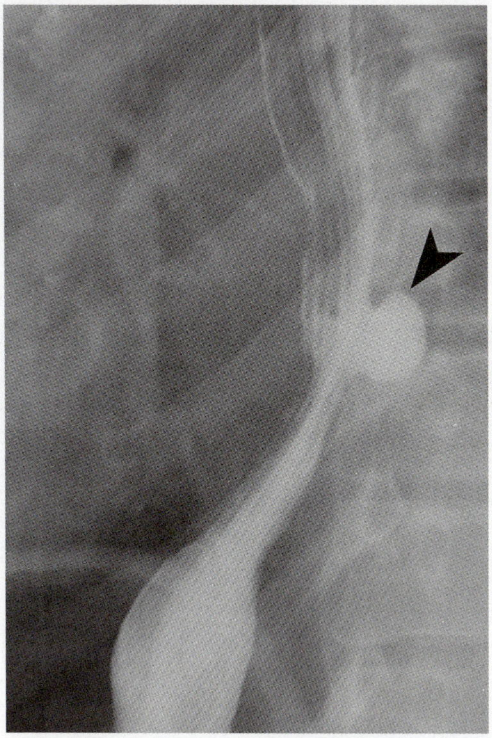

**FIG. 2.13 • Pulsion diverticula.** Spot image from barium esophagram shows thoracic esophageal pulsion diverticulum (*arrowhead*) with a wide neck.

been reported with nutcracker esophagus, achalasia, and other motility disorders.[7] Large epiphrenic diverticula can cause dysphagia, narrow the esophagus, or cause aspiration.[3,7]

*Aortopulmonary window diverticulum* occurs as the esophagus transiently protrudes into the aortopulmonary window.[7]

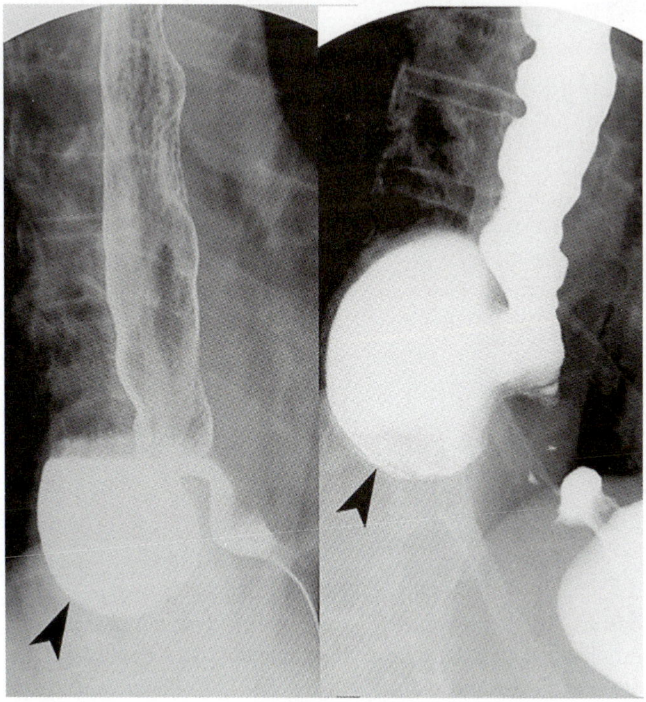

**FIG. 2.14 • Large epiphrenic diverticulum.** Spot images from barium esophagram show large epiphrenic diverticulum (*arrowheads*) and tertiary contractions in the thoracic esophagus.

## ESOPHAGEAL MOTILITY DISORDERS

Physiologically, the primary contraction propels the bolus through the esophagus, and the secondary contraction follows, which propels any remaining bolus from the thoracic esophagus.

Tertiary contractions are abnormal, nonpropulsive, transient, and intermittent contractions that are inconstant in location but not accompanied by symptoms. When seen in older patients, these are termed presbyesophagus.[8]

*Diffuse esophageal spasm* produces intermittent uncoordinated contractions of the mid- and distal esophageal smooth muscle, associated with chest symptoms. On esophagogram, it is typically described as corkscrew esophagus (Fig. 2.15).

*Achalasia* is an idiopathic type of esophageal dysmotility, which is characterized by loss of distal esophageal peristalsis and failure of the LOS relaxation. Achalasia is most common in middle age with equal incidence in men and women. There is an associated increased incidence of carcinoma in achalasia. The etiology of primary achalasia is unknown, although with some inflammatory degeneration of esophageal ganglion cells.[3] Affected individuals typically have long-standing dysphagia and slow progression of symptoms.

Secondary achalasia or pseudoachalasia is caused by pathologic causes of esophageal motility disorders often indistinguishable from primary achalasia. Malignancy (especially gastric cancer), Chagas disease, Sjögren, amyloidosis, sarcoidosis, and scleroderma are some of the causes for pseudoachalasia (Fig. 2.16).[9]

### Imaging Findings

Plain radiography shows absence of fundal gas shadow. Esophagram demonstrates dilated esophagus with uncoordinated, nonpropulsive, tertiary contractions (Fig. 2.17).

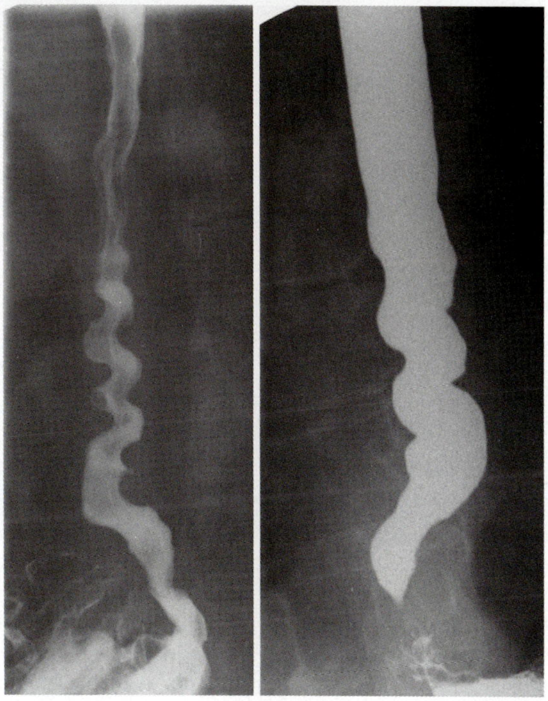

**FIG. 2.15 • Corkscrew esophagus.** Spot image from barium esophagram shows corkscrew appearance of the thoracic esophagus accounting for the patient's dysphagia.

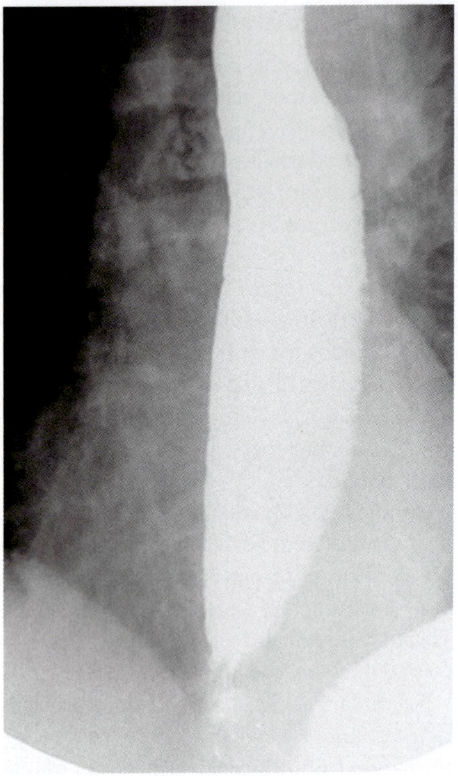

**A**

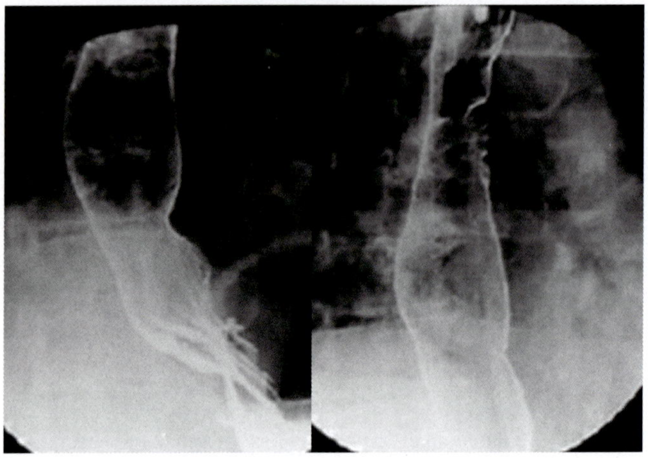

**B**

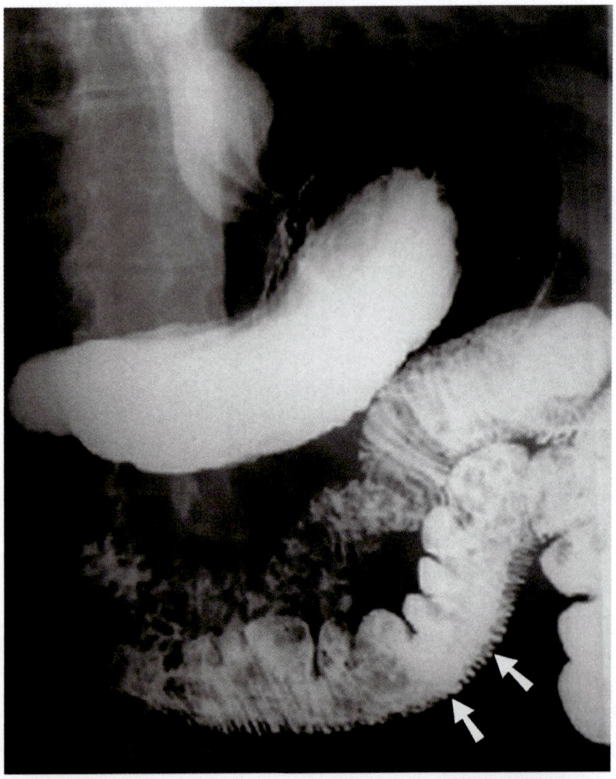

**C**

**FIG. 2.16 • Sjögren syndrome (A) and scleroderma (B,C).** **A:** Spot image from barium esophagram shows dilated atonic esophagus (due to decreased primary peristalsis) and delayed passage of bolus through the LOS. **B:** Spot images from barium esophagram show dilated esophagus with reduced peristalsis, which was seen at fluoroscopy. **C:** Spot image from the barium meal follow-through shows dilated jejunal loops with hidebound appearance (*white arrows*) and sacculations (*black arrow*) along the mesenteric border.

Incomplete LOS relaxation, not coordinated with esophageal contraction, gives the classic bird-beak sign (Figs. 2.17 to 2.19). There is failure of the normal peristalsis to clear the esophagus of barium, when the patient is in the recumbent position. In the standing position when the barium column is high enough, the hydrostatic pressure can overcome the LOS pressure allowing passage of the esophageal content. In advanced disease, the esophagus can become massively dilated and tortuous distally, also called sigmoid esophagus (Fig. 2.18).[3] In the advanced disease when the esophagus becomes atonic and aperistaltic, there is significant esophageal dilatation with retention of large amounts of food/fluid. Foamy esophagus in achalasia, with numerous tiny

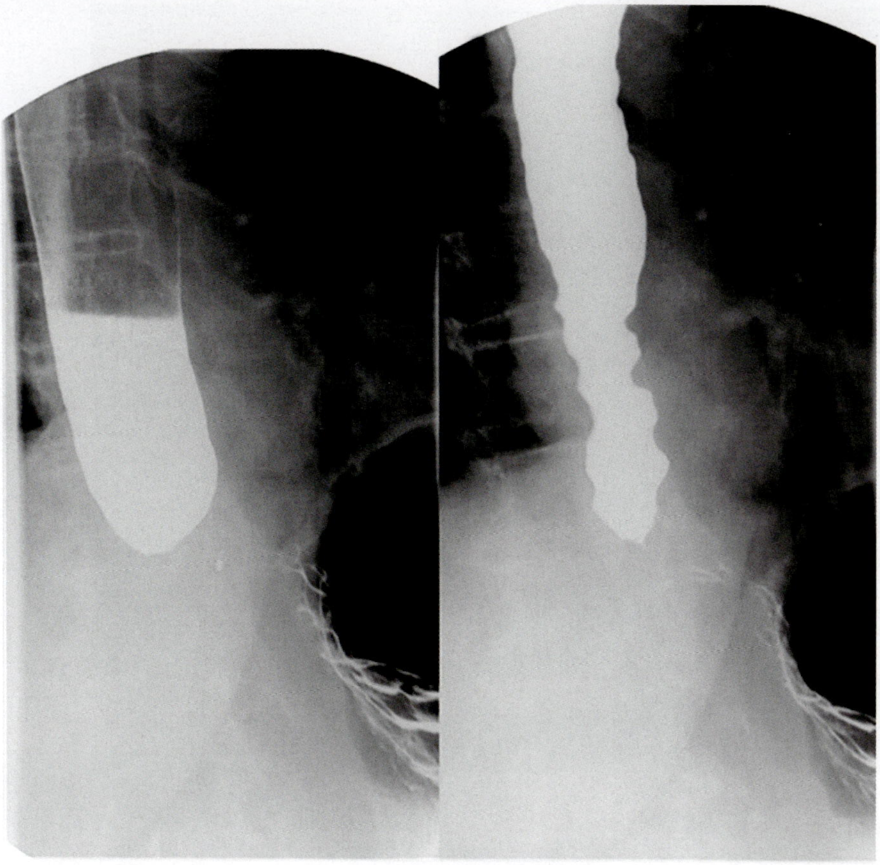

**FIG. 2.17 • Achalasia.** Spot images from barium esophagram demonstrate dilatation of the esophagus with a lack of relaxation of the LOS. Uncoordinated tertiary contractions are noted in the thoracic esophagus.

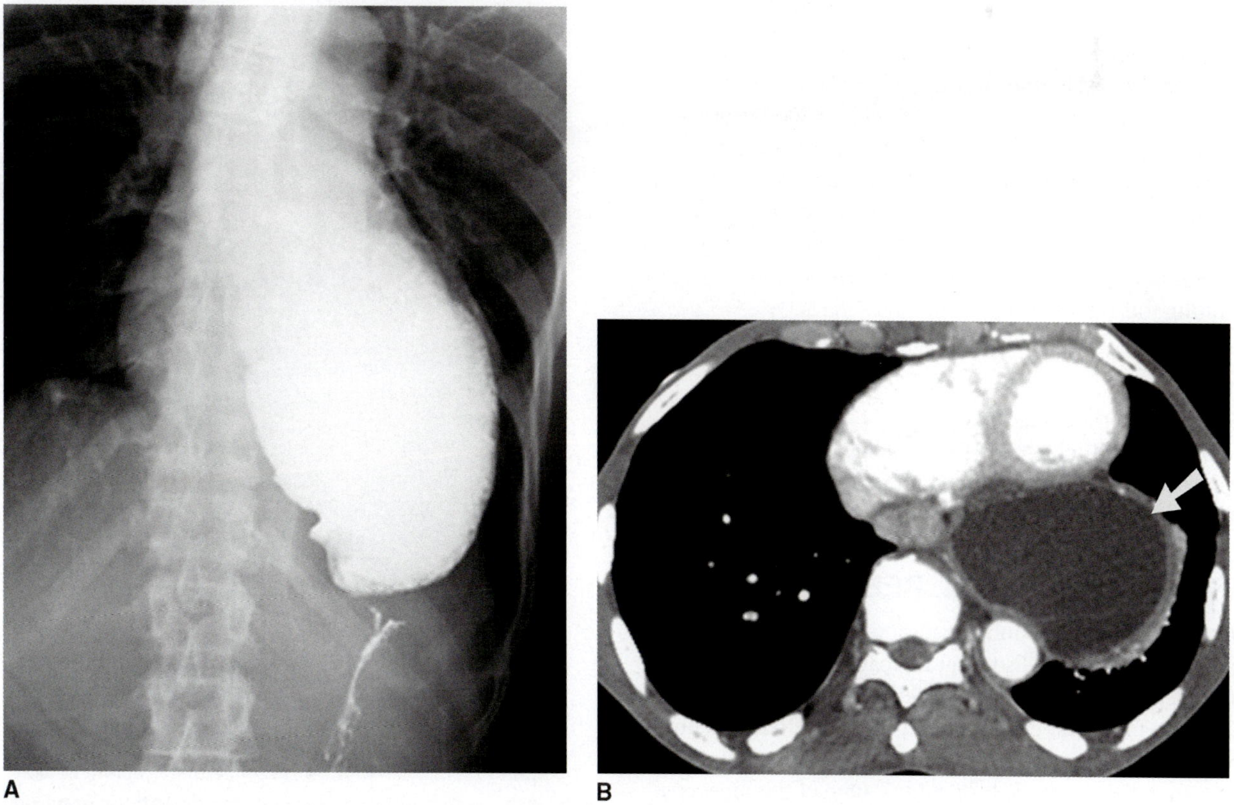

**FIG. 2.18 • Achalasia. A:** Spot image from barium esophagram shows massively dilated sigmoid-shaped atonic esophagus with bird-beak sign. **B:** The axial CT also demonstrates a massively dilated esophagus (*arrow*).

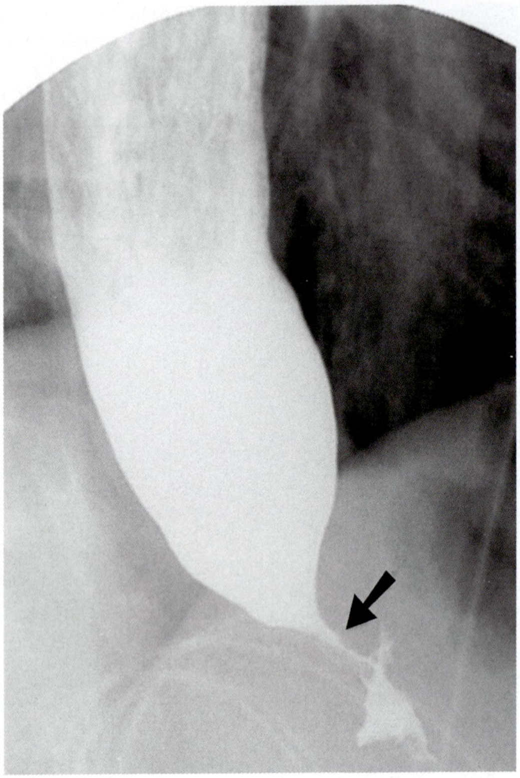


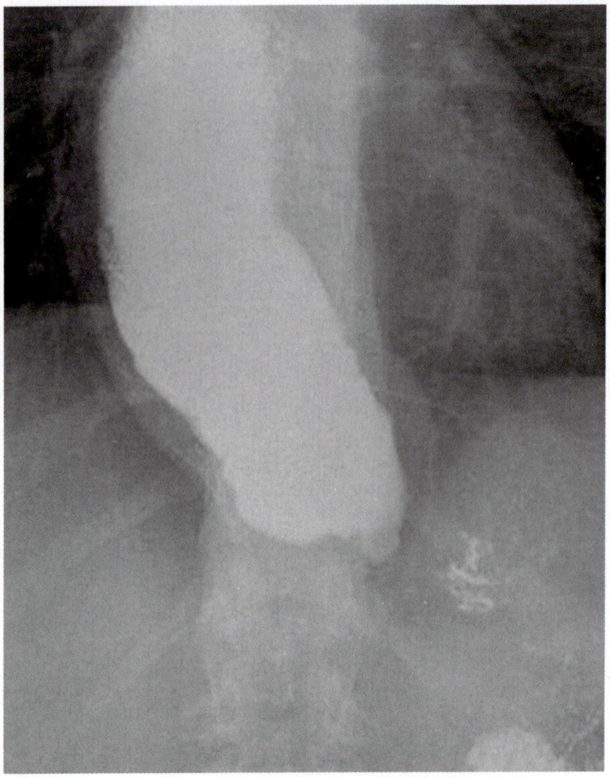


**FIG. 2.19 • Achalasia. A,B:** Spot images from barium esophagram show a grossly dilated esophagus in two different patients. Bird-beak appearance of the distal end of the esophagus (*arrow*) is well demonstrated in the first patient.

bubbles layering in the barium column, presumably results from candida infection due to long-standing stasis.[3] CT scan, although not commonly used for the diagnosis of achalasia, will also demonstrate esophageal dilatation with retention of food debris.

Secondary achalasia is also characterized by absent peristalsis in the esophagus and beak-like narrowing near the GE junction. In secondary achalasia caused by esophageal cancer at the GE junction, the length of the narrowed segment is larger, asymmetric, nodular, or ulcerated because of tumor infiltrating this region[9] (Fig. 2.20).

Differential diagnosis of achalasia

1. Chagas disease
2. Scleroderma (late stages)
3. Neoplasm at GE junction (pseudoachalasia)
4. Peptic stricture (10% to 20% of reflux esophagitis)
5. Intestinal pseudoobstruction

## GASTROESOPHAGEAL REFLUX DISEASE

*Reflux esophagitis* is the most common inflammatory disease involving the esophagus. Esophagram may be normal in patients with milder forms of esophagitis, which may be manifested on endoscopy as mucosal erythema and fragility. Double-contrast esophagrams are more sensitive in revealing mucosal abnormalities than the single-contrast study.[10] One of the most common signs of reflux esophagitis on double-contrast esophagram is a finely nodular or granular mucosal appearance, which is caused by mucosal edema and inflammation.[3,10] Shallow ero-

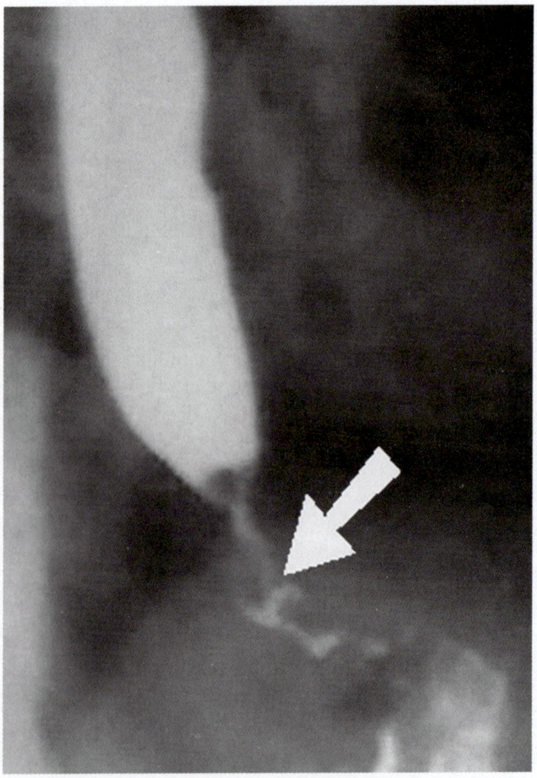

**FIG. 2.20 • Secondary achalasia due to distal esophageal carcinoma.** Spot image from barium esophagram shows dilated esophagus with asymmetric irregular narrowing at the lower end of the esophagus (*arrow*).

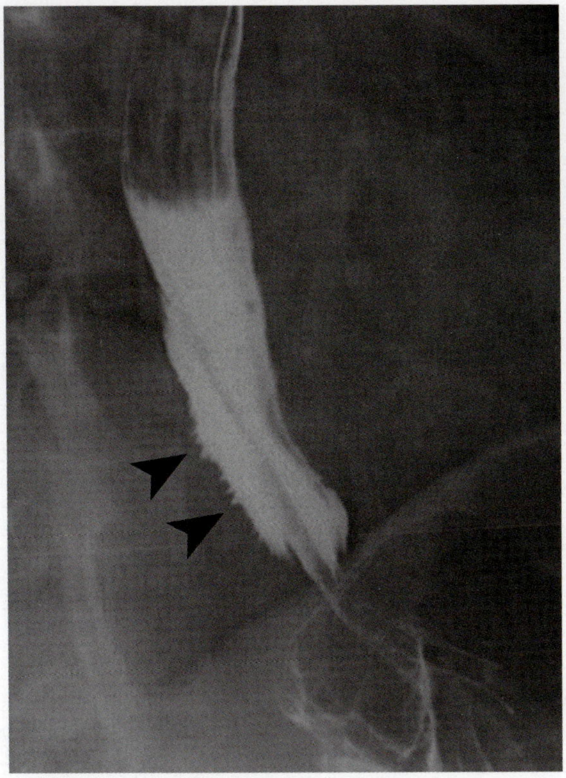

**FIG. 2.21 • Reflux esophagitis.** Spot images from barium esophagram show mucosal erosions (*arrowheads*) and mucosal fold prominence in the distal esophagus.

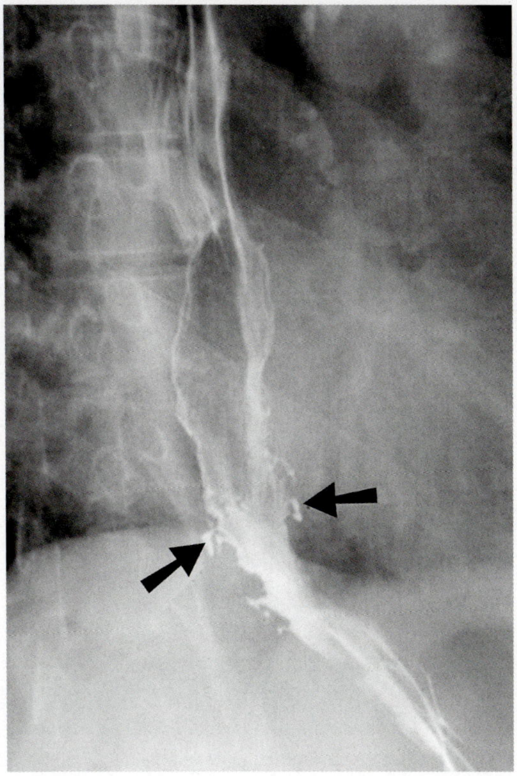

**FIG. 2.23 • Esophageal intramural pseudodiverticula in chronic reflux esophagitis.** Spot image of the barium esophagram shows multiple esophageal intramural pseudodiverticula seen as flask-shaped outpouchings (*arrows*) arising from the distal thoracic esophagus.

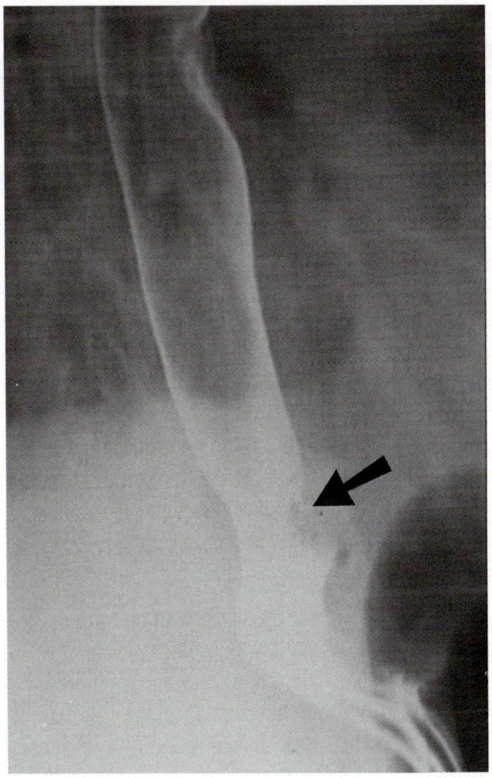

**FIG. 2.22 • Distal esophageal ulcer in reflux esophagitis.** Spot image from double-contrast barium esophagram shows punctate ulcer in the distal esophagus (*arrow*).

sions (Fig. 2.21) and ulcers in the distal esophagus with punctate, linear, or stellate configuration may be seen in the distal esophagus (Fig. 2.22). Dilated mural glands may be seen giving a pseudodiverticulosis appearance (Fig. 2.23). Patients with chronic reflux esophagitis may have a single enlarged fold arising from the gastric cardia, extending upward into the distal esophagus as a smooth, polypoid protuberance, also known as an inflammatory esophagogastric polyp.[3] Localized scarring from reflux esophagitis may appear as flattening, puckering, or sacculation of the adjacent esophageal wall, often associated with folds radiating toward the site of scarring. Further scarring will lead to circumferential stricture in the distal esophagus most often associated with hiatus hernia. Peptic strictures may manifest as short ring-like areas of narrowing that could be mistaken for Schatzki rings in patients with dysphagia.[3,10] Long-standing scarring can cause longitudinal shortening of the esophagus producing fixed transverse folds demonstrated by pooling of barium in between (Fig. 2.24). These folds should be differentiated from the thin transverse striations known as the feline esophagus often seen for brief intervals at fluoroscopy due to transient contraction of the longitudinally oriented muscularis mucosae and is often seen in patients with reflux (Fig. 2.25).

*Barrett esophagus* occurs due to columnar metaplasia as a result of long-standing chronic gastroesophageal reflux and reflux esophagitis. Barrett esophagus is a premalignant condition, which is associated with an increased risk of developing esophageal adenocarcinoma.[11,12] The classic findings on barium esophagram are mid- or high esophageal ulcer and web-like stricture.[11,12] A reticular mucosal pattern is also seen, which is the

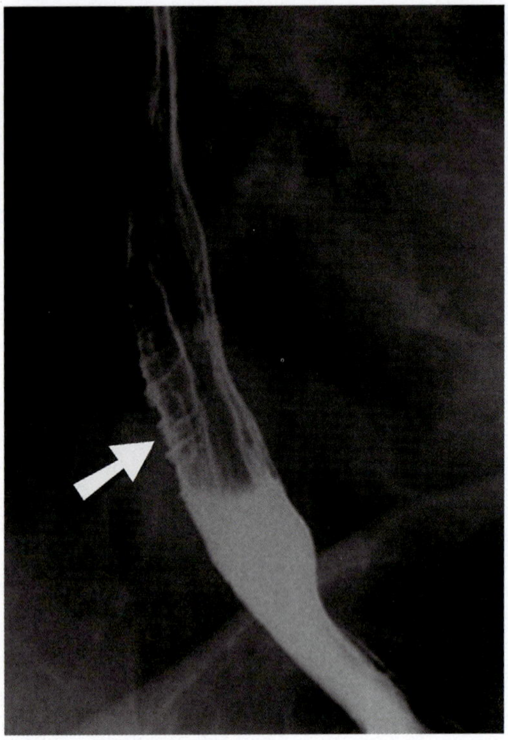

**FIG. 2.24 • Reflux esophagitis.** Spot image from double-contrast esophagram shows fixed transverse folds (*white arrow*) caused by longitudinal scarring of the distal esophagus.

characteristic pattern (Fig. 2.26). Barrett esophagus is most often associated with hiatus hernia.

Esophageal intramural pseudodiverticulosis is a condition characterized by multiple small outpouchings of the esophageal wall; representing dilated submucosal glands. It most commonly

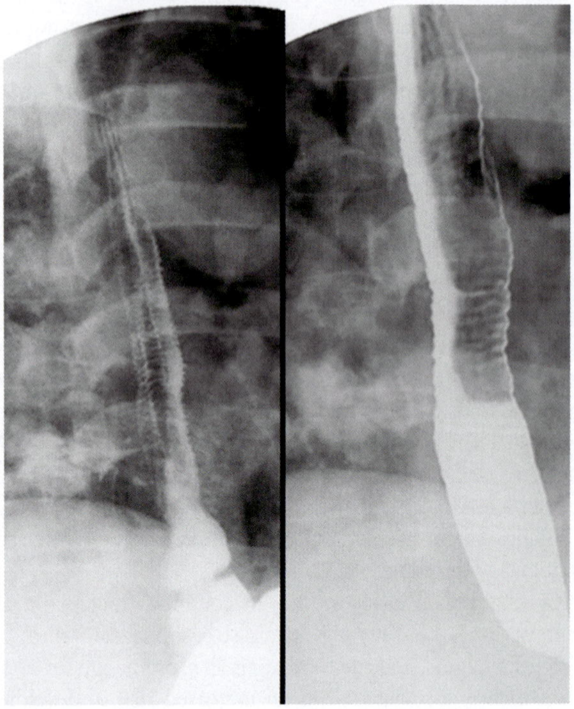

**FIG. 2.25 • Feline esophagus.** Spot images from barium esophagram study show thin transverse striations, which were seen for brief interval at fluoroscopy.

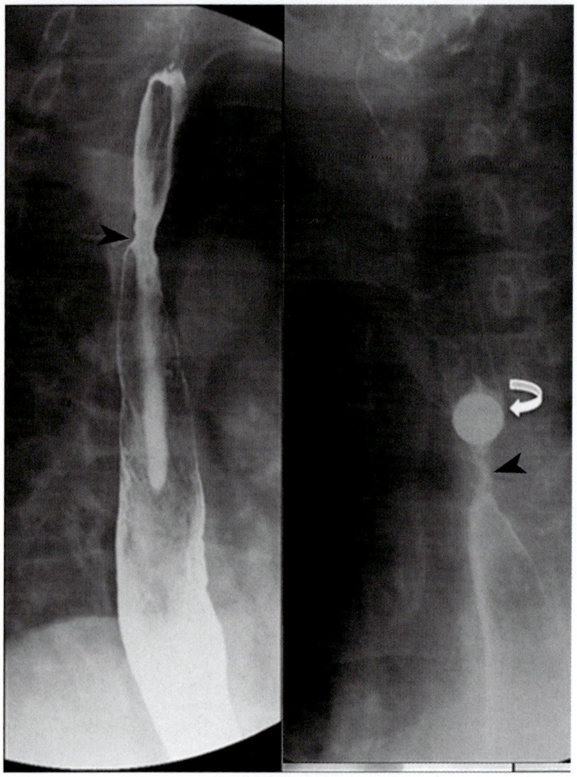

**FIG. 2.26 • Barrett esophagus.** Spot images of double-contrast barium esophagram show persistent high esophageal stricture (*arrowhead*). There is holdup of the barium tablet (*curved arrow*) at the level of stricture.

affects individuals in sixth and seventh decade of life. It is associated with chronic irritation from alcoholism, gastroesophageal reflux disease (GERD), diabetes, and candidiasis. On barium swallow, examination is seen as flask-shaped outpouchings (1 to 4 mm long) from the esophagus (Fig. 2.27). They may be associated with esophageal stricture, most commonly in the upper esophagus. Most of the patient's present with symptoms of dysphagia.

Differential diagnosis of esophageal stricture

1. Reflux esophagitis: distal esophagus
2. Drug-induced esophagitis: midesophagus
3. Radiation esophagitis: radiation portal (long segment)
4. Caustic esophagitis: upper or midesophagus (long segment)
5. Malignant stricture: more common in the distal esophagus
6. Epidermolysis bullosa dystrophica: upper thoracic or cervical esophagus
7. Erythema multiforme major: upper and midesophagus
8. Others: eosinophilic esophagitis, Crohn disease, achalasia, Chagas disease, scleroderma, and graft versus host disease

## ESOPHAGITIS

*Candida esophagitis* is the most common cause of infectious esophagitis particularly in AIDS and other immunocompromised patients presenting with odynophagia. Candida esophagitis can also result from local esophageal stasis caused by severe esophageal motility disorders such as achalasia and scleroderma.

On double-contrast esophagram, discrete longitudinally oriented linear or irregular plaque-like lesions separated by normal mucosa may be seen (Fig. 2.28). Small punctuate, round, or oval

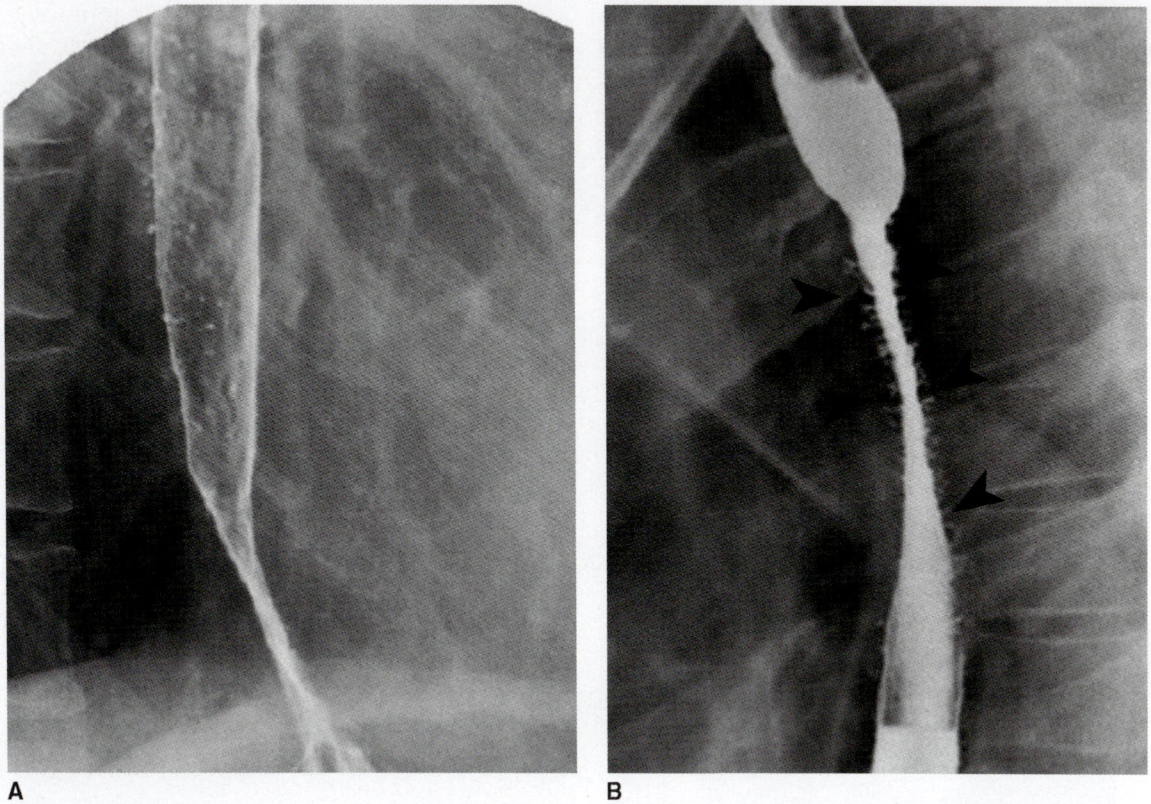


**FIG. 2.27 • Esophageal intramural pseudodiverticulosis. A:** Spot images from barium esophagram study in a patient with GE reflux show multiple small outpouchings from the esophagus, extending into the esophageal wall with lower esophageal stricture. **B:** Spot images from barium esophagram study in a patient with GE reflux show multiple small outpouchings (*arrowheads*) from the esophagus and a midesophageal stricture.

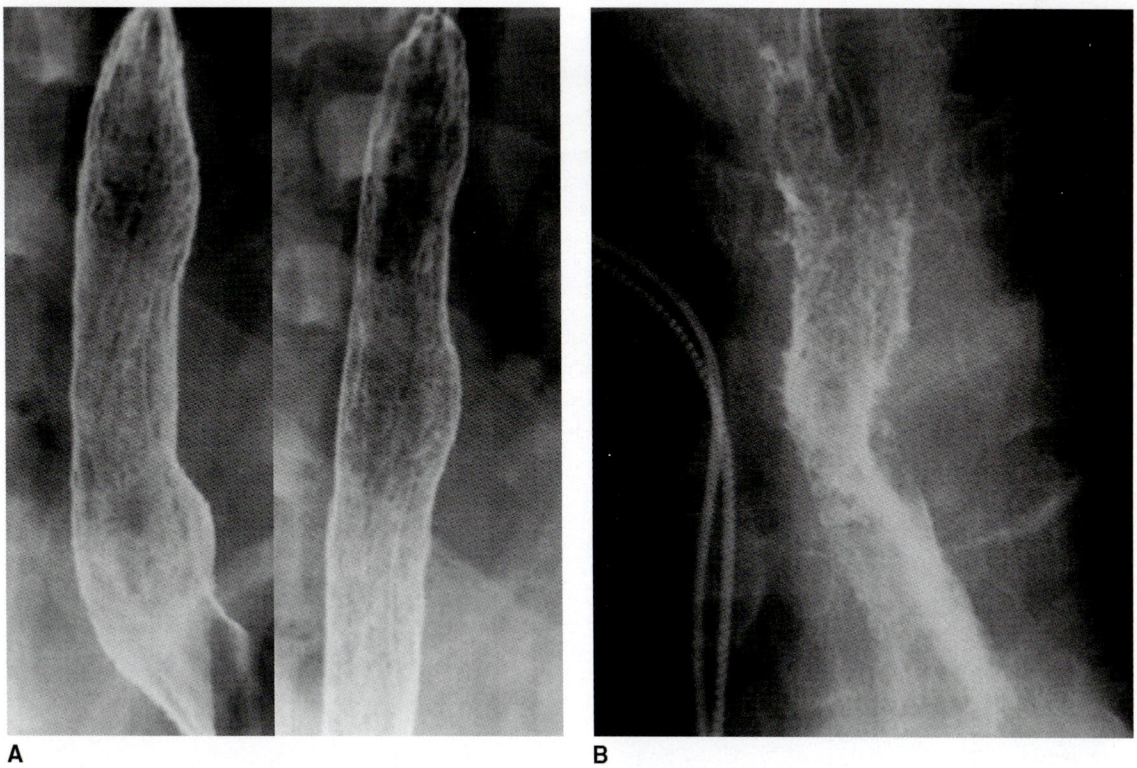


**FIG. 2.28 • Candida esophagitis. A:** Spot image of double-contrast esophagram shows discrete multiple longitudinally oriented linear, irregular plaque-like lesions giving a shaggy appearance due to trapping of barium in between. **B:** A spot image from barium esophagram in an immunocompromised patient shows extensive erosions and plaques. There is no normal mucosal lining seen in the esophagus.

ulcers may also be demonstrated.[3,13] In severe cases, irregular or shaggy appearance is seen due to innumerable coalescent pseudomembranes and plaques with contrast trapped in between.

Patients with severe esophageal motility disorders like achalasia or scleroderma may develop a foamy esophagus with numerous tiny bubbles layering out in the barium column, which is presumed to be due to superimposed candida infection from long-standing stasis.[3]

*Cytomegalovirus (CMV) esophagitis* is usually seen in patients with AIDS and a CD4 count of <200, present with giant ulcers. The ulcers may have an ovoid- or a diamond-shaped configuration surrounded by a thin radiolucent rim of edematous mucosa (Fig. 2.29A). Multiple small ulcers can also be seen in CMV esophagitis.[3,13]

*HIV esophagitis* causes giant ovoid- or diamond-shaped esophageal ulcers surrounded with edema indistinguishable

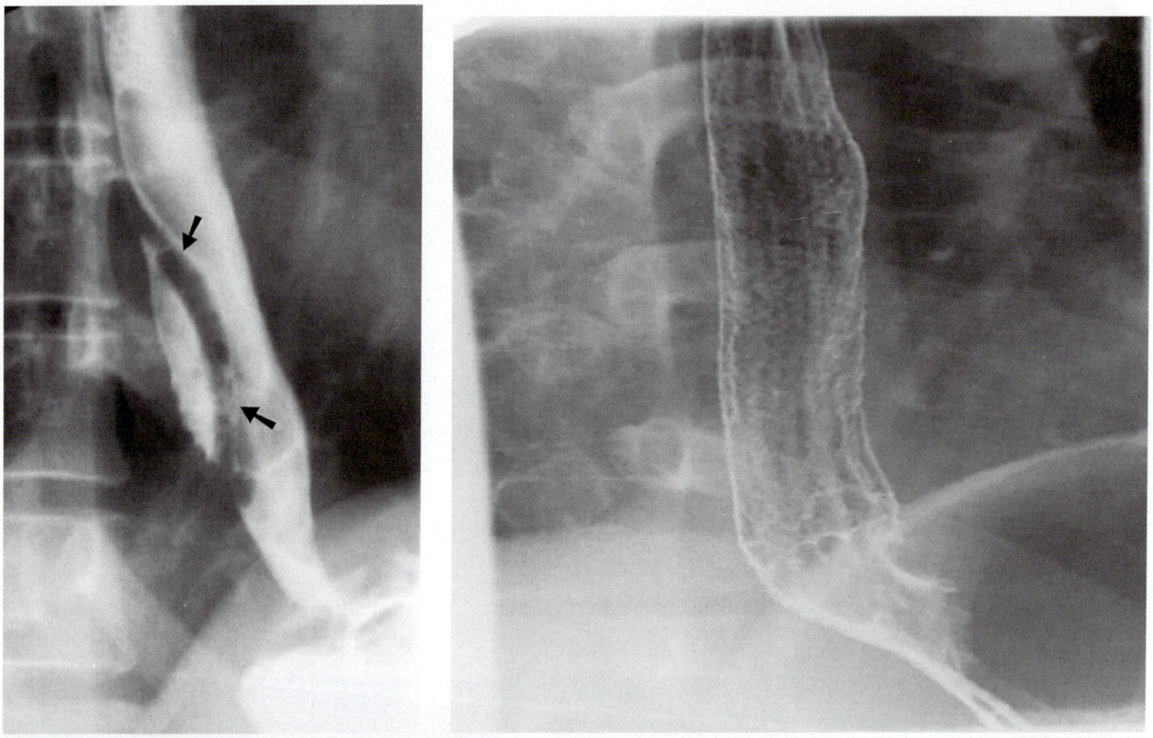

A B

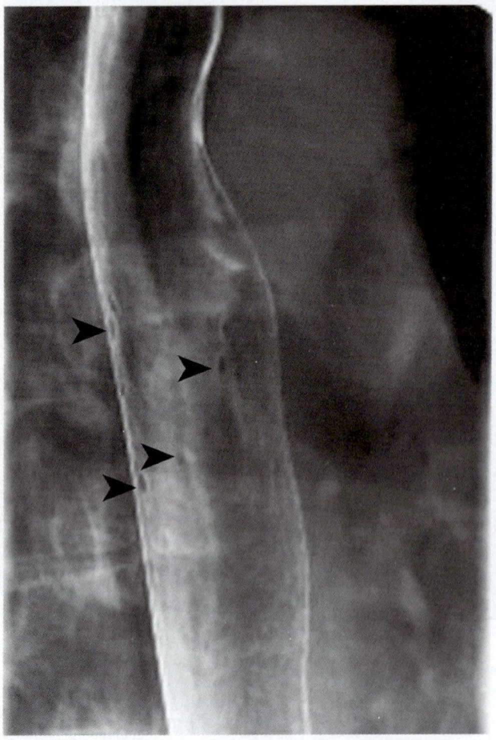

C

**FIG. 2.29 • CMV esophagitis, herpetic esophagitis, and glycogenic acanthosis. A:** CMV esophagitis—spot image of barium esophagram in an AIDS patient shows a giant esophageal ulcer with semilunar configuration with surrounding edema (*arrows*). **B:** Herpetic esophagitis: spot image of barium esophagram shows innumerable punctate ulcers without any plaques. In late stages, the esophagram is indistinguishable from candida esophagitis. **C:** Glycogenic acanthosis—double-contrast barium swallow shows multiple small filling defects (*arrowheads*) in the esophagus, which do not produce any symptoms.

from those caused by CMV esophagitis. Sometimes, HIV esophagitis can be associated with a cluster of small satellite ulcers. The diagnosis is established by obtaining endoscopic biopsy specimens, brushings, or cultures to rule out CMV as the cause of the ulcers. Unlike CMV ulcers, which are treated with antivirals, HIV-related esophageal ulcers usually heal markedly after treatment with oral steroids.[3,13]

*Herpes esophagitis* occurs mostly in immunocompromised patients; however, herpes esophagitis may occasionally develop as an acute self-limited disease in immunocompetent individuals. Herpes esophagitis results in the development of small mucosal vesicles that later rupture to form discrete punched-out ulcers. On double-contrast barium study, multiple small superficial ulcers are seen against the background of normal mucosa usually in the mid- to upper esophagus. The ulcers can also have a punctate, stellate, or ring-like configuration surrounded by radiolucent-raised edges of edema (Fig. 2.29B).[3,13]

*Tuberculous esophagitis* may occur from extension from caseous mediastinal lymph nodes or from the larynx, the pharynx, extension from tuberculous spondylitis, or hematogenous infection. Esophagram may demonstrate ulcers, strictures, or sinus tracts.[5]

*Glycogen acanthosis* is due to benign epithelial collections of glycogen producing small mucosal nodules, which are smooth and well defined. Glycogen acanthosis may be a degenerative process and produces no symptoms. On esophagram, it may mimic candida esophagitis; however, its nodules have a more rounded appearance as opposed to more linear appearing plaques in candidiasis (Fig. 2.29C).[3]

*Radiation esophagitis:* A radiation dose of 5,000 cGy or more to the mediastinum can cause severe injury to the esophagus. This usually occurs 2 to 4 weeks after the initiation of radiation therapy resulting in a granular appearance of mucosa due to edema and inflammation of the irradiated segment. Although most cases of acute radiation esophagitis are self-limited, some patients may have progressive dysphagia due to the development of radiation strictures 4 to 8 months after completion of radiation therapy. Radiation-induced strictures appear as smooth tapered areas of concentric narrowing confined to the radiation port (Fig. 2.30A).[3,5]

*Caustic esophagitis:* Accidental or intentional ingestion of lye or other caustic agents causes marked esophagitis leading to extensive stricture formation. Liquid lye causes a particularly severe form of caustic injury to the esophagus due to liquefactive necrosis. Unlike alkaline agents, which cause liquefactive necrosis, acid ingestion results in coagulative necrosis, forming a protective barrier and less severe damage. Endoscopy is initially performed after ingestion of a caustic agent to assess the extent and severity of esophageal injury.

If esophageal perforation is suspected, esophagram with water-soluble contrast material should be performed to document the presence of a leak, which may also reveal edema, spasm, and ulceration of the affected esophagus.[3,5] After the initial phase of esophagitis, follow-up barium studies will help to evaluate the

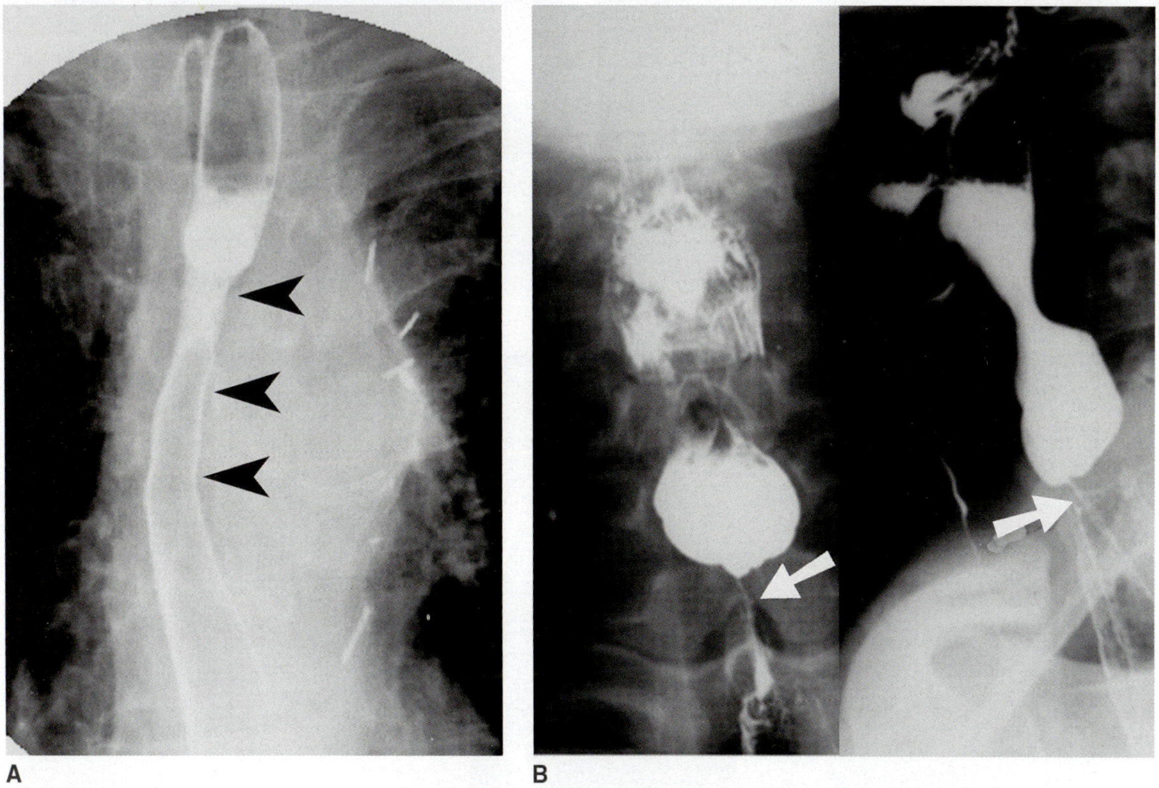


**FIG. 2.30 • Esophageal stricture from radiotherapy and caustic ingestion. A:** Single-contrast barium swallow demonstrates smooth, midesophageal narrowing without ulcerations or nodularity, secondary to past mediastinal radiation therapy for malignant neoplasm (*arrowheads*). **B:** A 35-year-old male had accidental ingestion of acid 6 months back and presenting with progressive dysphagia for 3 months. Spot image of barium esophagram demonstrates benign cervical esophageal stricture (*arrows*) with proximal dilatation.

length of developing strictures, which are usually long-segment concentric narrowing in the upper or midesophagus (Fig. 2.30B). New areas of mucosal irregularity or nodularity in a pre-existing chronic lye stricture should raise the suspicion of developing squamous cell carcinoma to which these patients are susceptible.[3,5]

*Other* causes of esophagitis include drug-induced esophagitis, Crohn disease, eosinophilic esophagitis, nasogastric intubation, and alkaline reflux esophagitis (due to reflux of pancreatobiliary secretions after partial or total gastrectomy). Some rare forms of esophagitis include chronic graft versus host disease, Behçet syndrome, and skin disorders such as epidermolysis bullosa dystrophica and pemphigoid.[5]

## ACUTE ESOPHAGEAL SYNDROMES

*Boerhaave syndrome* is a transmural or full-thickness perforation of the esophagus with rupture of the wall. This is seen with excessive vomiting and in eating disorders like bulimia. Rarely, it may be due to forceful coughing or obstruction by food. Chest radiographs may show pneumomediastinum and effusion.[14,15] Esophagram should be performed with water-soluble contrast media if leak is suspected (using barium incurs the theoretical risk of producing mediastinitis), which demonstrates contrast extravasation (Fig. 2.31A,B). Perforation is usually seen on the left side of the distal esophagus.[14]

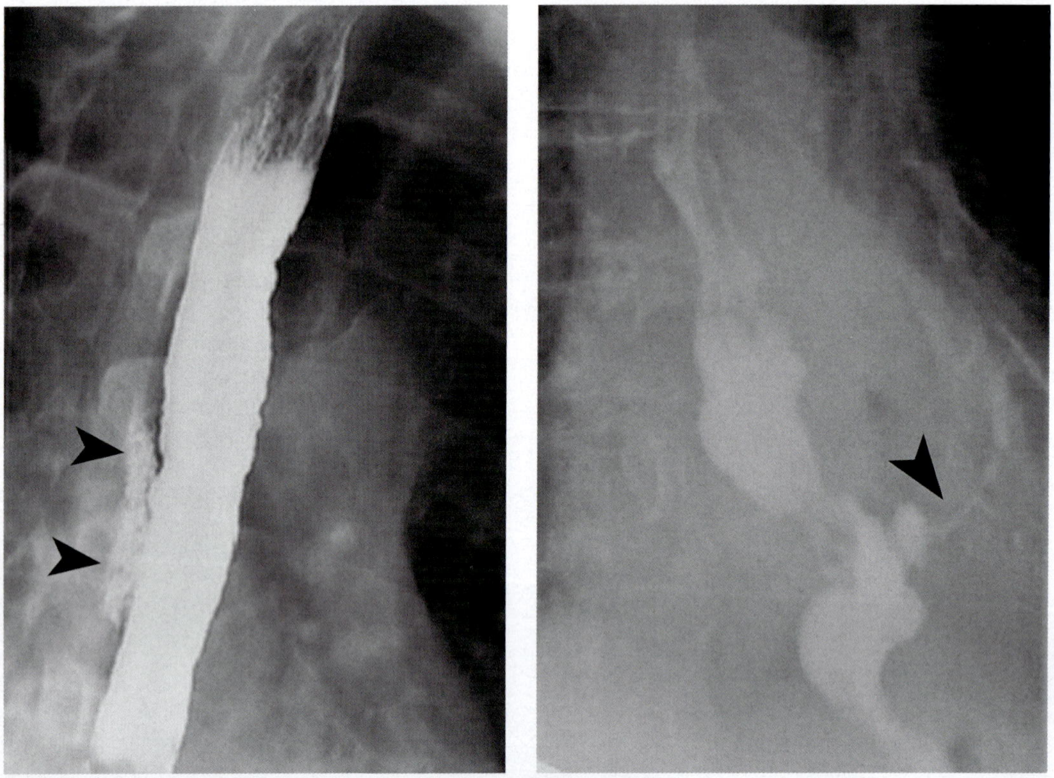

A B

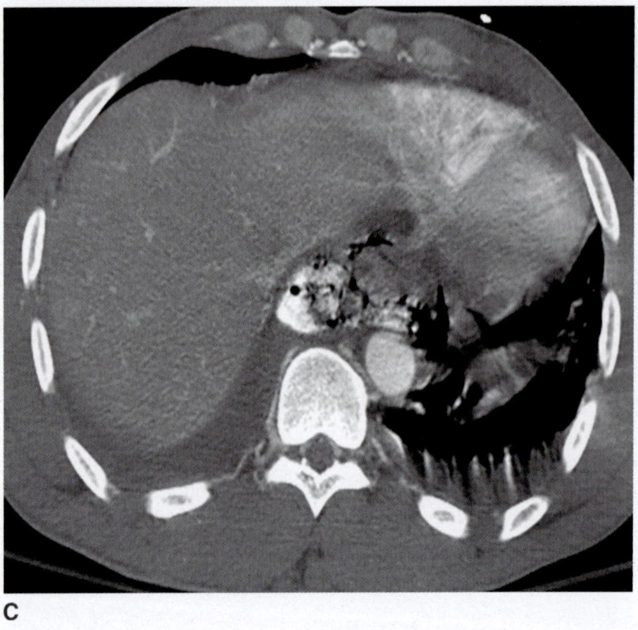

C

**FIG. 2.31 • Boerhaave syndrome. A:** Single-contrast Gastrograffin swallow study shows perforation in the midthoracic esophagus with leakage of contrast (*arrowheads*) outside the esophageal lumen. **B:** Single-contrast Gastrograffin swallow study shows perforation in the lower esophagus with formation of esophagobronchial fistula (*arrowhead*). **C:** Contrast-enhanced CT shows extraluminal air and contrast due to distal esophagus perforation.

CT scan can also confirm the diagnosis, which can detect small amounts of extraluminal gas or extravasation not visible on radiographs or esophagram (Fig. 2.31C).

*Mallory-Weiss tears* result from prolonged and forceful vomiting, coughing, and convulsions or as a result of excessive alcohol ingestion. This is a nontransmural (in contradistinction to Boerhaave) esophageal tear involving the mucous membrane at the junction of the esophagus and the stomach resulting in lacerations, which bleed. Patients present with bright red blood in vomitus or bloody stools. Barium esophagram may demonstrate linear mucosal tear near the GE junction. Mucosal tears may be found in the distal esophagus or gastric fundus or extend across the GE junction.

*Esophageal hematoma* is unusual and may be spontaneous or may have association with severe vomiting, instrumentation, trauma, anticoagulation, or bleeding disorders. Esophageal hematoma is a self-limiting condition, which usually resolves in 1 to 2 weeks with conservative treatment. Barium esophagram will demonstrate luminal narrowing with a flattened appearance, similar to any other submucosal pathology. Iatrogenic instrumentation tear may show a double lumen due to dissecting intramural hematoma. CT scan confirms the diagnosis of intramural hematoma, which will appear as a high-density intramural thickening.[16] Follow-up scan will show resolution on conservative management.

## BENIGN ESOPHAGEAL TUMORS

*Leiomyomas* are the most common benign submucosal tumor (50%) of the esophagus. These are usually asymptomatic but large tumors may cause dysphagia.

On plain radiographs, these tumors may be seen as a soft tissue density with obliteration or displacement of the azygoesophageal recess interface. On barium esophagram, leiomyoma manifests as a smooth submucosal mass etched in white, forming a right angle or a smaller obtuse angle with the adjacent esophageal wall when viewed in profile[3,17] (Fig. 2.32). It is difficult to distinguish these from other mesenchymal tumors like fibromas, neurofibromas, and hemangiomas. A calcified submucosal mass is most often a leiomyoma. CT scan further confirms finding by demonstrating a well-defined circumferential or multilobulated, sometimes circumferential, soft tissue mass without mucosal destruction or constricting luminal narrowing.[3,17]

*Fibrovascular polyps* are rare benign tumors consisting, as the name implies, of fibrous, vascular, and adipose tissue covered by squamous epithelium. Fibrovascular polyps usually arise near the level of the cricopharyngeus muscle and elongate inferiorly over a period of years.

On esophagram, it demonstrates as expansile, sausage-shaped masses, which expand the upper and middle esophageal lumen (Fig. 2.33A). On real-time fluoroscopy, the movement of the fibrovascular polyp may be demonstrated producing an inconstant position and shape.[3,17] On CT, these lesions may demonstrate fat attenuation or have a heterogeneous appearance depending on the content of adipose and fibrovascular tissue (Fig. 2.33B).

## ESOPHAGEAL CANCER

Esophageal cancer is one of the leading causes of cancer mortality. Most esophageal cancers are epithelial in origin involving the upper and midesophagus. Squamous cell carcinoma is the most common type (95%) of esophageal cancer, followed by adenocarcinoma, which usually occurs near the GE junction.

Alcohol abuse and tobacco are the most significant risk factors for the development of squamous cell carcinoma of the esophagus in the Western world. Other predisposing factors are achalasia, lye strictures, celiac disease, Plummer-Vinson

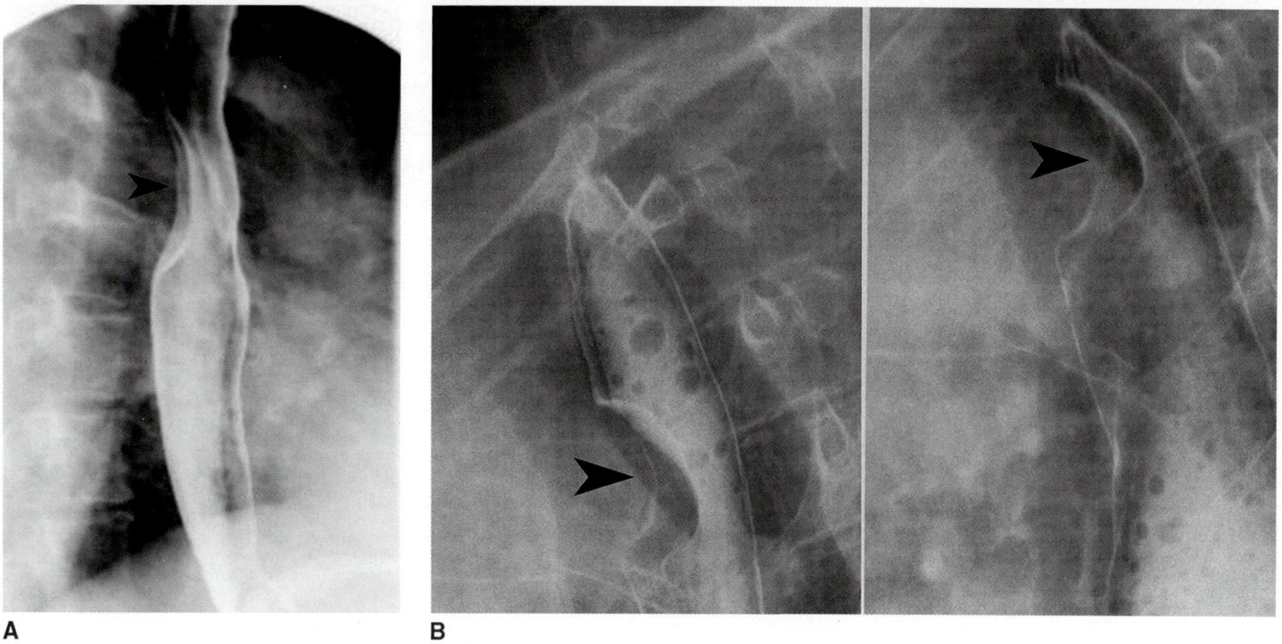



**FIG. 2.32 • Leiomyoma. A,B:** Double-contrast barium study demonstrates well-defined lobulated submucosal mass in the esophagus causing a smooth marginated oval filling defect (*arrowheads*) without obstruction. The margin of the filling defect forms obtuse angle with the esophageal wall.

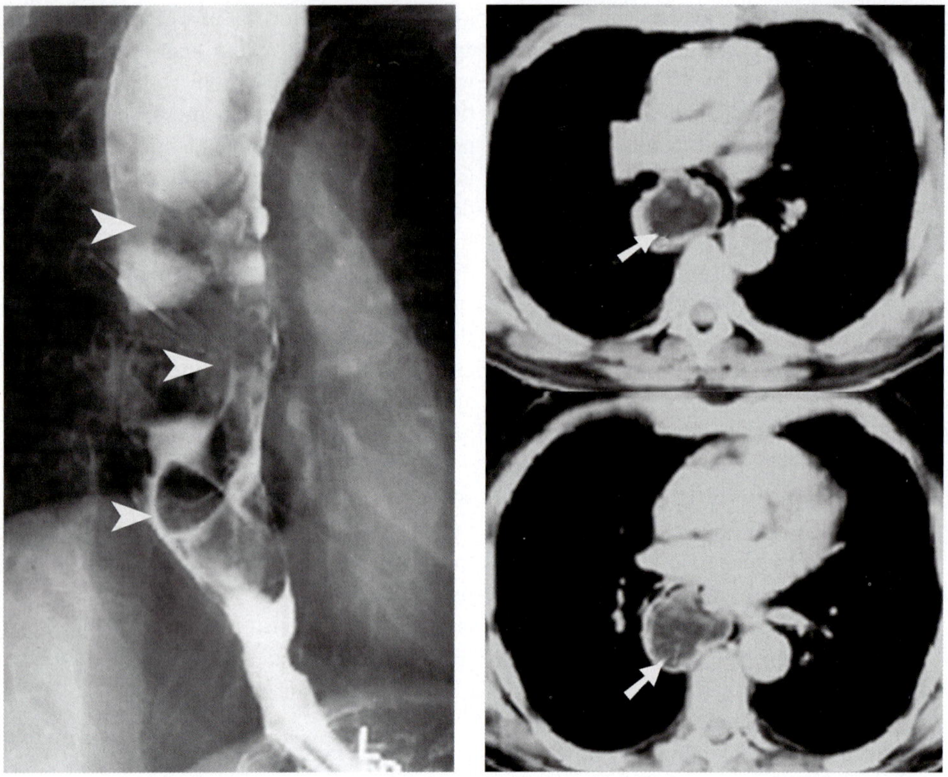

A B

**FIG. 2.33 ● Fibrovascular polyp. A:** Barium esophagram demonstrates large polypoid filling defect (*arrowheads*) with long pedicle expanding the esophageal lumen. **B:** Axial contrast-enhanced CT images show predominantly low density mass (*arrows*) with areas of fat attenuation and enhancing fibrovascular component within the esophagus with luminal expansion.

syndrome, and, arguably, eating pickled or fermented foods. Barrett's esophagus is columnar metaplasia of the squamous epithelium of the distal esophagus, usually related to GERD, and is considered a premalignant condition, predisposing to the development of adenocarcinoma of the esophagus. Unlike squamous cell carcinoma, which involves the upper and midesophagus, adenocarcinoma involves the lower esophagus and also has a marked tendency to invade the gastric cardia or fundus.

Patients with esophageal carcinoma usually present with dysphagia; however, this is a late finding after the tumor invades into the esophageal wall, periesophageal lymphatics, or other mediastinal structures (Table 2.1).

Table 2.1 **TNM STAGING OF ESOPHAGEAL CARCINOMA**

| T Staging | N Staging | M Staging |
|---|---|---|
| **Tx:** primary tumor cannot be assessed | **Nx:** regional nodes cannot be assessed | **Mx:** metastatic disease cannot be assessed |
| **T0:** no evidence of primary tumor | **N0:** no regional lymph node metastases | **M0:** no distant metastases |
| **Tis**: high-grade dysplasia | | |
| **T1:** invades lamina propria, muscularis mucosae, or submucosa<br>**T1a:** invades lamina propria or muscularis mucosae<br>**T1b:** invades submucosa | **N1:** 1–2 regional nodes involved | **M1:** distant metastases |
| **T2:** invades muscularis propria | **N2:** 3–6 regional nodes involved | |
| **T3:** invades adventitia | **N3:** >7 regional nodes involved | |
| **T4:** direct extension into adjacent structures<br>**T4a:** (resectable) invades the pleura, pericardium, or diaphragm.<br>**T4b:** (unresectable) invades other structures like the aorta or trachea | | |

## IMAGING

*Barium studies* are often used to evaluate esophageal carcinomas. On double-contrast barium esophagram, various radiologic types are described. *Early esophageal cancers* may appear as small, protuberant lesions less than 3.5 cm in size and may manifest as plaque-like lesions with flat central ulcers, sessile polyps with a smooth or lobulated contour, or focal irregularities of the esophageal wall. Wall flattening or irregularity within a pre-existing peptic stricture should raise suspicion for early carcinomas. Superficial spreading carcinoma is a form of early esophageal cancer, which is characterized by poorly defined confluent nodules or plaques. *Advanced esophageal carcinomas* can be infiltrating, polypoid, ulcerative, or varicoid lesions.[3,18] Infiltrating carcinomas on barium esophagram will manifest as irregular luminal narrowing with mucosal nodularity or ulceration and abrupt shelf-like borders[3,18]. Polypoid carcinomas appear as lobulated intraluminal masses or as polypoid-ulcerated masses (Figs. 2.34 and 2.35). Primary ulcerative carcinomas will appear as giant meniscoid ulcers surrounded by a radiolucent rind of tumor. Varicoid carcinomas are rare, and their appearance is due to submucosal spread of tumor, which produces thickened, tortuous, and longitudinal filling defects on the barium column. They have a fixed configuration unlike varices, which change in size and shape at fluoroscopy.

Esophageal cancers can spread to other parts from submucosal lymphatics and produce satellite metastases that may appear polypoid, plaque-like, or as ulcerated lesions separated by normal mucosa from the primary tumor. Subdiaphragmatic

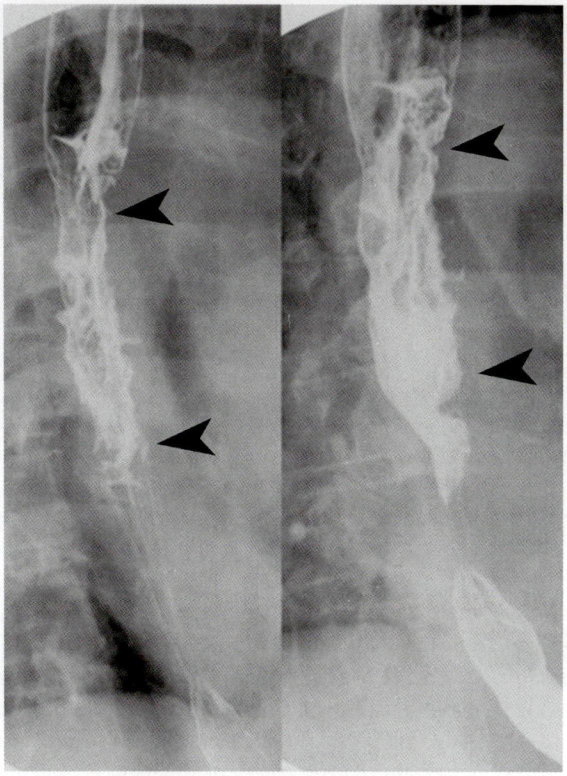

**FIG. 2.34 • Infiltrating esophageal carcinoma.** Spot images from double-contrast esophagram show advanced infiltrating carcinoma (*arrowheads*) as irregular area of narrowing, mucosal nodularity, and ulcerations in the midthoracic esophagus.

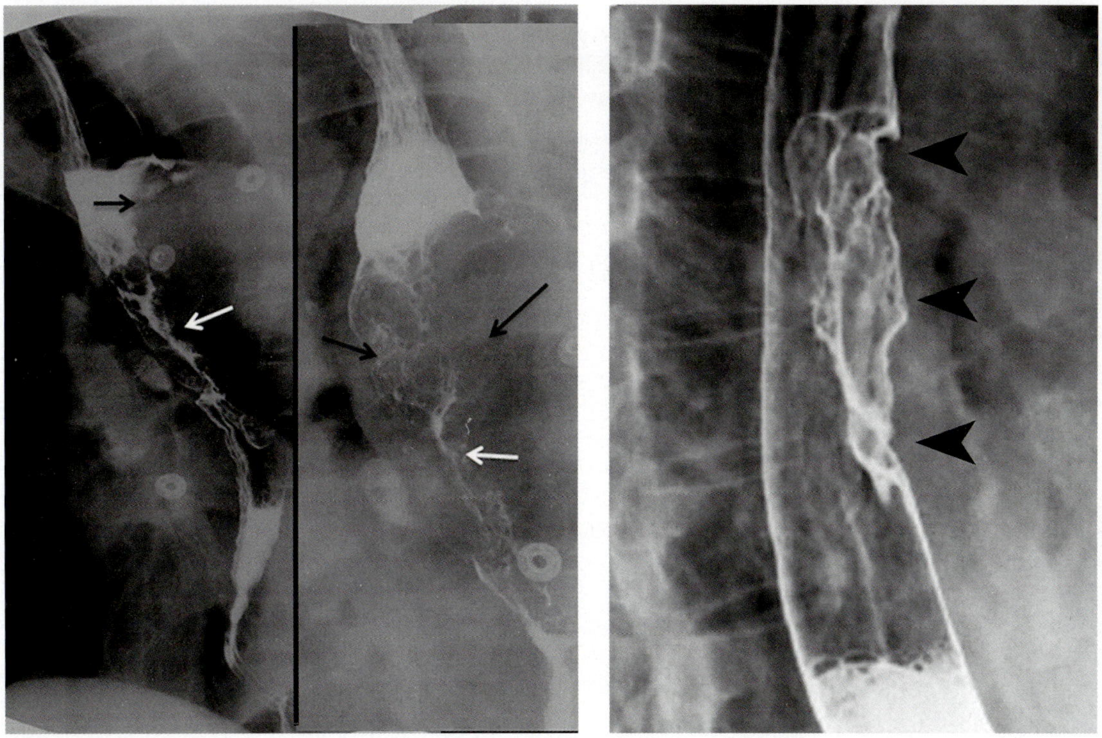

A B

**FIG. 2.35 • Advanced esophageal carcinoma. A:** Spot images from double-contrast barium esophagram show advanced esophageal carcinoma as polypoid mass (*black arrows*) with large areas of ulceration and mucosal irregularities (*white arrows*) in the midthoracic esophagus. **B:** Spot images from double-contrast barium esophagram show esophageal carcinoma as asymmetric irregular filling defect in the midthoracic esophagus with proximal shouldering (*arrowhead*).

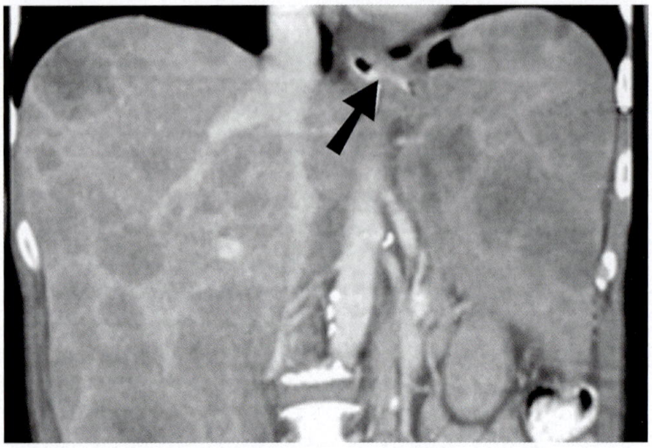

**FIG. 2.36 • Esophageal adenocarcinoma.** Coronal contrast-enhanced CT reformations show distal esophageal wall thickening (*arrow*), also involving the gastric cardia. There is hepatomegaly with multiple metastatic deposits.

tumor spread to the proximal stomach will appear as large submucosal masses with central ulcers.

*Endoscopic US* (EUS) is considered to be the most accurate imaging modality currently available for primary tumor staging in patients with esophageal cancer. The esophageal wall is visualized as five alternating layers of differing echogenicity, allowing accurate preoperative determination of the depth of tumor invasion.[18]

*CT imaging* is important for initial preoperative staging. For this purpose, the esophagus is divided into four regions: cervical, upper thoracic, midthoracic, and lower thoracic esophagus. The cervical esophagus begins at the level of the lower border of the cricoid cartilage and ends at the thoracic inlet. The upper thoracic esophagus begins at the thoracic inlet and ends at the level of the tracheal bifurcation; the midthoracic esophagus is the proximal portion of the esophagus between the tracheal bifurcation and the esophagogastric junction, while the lower thoracic esophagus is approximately 8 cm distal to the esophagus and includes the intra-abdominal portion and the esophagogastric junction. Esophageal cancer has an aggressive behavior and spreads by direct extension, lymphatic spread, and hematogenous metastasis (Fig. 2.36). Esophageal cancer spreads easily to adjacent structures due to lack of serosa and therefore an anatomical barrier. The CT criteria for local invasion include loss of fat planes between the tumor and adjacent structures in the mediastinum and displacement or indentation of other mediastinal structures. Aortic invasion is suggested if 90 degrees or more of the aorta is in contact with the tumor or if there is obliteration of the triangular fat space between the esophagus, aorta, and spine adjacent to the primary tumor.[18,19] Displacement of the trachea or bronchus, or indentation of the posterior wall of the trachea or bronchus by the tumor, also predicts tracheobronchial invasion (see Fig. 2.35). A tracheoesophageal or bronchoesophageal fistula can occur from tracheobronchial invasion (Fig. 2.37). Pericardial invasion is suspected if pericardial thickening, pericardial effusion, or indentation of the heart with loss of the pericardial fat plane is seen.[18,19]

*Positron emission tomography (PET)* is useful for the assessment of distant metastases and in restaging after neoadjuvant therapy.[18]

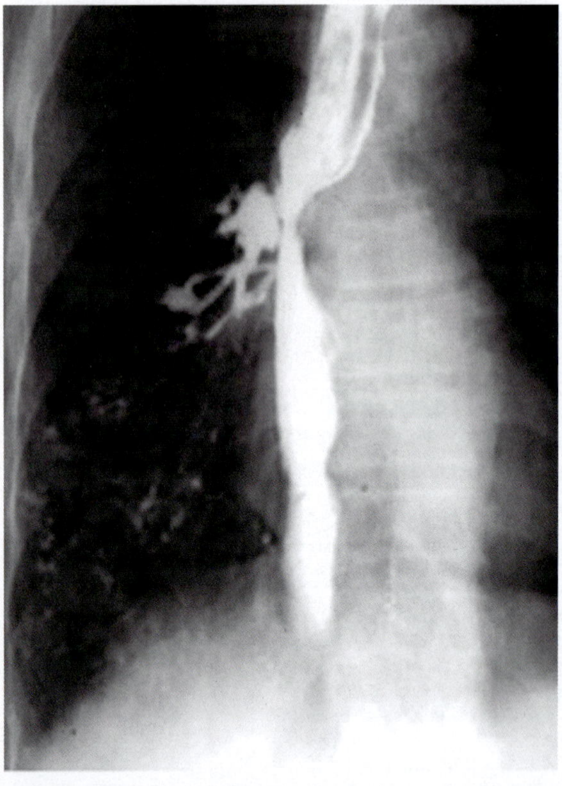

**FIG. 2.37 • Bronchoesophageal fistula in carcinoma esophagus.** Spot image of barium esophagram in the patient with carcinoma of the midthoracic esophagus shows bronchoesophageal fistula arising from the thoracic esophagus.

## References


1. Schatzki R. The lower esophageal ring: long term follow-up of symptomatic and asymptomatic rings. *Am J Roentgenol Radium Ther Nucl Med.* 1963;90:805–810.
2. Chen YM, Ott DJ, Gelfand DW, et al. Multiphasic examination of the esophagogastric region for strictures, rings, and hiatal hernia: evaluation of the individual techniques. *Gastrointest Radiol.* 1985;10:311–316.
3. Levine MS, Rubesin SE. Diseases of the esophagus: diagnosis with esophagography. *Radiology.* 2005;237:414–427.
4. Kahrilas PJ, Kim HC, Pandolfino JE. Approaches to the diagnosis and grading of hiatal hernia. *Best Pract Res Clin Gastroenterol.* 2008;22(4):601–616.
5. Karasick S, Lev-toaff AS. Esophageal strictures: findings on barium radiographs. *AJR Am J Roentgenol.* 1995;165(3):561–565.
6. Katsinelos P, Gkagkalis S, Chatzimavroudis G, et al. Recurrent esophageal web in Plummer-Vinson syndrome successfully treated with postdilation intralesional injection of mitomycin C. *Gastrointest Endosc.* 2012;75(5):1124.
7. Khan N, Ismail F, Van de Werke IE. Oesophageal pouches and diverticula: a pictorial review. *S Afr J Surg.* 2012;50(3):71–75.
8. DeVault KR. Presbyesophagus: a reappraisal. *Curr Gastroenterol Rep.* 2002;4(3):193–199.
9. Woodfield CA, Levine MS, Rubesin SE, et al. Diagnosis of primary versus secondary achalasia: reassessment of clinical and radiographic criteria. *AJR Am J Roentgenol.* 2000;175:727–731.
10. Creteur V, Thoeni RF, Federle MP, et al. The role of single- and double-contrast radiography in the diagnosis of reflux esophagitis. *Radiology.* 1983;147:71–75.
11. Gilchrist AM, Levine MS, Carr RF, et al. Barrett's esophagus: diagnosis by double-contrast esophagography. *AJR Am J Roentgenol.* 1988;150:97–102.

12. Yamamoto AJ, Levine MS, Katzka, DA, et al. Short-segment Barrett's esophagus: findings on double-contrast esophagography in 20 patients. *AJR Am J Roentgenol.* 2001;176(5):1173–1178.
13. Levine MS. Radiology of esophagitis: a pattern approach. *Radiology.* 1991;179(1):1–7.
14. Tonolini M, Bianco R. Spontaneous esophageal perforation (Boerhaave syndrome): diagnosis with CT-esophagography. *J Emerg Trauma Shock.* 2013;6(1):58–60.
15. Gimenez A, Franquet T, Erasmus JJ, et al. Thoracic complications of esophageal disorders. *Radiographics.* 2002;22:S247–S258.
16. Hong M, Warum D, Karamanian A. Spontaneous intramural esophageal hematoma (IEH) secondary to anticoagulation and/or thrombolysis therapy in the setting of a pulmonary embolism: a case report. *J Radiol Case Rep.* 2013;7(2):1–10.
17. Montesi A, Pesaresi A, Graziani L, et al. Small benign tumors of the esophagus: radiological diagnosis with double-contrast examination. *Gastrointest Radiol.* 1983;8:207–212.
18. Kim TJ, Kim HY, Lee KW, et al. Multimodality assessment of esophageal cancer: preoperative staging and monitoring of response to therapy. *Radiographics.* 2009;29(2):403–421.
19. Picus D, Balfe DM, Koehler RE, et al. Computed tomography in the staging of esophageal carcinoma. *Radiology.* 1983;146:433–438.

## SELF-ASSESSMENT QUESTIONS

1. Lateral view spot image of the barium esophagram is shown. What is the cause of the patient's dysphagia?

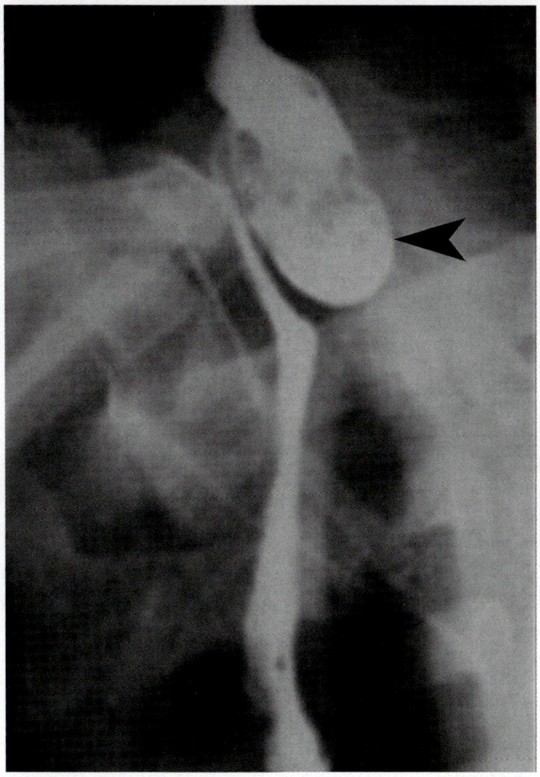

A. Killian-Jamieson diverticulum
B. Midesophageal diverticulum
C. Epiphrenic diverticulum
D. Zenker diverticulum

2. Spot image of the barium esophagram is shown. What is the cause of the patient's dysphagia?

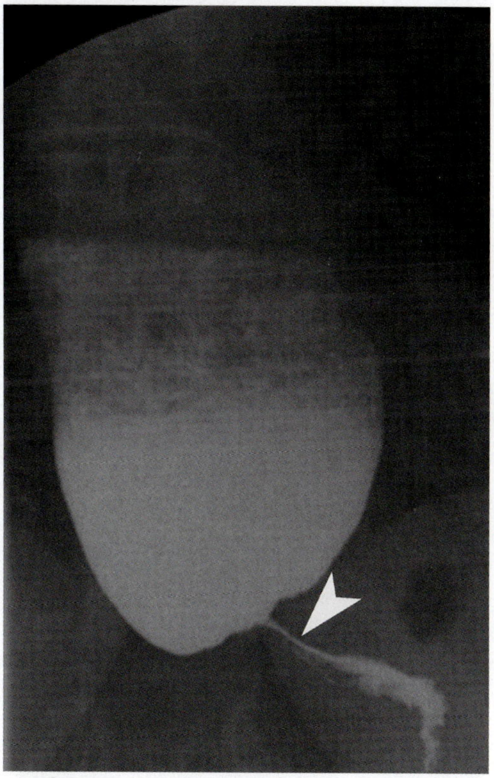

A. Hiatus hernia
B. Achalasia
C. Pseudoachalasia
D. Esophageal cancer

3. What does the black arrowhead on the double-contrast barium esophagram indicates?

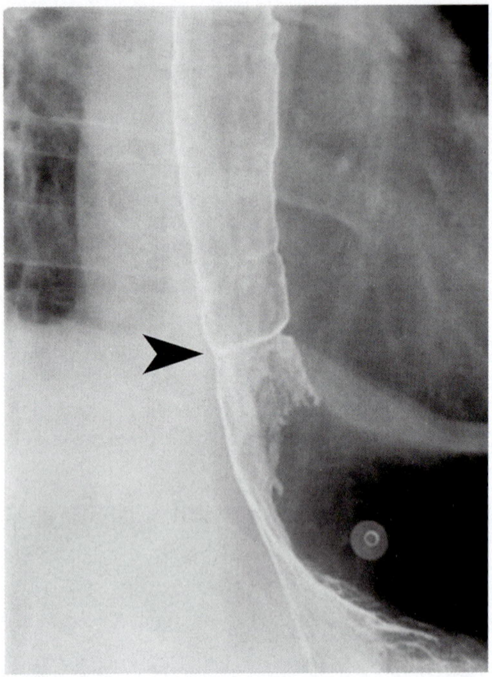

A. A ring
B. Z ring
C. B ring
D. Vestibule

4. What is the cause of dysphagia on the given barium esophagram?

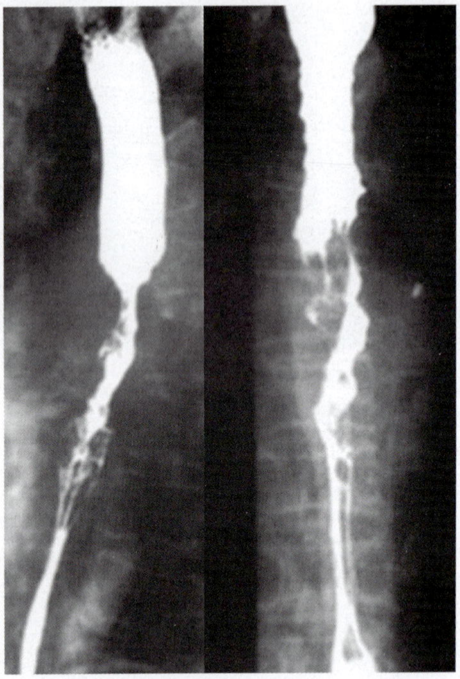

A. Benign esophageal stricture
B. Dilated intramural glands
C. Infiltrating esophageal carcinoma
D. Reflux esophagitis

5. What is the likely diagnosis in the patient presenting with chronic reflux disease?

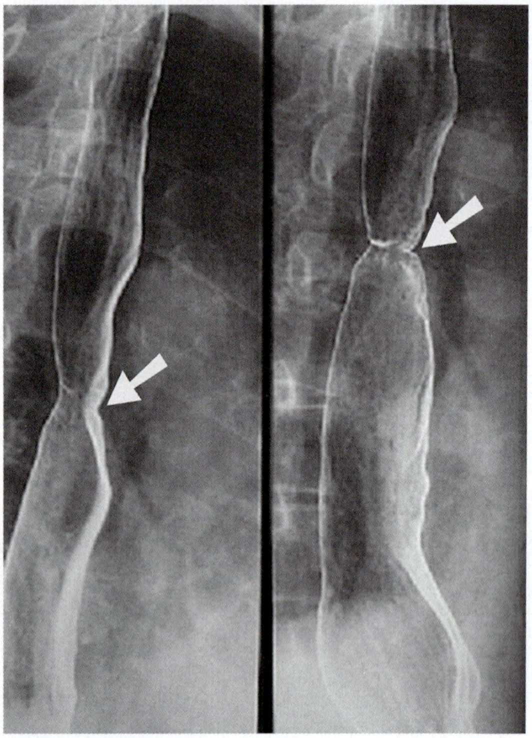

A. Candida esophagitis
B. Reflux esophagitis
C. Barrett esophagus
D. Malignant esophageal stricture

## *Answers to Self-Assessment Questions*

**1. D.** Zenker diverticulum. The barium swallow demonstrates a smooth pulsion diverticulum (arrowhead) protruding posteriorly from the hypopharynx and is consistent with Zenker diverticulum. Killian-Jamieson diverticulum arises below the upper esophageal sphincter and is directed anterolaterally.

**2. B.** Achalasia. Barium swallow demonstrates a grossly dilated esophagus with tight stricture (arrowhead) at the lower esophageal sphincter. Pseudoachalasia is the secondary type of achalasia, which can be due to tumor at the gastroesophageal junction.

**3. C.** The barium swallow depicts the B ring, which is a mucosal ring at the squamocolumnar junction or the Z line. It represents the lower boundary of the phrenic ampulla and is located 2 to 4 cm below the A ring.

**4. C.** Infiltrating esophageal carcinoma. The single-contrast barium swallow depicts a malignant stricture with proximal shouldering, mucosal irregularity, and filling defects. A benign stricture is typically long-segment stricture with smooth tapered margins and not nodular filling defects.

**5. C.** Barrett esophagus. The barium swallow depicts a benign stricture in the upper thoracic esophagus, often seen in patients with long-standing reflux disease.

# Stomach: Non-neoplastic Conditions 3A

*Caterina Missiroli and Ajay K. Singh*

## LEARNING OBJECTIVE

1. Show the barium as well as cross-sectional imaging appearance of principal nonneoplastic conditions of the stomach.

The stomach is a J-shaped hollow viscous organ in the left upper quadrant of the abdomen that is divided into five regions: cardia, fundus, body, antrum, and pylorus.[1,2] The lesser and greater curvatures outline the stomach medially and laterally. The gastric cardia is seen on the upper GI series as three or four stellate mucosal folds arising from the gastroesophageal junction. The gastric fundus is part of the stomach located cranial to the gastroesophageal junction. The gastric body extends from the gastric cardia to the curvature of the lesser curvature (incisura angularis). The gastric antrum is part of the stomach that extends from the incisura angularis to the pylorus.

The gastric wall consists of four concentric layers of tissue: mucosa, submucosa, muscularis propria, and serosa.[2] The mucosa is composed of the epithelium, lamina propria, and muscularis mucosa.

## UPPER GASTROINTESTINAL SERIES

Before the introduction of cross-sectional imaging, double-contrast barium examination was the primary imaging tool for the assessment of the stomach. The cross-sectional imaging techniques, in particular CT, allow detection of gastric wall as well as extragastric abnormalities. The mucosa is the layer detected by barium study and can be seen as gastric rugal folds (up to 5 mm thickness) and areae gastricae (1 to 5 mm) (Fig. 3A.1) on double-contrast studies.[1]

**Gastric rugal folds:**

- Composed of the gastric mucosa and submucosa
- Most prominent in the fundus and body
- Often absent in the gastric antrum
- Typically less than 5 mm in thickness in the distended stomach

**Areae gastricae:**

- Represents polygonal-shaped mucosa separated by grooves.
- Seen on the upper GI series as polygonal-shaped white lines that represent barium filling the groves surrounding the mucosal tufts.
- Typically 2 to 3 mm in diameter in the gastric antrum and up to 5 mm in diameter in the gastric body.
- Visualization is highest in the 70 plus age group (seen in three-fourths of patients).

Upper gastrointestinal series of the stomach may be performed in single- or double-contrast technique. Single-contrast radiography may be used to coat the mucosa for studying varices and to evaluate the stomach postoperatively (water-soluble contrast agent) at the beginning of the double-contrast exam.[2] Double-contrast technique uses barium and effervescent granules to optimize the demonstration of mucosal surface and the luminal contour, appearing as a smooth continuous line coated by barium. At the beginning of the exam, the radiologist investigates the position, shape, and size of the stomach and then he or she conducts the study of the luminal contour and the mucosal aspect. When viewed en face, the disruption of the normal areae gastricae is considered abnormal.[1]

The most important role of CT with intravascular administration of contrast agent is to show the extent of the disease beyond the gastric wall, where endoscopic ultrasonography (EUS) has limitation in panoramic visualization.[3,4] Dedicated CT protocols targeted to the study of the stomach involve gastric distension either with oral contrast (Gastrografin or similar) and water or air (CT gastrography).[4] Adequate gastric distension is the basis of CT imaging and can be obtained by effervescent granules, followed by prone and supine scanning, with the second series acquired in portal venous phase.[4]

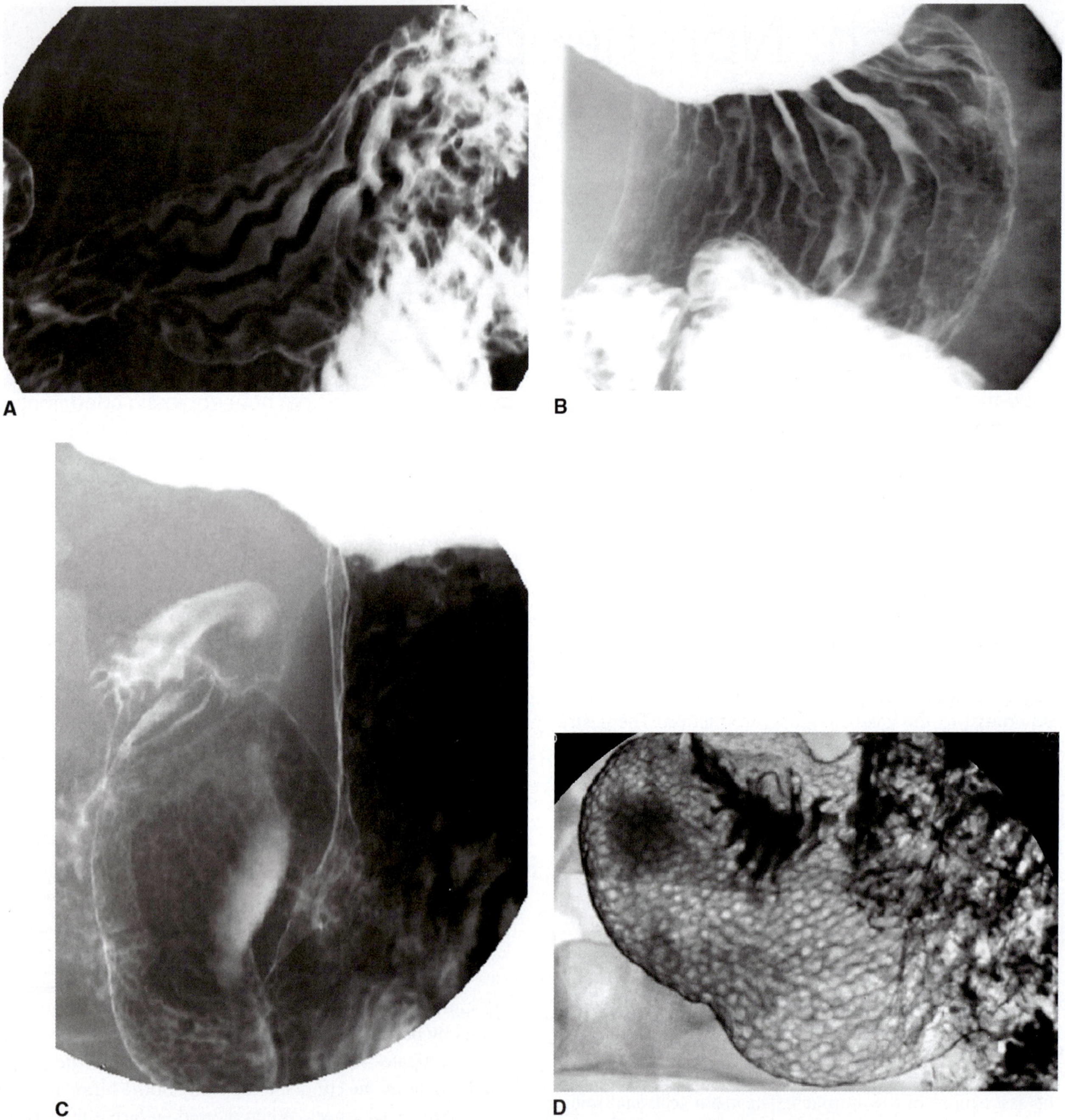

**FIG. 3A.1 • Gastric rugal folds and areae gastricae anatomy. A:** Double-contrast upper GI study demonstrates normal gastric rugal folds in the gastric body, running parallel to the long axis of the stomach. **B:** Prominent gastric rugal folds with some prominence of the areae gastricae in a patient with gastritis. **C:** Double-contrast study demonstrates prominent areae gastricae, most prominently in the gastric antrum in a patient with gastritis. **D:** Markedly prominent areae gastricae in the gastric antrum in a patient with acute gastritis.

CT imaging of the gastric wall is most frequently used for the detection of malignant lesions. The gastric wall thickness on CT of greater than 5 mm can be considered abnormal, but a threshold of 1 cm increases the positive predictive value in detecting malignant or potentially malignant conditions.[3,5]

## GASTRITIS

This term refers to a wide variety of inflammatory pathologies involving the gastric mucosa. The mucosal aspect findings are different according to type and evolution of the pathology, including striations, enlarged areae gastricae, nodules, thickened folds, mucosal erosions, and ulcerations.[1,2]

*Helicobacter pylori* is a helix-shaped gram-negative bacillus infecting the stomach wall in 50% of the Americans and primarily involving the antrum. It is not completely understood how *H. pylori* causes mucosal ulcers, but its presence has been documented in almost 80% of the patients with gastric ulcer.[1,6] When chronic, this type of gastritis may cause bleeding, obstruction, and perforation. The most important alterations of the mucosal surface due to this bacillus are thickened rugal folds (greater than 5 mm), nodularity, enlarged areae gastricae, erosions, ulcers, antral narrowing, and polyps.[1,2] The thickened folds are usually longitudinal or transverse in orientation, and they are found in about 90% of the patients.[6] Typical *H. pylori* gastritis causes hypertrophic antral-pyloric folds, seen as a smooth defect in the submucosal layer extending from the antrum to the pylorus. Disruption of the normal areae gastricae is seen in about 33% of the patients with *H. pylori* gastritis, in which the tufts are more prominent but not always larger.[6] These findings are not seen in atrophic gastritis, when folds are smaller or absent. Linear or serpentine erosions, which are focal areas of mucosal necrosis limited to the epithelium or lamina propria, without involving the submucosa, are pathognomonic for NSAID-induced gastritis. Erosions are seen as tiny, punctuate, round, stellate, or linear barium collection with surrounding radiolucent halo of edematous mucosa, usually involving the greater curvature of the gastric antrum.[6]

On CT imaging, the two patterns include circumferential antral wall thickening and thickening of the posterior gastric wall along the greater curvature, with or without ulceration (Fig. 3A.2).

Differentiating ulcer from erosion is not easy, but a lesion greater than 2 mm in depth is conventionally called an ulcer. Ulcer is a crater extending into the gastric wall beyond the mucosa. On the nondependent wall, the ulcer is seen as a ring of barium that coats the edge of the crater. On the dependent wall, it is demonstrated as a barium-filled crater.[2] An ulcer is seen en face as a distinct collection of barium, most often in a round configuration. In profile, an ulcer crater will project outside the expected outline of the gastric mucosal lining (Figs. 3A.3 to 3A.6). Hampton line is a thin, radiolucent line across the mouth of the ulcer, due to the overhanging mucosa at the margin of the ulcer crater. Ulcer collar and ulcer mound are characterized by progressive edema of the overhanging mucosa, resulting in thicker lucent line. Severe edema of the overhanging mucosa can cause crescent sign due to the trapped barium between the base of the ulcer and overhanging mucosa. On double-contrast study, the ulcer crater may be empty, and the peripheral outline of the crater may be visualized as a rim.

**Features of benign ulcers:**

- Ninety-five percent of gastric ulcers are benign.
- Most cases are located along the lesser curvature or posterior wall of the stomach (gastric fundus ulcers are mostly malignant).
- Most ulcers are less than 1 cm in diameter.
- Most are solitary (20% are multiple).
- They are round or ovoid in configuration but may also be serpentine, rectangular, flame shaped, or rod shaped.
- They are characterized with ulcer mound, ulcer collar, and Hampton line.
- Radiating mucosal folds extend to the edge of the ulcer crater.
- They have thin and smooth mucosal folds (irregularity or nodularity of mucosal folds indicates malignancy).

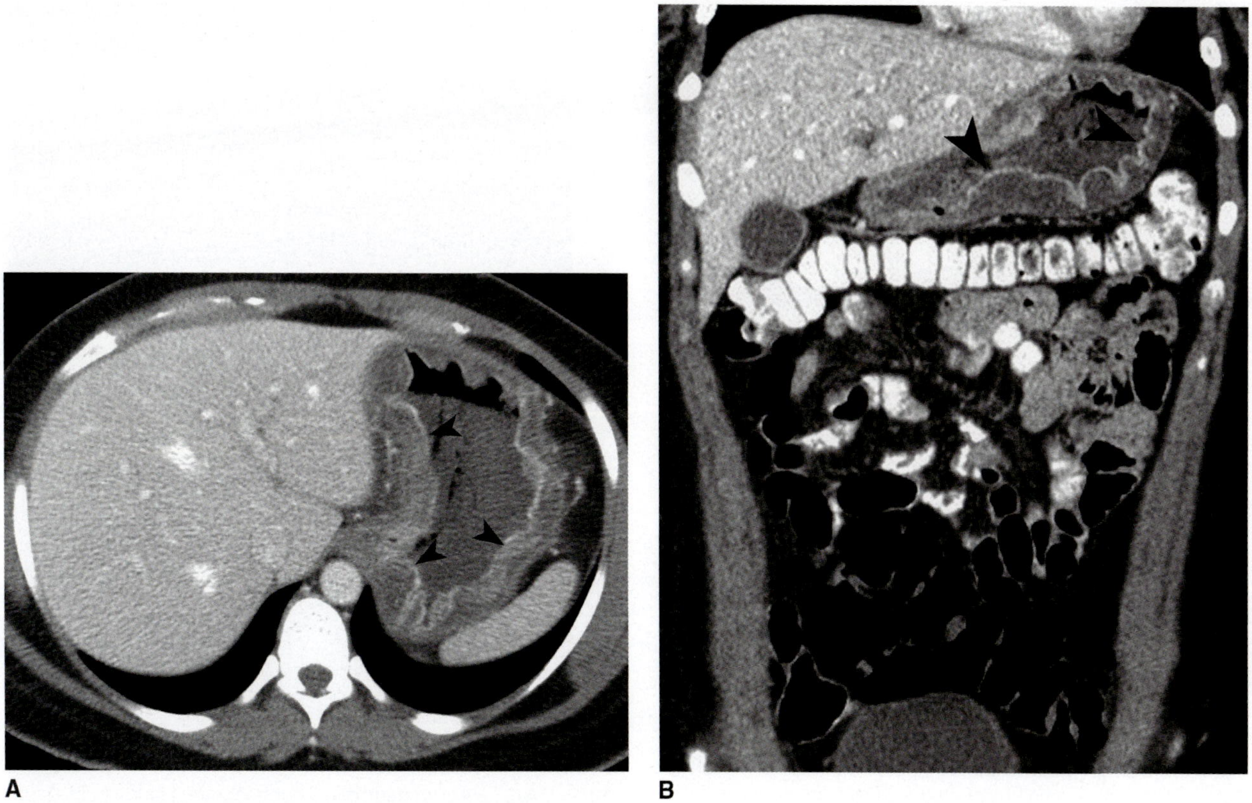

A B

**FIG. 3A.2 • Acute gastritis.** Axial **(A)** and coronal **(B)** CT images of the upper abdomen demonstrate extensive gastric wall thickening (*arrowheads*) with mucosal enhancement and submucosal edema.

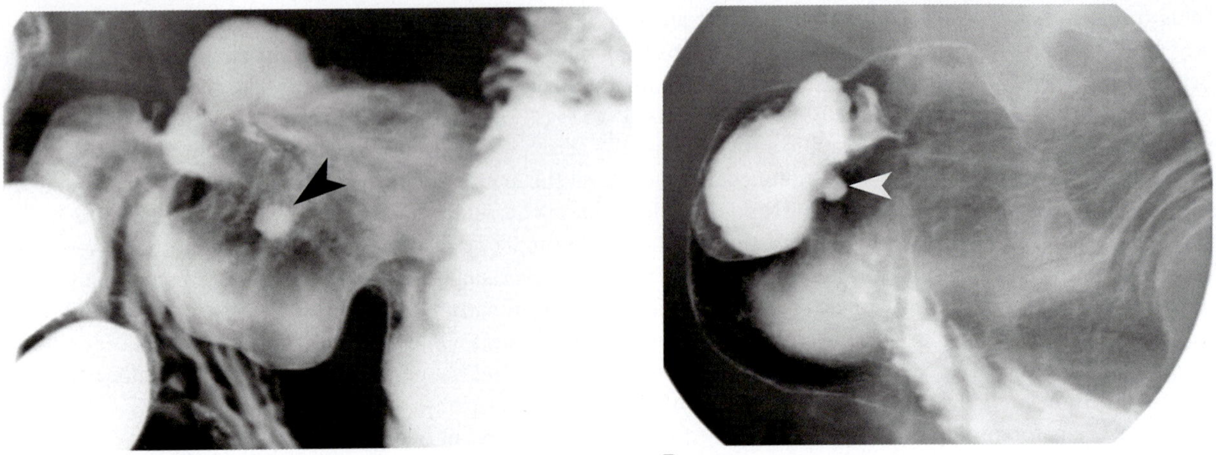

A B

**FIG. 3A.3 • Benign gastric ulcer. A, B:** En face and tangential spot fluoroscopy images of the gastric ulcer demonstrate collection of contrast in the ulcer crater (*arrowhead*) with surrounding edema in the gastric antrum. No mucosal nodularity is identified to indicate the presence of underlying malignancy.

## ACUTE EROSIVE GASTRITIS

Aspirin and other nonsteroidal anti-inflammatory drugs are the most frequent agents causing this gastropathy: alcohol, chemotherapeutic agents, cocaine use, uremia, radiation therapy, and infections being the other causes of this condition. NSAIDs cause acute and chronic gastritis by breaking the mucosal barrier and generating mucosal hypoxia, resulting in focal necrosis of the epithelium and alterations of the lamina propria, such as hemorrhage, edema, and vascular dilatation.[1,6]

The intraluminal aspect of the stomach is similar to the *H. pylori* gastritis, but characteristic findings are erosions, generally multiple and varioliform.[1,2] In chronic gastritis, there is atrophy of the mucosa, and the areae gastricae are usually small or absent.[1]

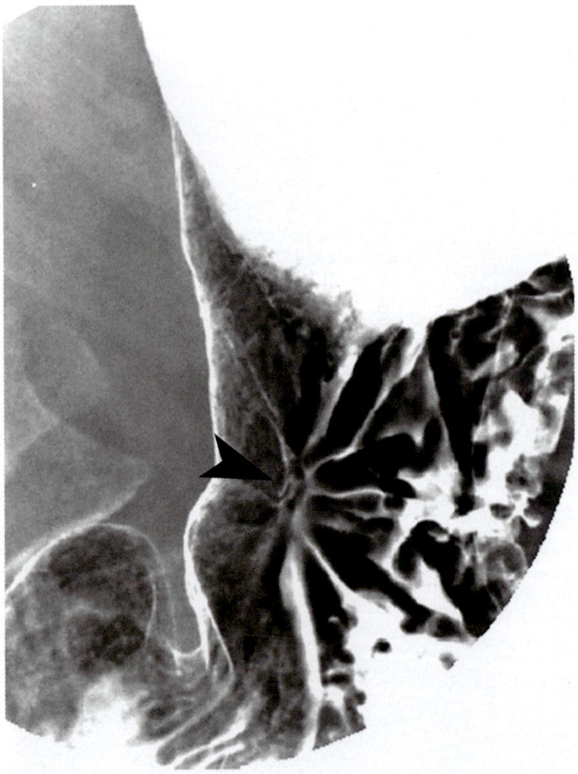

**FIG. 3A.4 • Benign gastric ulcer.** Double-contrast study of the stomach demonstrates small ulcer crater in the dependent wall of the gastric body with radiating gastric folds extending to the edge of the ulcer crater (*arrowhead*).

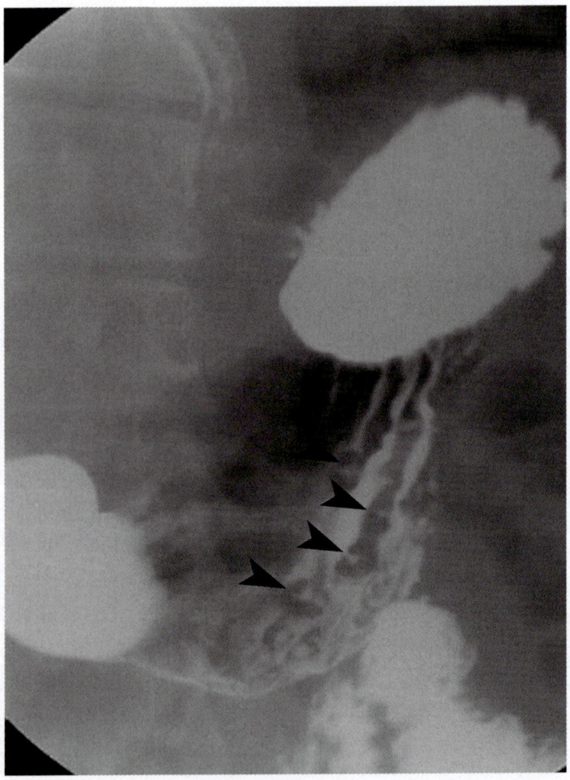

**FIG. 3A.5 • Acute gastritis.** Double-contrast study of the stomach demonstrates multiple focal ulcerations in the gastric body, indicated by central ulcer craters (*arrowheads*) and surrounding edema.

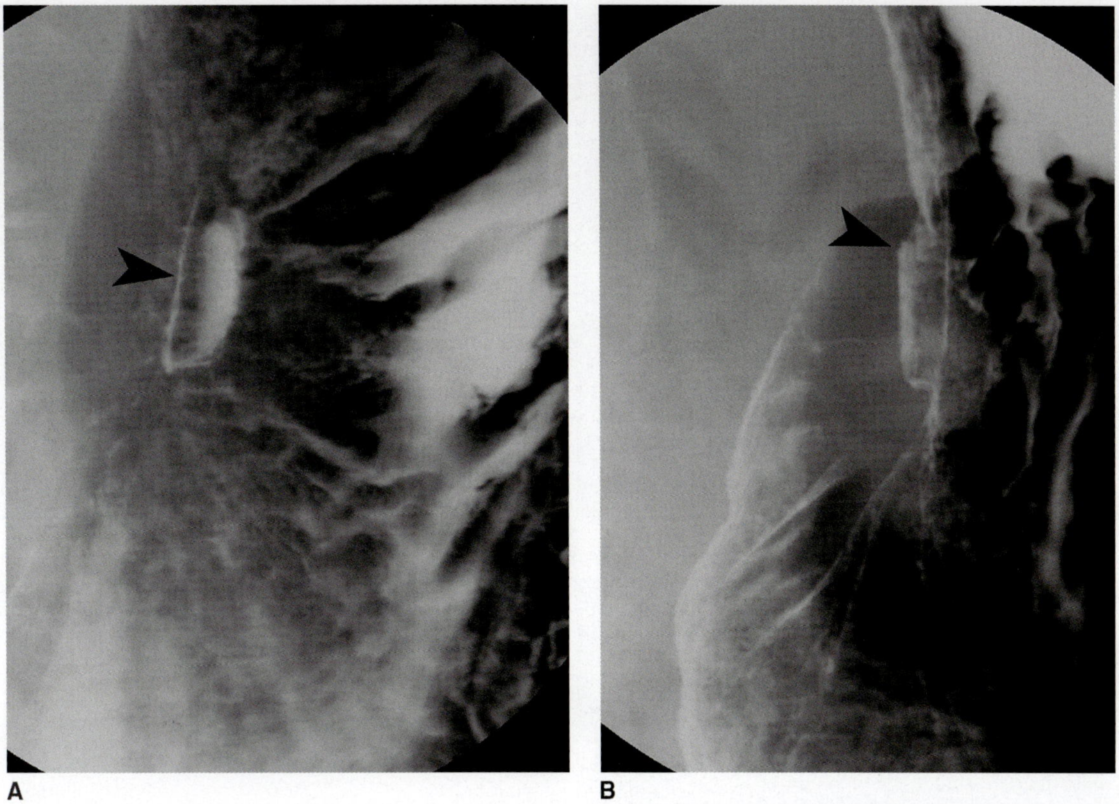


**FIG. 3A.6 • Benign gastric ulcer. A:** En face spot double-contrast image of the stomach demonstrates an ulcer crater (*arrowhead*) containing radiopaque contrast along the dependent wall of the gastric body with radiating mucosal folds extending to the edge of the ulcer crater. **B:** Tangential view demonstrates the ulcer crater (*arrowhead*), which does not appear to extend beyond the gastric serosa.

## EMPHYSEMATOUS GASTRITIS

It is a severe form of phlegmonous gastritis, which is characterized by the presence of intramural air. Images of infectious origin can be associated with streptococci, *E. coli*, enterobacter, or pseudomonas infections. Predisposing factors for emphysematous gastritis include gastroenteritis, nonsteroidal anti-inflammatory drug intake, diabetes, alcohol abuse, recent surgery, leukemia, and adenocarcinoma of the stomach. The condition has high mortality and needs urgent surgery. Gastric emphysema and cystic pneumatosis also are characterized by the presence of air in the wall of the stomach but are of noninfectious origin (Fig. 3A.7).

## MÉNÉTRIER DISEASE

Giant hypertrophic gastritis is a rare acquired chronic disease that is seen most commonly in middle-aged adults.[2,5] The cause is unknown. Although this disease is considered more prevalent in the fundus and body, with sparing of the antrum, it has been demonstrated that the folds alterations are diffuse in almost 50% of the patients.[1] Diffuse hyperplasia of mucous cells of the gastric surface generates a cerebriform prominence of mucosal folds. There is increased prevalence of gastric carcinoma in patients with Ménétrier disease.

On double-contrast barium study, there are thickened rugal folds, most commonly in the distal stomach (Fig. 3A.8A). Hypersecretion results in dilution of the barium and poor mucosal coating.[2] CT imaging may allow the diagnosis, better if performed in combination with enteroclysis (water distension of the stomach), demonstrating diffusely thickened irregular cerebriform gastric folds, and mucosal erosions (Fig. 3A.8B). There is no adjacent lymphadenopathy and no extragastric involvement with smooth serosal outline.[5] The differential diagnosis of gastric rugal folds includes peptic ulcer disease, Z-E syndrome, gastric varices, infection, corrosive agents, radiation, pancreatitis, lymphoma, and adenocarcinoma (Figs. 3A.9 and 3A.10).

## OTHER GASTRITIS

Crohn gastritis is localized in the distal stomach, most commonly in the gastric antrum. Earliest findings include apthoid ulcers in the gastric antrum. It is characterized by narrowing of the lumen, wall thickening, ulcerations, and fistulas.[2]

Atrophic gastritis is a chronic autoimmune condition that destroys the fundal mucosa and is associated with pernicious anemia. Abnormal pattern of the mucosa shows decreased or absent folds in the fundus and body, tube-shaped stomach, and small or absent areae gastricae.[2]

## LYMPHOID HYPERPLASIA

Lymphoid tissue is absent in the stomach at birth, but the presence of chronic *H. pylori* infection leads to colonization of the mucosa by lymphatic cells (mucosa-associated lymphoid tissue, MALT) and development of this pathologic condition, which predisposes to the development of MALT lymphoma

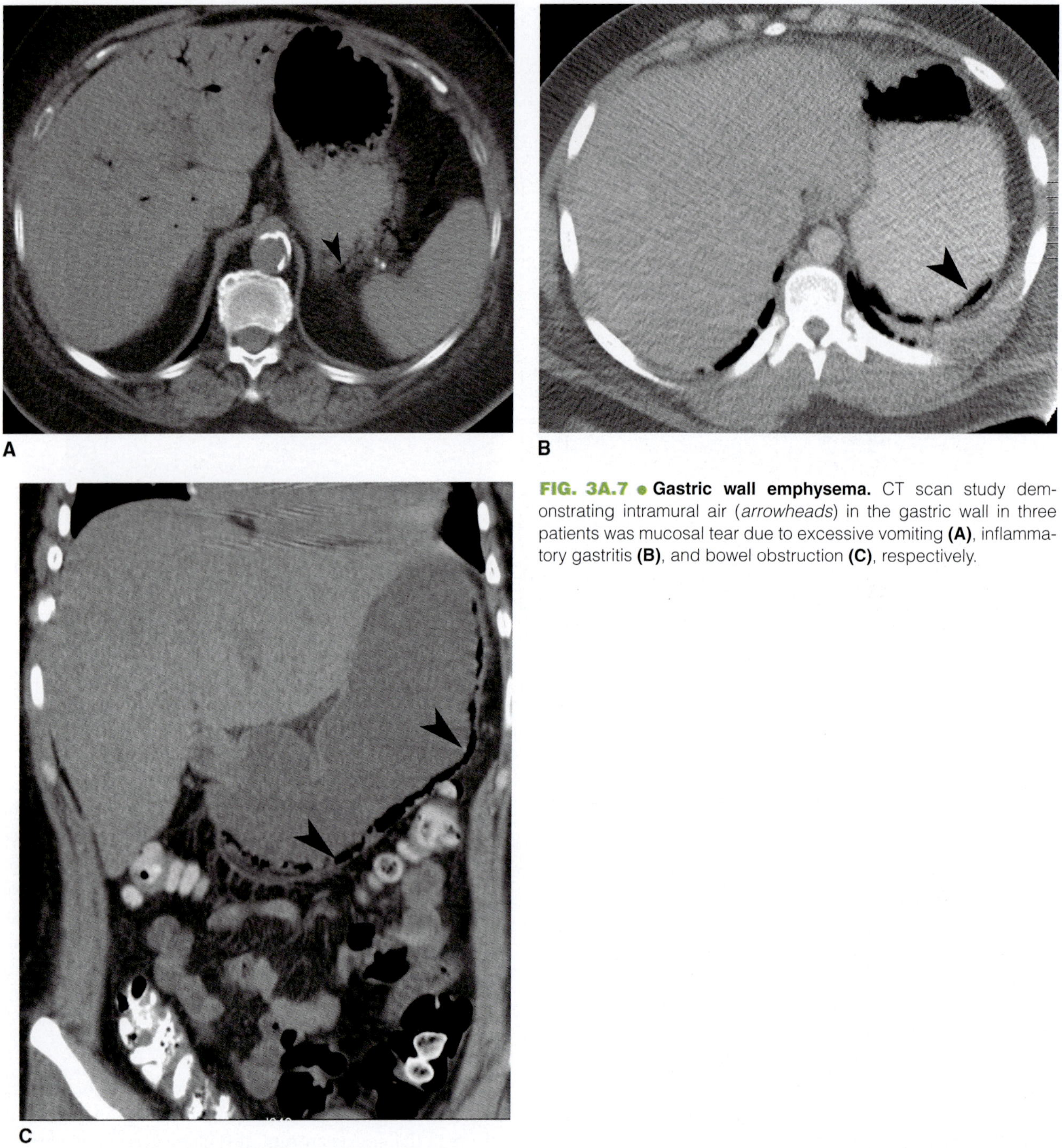


**FIG. 3A.7 • Gastric wall emphysema.** CT scan study demonstrating intramural air (*arrowheads*) in the gastric wall in three patients was mucosal tear due to excessive vomiting **(A)**, inflammatory gastritis **(B)**, and bowel obstruction **(C)**, respectively.

(low-grade B-cell lymphoma).[7] On UGI study, the mucosa of the stomach shows innumerable small round uniform (1 to 3 mm) nodules present on the luminal aspect.[1,7]

## DIVERTICULA

These are sac-shaped gastric outpouching seen in 0.02% to 2.6% of the patients, more commonly in elderly females. It is congenital in 70% and acquired in 30% of the cases. The acquired diverticula are pulsion diverticula, resulting from mucosal herniation through the gaps present in the muscularis layer of the gastric wall. The congenital diverticula are true diverticula, containing all the gastric wall layers, most commonly arising from the posterior wall of the fundus or cardia.[8] Acquired diverticula are pseudodiverticula and usually situated in the antrum.[8]

On UGI study, they are 1- to 10-cm diameter contrast-filled sacs with smooth contour (Fig. 3A.11A).[1,8] On CT, they can be seen as thin-walled fluid density lesions with air-fluid level situated in the left paravertebral space, between the stomach, spleen, left adrenal gland, and left diaphragm (Fig. 3A.11B).[8] On MR imaging, they may be seen as fluid-filled cystic lesion with thin wall in relation to the gastric cardia. Because of their location and the morphology, diverticula may mimic cystic lesion of the left adrenal gland, pancreatic pseudocyst, or gastric wall duplication cyst.

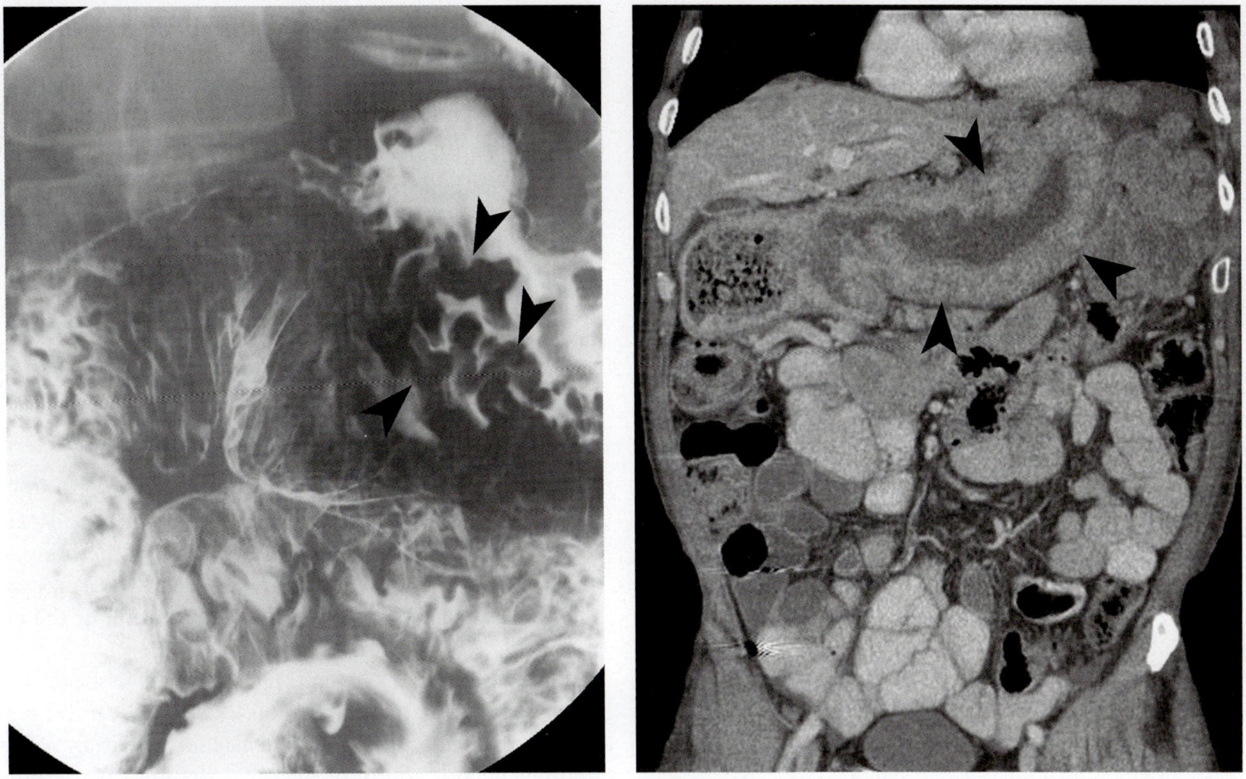

A B

**FIG. 3A.8 • Gastric rugal fold thickening. A:** Double-contrast UGI study demonstrates prominent gastric rugal folds (*arrowheads*) in the gastric antrum. **B:** CT coronal reformation demonstrates prominent gastric wall thickening (*arrowheads*) in the stomach. The patient also has exophytic leiomyosarcoma, not seen on this image.

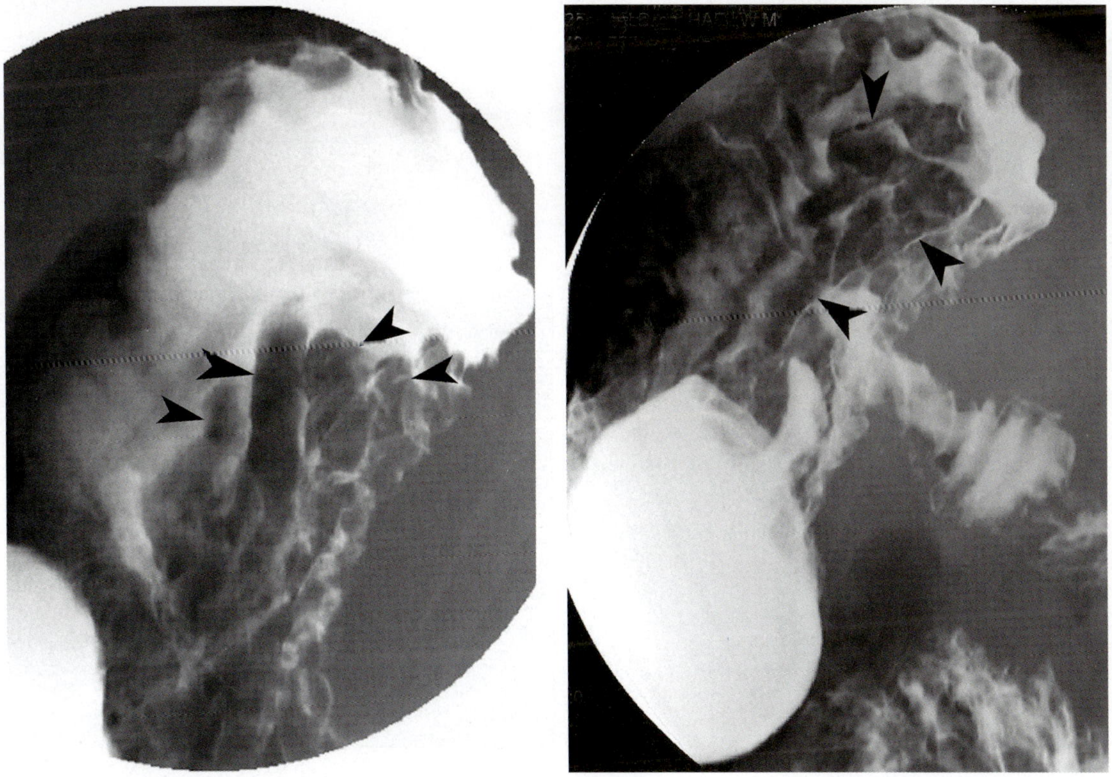

A B

**FIG. 3A.9 • Gastric varices. A, B:** Double-contrast upper GI study in a patient with splenic vein thrombosis caused by pancreatic cancer demonstrates extensive submucosal linear filling defects (*arrowheads*) in the stomach, caused by gastric varices.

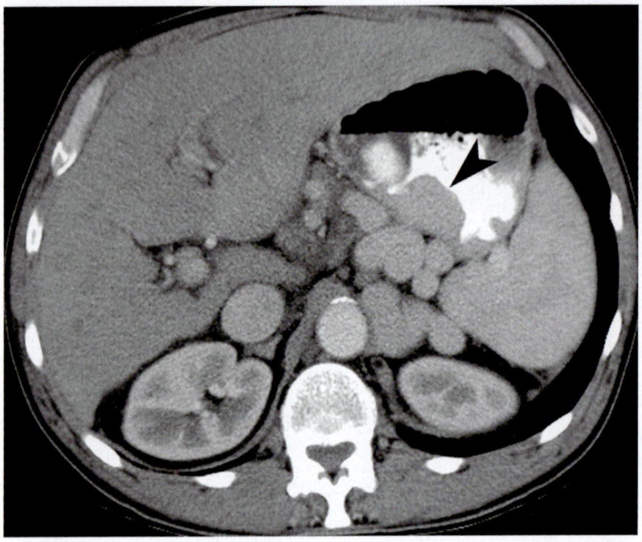

**FIG. 3A.10 • Gastric varices.** Contrast-enhanced CT scan study in a cirrhotic patient demonstrates multiple prominent gastric varices, one of which is seen to produce a submucosal mass (*arrowhead*) in the posterior wall of the gastric body.

## POLYPS

Small intraluminal protrusions from the mucosal surface, either sessile or pedunculated, are called polyps. Polyps are seen on UGI study as smooth, nodular, or lobulated sessile or pedunculated filling defect.[1]

Hyperplastic polyps are the most common and are typically smooth or lobulated, sessile, less than 1 cm in size, multiple, and located in the body or antrum (Fig. 3A.12). Adenomatous polyps are uncommon, larger than 1 cm in size, sessile or pedunculated, and single. Fundal gland polyps are multiple, smooth surfaced, sessile, smaller than 1 cm, and located in the fundus. Retention polyps or juvenile polyps are solitary or multiple and related to the Cronkite-Canada syndrome.[1] Hamartomatous polyps are typical of Peutz-Jeghers syndrome and have no malignant degeneration.[2]

## HETEROTOPIC PANCREAS

Lobules of pancreatic tissue are found in 0.5% to 13% of autopsies, usually located in the gastric antrum, especially in the greater curvature (less frequently in the body), and are up to 5 cm in size. They are covered by normal gastric mucosa, usually with the central umbilication of the excretory duct.[2,4,9]

On UGI study, the heterotopic pancreatic tissue appears as smooth, broad-based, intramural lesion with central umbilication, manifested by a central collection of barium.[9] The CT findings include round or oval mass within the gastric wall, with variable postcontrast enhancement (from higher than pancreas to nonenhanced, simulating a cyst).[4,9]

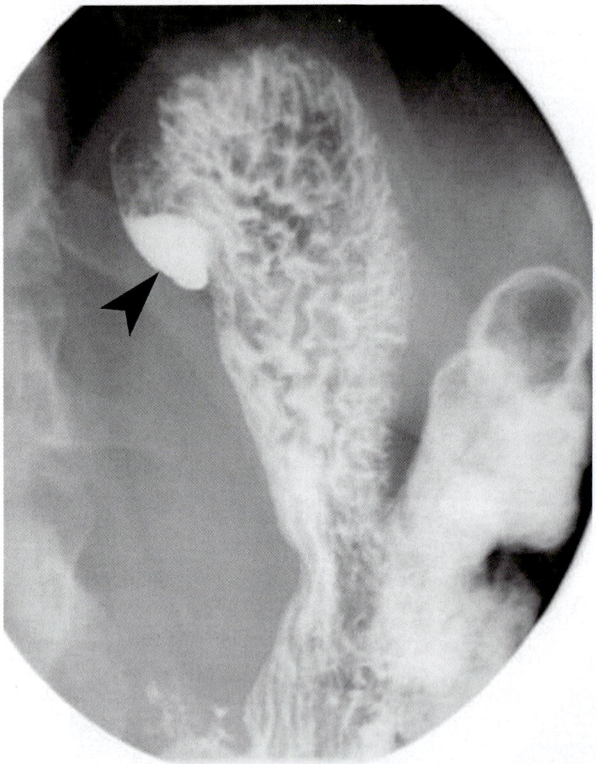

A

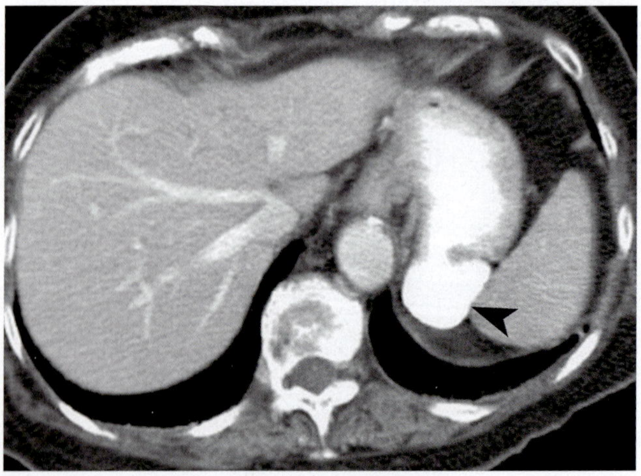

B

**FIG. 3A.11 • Gastric diverticulum. A:** Double-contrast study of the stomach demonstrates contrast-containing gastric diverticulum (*arrowhead*) seen on the posteromedial aspect of the gastric cardia. **B:** Axial contrast-enhanced CT scan study of the same patient demonstrates a contrast-containing gastric diverticulum (*arrowhead*) arising on the posterior aspect of the gastric cardia.

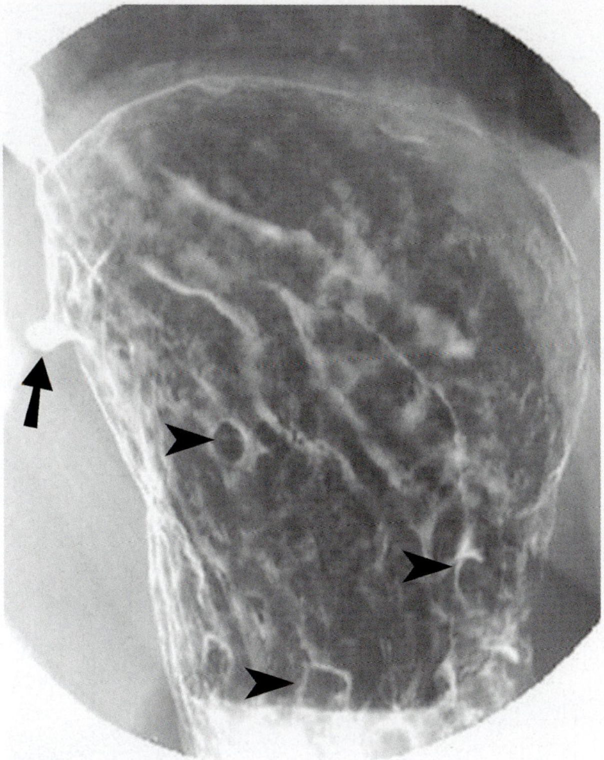

A

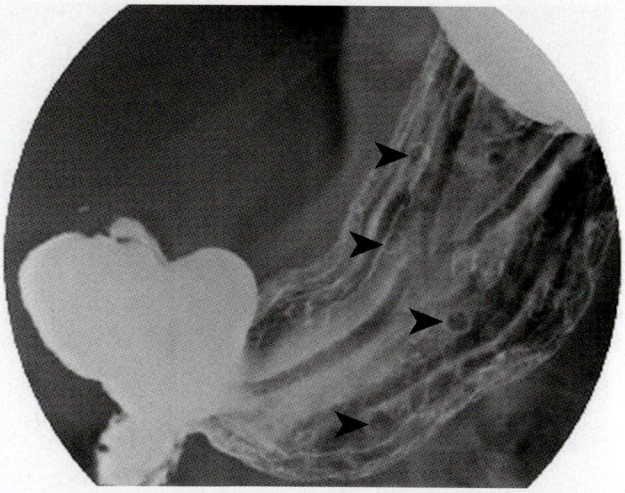

B

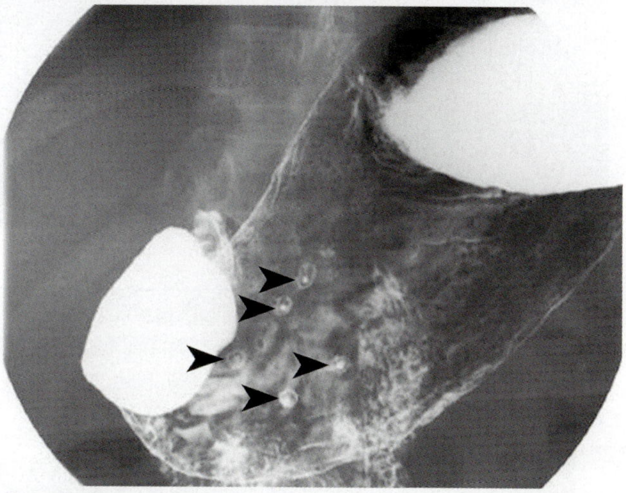

C

**FIG. 3A.12 • Gastric polyps. A–C:** Double-contrast upper GI study demonstrates multiple subcentimeter polyps (*arrowheads*) identified in the gastric fundus **(A)** and body **(B–C)**. There is a 1.5-cm gastric diverticulum that is seen in the first patient (*arrow*) (A).

## SARCOIDOSIS

Sarcoidosis typically involves the lungs but can also affect the abdomen (liver, spleen, lymph nodes, bowel).[10] The stomach is the most frequently involved site in the gastrointestinal tract and usually is associated with pulmonary involvement.[10] For the diagnosis, biopsy and culture are required, both for the diagnosis and to rule out malignancy. Gastric sarcoidosis may occur in association to other diffuse conditions and usually is characterized by granulomatous gastritis; frequently, it may diffuse fold thickening identical to Ménétrier disease and gastric antral narrowing similar to scirrhous carcinoma.[10]

**Differential diagnosis of gastric antral narrowing:**

1. Peptic ulcer disease
2. Neoplasm
3. Caustic ingestion
4. Radiation
5. Granulomatous conditions (sarcoidosis, Crohn disease, syphilis, and tuberculosis)

## HYPERTROPHIC PYLORIC STENOSIS

This condition is characterized by hypertrophy of the pyloric canal musculature, resulting in gastric outlet obstruction, most commonly in less than 3-month-old males.

Plain radiograph may show distended stomach with paucity of gas in the distal bowel loops (Fig. 3A.13A). On barium study, the imaging findings include delayed gastric emptying and elongated pyloric canal (string sign). Double-track sign refers to more than one linear tract of contrast in the pyloric canal separated by redundant mucosa. The shoulder sign and mushroom sign refer to the indentation of pyloric hypertrophic musculature into the gastric antrum and duodenal bulb, respectively (Fig. 3A.13B). The beak sign refers to beak-shaped configuration of the proximal end of the pyloric canal, caused by muscular hypertrophy.

Ultrasound is the imaging modality of choice because of its ability to directly visualize the hypertrophic pyloric musculature. The hypertrophic pyloric canal musculature is hypoechoic with central hyperechogenicity of the mucosa on cross section. The thickness of the pyloric canal musculature

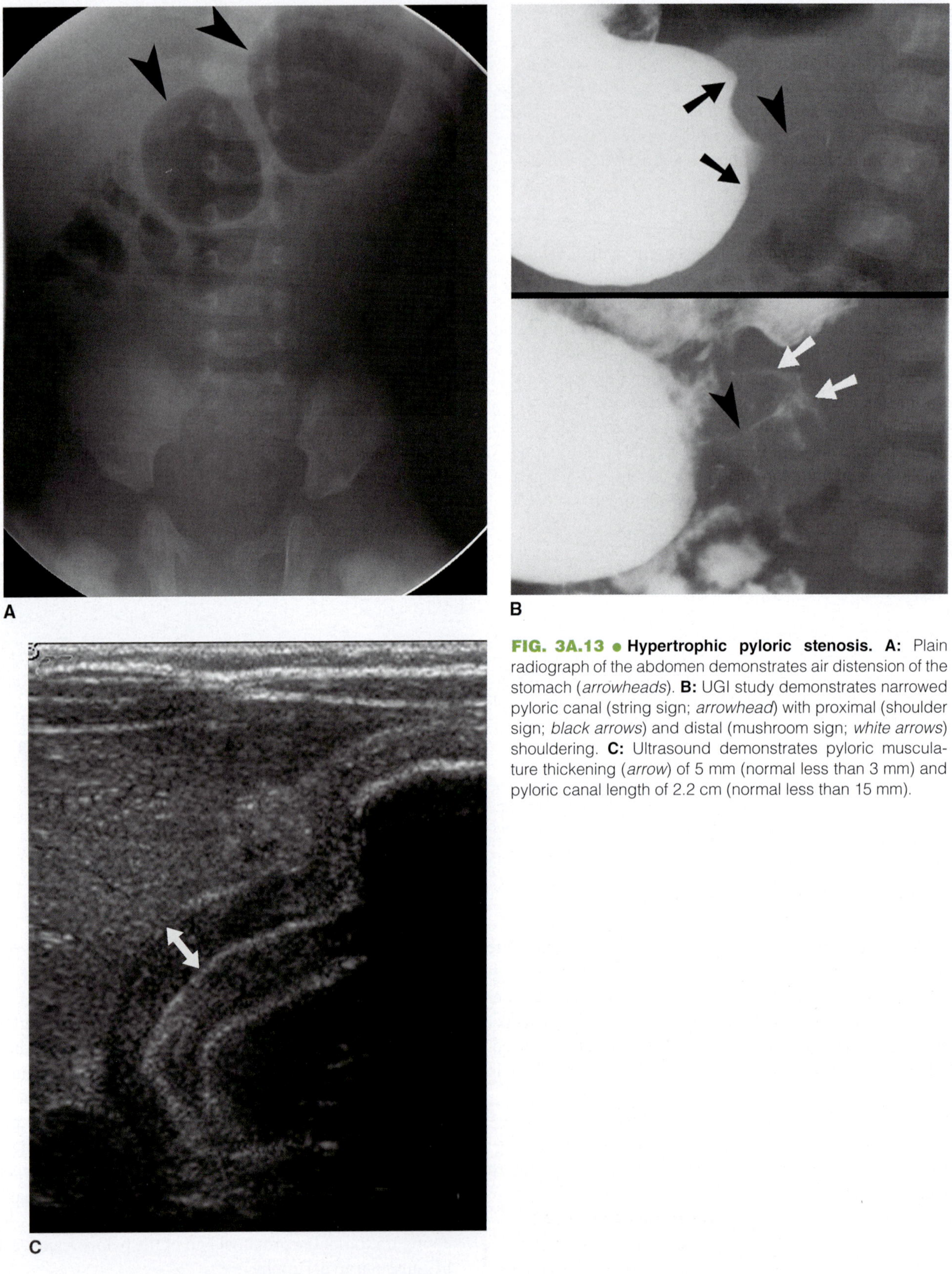

**FIG. 3A.13 • Hypertrophic pyloric stenosis. A:** Plain radiograph of the abdomen demonstrates air distension of the stomach (*arrowheads*). **B:** UGI study demonstrates narrowed pyloric canal (string sign; *arrowhead*) with proximal (shoulder sign; *black arrows*) and distal (mushroom sign; *white arrows*) shouldering. **C:** Ultrasound demonstrates pyloric musculature thickening (*arrow*) of 5 mm (normal less than 3 mm) and pyloric canal length of 2.2 cm (normal less than 15 mm).

on cross section is normally less than 3 mm, and the length of the muscle is less than 15 mm (Fig. 3A.13C). In patients with hypertrophic pyloric stenosis, the thickness of the wall is 3 mm or more, and the lumen of the pyloric canal fails to distend.

## GASTRIC BEZOAR

Bezoar is accumulation of ingested foreign material in the gastrointestinal tract. The stomach is the most common location, and the condition is most often seen in patients with prior gastric surgery. The different types of bezoars include trichobezoar (hair), phytobezoar (fruits and vegetables), lactobezoar (milk proteins), and pharmacobezoar (medications).[11,12] Rapunzel syndrome is characterized by ingestion of hair, leading to trichobezoar formation in the stomach and proximal small bowel.

On plain radiography, bowel obstruction can be diagnosed but bezoar not usually identified (Fig. 3A.14A). Sonography can also be used to diagnose bowel obstruction in patients with bezoar. Sonographic finding of intraluminal mass with hyperechoic arc along the anterior surface with distal acoustic shadowing is suggestive of bezoar (Fig. 3A.14B). The sharp distal acoustic shadowing from bezoar is different from dirty shadowing caused by ingested food and gas in the stomach. The CT findings include demonstration of a well-defined oval intraluminal mass with gas bubbles retained within the interstices of the bezoar (Figs. 3A.14 to 3A.16). The other findings include dilated small bowel loop proximal to the bezoar with decompressed distal bowel loops.

## GASTRIC VOLVULUS

The stomach is the less commonly affected side of volvulus compared to small bowel or large bowel volvulus. It can be identified by the Borchardt triad, which consists of epigastric pain, intractable retching, and inability to pass an esophagogastric tube into the stomach.

The two types of gastric volvulus are organoaxial type and mesenteric axial type, which are less common forms of the volvulus (Fig. 3A.16). Organoaxial volvulus accounts for two-thirds of cases of gastric volvulus and involves stomach rotation along its long axis, with the greater curvature located more cranial to the lesser curvature (Fig. 3A.17). This is most often seen in patients with paraesophageal hernia and is less likely to cause vascular compromise. There is gastric outlet obstruction if the rotation is more than 180 degrees. The rotation of the stomach is along a line along the long axis of the stomach, which connects the gastric cardia with the pylorus.

The mesentericoaxial volvulus is more likely to present with chronic symptoms compared to organoaxial volvulus and is less likely to be associated with diaphragmatic defects. The twist of the stomach is along a plane running from the lesser curvature to the greater curvature of the stomach. The mesentericoaxial volvulus is characterized by gastric rotation along its short axis, resulting in displacement of the gastric antrum above the gastroesophageal junction. This volvulus is more common in children and usually produces twist less than 180 degrees.

## LAPAROSCOPIC ADJUSTABLE GASTRIC BANDING

Laparoscopic adjustable gastric banding is the second most common procedure performed for management of morbid obesity and was approved by the FDA in 2001. In this procedure, the stomach is divided into two bulges by placing gastric band 2 cm caudal to the gastroesophageal junction.[13] The gastric pouch volume is approximately 15 mm. The band

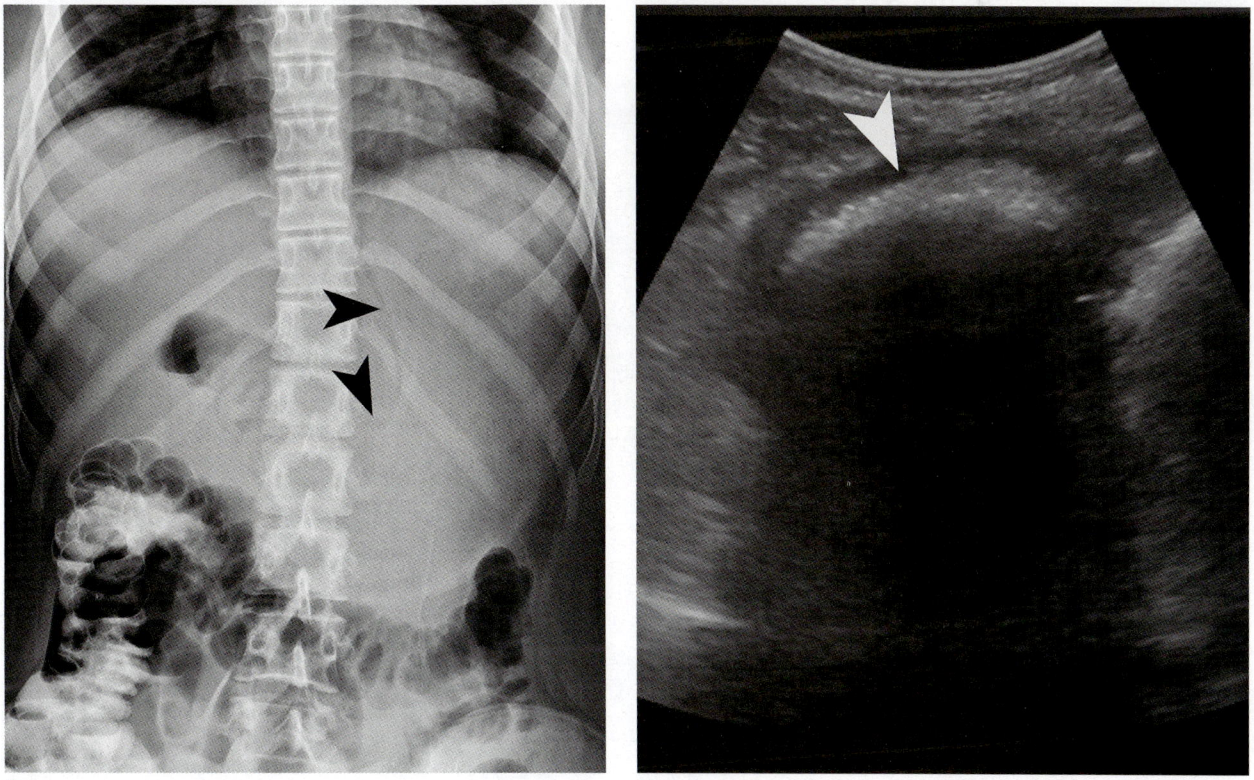

A B

**FIG. 3A.14 • Gastric trichobezoar. A:** Plain x-ray of the abdomen demonstrates the gastric trichobezoar, outlined by air (*arrowheads*) between the bezoar and gastric wall. **B:** Ultrasound of the trichobezoar demonstrates the anterior echogenic margin (*arrowhead*) of the bezoar, causing distal acoustic shadowing.

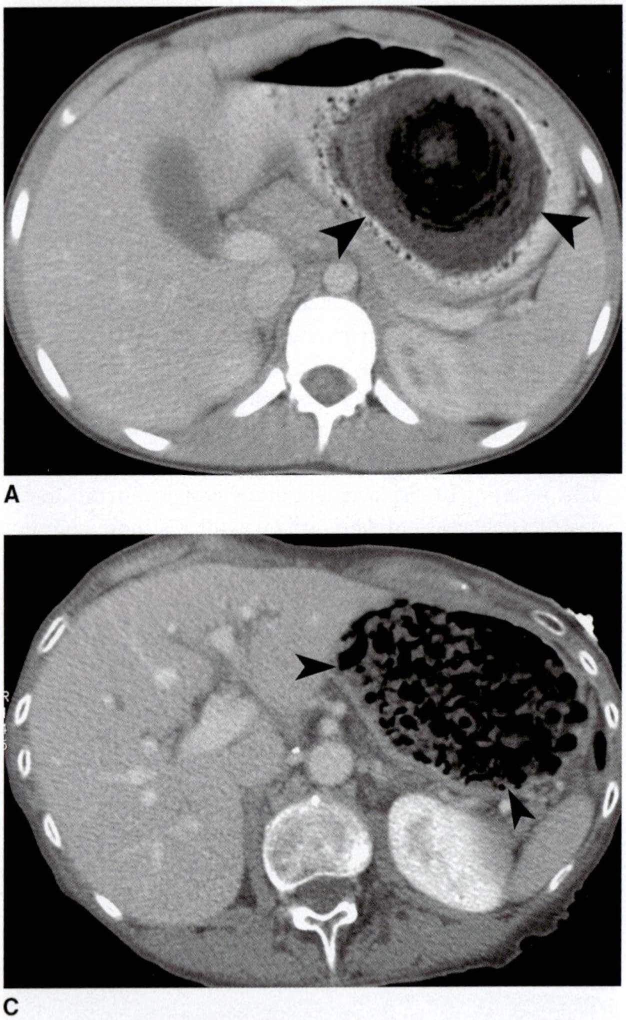

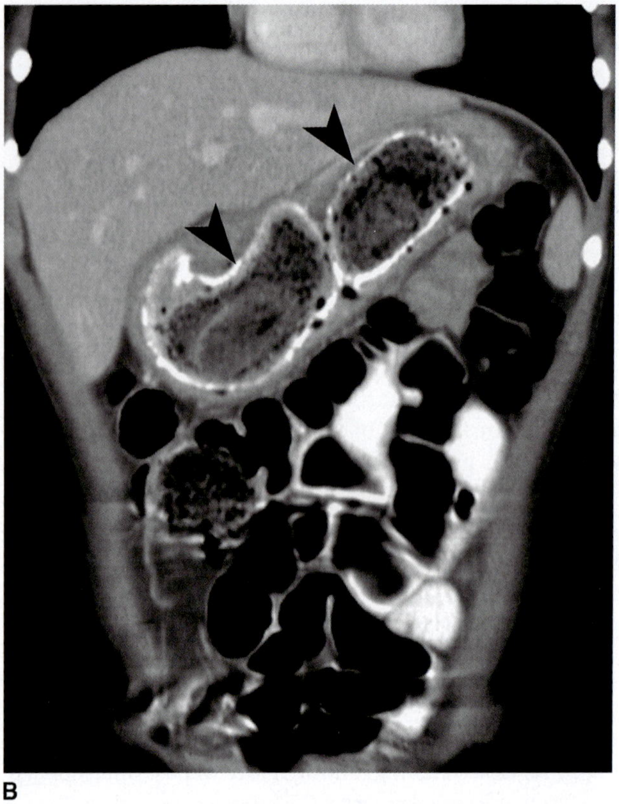

**FIG. 3A.15 • Gastric trichobezoar (A–B) and pharmacobezoar (C). A, B:** Axial and coronal contrast–enhanced CT images demonstrate mottled air density of the trichobezoar (*arrowheads*), in the gastric fundus, body, and antrum. **C:** Axial contrast-enhanced CT demonstrates the stomach lumen filled with Procardia medication tablets (*arrowheads*).

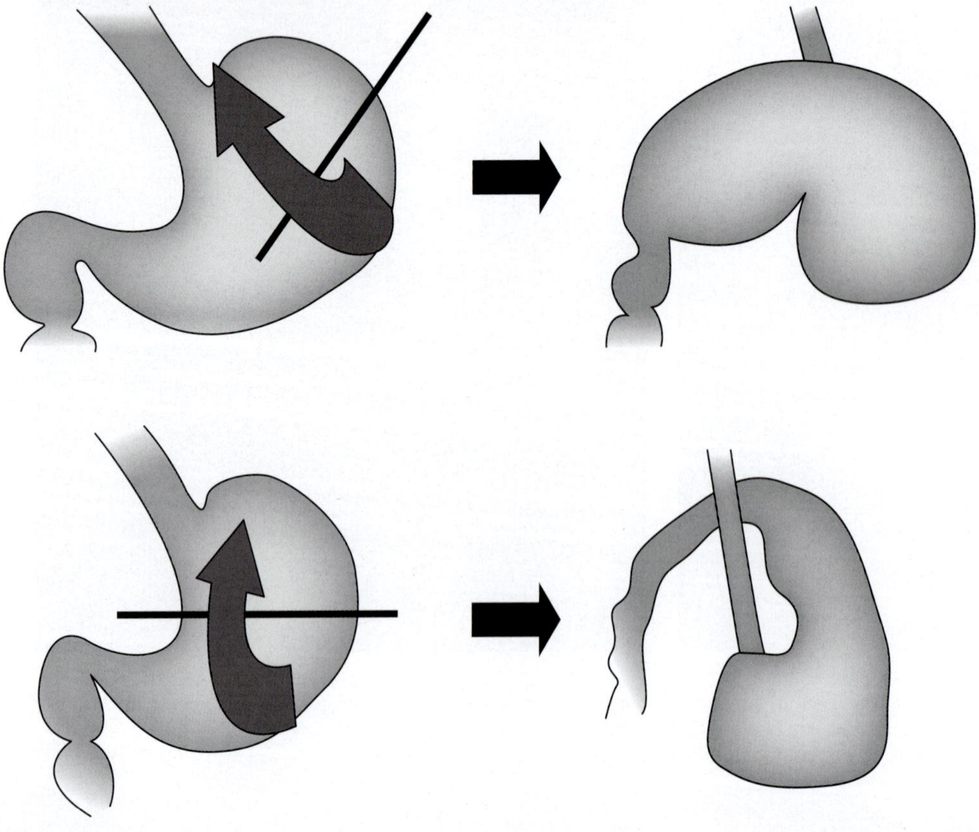

**FIG. 3A.16 • Gastric volvulus.** Schematic diagram depicts organoaxial and mesentericoaxial volvulus of the stomach.

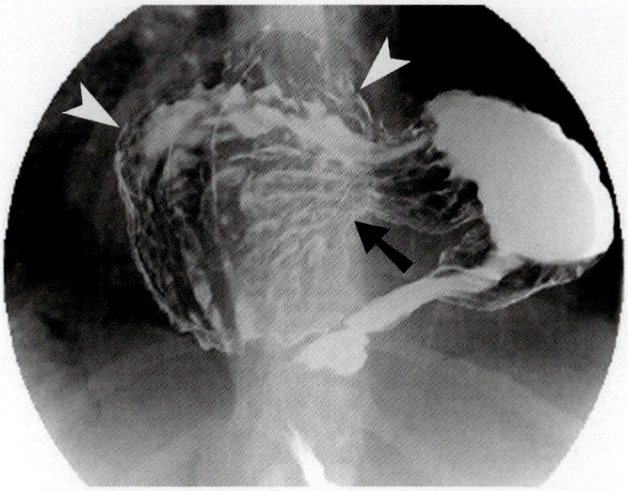

**FIG. 3A.17 • Gastric volvulus (organoaxial type).** Upper GI study demonstrates intrathoracic herniation of the stomach, with the greater curvature (*arrowheads*) located more cranial to the level of the lesser curvature (*arrow*). These findings are consistent with organoaxial volvulus.

diameter can be adjusted using a subcutaneous port placed in the abdominal wall connected to the inner portion of the band. Preoperatively, a barium esophagram is performed to demonstrate the normal anatomy of the esophagus and stomach.

The angle formed by the long axis of the gastric band and vertical line running through the spine is known as the phi angle and ranges from 4 to 58 degrees (Fig. 3A.18). The lap band has a rectangular appearance on the AP radiographic assessment. The gastric pouch is usually less than 4 cm wide and the stoma less than 4 mm wide. Fluoroscopy evaluation with contrast can be performed to evaluate the postsurgical complications of this procedure.

*Complications* (Figs. 3A.19 and 3A.20): Stomal stenosis is the most commonly encountered complication and manifests with abdominal pain, vomiting, and nausea. On esophagram study, there is narrowing of the stoma with delayed passage of contrast through the stoma. Chronic stomal stenosis can result in dilatation of the gastric pouch and is seen in 3% to 8% of the patients.

Slippage of gastric band is a complication, which can be seen in 4% to 13% of the patients. The slippage of the gastric band is most commonly posterior (82%) and less commonly anterior (18%). Posterior slippage of the band results in craniocaudal herniation of the posterior gastric wall, and anterior slippage of the band results in downward displacement of the band over the anterior gastric wall. Gastric band slippage is seen on barium study as horizontal orientation of the gastric band and stomal stenosis. The gastric pouch is usually posterior and inferior in patients with posterior slippage, while it is anterior and superior in anterior slippage. Less common complications include gastric perforation, laparoscopic band erosion, malfunction of the catheter, and infections.

## ROUX-EN-Y GASTRIC BYPASS

Roux-en-Y gastric bypass has become the procedure of choice for surgical management of morbid obesity in North America. It is performed in patients with a body mass index of more than 40 or in patients with a body mass index of more than 35 with associated comorbidities.

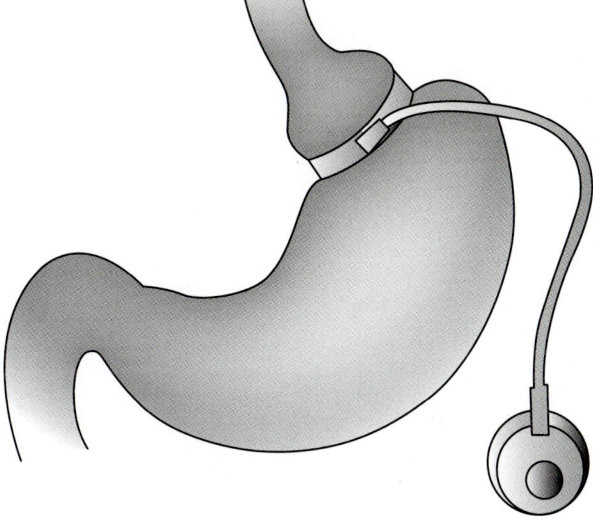

A

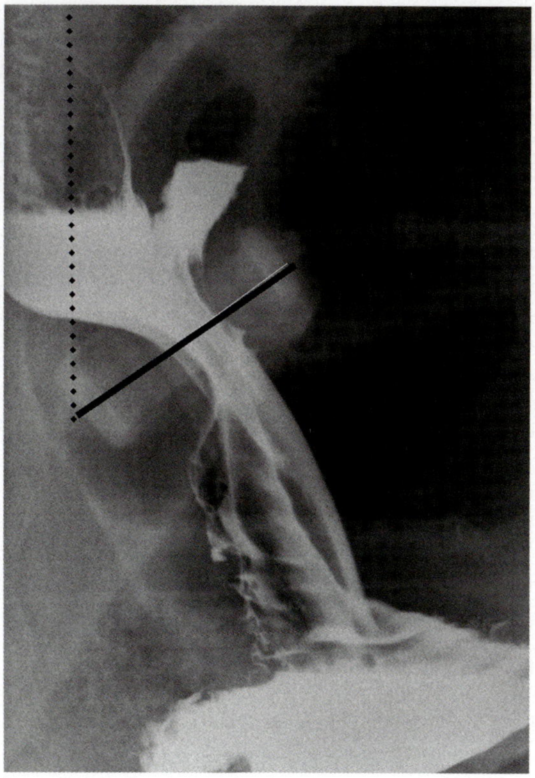

B

**FIG. 3A.18 • Gastric lap band anatomy. A:** Diagram indicates the gastric anatomy after placement of a lap band. The lap band is typically approximately 45 degrees to the horizontal plane and produces a gastric pouch proximal to the band. **B:** Normal orientation of the lap band is seen on this single-contrast upper GI study.

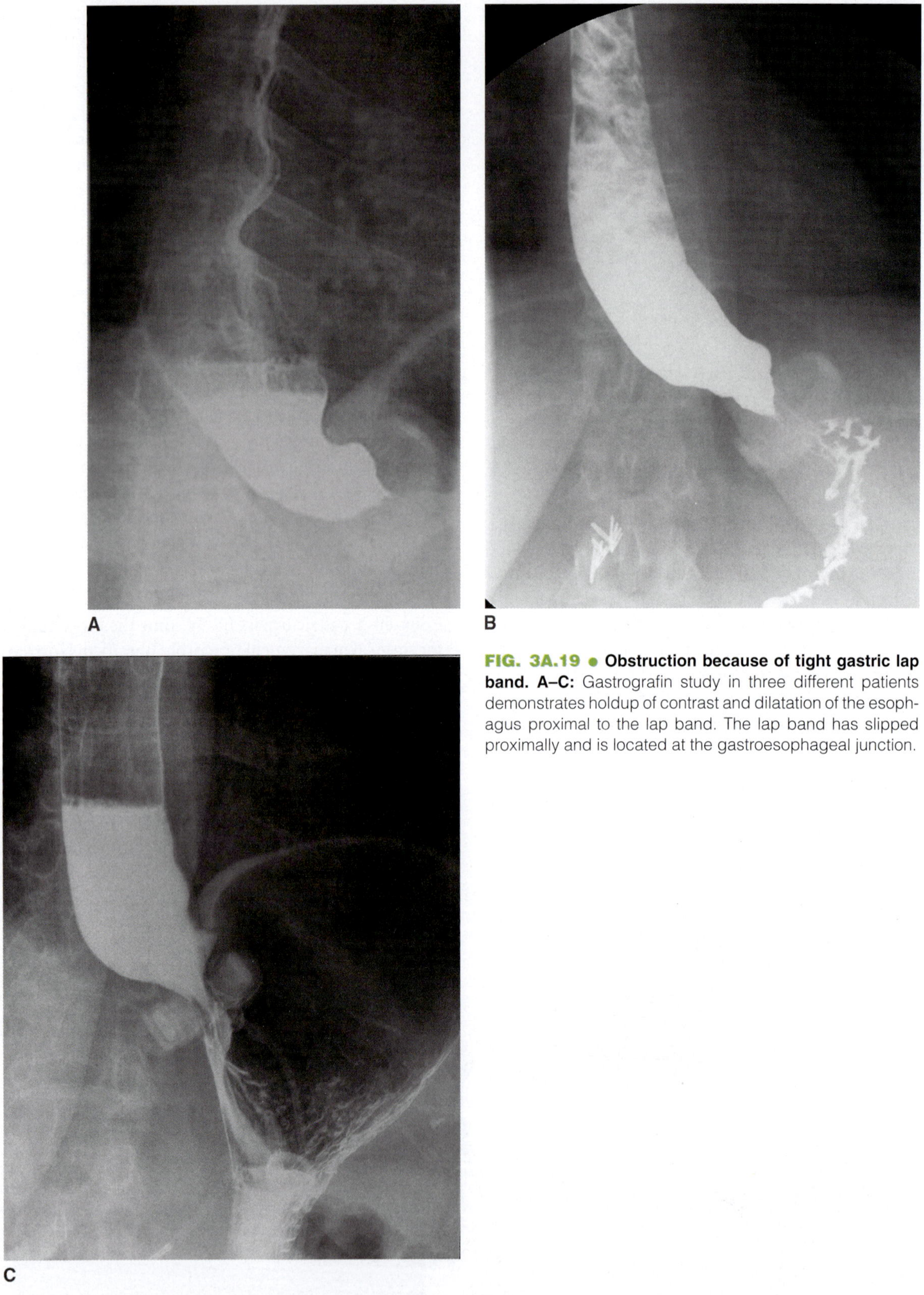

**FIG. 3A.19 • Obstruction because of tight gastric lap band. A–C:** Gastrografin study in three different patients demonstrates holdup of contrast and dilatation of the esophagus proximal to the lap band. The lap band has slipped proximally and is located at the gastroesophageal junction.

The Roux-en-Y gastric bypass is performed laparoscopically using open surgical technique. Preoperatively, ultrasound is performed in all patients to evaluate for gallstones, for which cholecystectomy can be performed during the gastric bypass surgery. Postoperatively, the patients are evaluated with water-soluble contrast study on day 1 to screen for leak or bowel obstruction.[14]

Roux-en-Y gastric bypass surgery involves the creation of a 30-mL gastric pouch that is excluded from remainder of the stomach (Fig. 3A.21). The gastric pouch is anastomosed

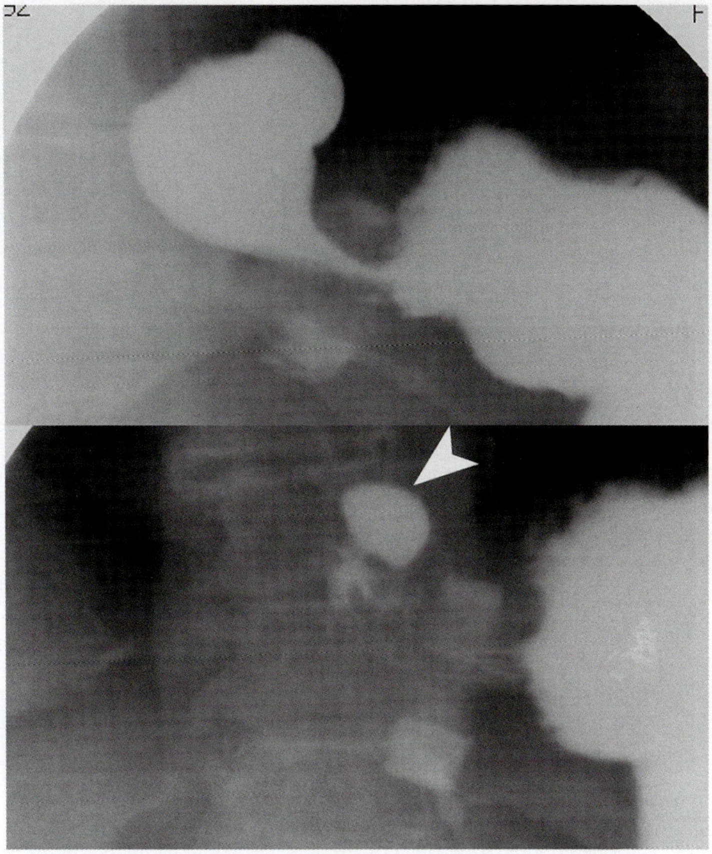

**FIG. 3A.20 • Pulsion diverticulum.** Single-contrast upper GI study demonstrates a pulsion diverticulum (*arrowhead*) from the left wall of the gastric pouch.

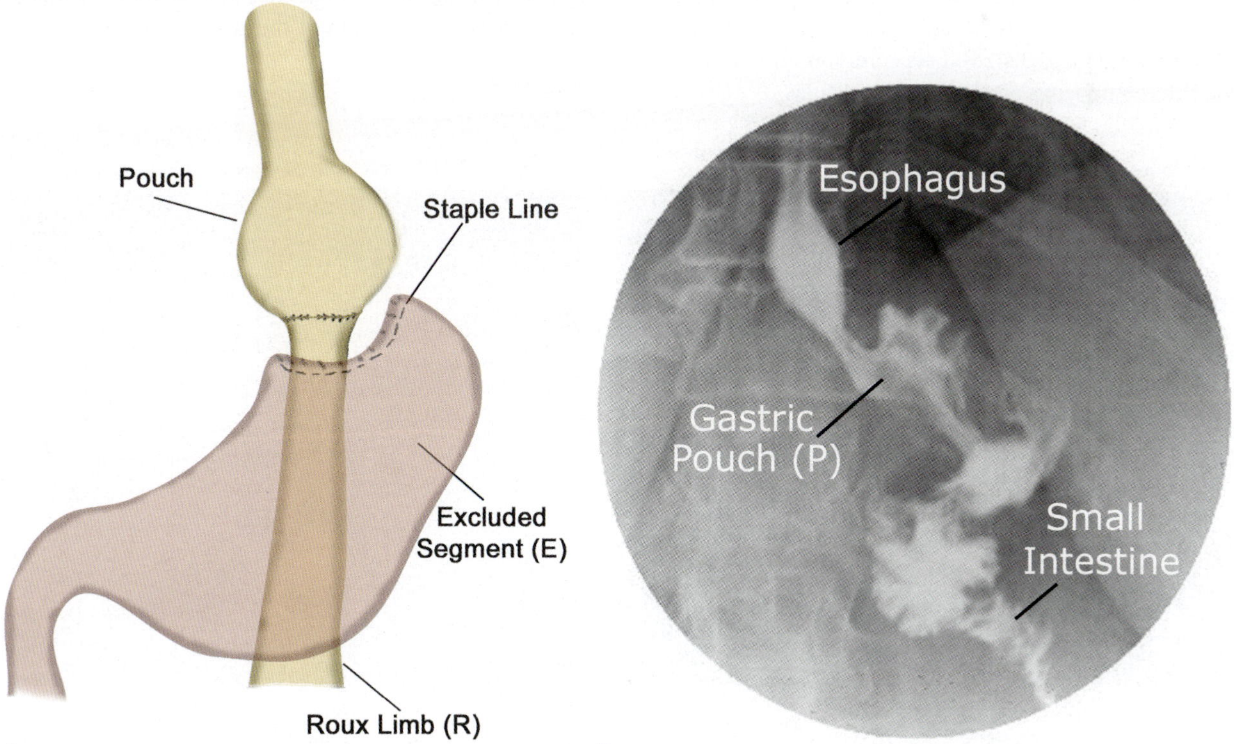


A B

**FIG. 3A.21 • Anatomy after gastric bypass surgery. A:** Schematic diagram demonstrates normal anatomy after gastric bypass surgery. The gastric pouch communicates with the Roux limb, while the excluded stomach drains through the duodenum and Roux-en-Y anastomosis. **B:** Single-contrast Gastrografin study demonstrates normal anatomy after gastric bypass surgery. There was free flow of contrast seen from the esophagus, through the gastric pouch into the small bowel.

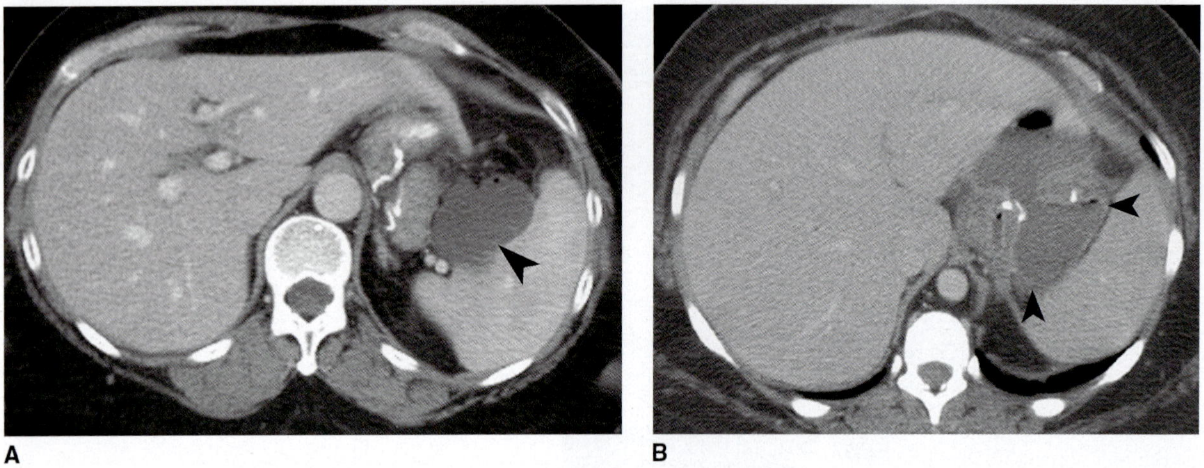

**FIG. 3A.22 • Postoperative collection. A:** Postoperative seroma—axial contrast CT of the upper abdomen demonstrates a 6-cm diameter postsurgical seroma (*arrowhead*) located lateral to the excluded stomach. **B:** Postoperative gastric perforation—axial contrast-enhanced CT scan study demonstrates defect in the posterior gastric wall, communicating with a collection (*arrowheads*) located medial to the spleen.

to a 1-to 1.5-m–long Roux-en-Y loop of the small bowel. This loop is brought to the gastric pouch through the transverse mesocolon in a retrogastric and retrocolic position. The distal Roux-en-Y limb is anastomosed to the distal jejunum.

The frequency of anastomotic leak is less than 3% and can be due to breakdown of the gastrojejunostomy or jejunojejunostomy anastomosis. A CT scan study can demonstrate extragastric bowel contents or abscess formation (Figs. 3A.22 and 3A.23). Fistula formation can be due to staple line breakdown and most commonly leads to gastrogastric communication (Figs. 3A.24 and 3A.25). Less common types of fistula include enterocutaneous or enterogastric fistulas.

Bowel obstruction can be the result of postoperative edema or internal hernia (Figs. 3A.26 to 3A.29). Delayed obstruction is due to adhesions, anastomotic stricture, or internal hernia. Other complications of gastric bypass surgery include stomal stenosis, gastritis, anastomotic ulcers, iron deficiency, and vitamin $B_{12}$ deficiency.

Other postsurgical conditions of the stomach include Billroth 1 and 2. Billroth 1 is characterized by resection of the pylorus, followed by gastroduodenostomy. Billroth 2 is characterized by resection of the gastric antrum, followed by gastrojejunostomy.

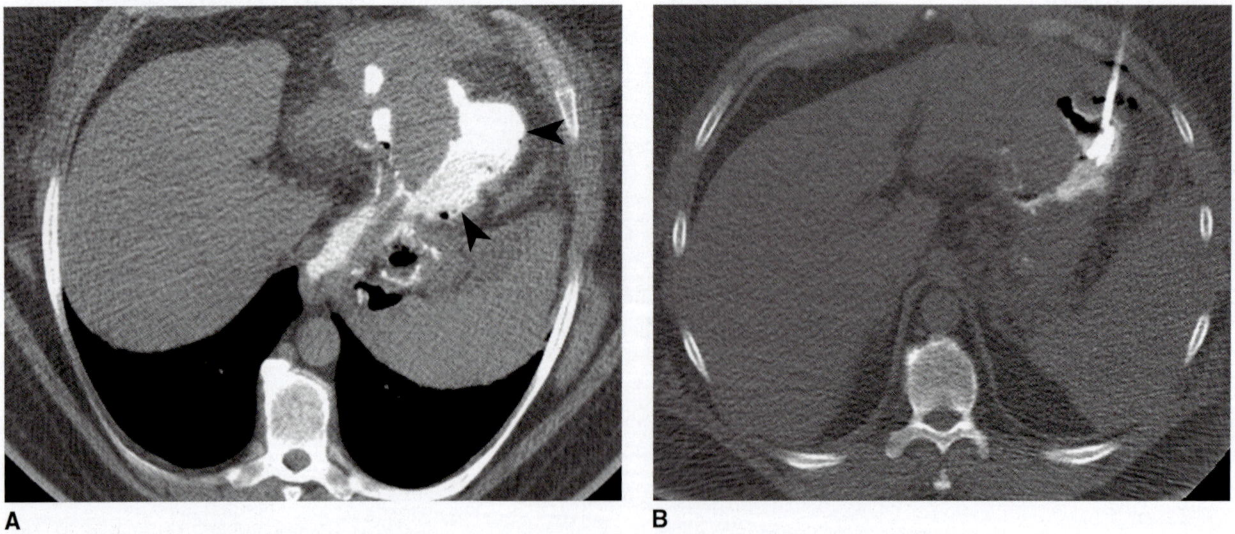

**FIG. 3A.23 • Gastric perforation. A:** Axial CT scan study demonstrates frank communication of the stomach with a collection (*arrowheads*) in the left upper quadrant of the abdomen. **B:** Axial CT scan study after placement of a pigtail drainage catheter demonstrates decrease in the size of the collection.

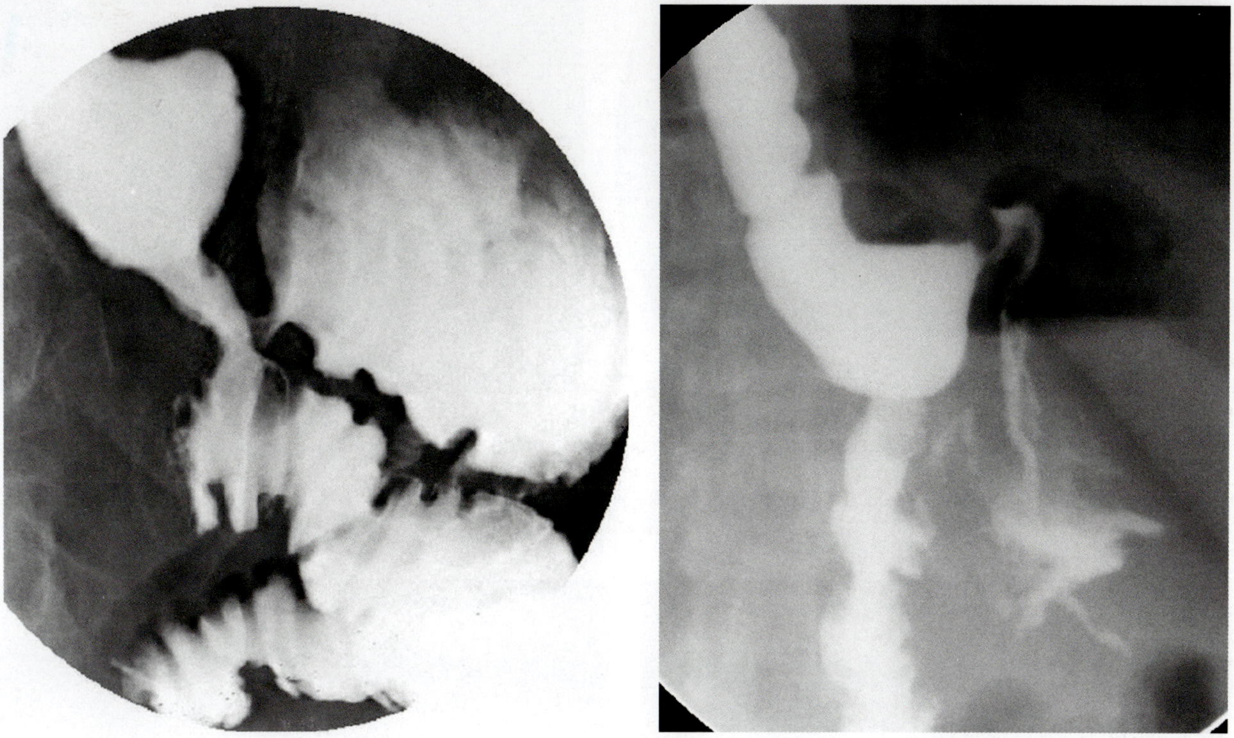

A B

**FIG. 3A.24 • Gastrogastric fistula. A, B:** Single-contrast upper GI study demonstrates frank communication of the gastric pouch with the excluded stomach.

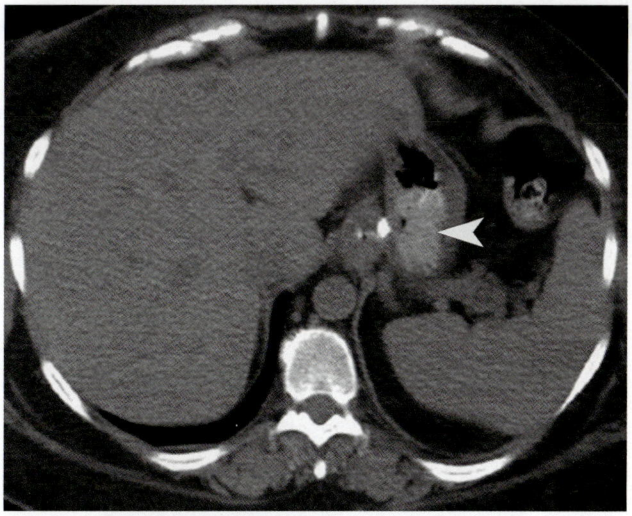

**FIG. 3A.25 • Gastrogastric fistula.** Noncontrast CT scan study of the abdomen demonstrates oral contrast in the gastric pouch as well as excluded stomach (*arrowhead*), indicating the presence of a fistulous communication.

## CORROSIVE INJURY

Ingestion of corrosive agents such as lye or dishwasher detergent causes acute inflammatory injury in the upper gastrointestinal tract. Eighty percent cases of accidental ingestion occur in children. The injury from caustic ingestion causes acute necrosis, ulceration, granulation, and stricture formation. Liquid alkali has no taste or odor and is easily ingested, causing severe injury to the esophagus and stomach. Lye ingestion can cause thrombosis of blood vessels, necrosis of cells, fatty saponification (less than 3 days), sloughing of the mucosa (less than 7 days), and stricture formation (after 3 weeks).

Injection of acidic agents causes less severe injury compared to an alkali agent. Acid ingestion in the stomach causes coagulative necrosis, which produces a protective barrier with predilection of the gastric antrum. Since caustic agent tends to flow down the lesser curvature of the stomach, it sustains the most damage.

The imaging findings on UGI study include thickened folds, ulcerations, spasm, atony, intramural gas, and perforation. In a few weeks, there is narrowing and stricture formation in the distal stomach, most often in the antrum (Fig. 3A.30).

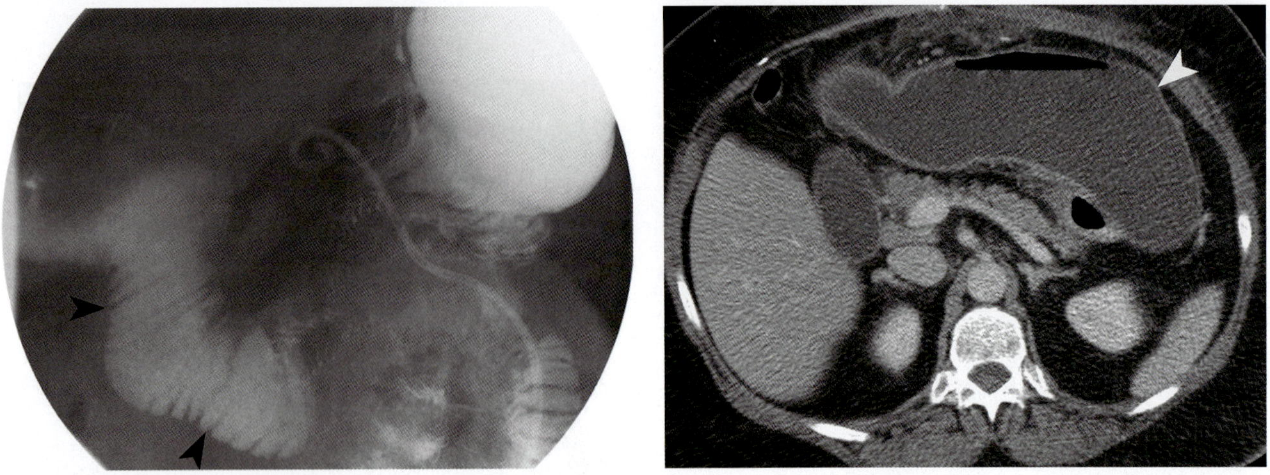

A B

**FIG. 3A.26 • Gastric obstruction. A:** Gastrografin study demonstrates dilated stomach and duodenum (*arrowheads*) with the site of obstruction at the level of the duodenojejunal junction. A catheter is located in the excluded stomach for decompression of the gastric lumen. **B:** Axial contrast-enhanced CT scan study of the same patient demonstrates dilatation of the stomach (*arrowhead*) as well as the duodenum.

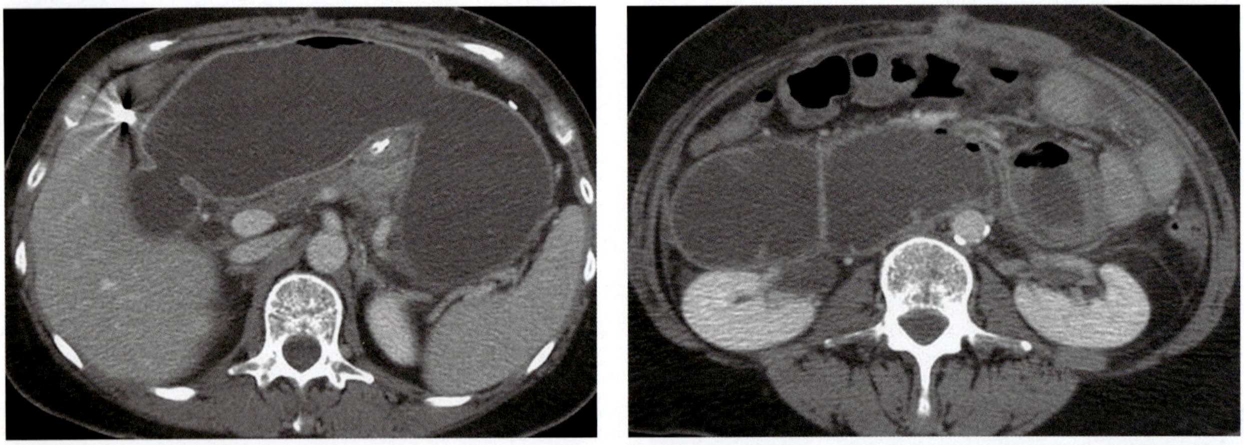

A B

**FIG. 3A.27 • Gastric obstruction. A, B:** Contrast-enhanced CT scan study shows distention of the excluded stomach as well as the duodenum due to obstruction located at the anastomosis with jejunum.

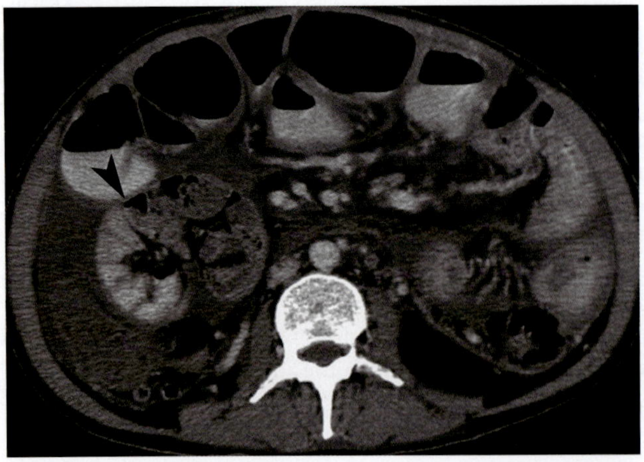

**FIG. 3A.28 • Internal hernia.** Axial contrast-enhanced CT scan study of the abdomen demonstrates an oval cluster of bowel loops (*arrowhead*) in the right abdomen with smooth outline, consistent with internal hernia.

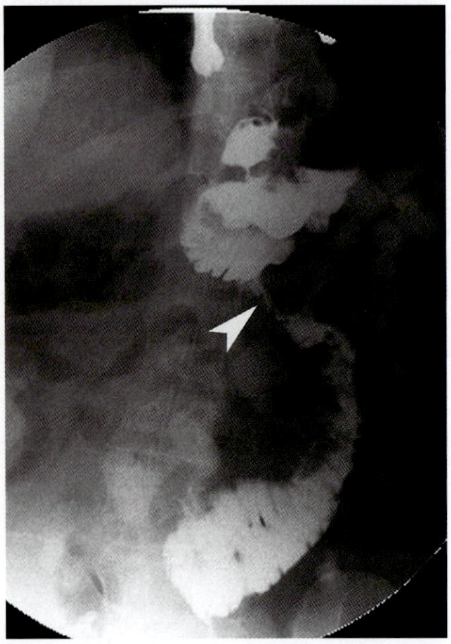

**FIG. 3A.29 • Jejunal stricture.** UGI study demonstrates a stricture (*arrowhead*) formation 10 cm beyond the gastrojejunostomy anastomosis site.

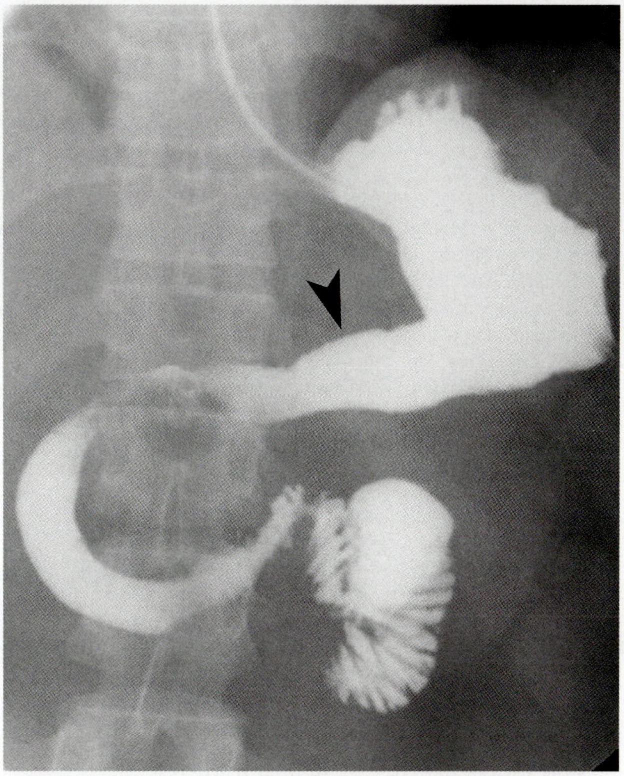

A

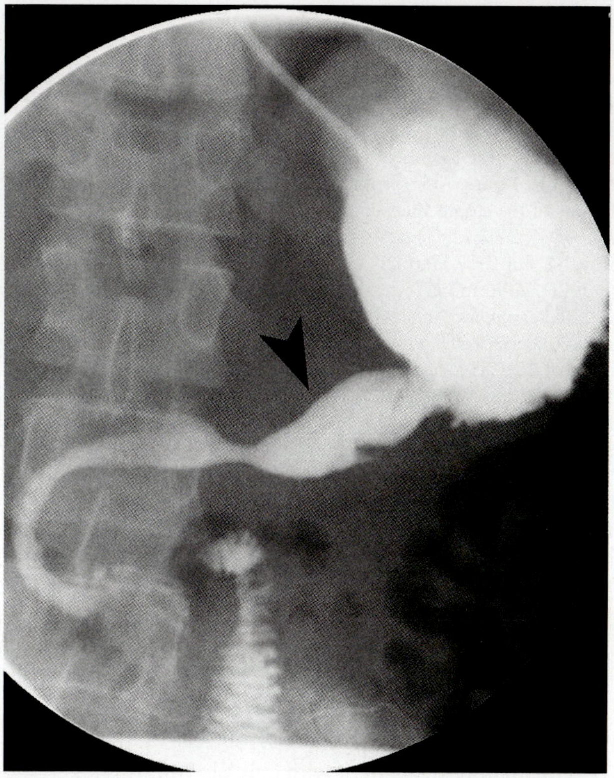

B

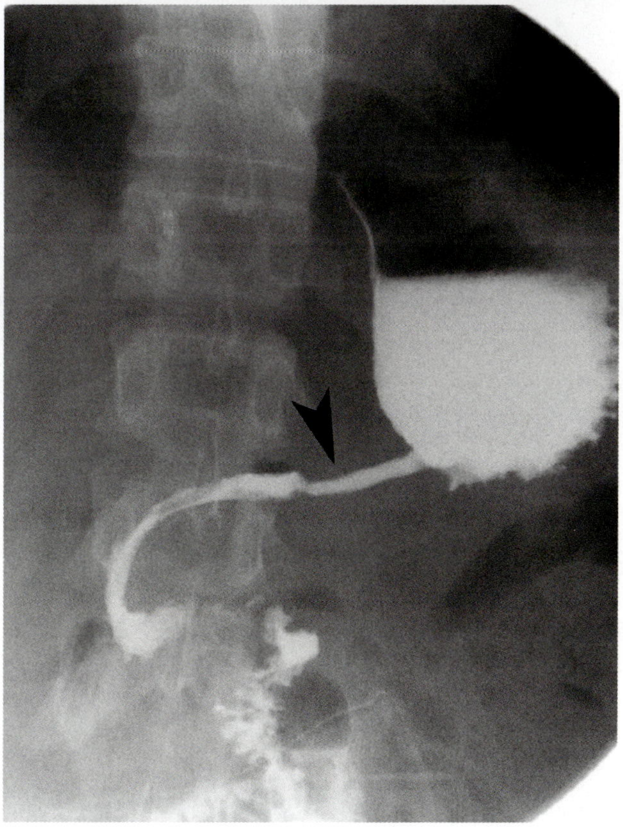

C

**FIG. 3A.30 • Caustic ingestion injury. A–C:** Barium swallow and study performed at 2, 4, and 7 weeks after caustic injection demonstrate progressive stricture formation in the gastric antrum (*arrowhead*) and duodenum. The first barium study also demonstrates edema in the gastric fundus and body, which resolved on follow-up studies.

## References


1. Rubesin SE, Levine MS, Laufer I. Double-contrast upper gastrointestinal radiography: a pattern approach for diseases of the stomach. *Radiology*. 2008;246(1):33–48.
2. Brant WE, Helms CA. *Fundamentals of Diagnostic Radiology*. Philadelphia, PA: Lippincott Williams & Wilkins; 1999.
3. Insko EK, Levine MS, Birnbaum BA, et al. Benign and malignant lesions of the stomach: evaluation of CT criteria for differentiation. *Radiology*. 2003;228(1):166–171.
4. Kim JH, Eun HW, Goo DE, et al. Imaging of various gastric lesions with 2D MPR and CT gastrography performed with multidetector CT. *Radiographics*. 2006;26(4):1101–1116.
5. Fiori R, Velari L, Di Vito L, et al. Menetrier's disease diagnosed by enteroclysis CT: a case report and review of the literature. *Abdom Imaging*. 2011;36:689–693.
6. Rubesin SE, Furth EE, Levine MS. Gastritis from NSAIDs to *Helicobacter pylori*. *Abdom Imaging*. 2005;30:142–159.
7. Torigian DA, Levine MS, Gill NS, et al. Lymphoid hyperplasia of the stomach: radiographic findings in five adult patients. *AJR Am J Roentgenol*. 2001;177:71–75.
8. Schramm D, Bach AG, Zipprich A, et al. Imaging findings of gastric diverticula. *Scientific World J*. 2014; Article ID 923098, http://dx.doi.org/10.1155/2014/923098.
9. Park SH, Han JK, Choi BI, et al. Heterotopic pancreas of the stomach: CT findings correlated with pathologic findings in six patients. *Abdom Imaging*. 2000;25:119–123.
10. Farmann J, Ramirez G, Rybak B, et al. Gastric sarcoidosis. *Abdom Imaging*. 1997;22:248–252.
11. Guzmán E, Montes P, Del Carmen Chávez R, et al. Education and imaging. Gastrointestinal: gastric trichobezoar. *J Gastroenterol Hepatol*. 2013; 28(6):902.
12. Iwamuro M, Okada H, Matsueda K, et al. Review of the diagnosis and management of gastrointestinal bezoars. *World J Gastrointest Endosc*. 2015;7(4):336–345.
13. Sonavane SK, Menias CO, Kantawala KP, et al. Laparoscopic adjustable gastric banding: what radiologists need to know. *Radiographics*. 2012;32(4):1161–1178.
14. Park HJ, Hong SS, Hwang J, et al. Mini-gastric bypass to control morbid obesity and diabetes mellitus: what radiologists need to know. *Korean J Radiol*. 2015;16(2):325–333.


## SELF-ASSESSMENT QUESTIONS

1. What is the cause of the patient's symptoms on the coronal CT reformation in a patient with chronic vomiting?

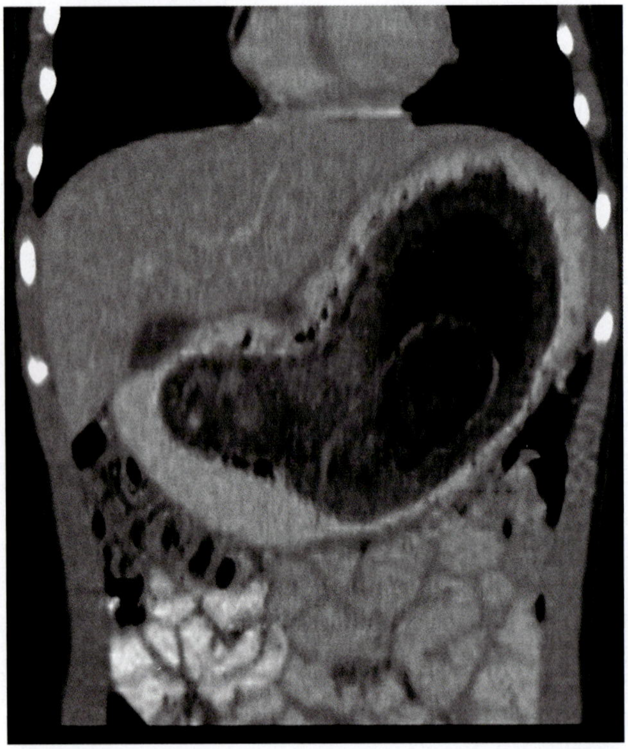

A. Intussusception
B. Gastric volvulus
C. Bezoar
D. Gallstone ileus

2. What is the most significant upper GI study finding responsible for the patient's abdominal pain?

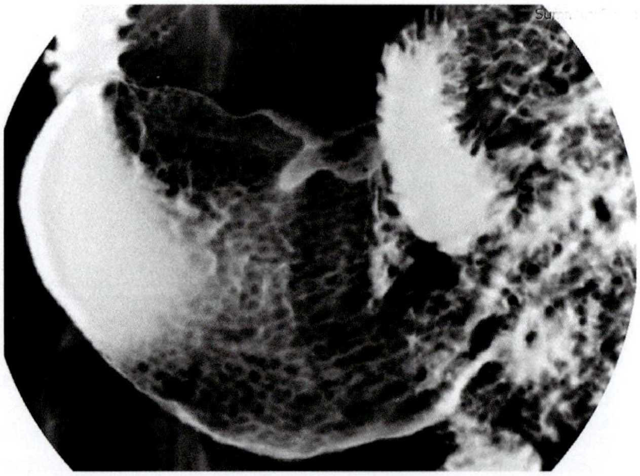

A. Prominent gastric rugal folds
B. Prominent area gastrica
C. Gastric wall ulcerations
D. Gastric wall polyps

3. Is pyloric muscle thickness of 7 mm seen on US normal?

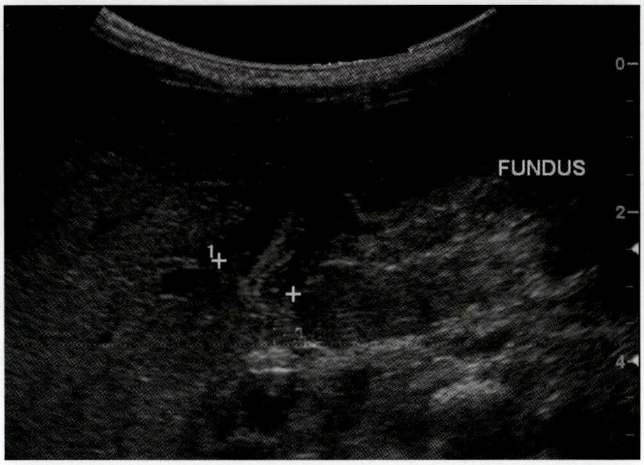


A. Yes
B. No
C. Always

## *Answers to Self-Assessment Questions*

**1. C.** Bezoar. Coronal CT reformation demonstrates large filling well-defined oval intraluminal mass with central low density (from gas bubbles retained within the interstices of the bezoar).

**2. B.** Prominent area gastrica. The double-contrast view of the gastric antrum depicts enlarged and prominent area gastrica (normal area gastrica is typically 2 to 3 mm in diameter in the gastric antrum).

**3. B.** No. The thickness of the pyloric canal musculature is normally less than 3 mm and the length of the muscle is less than 15 mm.

# Stomach: Neoplastic Conditions 3B

*Caterina Missiroli and Ajay K. Singh*

## LEARNING OBJECTIVE

1. Describe the important benign and malignant neoplastic condition of the stomach and their imaging features.

Gastric cancer is the 15th month most common type of cancer in the United States and is also the third most common cause of cancer in the world (after lung, breast, and colorectal cancers). Approximately 80% of the gastric cancers are located in the middle (40%) or lower (40%) stomach.

Esophagogastroduodenoscopy is the first-line investigation in diagnosing gastric cancer and involves biopsy of at least six sites. Carcinoembryonic antigen (CEA), which is elevated in 50% cases, and cancer antigen (CA 19-9), which is elevated in about 20% of the cases, are not sensitive enough in the diagnosis of gastric cancer. Upper gastrointestinal series is typically performed when endoscope cannot be passed due to obstructing gastric mass.

## IMAGING

### Upper Gastrointestinal Series

It is performed most optimally in double-contrast technique to allow the evaluation of the mucosal abnormalities and demonstrates cancers, nodules, ulcers, polyps, and masses.[1]

*Nonuniform nodules* are irregular in outline, disrupting the smooth mucosal surface or areae gastricae of the stomach. They are usually detected in metaplasia, malignancy, and inflammatory diseases. The most important tumors manifesting with nodular pattern are MALT lymphoma and, rarely, superficial spreading carcinoma.[1] Uniform nodules are 1- to 2-mm diameter nodules and are seen with lymphoid hyperplasia.

*Ulcers* are important because of their relationship with early gastric cancer and tumors. Unlike erosions (1 to 2 mm in depth), which do not penetrate the muscularis mucosa and submucosa, an ulcer penetrates into the submucosa. To distinguish a benign ulcer from a malignant one is the most important challenge for radiologist (Table 3B.1). In profile view, visualization of Hampton line, which indicates thin radiolucent line traversing the base of the ulcer crater due to undermining of the mucosa, is diagnostic of benign ulcers. Malignant ulcers, which represent crater formation within the tumor mass, are surrounded by irregular mucosal folds, nodularity, and mucosal irregularity (Figs. 3B.1 and 3B.2). The base of the ulcer crater within a neoplastic mass may not project outside the expected outline of the gastric lumen.

A gastric polyp arising from the mucosa may have a small, lobular or nodular outline on double-contrast study. Space-occupying lesions arising from the submucosa have a smooth outline on double-contrast study. When seen in profile, submucosal lesions form right angle or obtuse angle with the adjacent gastric wall.

Submucosal masses are round or ovoid, well-delimited, and increased in opacity, and about 50% of them have a central area of necrosis, seen as "bull's-eye" lesion on double-contrast study.[1] When viewed in profile, they typically form obtuse or right angle with the gastric wall (Fig. 3B.3). Gastrointestinal stromal tumors (GISTs) are the most common benign submucosal tumors in the stomach.

The differential diagnosis of gastric submucosal mass:

1. GIST (most common)
2. Lipoma
3. Leiomyoblastoma
4. Hemangioma
5. Schwannoma
6. Nonneoplastic causes: lymphangioma, inflammatory fibroid polyp, ectopic pancreas, granular cell tumor, and Brunner cell hamartoma

Table 3B.1 **IMAGING FEATURES OF BENIGN AND MALIGNANT GASTRIC ULCERS**

| Features | Benign Ulcer | Malignant Ulcer |
|---|---|---|
| Margins | Smooth | Irregular |
| Mass effect | None | Yes |
| Nodularity | None | Yes |
| Hampton line | Yes | None |
| Location | Lesser curvature<br>Posterior wall | – |
| Edge | Sharp, rounded | Elevated, asymmetric |
| Gastric folds | Converging | Thickened, nodular, distorted |

## Cross-Sectional Imaging

Evaluation with computed tomography technique with multidetector scanners involves two different techniques, CT with double-contrast agents and CT gastrography. CT virtual endoscopy (VE) allows detection of mucosal and submucosal alterations just like endoscopy with the additional advantage of allowing extragastric abnormalities.[2–5] The advantages of the VE include the noninvasive technique and visualization of blind areas not possible on endoscopy. VE limitations are the radiation exposure and inability to obtain histologic samples. This type of CT may be useful to a first-step evaluation of the stomach to avoid unnecessary endoscopies. T- and N-staging are the principal targets of CT imaging, and the intravenous administration of contrast agent (late arterial, venous, and late scanning at 40, 75, and 150 seconds, respectively) is useful to detect the difference among the various types of tumors.[4,6] In the TNM staging (Table 3B.2), T1 is tumor invasion of the lamina propria, muscularis mucosa, or submucosa. T2 is invasion of the muscularis propria, T3 is invasion of the subserosal connective tissue, and T4 is invasion of the serosa (visceral peritoneum or adjacent organs). Another important role of CT examination is in the evaluation after surgical or palliative treatment, to investigate early complications and to follow-up after gastric surgery.[7]

MR is not routinely used as first-line imaging modality but can be used for local staging (T) and lymph nodal involvement. To avoid difficulty in interpreting the significance of wall thickness, usually, the stomach is distended by water and muscles transiently paralyzed with antiperistaltic agents. The main sequences in use are T1-weightened spoiled gradient echo (T1-SGE) with or without fat suppression both before and after intravenous administration of gadolinium. Either half-Fourier acquisition snapshot turbo spin echo or true fast imaging with steady-state precession sequence may be used because of the short imaging time. MRI accuracy in detecting wall involvement and peritoneal infiltration ranges from 73% to 88%. N-staging uses size of the lymph node as diagnostic criteria for involvement, similar to CT, with low accuracy (55% to 65%). The limitations of MR are motion artifacts due to breathing and peristalsis, different wall thickness relative to different degree of gastric distension, and limited accuracy for

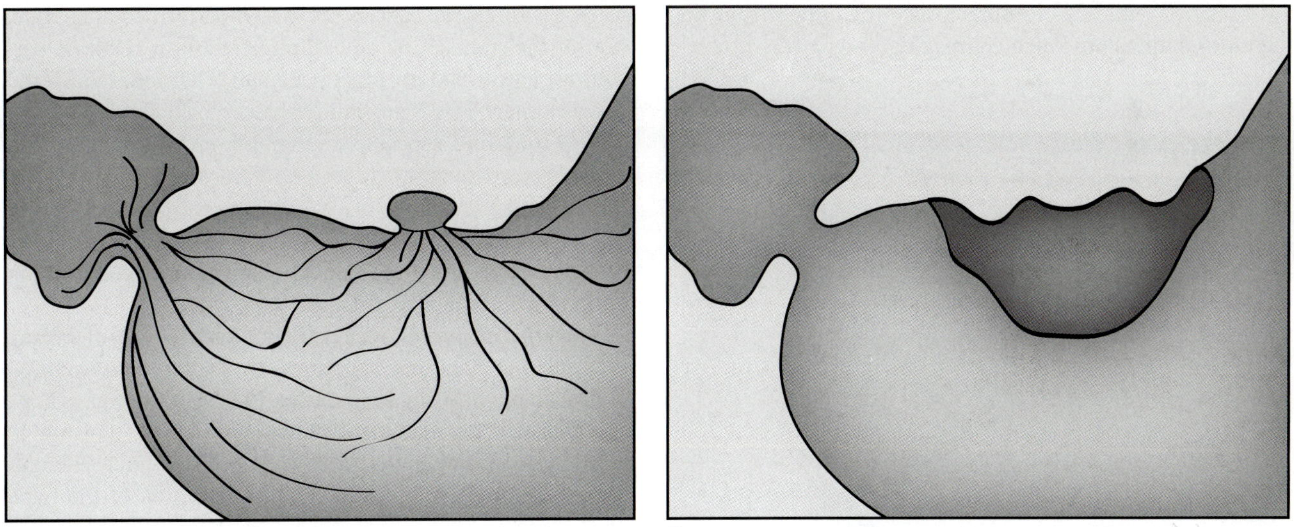

A B

**FIG. 3B.1 • Schematic diagram representing the upper GI study imaging features of benign and malignant gastric ulcer. A:** Benign gastric ulcer—the ulcer crater protrudes outside the luminal outline of the gastric wall. There are radiating mucosal folds seen extending to the edge of the ulcer crater with smooth (no nodularity) mucosal folds. A Hampton line across the mouth of the ulcer crater represents undermining of the gastric mucosa. **B:** Malignant ulcer—there is nodularity of the mucosal folds surrounding the ulcer crater. Since the ulcer may be located within the intraluminal gastric mass, the base of the ulcer crater fails to project beyond the luminal aspect of the gastric wall. Carmen meniscus sign is due to a large flat malignant gastric ulcer with heaped up margins. On barium study, the ulcer will appear always convex toward the lumen of the stomach. Kirklin meniscus complex represents Carmen meniscus sign along with radiolucent elevated edges of the ulcer.

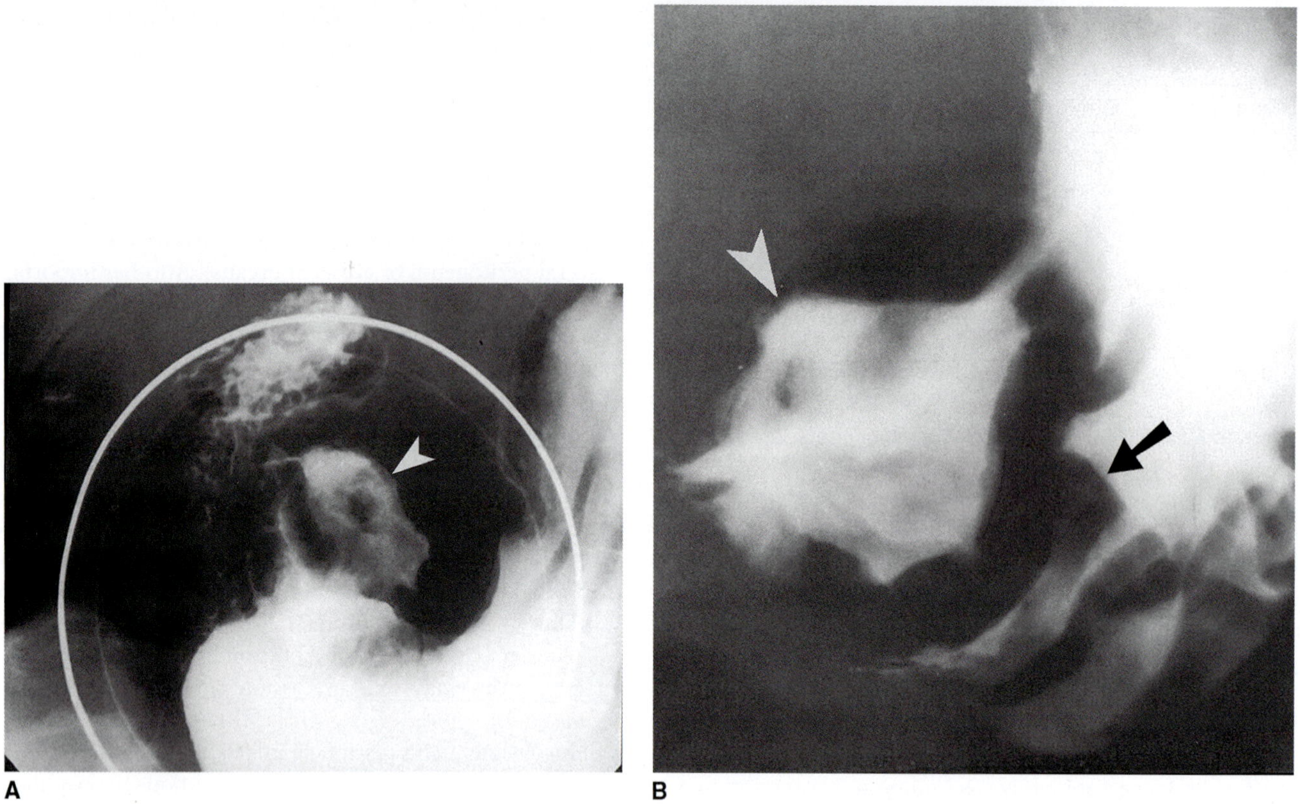

**FIG. 3B.2 • Malignant gastric ulcer. A, B:** Single-contrast UGI study demonstrates malignant gastric ulcer crater (*arrowhead*) surrounded by nodular ulcer mound (*arrow*).

N-staging. The advantages of MR compared to other imaging techniques include high soft tissue contrast, availability of fluid-sensitive sequences to differentiate the lumen from the mucosa, and diffusion-weighted imaging.[8,9]

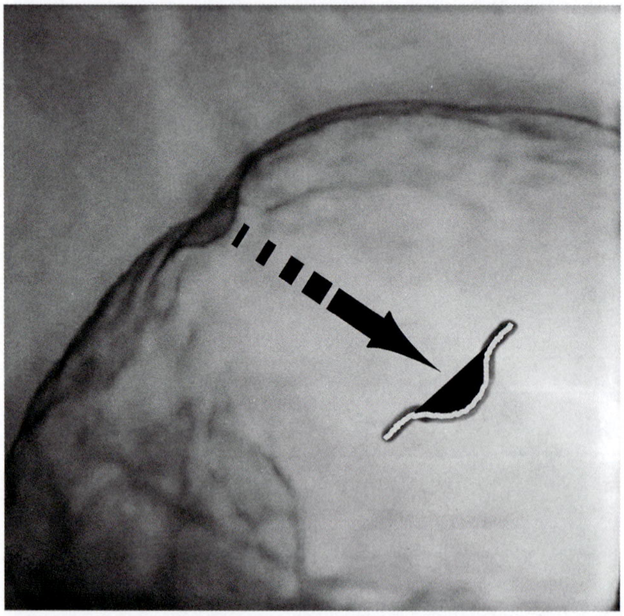

**FIG. 3B.3 • Sessile polyp.** Double contrast upper GI study demonstrates a smooth hemispherical filling defect in the gastric fundus with obtuse margins with the luminal aspect of the gastric wall.

Ultrasonography use has been mostly associated with endoscopy, but recently, some studies do use transabdominal US in patient with gastric cancer. US can be performed after distension of the stomach by oral administration of cellulose-based contrast agent (500 mL) that generates a homogeneous echoic gastric lumen. This US technique has a sensitivity ranging from 77% to 100% and a specificity ranging from 94% to 100%.[10]

## GASTRIC POLYP

Gastric polyps constitute half of benign gastric neoplasm, seen in up to 2% of double-contrast study.

*Hyperplastic polyps*, which are nonneoplastic proliferations of branching glandular structures, are the most common type of gastric polyp. They account for 75% to 90% of gastric polyps and have no malignant potential. They are typically less than 1 cm in diameter and have smooth or finely lobulated outline (Figs. 3B.3 and 3B.4). More than 30% of the hyperplastic polyps are multiple and are most commonly located in the gastric body or fundus. They arise in patients with chronic gastritis and therefore more commonly seen in patients with synchronous gastric carcinoma and gastric dysplasia. Ten to twenty-five percent of patients with hyperplastic polyps can have synchronous gastric carcinoma.

*Fundic gland polyps* are the second most common type of polyps except in Western countries where *H. pylori* is less prevalent and where fundic gland polyps are the most common type of gastric polyp. They are most common in middle-aged

Table 3B.2 **TNM STAGING OF GASTRIC NEOPLASM (AMERICAN JOINT COMMITTEE ON CANCER STAGING SYSTEM)**

| | T | N | M | Treatment |
|---|---|---|---|---|
| Stage 0 | IS | 0 | 0 | Subtotal/total gastrectomy |
| Stage IA | 1 | 0 | 0 | Gastrectomy + lymphadenectomy |
| Stage IB | 1<br>2 | 1<br>0 | 0<br>0 | Gastrectomy + lymphadenectomy |
| Stage II | 1<br>2<br>3 | 2<br>1<br>0 | 0<br>0<br>0 | Gastrectomy + lymphadenectomy |
| Stage IIIA | 2<br>3<br>4 | 2<br>1<br>0 | 0<br>0<br>0 | Radical surgery + lymphadenectomy +/– chemotherapy |
| Stage IIIB | 3 | 2 | 0 | Radical surgery + lymphadenectomy +/– chemotherapy |
| Stage IV | 4<br>1<br>2<br>3<br>4<br>4<br>1/2/3/4 | 1<br>3<br>3<br>3<br>2<br>3<br>1/2/3 | 0<br>0<br>0<br>0<br>0<br>0<br>1 | Chemotherapy or Palliative |

Stage 0 = No lesion/involvement.
Tis = In situ.
T1 = Tumor invades lamina propria or submucosa.
T2 = Muscularis propria or subserosa.
T3 = Penetrates serosa and no other structures.
T4 = Involves adjacent structures.
N1 = 1–6 regional lymph nodes involved.
N2 = 7–15 regional lymph node.
N3 = More than 15 regional/other lymph nodes.
M1 = Distant metastases.

women. Similar to hyperplastic polyp, they have no malignant potential. They are usually sessile, subcentimeter polyps located in the fundus and upper gastric body. These are often multiple (up to 50%) and have association with adenomatosis polyposis syndrome (Fig. 3B.5A, B).

*Adenomatous polyps* are less common than hyperplastic and fundic gland polyps. These have malignant potential and may progress to carcinoma. Adenomatous polyps more than 2 cm in diameter have in situ carcinoma or invasive carcinoma in more than 50% of the cases. Adenomatous polyps, which cause symptoms, are typically more than 1 cm in diameter and may be sessile or pedunculated. On double-contrast UGI study, a polyp more than a centimeter in diameter requires biopsy confirmation to rule out the possibility of an adenoma (Fig. 3B.5C). Multiple polyps less than a centimeter in size are most often hyperplastic and may not require endoscopy or biopsy confirmation.

Imaging findings of gastric polyps:

- On dependent wall, hyperplastic polyps are seen as smooth, sessile, subcentimeter nodular filling defects.
- On nondependent wall, hyperplastic polyps are seen as ring shadows, etched in white with hanging barium droplet or stalactite.
- Fundic gland polyps are similar to hyperplastic polyp on imaging and are more likely to be multiple.
- Adenomatous polyps are seen as more than 1-cm diameter, sessile or pedunculated, and often lobulated filling defects in gastric antrum. Pedunculated polyps can be seen as two concentric rings (Mexican hat sign) when viewed en face, produced by the stalk (inner ring) and head (outer ring).

## MALIGNANT NEOPLASTIC PATHOLOGIES OF THE STOMACH

The different types of gastric malignancies include:

1. Adenocarcinoma (90%)
2. Lymphoma (5%)

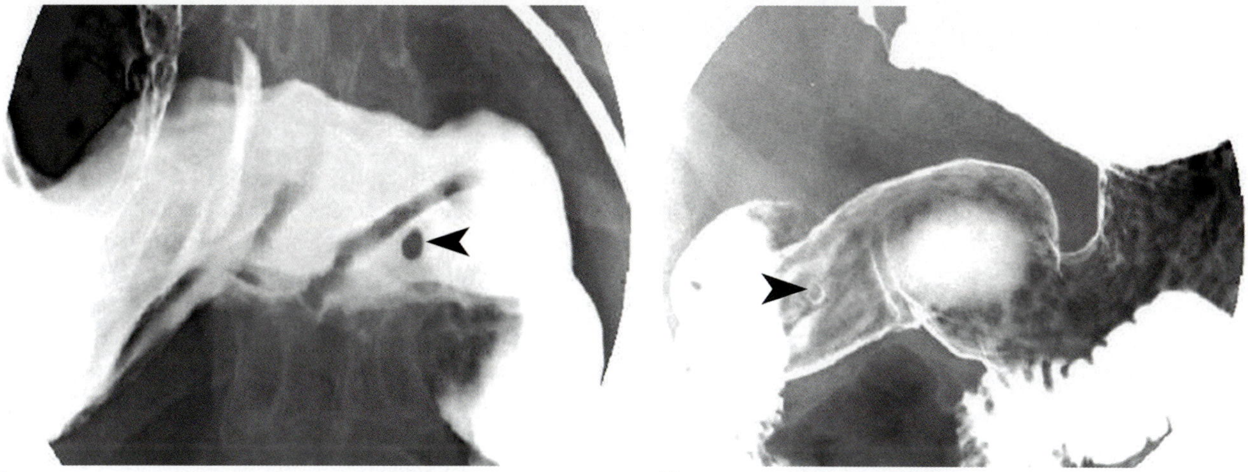

A B

**FIG. 3B.4 • Solitary gastric antral polyp.** Single- and double-contrast images of the gastric antrum demonstrate oval polypoidal filling defect in the anterior wall of the gastric antrum. On prone single-contrast view **(A)**, the polyp is seen as a filling defect (*arrowhead*) in a pool of radiopaque barium. On the supine double-contrast view **(B)**, the polyp is seen as a filling defect outlined by rim of barium (*arrowhead*).

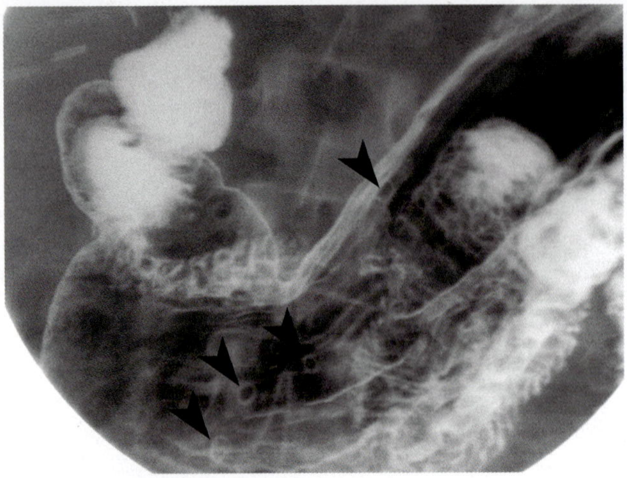

A

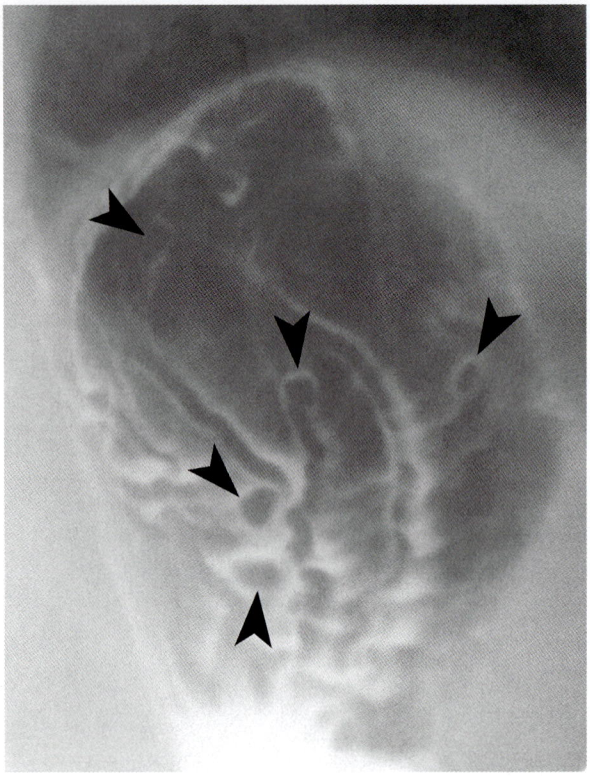

B

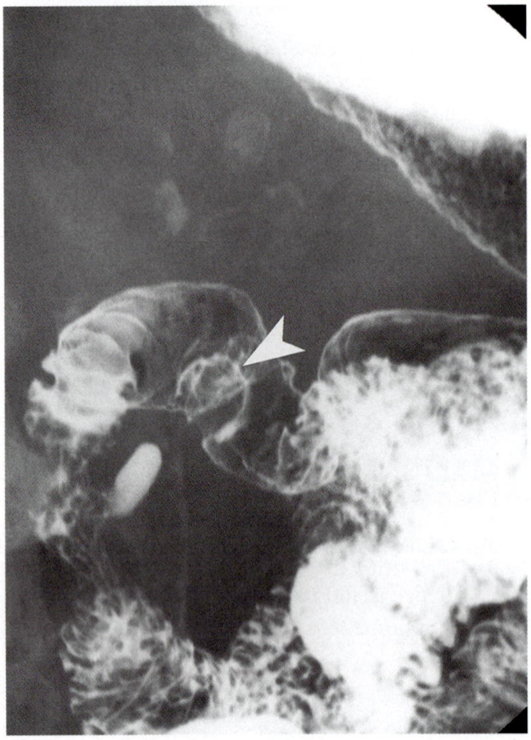

C

**FIG. 3B.5 • Hyperplastic gastric polyps. A–C:** Double-contrast UGI series in three patients demonstrating multiple subcentimeter polyps Q2 (*arrowheads*) seen as smooth round filling defects outlined by barium.

3. Gastrointestinal stromal tumor (2%)
4. Carcinoid (1%)
5. Adenoacanthoma (1%)
6. Carcinoid (1%)
7. Squamous cell carcinoma (1%)

## ADENOCARCINOMA

Adenocarcinoma of the stomach accounts for about 90% to 95% of the total gastric carcinomas.[7,8,11,12] Other cancer histologies include diffuse anaplastic cancer, squamous cell cancer, and other rare tumors. *H. pylori* infection has been demonstrated in half of gastric cancers and is the most important risk factor, especially when associated with gastric ulcer.[7,12] The other predisposing factors for adenocarcinoma include smoking, polyps, pernicious anemia, atrophic gastritis, pernicious anemia, gastrojejunostomy, and diet (nitrates, nitrites, salted/smoked foods). The age range of prevalence is 50 to 70 years, with male predominance.

Based on whether muscularis propria is invaded, gastric carcinoma can be classified as early or advanced gastric carcinoma. Most gastric carcinomas have invaded the muscularis propria at the time of diagnosis and are advanced gastric carcinomas.

Early gastric cancer:

- Tumor limited to the mucosa and submucosa of the stomach, regardless the presence of lymph nodal or distant metastasis.
- The high survival at 5 years (85% to 100%).

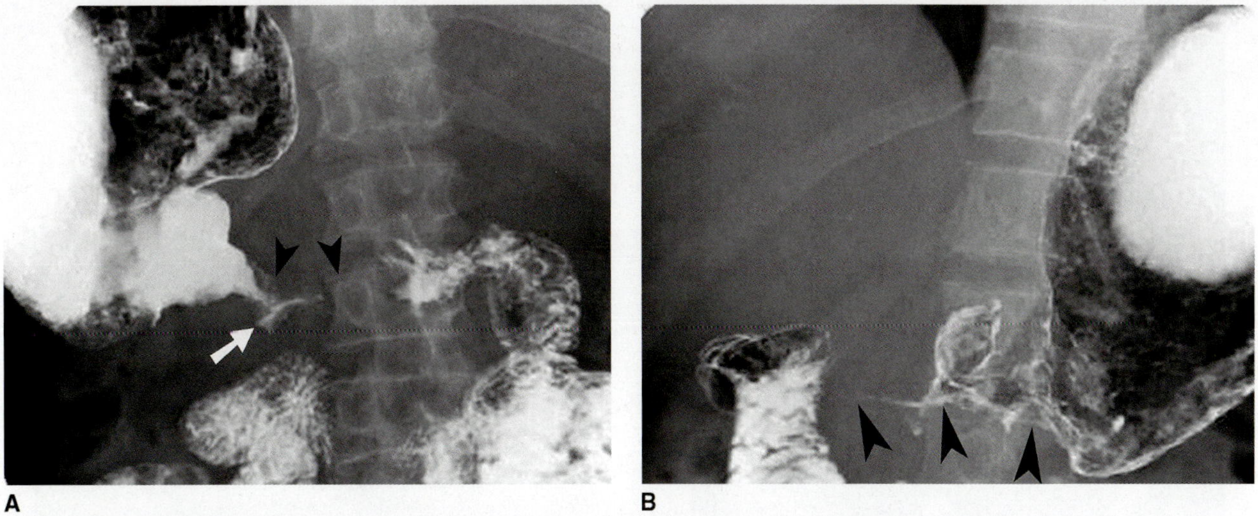


**FIG. 3B.6 • Gastric outlet obstruction caused by gastric adenocarcinoma. A, B:** Single- and double-contrast images of the gastric antrum demonstrates irregular, eccentric stricture (*arrowheads*) with areas of mucosal irregularity and ulceration (*arrow*) caused by gastric adenocarcinoma involving the antrum and pylorus.

- On UGI study, it can have variable appearance, including protruded polypoidal mass and ulcerating lesions.
- At CT gastroscopy and multiplanar reconstructions, EGC may be assessed with high accuracy (80% to 85%), but this technique is at the moment in used more frequently for the evaluation of the tumor extension and preoperative planning rather than for the T-staging.[11,12]

On UGI study, adenocarcinoma may present as a polypoid, plaque-like, or ulcerative lesion (Fig. 3B.6).[12,13] Ulcerated cancer has the characteristic of a malignant ulcer (see Table 3B.1) located in a mass lesion. Infiltrating tumor may generate diffuse wall infiltration by undifferentiated cells (scirrhous carcinoma), rigid and thick wall with narrowed lumen (*linitis plastica* or *water-bottle stomach*), or superficial spreading with mucosal and submucosal involvement (nodular and/or ulcerated) (Figs. 3B.7 to 3B.9).[7,12]

On CT, detection of wall thickening of more than 1 cm has high sensitivity but low specificity. Gastric carcinoma

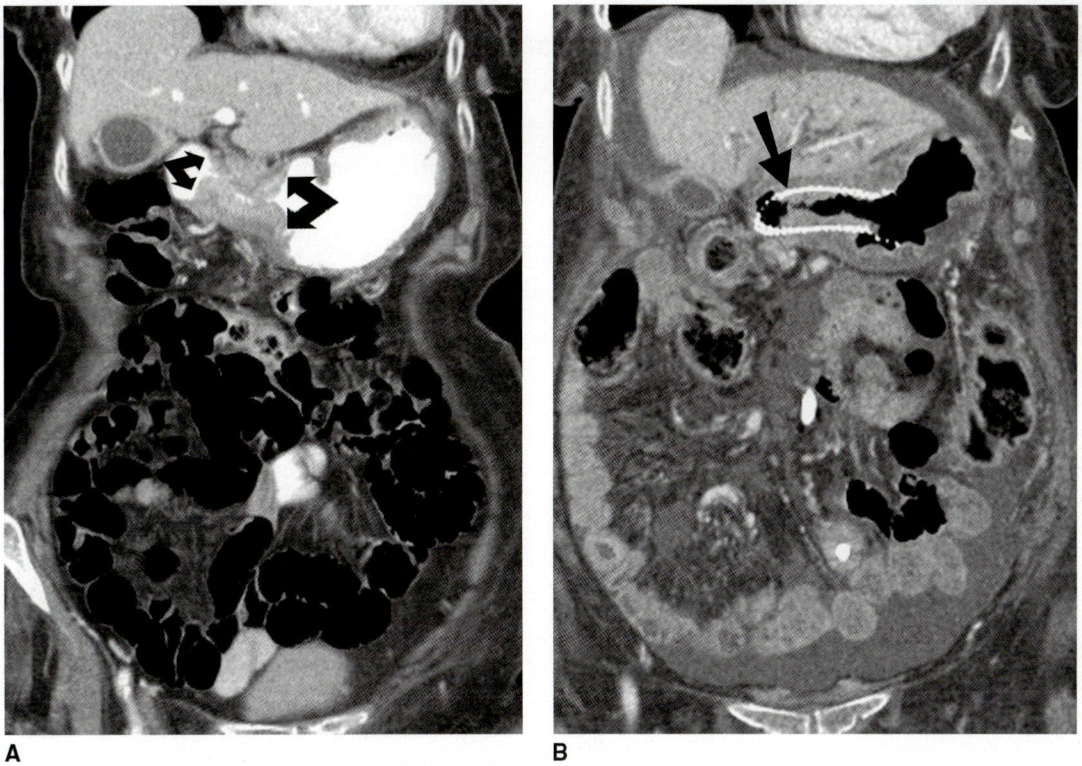


**FIG. 3B.7 • Gastric carcinoma with gastric outlet obstruction. A:** Coronal CT reformation demonstrates segmental gastric antral wall thickening causing marked narrowing of the gastric lumen. There is proximal as well as distal shouldering (*double arrows*). **B:** Coronal CT reformation after wallstent (*arrow*) placement shows improved caliber of the gastric antrum.

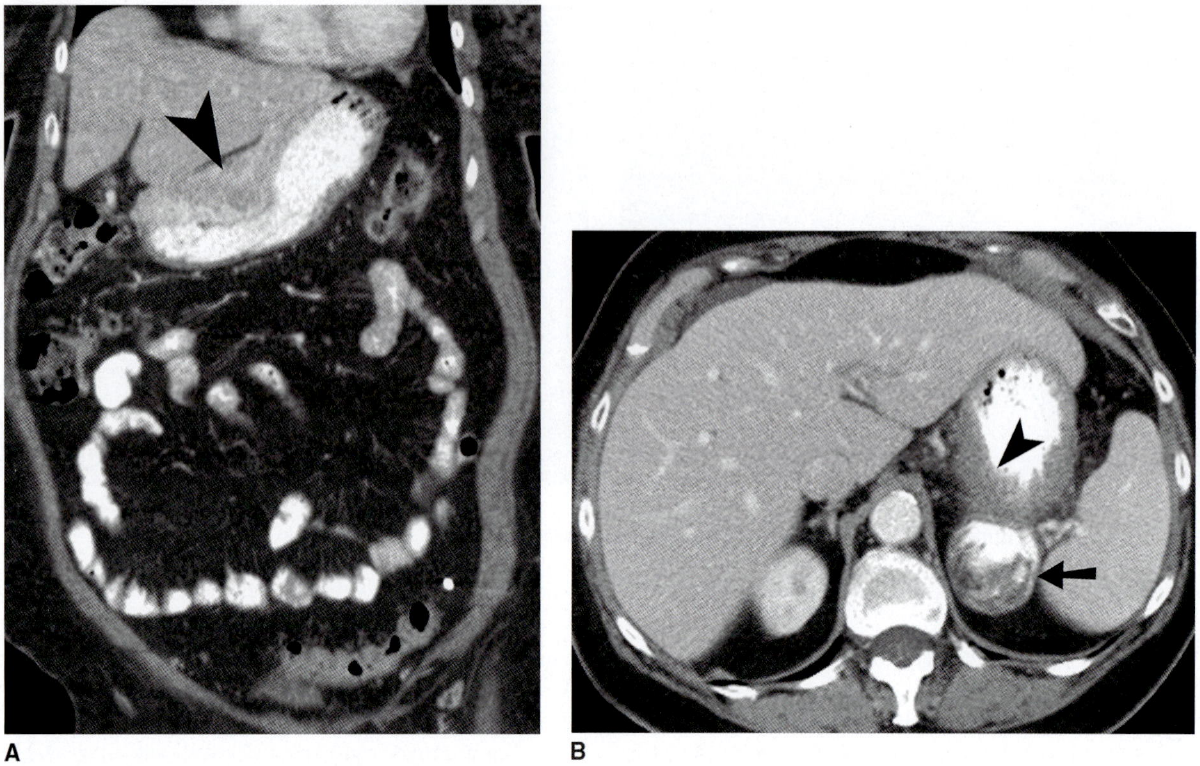


**FIG. 3B.8 • Adenocarcinoma of the stomach. A:** Coronal CT reformation demonstrates marked thickening of the gastric antral wall (*arrowhead*) due to adenocarcinoma of the stomach, causing narrowing of the gastric body. **B:** Axial contrast-enhanced CT scan study demonstrates thickening of the gastric fundal wall (*arrowhead*) located anterior to an incidentally seen gastric diverticulum lateral (*arrow*).

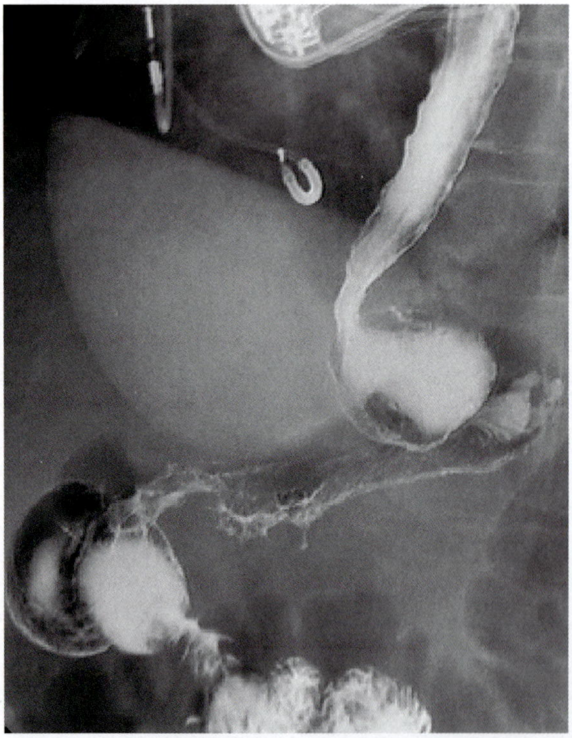

**FIG. 3B.9 • Adenocarcinoma of the stomach with linitis plastic.** Double-contrast upper GI study demonstrates diffuse narrowing of the gastric lumen caused by infiltrating mass involving the gastric body and antrum. A focal deep ulcer is seen along the greater curvature of the stomach.

can be seen on CT as polypoidal, fungating, ulcerating, or infiltrating mass, which enhances more with tightly aggregated cells. CT is performed after diagnosing adenocarcinoma of the stomach to evaluate for tumor spread through the gastric wall to the perigastric fat, adjacent organs (pancreas and spleen), peritoneal cavity, lymph nodes, and distant organs (liver, adrenal glands, ovaries; colon, uterus, bone, and lung) (Fig. 3B.10).[7,12]

Differential diagnosis of gastric carcinoma:

1. Gastric carcinoma (most common)
2. Metastatic breast cancer, pancreatic carcinoma, and omental metastases
3. Non-Hodgkin lymphoma (NHL)
4. Nonneoplastic causes (caustic ingestion, pancreatitis, peptic ulcer disease, radiation, Crohn disease, sarcoidosis, syphilis, tuberculosis)

## LYMPHOMA

Gastric lymphomas account for up to 5% gastric malignancies and represent the most common site of extranodal lymphoma. The stomach is the most common gastrointestinal site for lymphomas, with 80% being NHL.[7,12,13] MALT lymphomas are low-grade lymphomas, which account for majority of gastric lymphomas.

On UGI study, lymphoma can appear as polypoidal, ulcerated mass, bulky mass, multiple nodules with bull's-eye

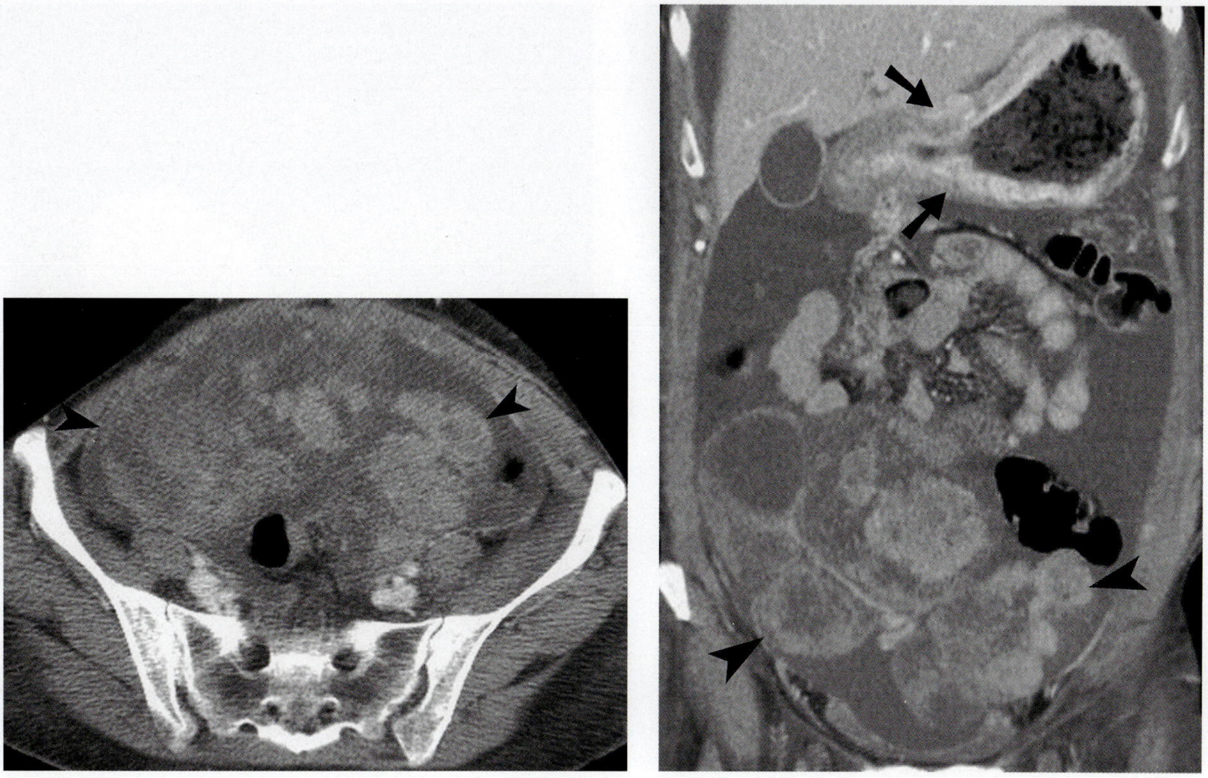

A B

**FIG. 3B.10 • Krukenberg tumor. A, B:** Axial and coronal CT demonstrate large lobulated bilateral ovarian (*arrowheads*) mass lesions secondary to peritoneal metastasis from the patient's gastric cancer (*arrows*).

appearance, confluent nodules, and, rarely, linitis plastic.[1,12] On CT, the main findings suspected for lymphoma are the presence of multiple areas of wall thickening (diffuse or segmental; average size 5 cm) with or without ulcerations, absence of perigastric involvement, and the presence of bulky adenopathy (Figs. 3B.11 to 3B.13).[7,12,13]

MALT lymphoma has better prognosis (62% to 90% at 5 years) than adenocarcinoma, because of the rarity of adenopathy or extragastric involvement.[12,13]

Gastric carcinoma versus gastric lymphoma on imaging:

- Lymphoma associated with thicker gastric wall and more uniform enhancement
- Lymphoma more likely to be multiple and less likely to cause gastric outlet obstruction
- Gastric carcinoma more likely to extend outside the stomach and usually causes more local lymphadenopathy (vs. lymphoma, which can cause systemic lymphadenopathy)

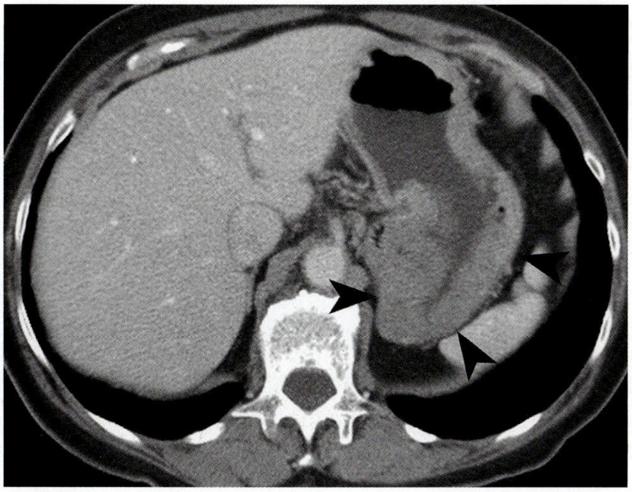

**FIG. 3B.11 • Gastric lymphoma.** Axial contrast-enhanced CT demonstrates marked thickening of the gastric rugal folds on the posterior aspect of the gastric body and fundus (*arrowheads*).

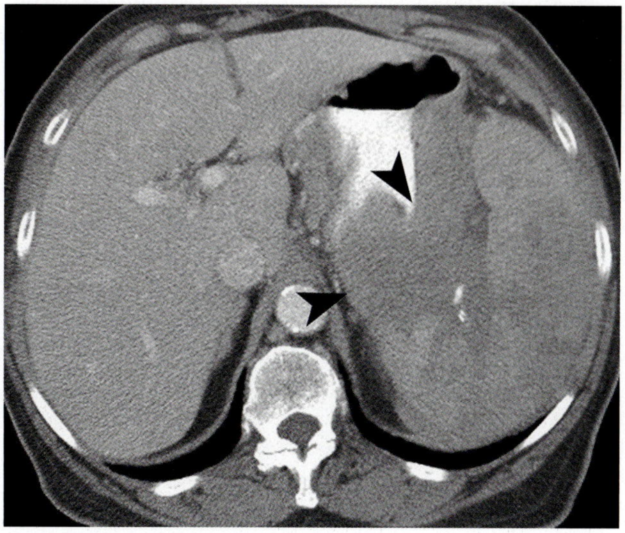

**FIG. 3B.12 • Gastric lymphoma.** Axial contrast-enhanced CT scan study demonstrates marked thickening of the posterior gastric wall (*arrowheads*) with extragastric extension of the lymphomatous disease into the splenic hilum.

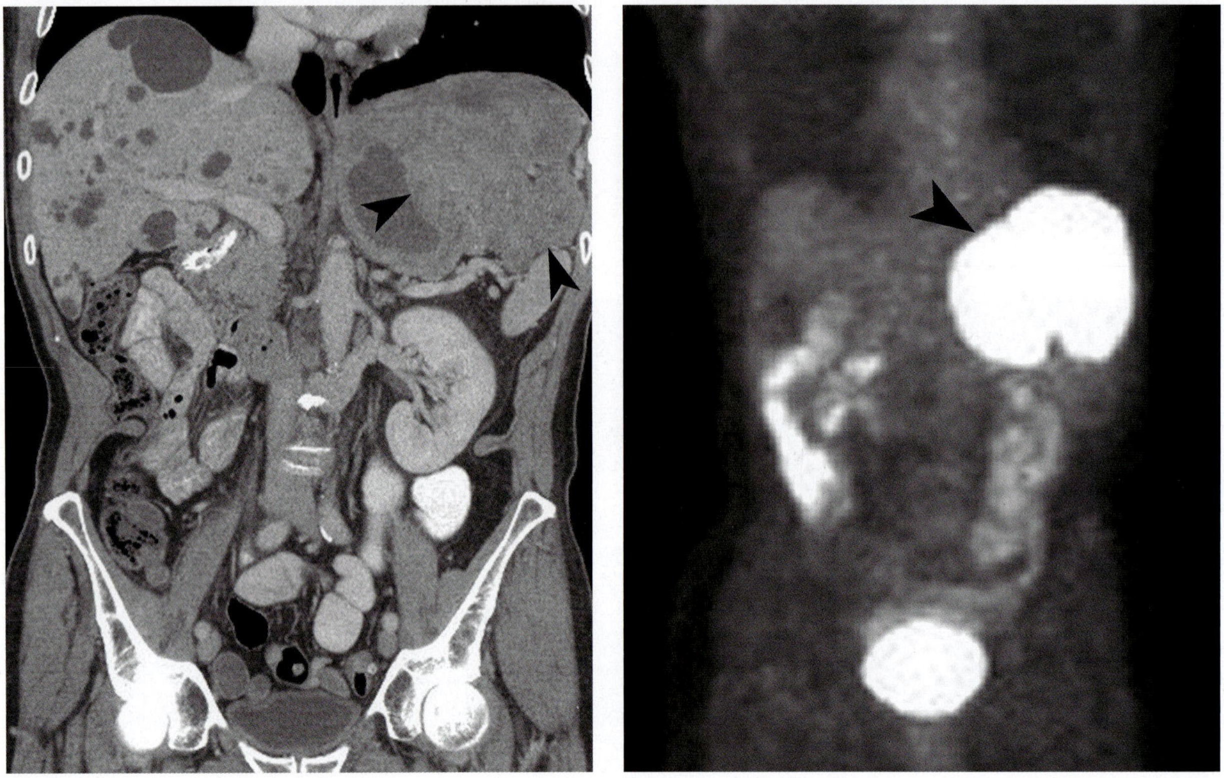

A B

**FIG. 3B.13 • Gastric lymphoma. A:** Coronal CT reformation demonstrates gross thickening of the gastric fundal wall (*arrowheads*) from lymphomatous disease extending in the left subdiaphragmatic region. The spleen is displaced caudally by the mass. **B:** PET scan demonstrates hypermetabolic lymphoma in the left upper quadrant (*arrowhead*) of the abdomen.

## GASTROINTESTINAL STROMAL TUMOR

GIST of the stomach accounts for 2% to 3% of gastric malignancies and represents the most common gastrointestinal location of mesenchymal cells tumors. Approximately 90% of gastric GISTs are benign lesions. They arise from intestinal cells of Cajal and are endogastric (intramural) in 80% cases, exogastric (15%; grow exophytic), or dumbbell lesions (5%). They may invade the adjacent organs and spread through the hematologic route, most frequently to the liver, peritoneum, and lung. Lymph nodal involvement is less frequent.[13–15]

Radiologic appearances of GIST can vary depending on tumor size and morphology (intramural or exophytic). The intramural GIST is usually smooth, well circumscribed, and etched in white submucosal mass with obtuse or right angle with the gastric wall (Fig. 3B.5). The exophytic type and larger GIST often have areas of hemorrhage, necrosis, or cystic degeneration (Figs. 3B.14 and 3B.15). One-half of the lesions greater than 2 cm develop ulcerations, and small tumors (less than 4 to 5 cm) are usually less invasive than larger tumors.

Leiomyoma and leiomyosarcoma arise from the smooth muscle tissue of the gastric wall. They have been considered stromal tumors in the past until the finding of the mesenchymal precursors of the GIST. Usually (90%), these tumors are located in the fundus or the body of the stomach.[14] Leiomyoma is benign, small, smooth, and homogeneous, while leiomyosarcoma is large (greater than 5 to 10 cm), irregular in enhancement with frequent central hypodensity due to hemorrhage and necrosis, and often exophytic (Fig. 3B.16). On UGI study, leiomyoma and leiomyosarcoma may appear as submucosal mass, with larger lesions demonstrating central bull's-eye ulcerations.

## CARCINOID

Carcinoids are well-differentiated neuroendocrine tumors originating from the endocrine system (Kulchitsky cells). They usually occur in the gastrointestinal tract (67%), but can less commonly originate from the tracheobronchial system (24%). The small bowel is the most frequent site of origin in GI carcinoid, followed by the rectum, appendix, and stomach (rare, 1.8% of gastric malignancies). Histology classifies the carcinoid tumors in three types: types 1 and 2 are associated to hypergastrinemia, a hormone that promotes the proliferation of the carcinoid cells and the development of multiple tumors.[15,16] The origin of the tumor is from the mucosa, but often, the mass involves the submucosa.[16] The principal characteristic of type 1 carcinoid of the stomach is benignity with rare distant extension into the liver and lymph nodes. Type 2

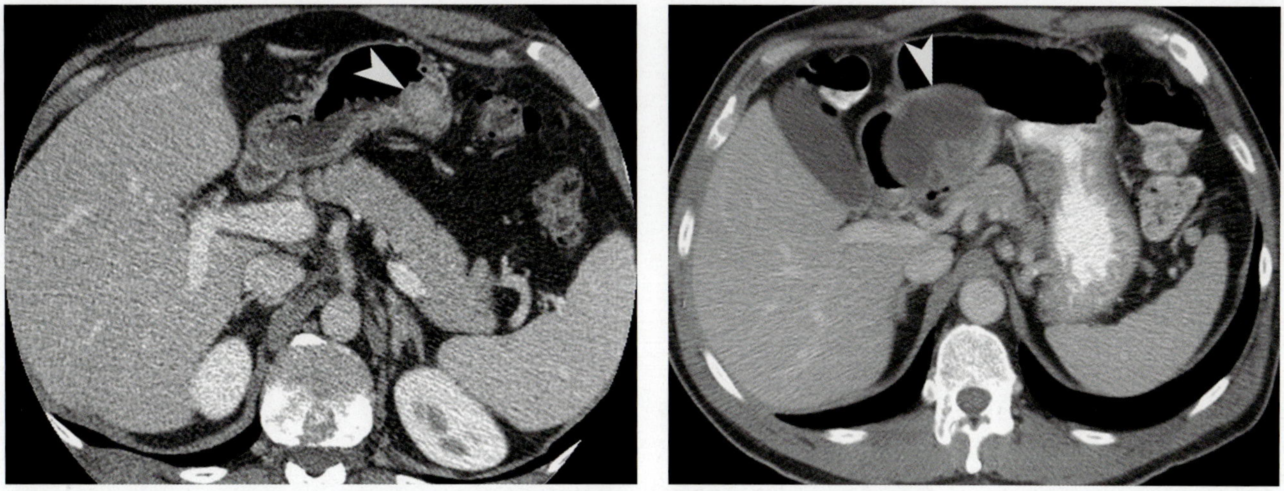

A B

**FIG. 3B.14 • Gastrointestinal stromal tumor. A:** Axial contrast-enhanced CT shows a 3-cm, focal submucosal mass in the wall of proximal gastric body (*arrowhead*) without any extragastric extension of the disease process. **B:** Axial contrast-enhanced CT shows a 7-cm diameter heterogeneous density mass (*arrowhead*) seen in the posterior wall of the gastric antrum with areas of necrosis in it.

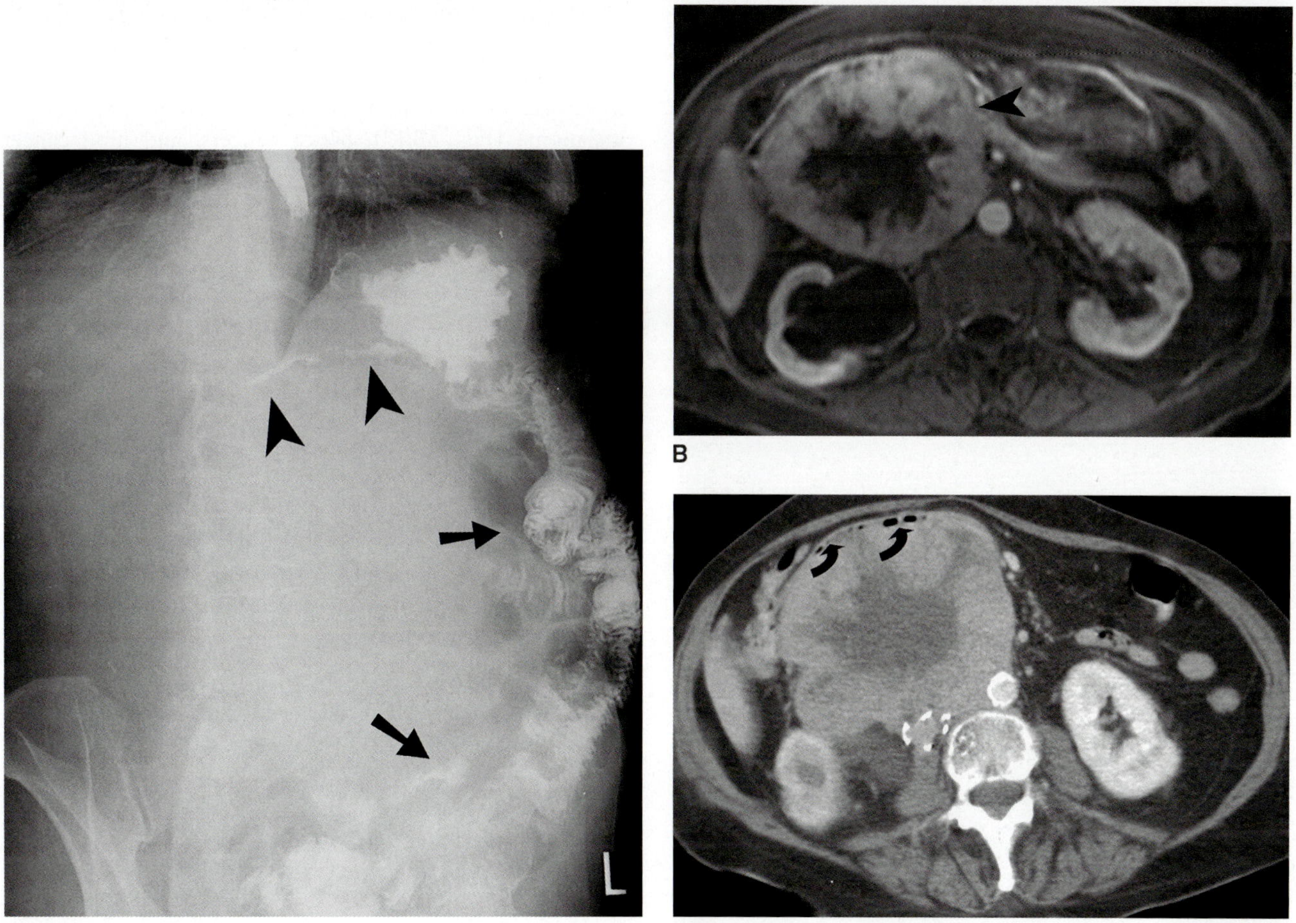


B

A C

**FIG. 3B.15 • Malignant gastrointestinal stromal tumor. A:** Upper GI study demonstrates marked narrowing of the gastric body and antrum (*arrowheads*) due to the large mass, which is also displacing the small bowel loops (*arrows*) to the left side. **B, C:** Postgadolinium T1-weighted MR and axial postcontrast CT image demonstrate large exophytic gastric mass (*arrowhead*) lesion with central necrosis arising from the posterior gastric antral wall (*curved arrows*).

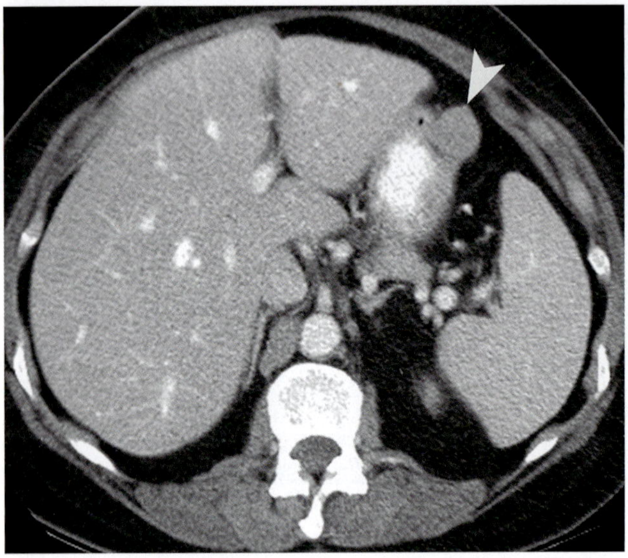

**FIG. 3B.16 • Gastric leiomyoma.** Axial contrast-enhanced CT scan study demonstrates a 2.5-cm diameter submucosal mass (*arrowhead*) in the gastric fundus.

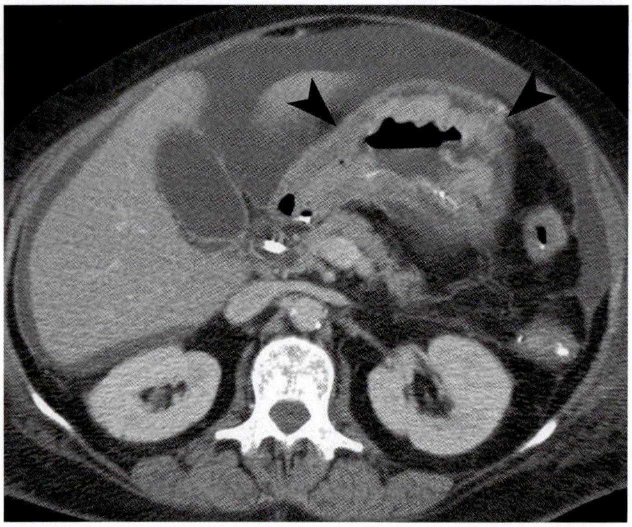

**FIG. 3B.18 • Linitis plastica.** Contrast-enhanced CT demonstrates narrowing of the gastric lumen and diffuse gastric wall thickening (*arrowheads*) caused by gastric wall infiltration from breast cancer.

tumors are less frequent (5% to 10%) and are associated with multiple endocrine neoplasia syndrome type 1. Type 3 carcinoids are uncommon (13%) sporadic tumors and are not associated with hypergastrinemia.

On imaging, type 1 carcinoid tumors usually appear as multiple polypoid lesions less than 2 cm in diameter in the fundus or body of the stomach, often detected in patients with no symptoms. Type 2 carcinoids manifest as multiple masses with diffuse gastric wall thickening and frequent nodal involvement. Type 3 carcinoids often present as one large solitary submucosal ulcerated lesion with frequent distant metastases.

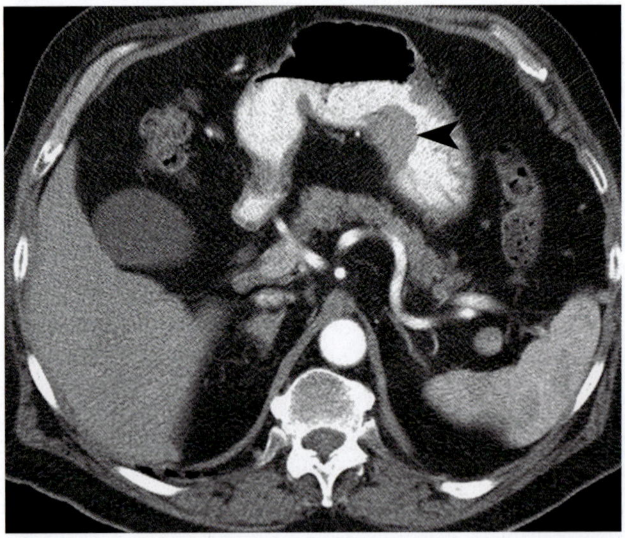

**FIG. 3B.17 • Melanoma metastasis to the stomach.** Axial contrast-enhanced CT study of a patient with metastatic disease from the melanoma demonstrates a solitary 3.5-cm mass (*arrowhead*) in the posterior gastric body.

## OTHER TUMORS AND METASTASIS

Other types of tumors of the stomach include lipomas, glomus tumor, hemangioma, and plexiform fibromyxoma, each accounting for 1% to 3% of benign gastric tumors.[15,17] Metastasis to the stomach can be seen in patients with melanoma (Fig. 3B.17), breast cancers, and lung cancers, causing submucosal multiple nodules or multiple ulcerated masses. Breast cancer metastases to the stomach can cause linitis plastic (Fig. 3B.18).[17]

### References


1. Rubesin SE, Levine MS, Laufer I. Double-contrast upper gastrointestinal radiography: a pattern approach for diseases of the stomach. *Radiology*. 2008;246(1):33–48.
2. Kim HJ, Eun HW, Goo DE, et al. Imaging of various gastric lesions with 2D MPR and CT gastrography performed with multidetector CT. *Radiographics*. 2006;26:1101–1118.
3. Inamoto K, Kouzai K, Ueeda T, et al. CT virtual endoscopy of the stomach: comparison study with gastric fiberscopy. *Abdom Imaging*. 2005;30:473–479.
4. Chen CY, Hsu JS, Wu DC, et al. Gastric cancer: preoperative local staging with 3D multi-detector row CT—correlation with surgical and histopathologic results. *Radiology*. 2007;242(2): 472–482.
5. Lee IJ, Lee JM, Kim SH, et al. Diagnostic performance of 64-channel multidetector CT in the evaluation of gastric cancer: differentiation of mucosal cancer (T1a) from submucosal involvement (T1b and T2). *Radiology*. 2010;255(3):805–815.
6. Kumano S, Murakami T, Kim T, et al. T staging of gastric cancer: role of multi-detector row CT. *Radiology*. 2005;237:961–966.
7. Fishman EK, Urban BA, Hruban RH. CT of the stomach: spectrum of disease. *Radiographics*. 1996;16:1035–1054.
8. Motohara T, Semelka RC. MRI in staging of gastric cancer. *Abdom Imaging*. 2002;27:376–383.
9. Sheybani A, Menias CO, Luna A, et al. *Abdom Imaging* [published online September 27, 2014]. doi:10.1007/s00261-014-0251-5.
10. Liu Z, Guo J, Sun S, et al. Evaluation of transabdominal ultrasound after oral administration of an echoic cellulose-based gastric ultrasound contrast agent for demonstrating small gastric subepithelial masses. *Abdom Imaging*. 2014;39:424–431.

11. Shen YL, Kang HK, Jeong YY, et al. Evaluation of early gastric cancer at multidetector CT with multiplanar reformation and virtual endoscopy. *Radiographics*. 2011;31:189–199.
12. Brant WE, Helms CA, eds. *Fundamentals of Diagnostic Radiology*. Philadelphia, PA: Lippincott Williams & Wilkins; 1999.
13. Burkill GJ, Badran M, Al-Muderis O, Meirion Thomas J, Judson IR, Fisher C, Moskovic EC. Malignant gastrointestinal stromal tumor: distribution, imaging features, and pattern of metastatic spread. *Radiology*. 2003;226(2):527–532.
14. Horton KM, Fishman EK. Current role of CT in imaging of the stomach. *Radiographics*. 2003;23:75–87.
15. Kim HC, Lee JM, Kim KW, et al. Gastrointestinal stromal tumors of the stomach: CT findings and prediction of malignancy. *AJR Am J Roentgenol*. 2004;83:893–898.
16. Kang HV, Menias CO, Gaballah AH, et al. Beyond the GIST: mesenchymal tumors of the stomach. *Radiographics*. 2013;33:1673–1690.
17. Binstock AJ, Johnson CD, Stephens DH, et al. Carcinoid tumors of the stomach: a clinical and radiographic study. *AJR Am J Roentgenol*. 2001;176:947–951.

## SELF-ASSESSMENT QUESTIONS

1. Diagnostic imaging tools are relevant in preoperative study of the stomach. Which is the most useful for the N-/M-staging?
   A. CT
   B. Endoscopy
   C. Double-contrast radiography
   D. Ultrasonography
   E. Magnetic resonance

2. What is the cancer type which is most likely to cause the imaging appearance shown on the upper GI study?

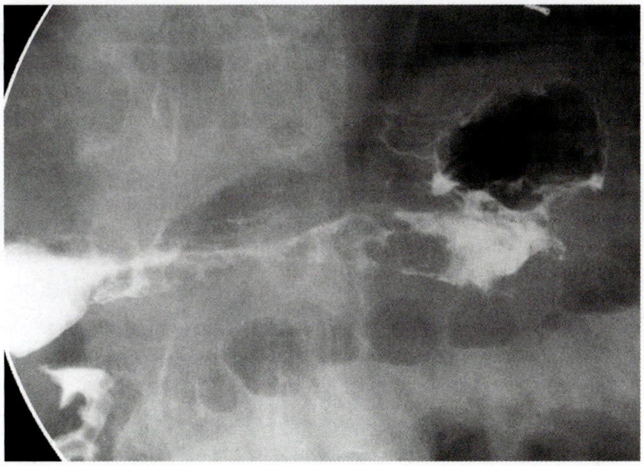

   A. Lymphoma
   B. Prostate cancer
   C. Leukemia
   D. Breast cancer

### Answers to Self-Assessment Questions

**1. A.** CT is useful to evaluate for gastric tumor spread to the perigastric fat, adjacent organs (pancreas and spleen), peritoneal cavity, lymph nodes, and distant organs (liver, adrenal glands, ovaries; colon, uterus, bone, and lung).

**2. D.** Breast cancer. The upper GI series depicts diffuse narrowing of gastric lumen and wall infiltration, consistent with linitis plastica appearance. Breast cancer metastasis is most likely to create this appearance.

# Duodenum 4A

*Ajay K. Singh*

## LEARNING OBJECTIVE

**1.** Describe the important neoplastic and nonneoplastic conditions of the duodenum.

The duodenum is the shortest and widest segment of the small bowel, measuring 25 cm in length. It extends from the pyloric canal to the ligament of Treitz, measuring up to 3.5 cm in diameter. It is a retroperitoneal structure except the duodenal bulb, which is intraperitoneal. The duodenojejunal junction is located to the left of midline, except in patients with malrotation of the small bowel.

## DUODENAL ATRESIA

This is a congenital condition resulting in a complete absent segment of the duodenum, often replaced with a fibrous cord. One-fourth of the cases are associated with Down syndrome. The obstruction is just beyond the ampulla of Vater. The condition can be diagnosed in utero using US where it is seen as fluid containing dilated stomach and duodenum (double bubble sign), with associated polyhydramnios (Fig. 4A.1). On plain abdominal radiography, double bubble sign refers to air-distended stomach and duodenum, with absence of air in the distal bowel (Fig. 4A.2).[1]

## DUODENAL DIAPHRAGM AND WEB

These are most commonly seen in the second portion of the duodenum and can be seen on the upper GI study as transversely oriented, thin lucent line with proximal duodenal distention. The Windsock sign is seen on the upper GI series as barium-filled sac located within the duodenal lumen, surrounded by a lucent line that represents the stretched duodenal web or diaphragm (Fig. 4A.3).

## ANNULAR PANCREAS

Annular pancreas is characterized by a ring of pancreatic tissue that encircles the second portion of the duodenum. It most commonly presents in infancy and fourth decade of life and can be associated with bowel malrotation, duodenal web, and Schatzki ring. Annular pancreas is believed to be due to persistence of the two ventral buds, resulting in encircling pancreatic tissue around the duodenum. It may cause duodenal stenosis, which is the common mode of presentation in infancy. Pancreatitis is the most common mode of presentation in adults (third to sixth decades). On the upper GI study, it can be seen as a narrowing of the second portion of the duodenum. The presence of pancreatic tissue posterolateral to the second part of the duodenum has high sensitivity (92%) for the diagnosis of annular pancreas. There is high rate of pancreatic divisum (37%) and chronic pancreatitis (48%) (Figs. 4A.4 and 4A.5).[2–4]

## DUODENAL DIVERTICULITIS

The duodenum is the second most common site of diverticulosis after the colon. Diverticula of the duodenum are false diverticula, most commonly seen along the medial border of the second portion of the duodenum, in the periampullary region. They are seen in up to one-sixth of the upper GI study and are seen as smooth outpouchings along the medial border of the second portion of the duodenum. Incidentally seen diverticula have no irregularity of the outline, which allows differentiation from an ulcer crater. Uncommonly, these duodenal diverticula may become inflamed and result in diverticulitis, bleeding, pancreatitis, or bowel obstruction.[5–7]

Duodenal diverticulitis is a rare complication of small bowel diverticulosis. Jejunoileal diverticula are four times more likely to develop complications and 18 times more likely to develop perforation than duodenal diverticula.[7] Duodenal diverticulitis can be secondary to food stasis, enterolith, gallstone, or ulceration. Approximately 1 in 20 patients with duodenal diverticula are clinically symptomatic, most commonly secondary to perforation, hemorrhage, and diverticulitis.

The findings of duodenal diverticulitis on CT include the demonstration of inflammatory changes around a diverticulum which can be recognized by the presence of air, oral contrast, or air–fluid level in the duodenal diverticulum (Fig. 4A.6). Duodenal diverticulitis should be in the differential diagnosis in patients with peripancreatic inflammatory changes with normal serum amylase levels.

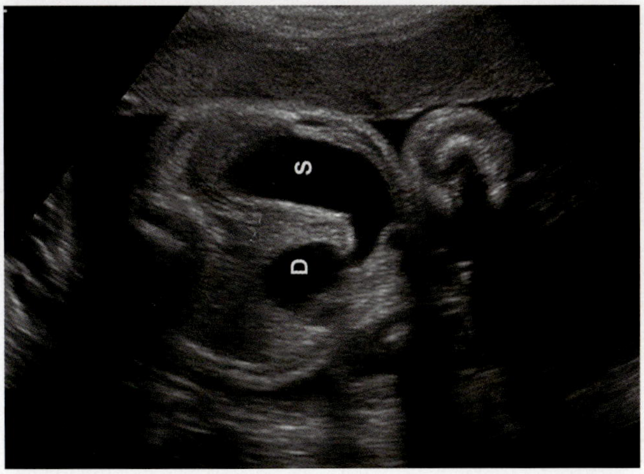


**FIG. 4A.1 • Duodenal atresia.** Prenatal US study demonstrates dilatation of the stomach (S) and duodenum (D) secondary to duodenal atresia.

## DUODENITIS

Duodenitis refers to inflammation of the duodenal mucosa and is a condition which is much more common than duodenal ulcer. The cause of duodenitis is not entirely clear but may be related to gastric hyperacidity or *Helicobacter pylori* infection. The radiologic features of duodenitis are similar to gastritis and includes thickening of the mucosal fold, nodularity, and mucosal erosions. The mucosal folds are thicker than 4 mm on the upper GI study in patients with duodenitis. Nodular filling defects and nodular folds are the second most common imaging finding of duodenitis (Fig. 4A.7).[8]

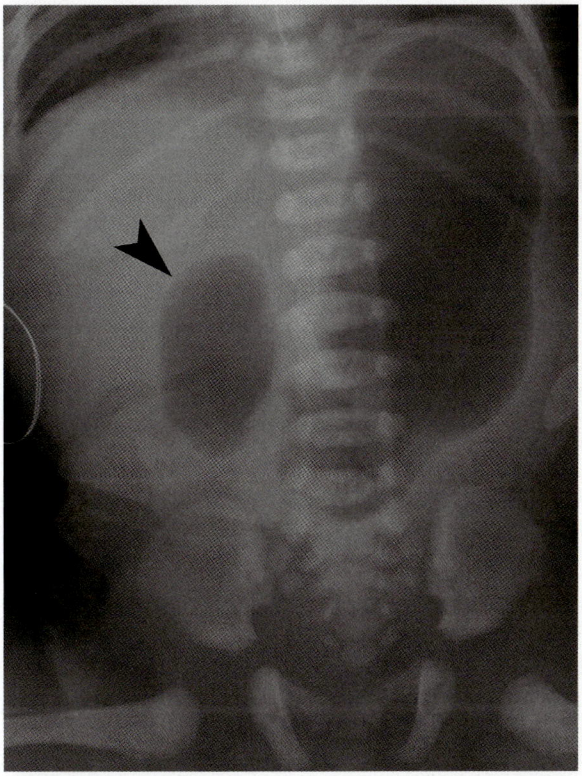

**FIG. 4A.2 • Duodenal atresia.** Supine film of the abdomen demonstrates gross distention of the stomach and duodenum (*arrowhead*) with air. There is no air identified in the distal small bowel or colon.

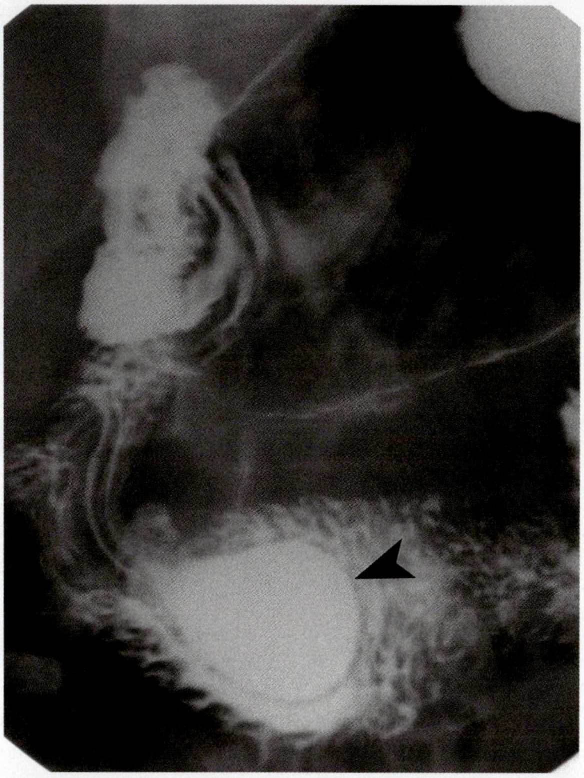

**FIG. 4A.3 • Duodenal web.** The upper GI study in a young adult patient demonstrates pear-shaped collection (*arrowhead*) of contrast outlined by a smooth radiolucent line which represents the stretched duodenal web, extending into the distal duodenum.

Crohn disease involvement of the duodenum is most commonly associated with the involvement of the gastric antrum. The imaging findings include aphthous ulcers in early stages, followed by thickened mucosal folds, ulceration, cobblestoning, and asymmetric scarring (Fig. 4A.8).

## DUODENAL ULCERS

Approximately 10% of the western population has peptic ulcers, duodenal ulcers being more common than gastric ulcers. Unlike gastric ulcers, duodenal ulcers are almost always benign. On imaging, the duodenal ulcers are often round, oval, or linear in configuration, mostly less than 1 cm in diameter and located in the duodenal bulb (90% of the duodenal ulcers). One-sixth of the duodenal ulcers are multiple, most of which are located within the duodenal bulb. Unlike gastric ulcers that usually do not occur in the anterior wall, up to 50% of the duodenal ulcers are located in the anterior wall of the duodenal bulb. The ulcers are often surrounded by edematous mound of mucosa and radiating folds extending to the edge of the ulcer crater (Fig. 4A.9). Anterior duodenal wall ulcers are difficult to detect on double contrast views, and therefore, the compression views of the bowel are often required to fill the ulcer crater.

Ulcers beyond the duodenal bulb are not common; most often located in the medial wall of the second portion of the duodenum and should raise the possibility of Zollinger-Ellison

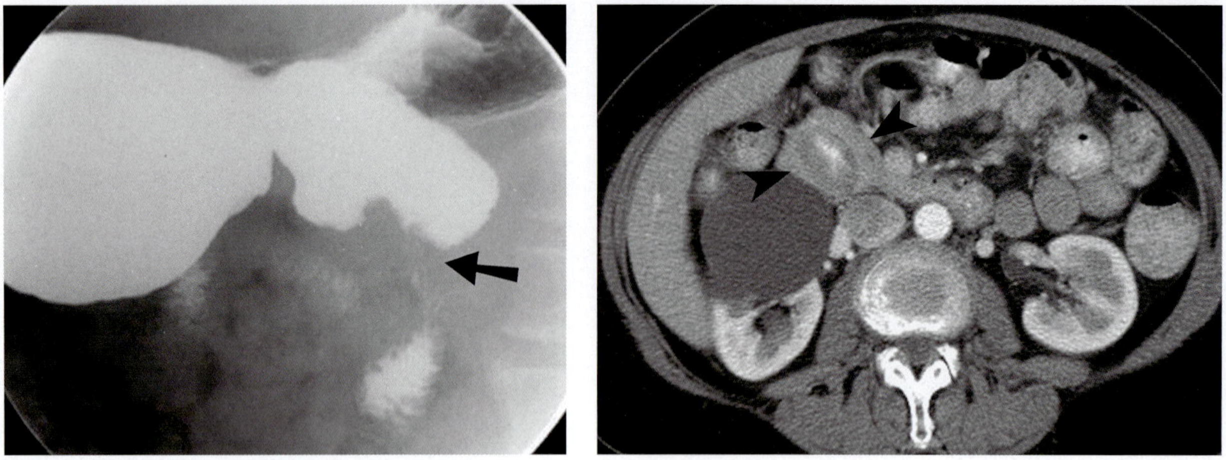

A B

**FIG. 4A.4 • Annular pancreas. A:** The upper GI study in a patient with annular pancreas demonstrates narrowing of the second portion of the duodenum with dilatation of the proximal duodenum (*arrow*). **B:** Contrast-enhanced CT scan study of a patient with annular pancreas demonstrates a soft tissue rind (*arrowheads*) seen around the second portion of the duodenum.

syndrome. Multiplicity of duodenal ulcer should also raise the possibility of Zollinger-Ellison syndrome.

Duodenal ulcers responded well to medical management and do not usually require a follow-up imaging because of the negligible malignant potential. The ulcers can sometimes heal with scarring, giving a cloverleaf deformity.

## ZOLLINGER-ELLISON SYNDROME

This condition is characterized by hypersecretion of gastric acid secondary to a gastrinoma. Seventy-five percent of the gastrinomas are located in the pancreas and 15% in the duodenum. More than 90% of the gastrinomas are located in the gastrinoma triangle which is located between:

1. Confluence of cystic and common bile duct
2. Junction of second and third portion of the duodenum
3. Junction of neck and body of the pancreas

Majority of the gastrinomas have malignant potential, metastasizing in up to 50% cases at the time of the diagnosis, most often to the liver. The frequency of gastrinoma is increased in patients with multiple endocrine neoplasia type I,

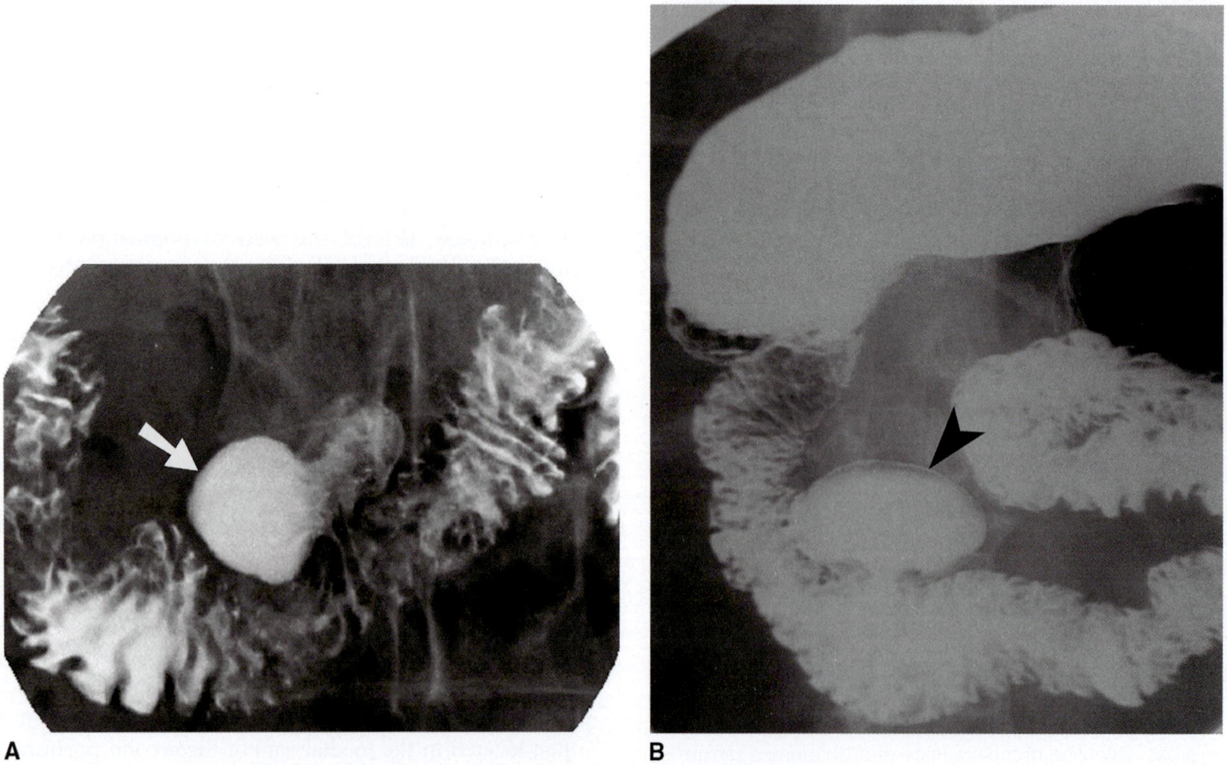

A B

**FIG. 4A.5 • Duodenal diverticulum. A, B:** The upper GI study in two patients demonstrating pseudodiverticulum (*arrowhead* and *arrow*) arising on the mesenteric aspect of the third portion of the duodenum.

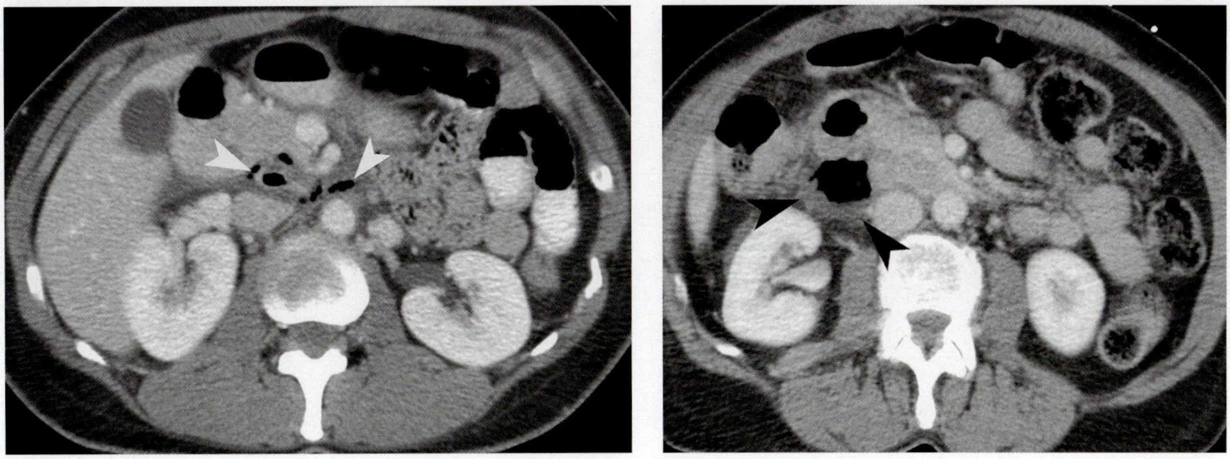

A B

**FIG. 4A.6 • Duodenal diverticulitis. A:** Contrast-enhanced CT scan study of a patient with perforated duodenal diverticulitis demonstrating multiple foci of extraluminal air (*arrowheads*) located around a duodenal diverticulum with surrounding inflammation. **B:** Axial contrast-enhanced CT scan study of the upper abdomen demonstrates inflamed diverticulum with thickened walls (*arrowheads*).

where they are associated with parathyroid, pituitary, and adrenal gland tumors.

The findings on the upper GI study include dilution of the barium caused by a large volume of acid in the stomach and duodenum, resulting in poor mucosal coating by the barium. There is prominence of the mucosal folds in the stomach, duodenum, and jejunum. Although majority of the ulcers are located in the stomach or duodenal bulb, approximately one-fourth of the ulcers are located in the postbulbar region and should raise the possibility of Zollinger-Ellison syndrome (Fig. 4A.10).

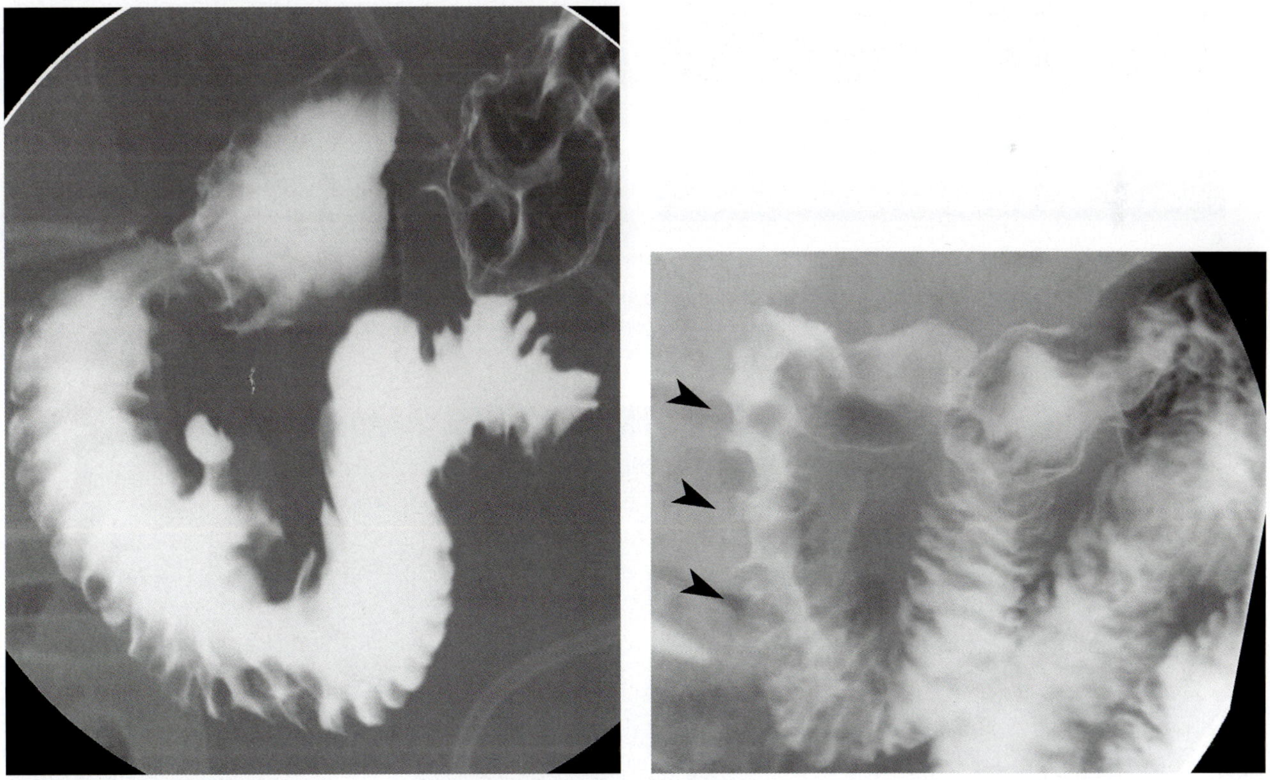

A B

**FIG. 4A.7 • Inflammatory duodenitis. A:** Single contrast upper GI study demonstrates mucosal fold thickening in the duodenum. Incidental note is made of a diverticulum seen arising on the medial aspect of the second portion of the duodenum. The patient also has gross nodular mucosal thickening in the gastric antrum from a known adenocarcinoma of the stomach. **B:** The upper GI study demonstrates extensive mucosal fold thickening (*arrowheads*) predominantly involving the second portion of the duodenum.

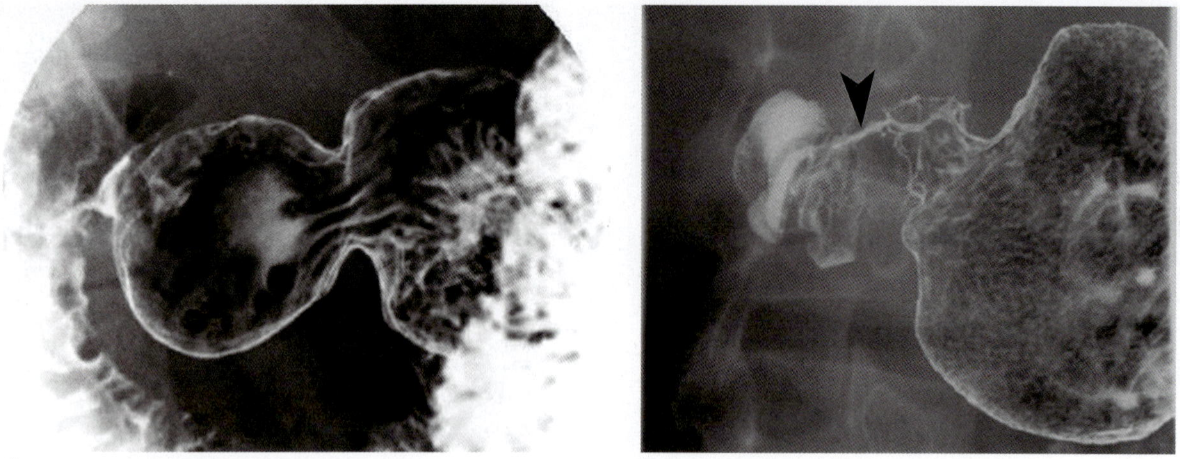

A B

**FIG. 4A.8 • Crohn disease. A:** The upper GI study demonstrates multiple aphthous ulcers in the gastric antrum in a patient with early Crohn disease. There is also mucosal thickening seen on the medial aspect of the second portion of the duodenum. **B:** The upper GI study in a patient with chronic Crohn disease demonstrating stricture formation in the distal stomach and proximal duodenum. There are mucosal ulcerations seen in the stomach, proximal to the stricture (*arrowhead*) site.

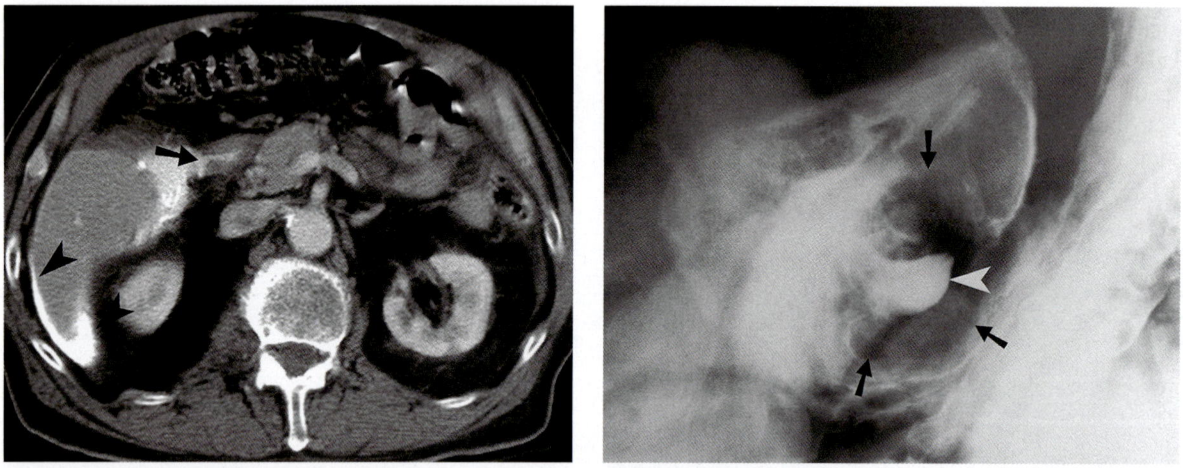

A B

**FIG. 4A.9 • Duodenal ulcer. A:** Axial contrast-enhanced CT scan study demonstrates duodenal perforation (*arrow*) with leakage of oral contrast into the Morison pouch and perihepatic region (*arrowheads*). **B:** The upper GI study demonstrates ulcer crater (*arrowhead*) in the proximal duodenum, surrounded by ulcer mound composed of mucosal edema (*arrows*).

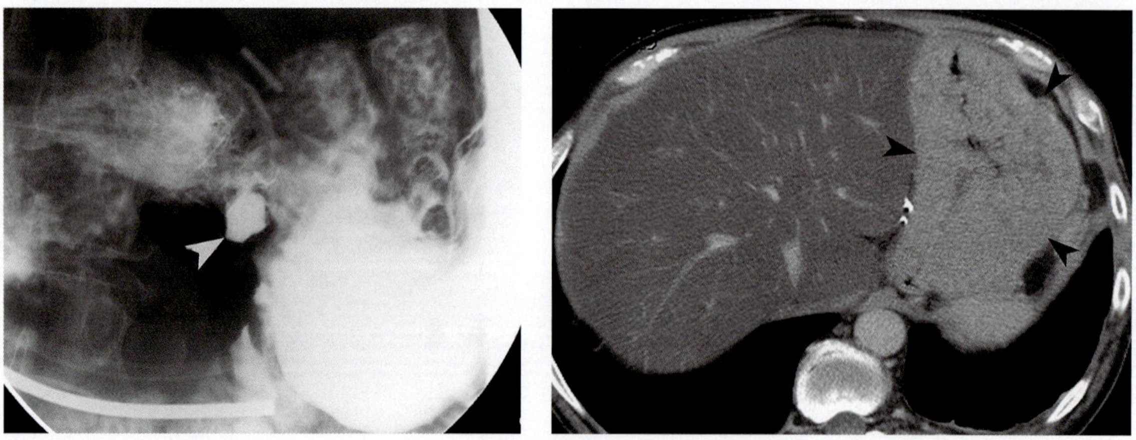

A B

**FIG. 4A.10 • Zollinger-Ellison syndrome. A:** The upper GI study demonstrates large ulcer crater (*arrowhead*) at the junction of the gastric pylorus and base of the duodenum in a patient with gastrinoma. **B:** Axial contrast-enhanced CT scan study demonstrates extensive gastric rugal fold thickening (*arrowheads*).

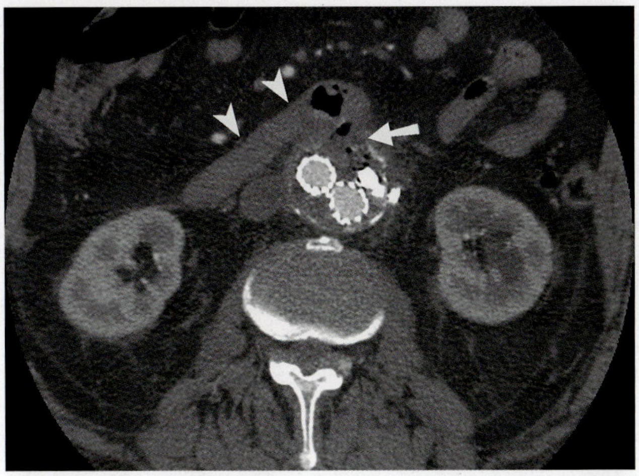

**FIG. 4A.11 • Aortoenteric fistula.** Axial contrast-enhanced CT scan study demonstrates communication between the infrarenal abdominal aorta (*arrow*) with the duodenum (*arrowheads*). Multiple foci of air are identified in the aortic aneurysm sac, surrounding the recently placed endovascular stent graft.

## AORTOENTERIC FISTULA

This is a rare pathology related to communication of the aorta with bowel lumen. Most often the fistula is from the abdominal aorta to the third part of the duodenum. It is usually seen after aortic aneurysm repair, most often resulting in communication near the proximal end of the graft with the adjacent bowel loop.

The most direct CT finding is the active extravasation of contrast from the aorta into the bowel lumen. The other imaging findings include presence of bowel gas in or around the aorta. There is typically anatomical fat plane loss around the aorta, perigraft inflammation, and fluid or air collection[9,10] (Fig. 4A.11).

## PARADUODENAL HERNIA

Among the internal hernias, the most common ones are paraduodenal hernia (53%) and pericecal hernia (13%).[11] Paraduodenal hernia is a type of internal hernia, characterized by extension of the small bowel loops either into the fossa of Landzert (on the left) or into the fossa of Waldeyer (on the right). The left paraduodenal hernia is three times more common than the right paraduodenal hernia, accounting for approximately 40% of all internal hernias. Left paraduodenal hernia extends into the left upper quadrant, lateral to the fourth portion of the duodenum, and posterolateral to the inferior mesenteric vein. The right paraduodenal hernia extends lateral and inferior to the second portion of the duodenum and posterior to the superior mesenteric artery (SMA).[11–14]

On cross-sectional imaging, the paraduodenal hernias are seen as an encapsulated cluster of small bowel loops located either lateral to the ascending duodenum (left paraduodenal hernia) or caudal to the third portion of the duodenum (right paraduodenal hernia) (Fig. 4A.12).

## DUODENAL TRAUMA

Duodenal injury is commonly due to the direct compression of the duodenum against the spine, either by a steering wheel (adults) or bicycle handlebar (children). Duodenal rupture most often involves the second portion of the duodenum, and duodenal hematoma most often involves the third portion of the duodenum. Duodenal rupture, which can be diagnosed by the presence of extraluminal air or contrast outside the duodenal lumen, requires emergent surgery (Fig. 4A.13).

Duodenal hematoma is characterized by submucosal hematoma in the distal duodenum and can be diagnosed on CT or MR (Figs. 4A.14 and 4A.15). It is more common in

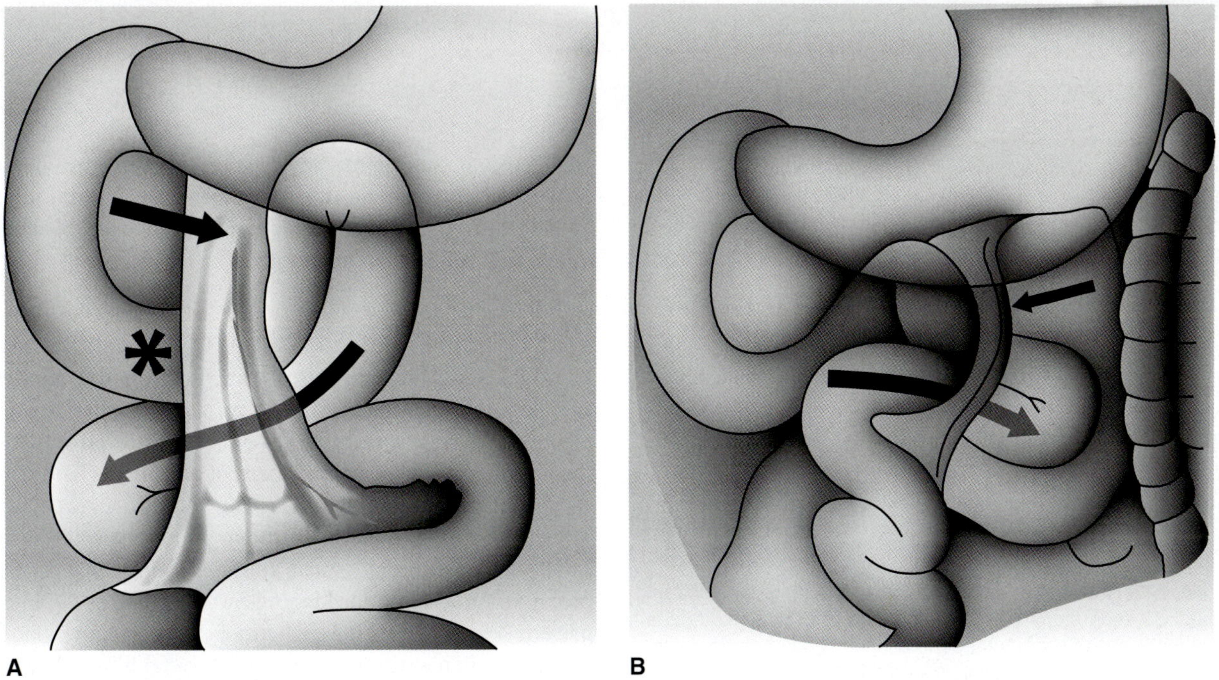


**FIG. 4A.12 • Paraduodenal hernia.** Schematic diagram demonstrating right paraduodenal hernia **(A)** and left paraduodenal hernia **(B)**.

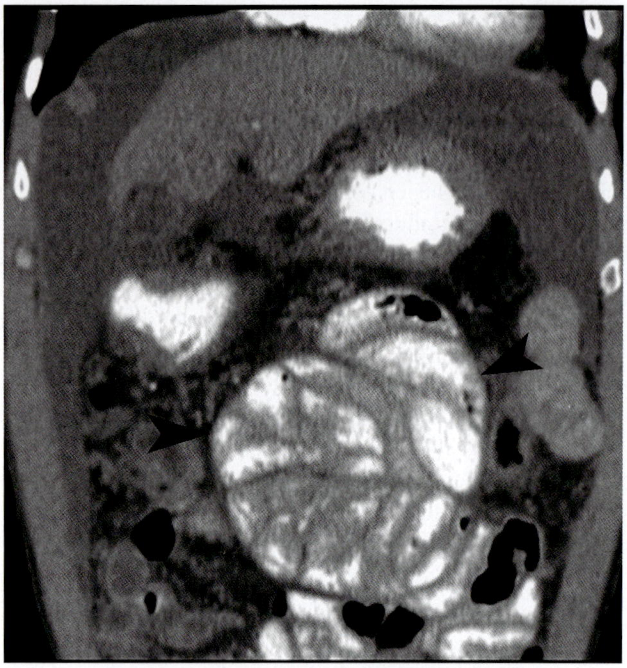

C

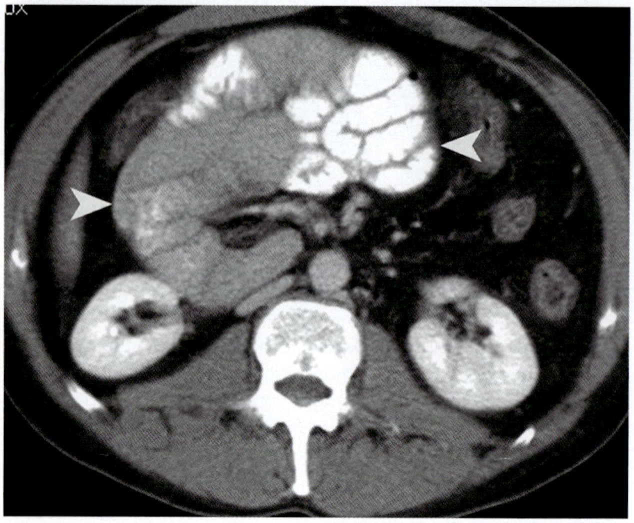

D

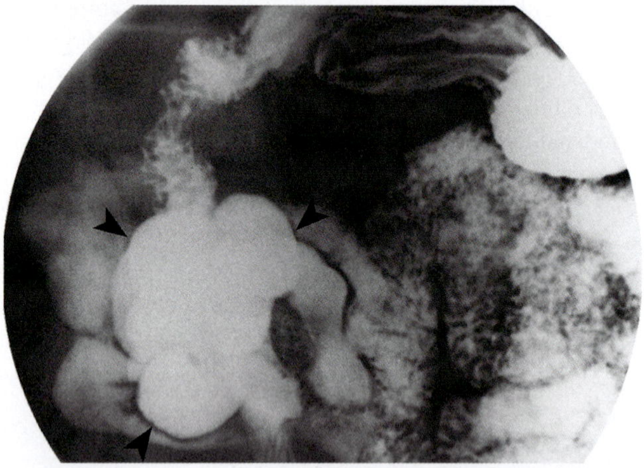

E

**FIG. 4A.12 •** (*Continued*) **C:** Coronal CT reformation demonstrates clustering of small bowel (*arrowheads*) located to the left of midline in a patient with left paraduodenal hernia. **D:** Contrast-enhanced CT scan study of a patient with a right paraduodenal hernia demonstrates clustering of small bowel loops (*arrowheads*), caudal to the second portion of the duodenum. **E:** The upper GI study demonstrates right paraduodenal hernia (*arrowheads*) located caudal to the C-loop of the duodenum.

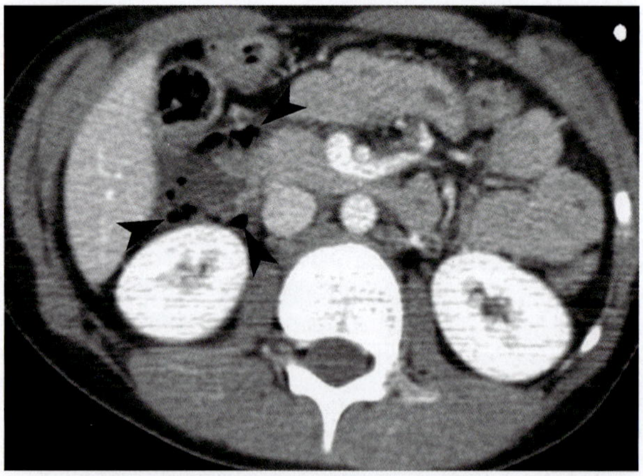

**FIG. 4A.13 • Traumatic duodenal perforation.** Axial contrast-enhanced CT scan study demonstrates fluid and air (*arrowheads*) adjacent to the site of transmural perforation of second portion of the duodenum. The site of perforation is located on the lateral aspect of the second portion of the duodenum.

children and thin young adults. These patients are managed conservatively with nasogastric tube and IV fluid therapy. One-third of the patients show evidence of bowel obstruction due to the submucosal hematoma.

## GLAND HYPERPLASIA

Brunner glands secrete mucus that protects the duodenum against the gastric acids. They can undergo hyperplasia in response to acidity, resulting in either diffuse prominence of the Brunner gland or enlargement of a solitary gland. It most commonly occurs in the middle age, with no sex predilection.

On the upper GI study, Brunner gland hyperplasia is typically seen as multiple small rounded filling defects in the proximal duodenum, producing Swiss cheese or cobblestone pattern (Fig. 4A.16). Enlargement of single Brunner gland can result in solitary submucosal or polypoidal filling defect. The differential diagnosis of Brunner gland hyperplasia includes

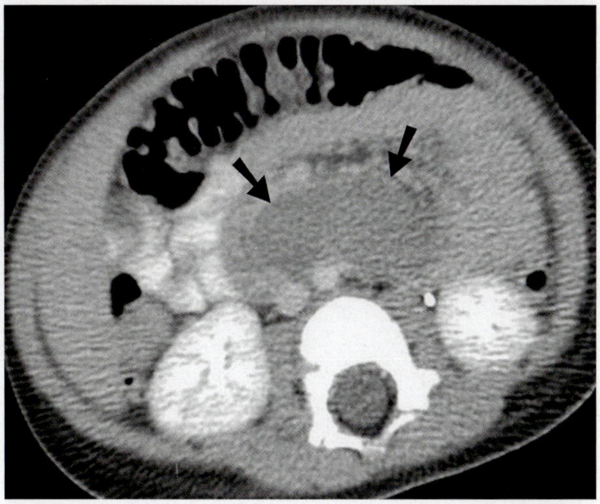

A

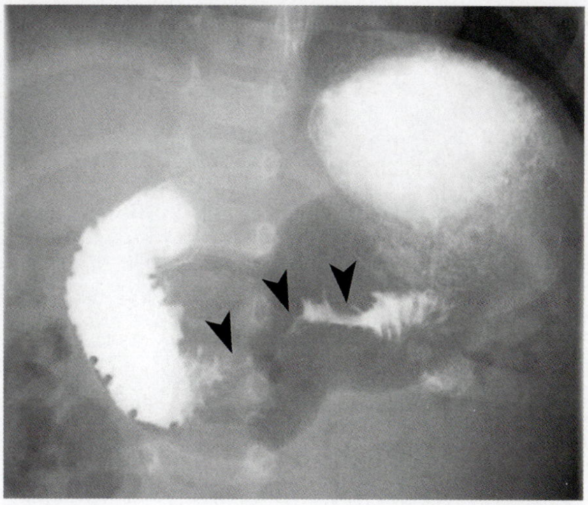

B

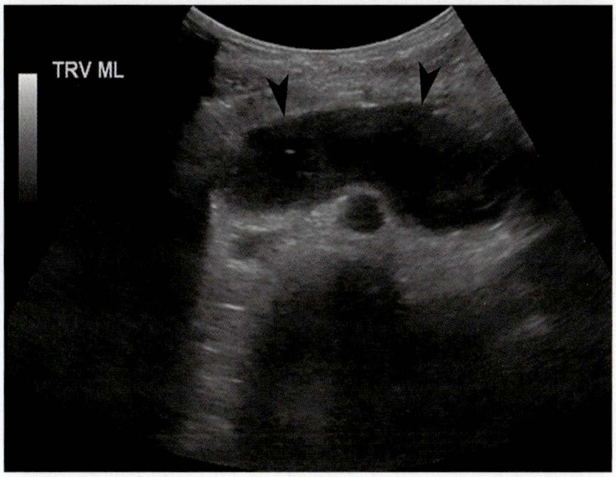


C

**FIG. 4A.14 • Posttraumatic duodenal hematoma. A:** Axial contrast-enhanced CT scan study in an infant demonstrates submucosal hematoma (*arrows*) located in the third and fourth portion of the duodenum. **B:** The upper GI study of the same patient demonstrates luminal narrowing (*arrowheads*) caused by submucosal hematoma in the third and fourth portion of the duodenum, which was treated conservatively. **C:** US study of the upper abdomen demonstrates the hypoechoic kidney-shaped hematoma (*arrowheads*) located in the third and fourth portion of the duodenum.

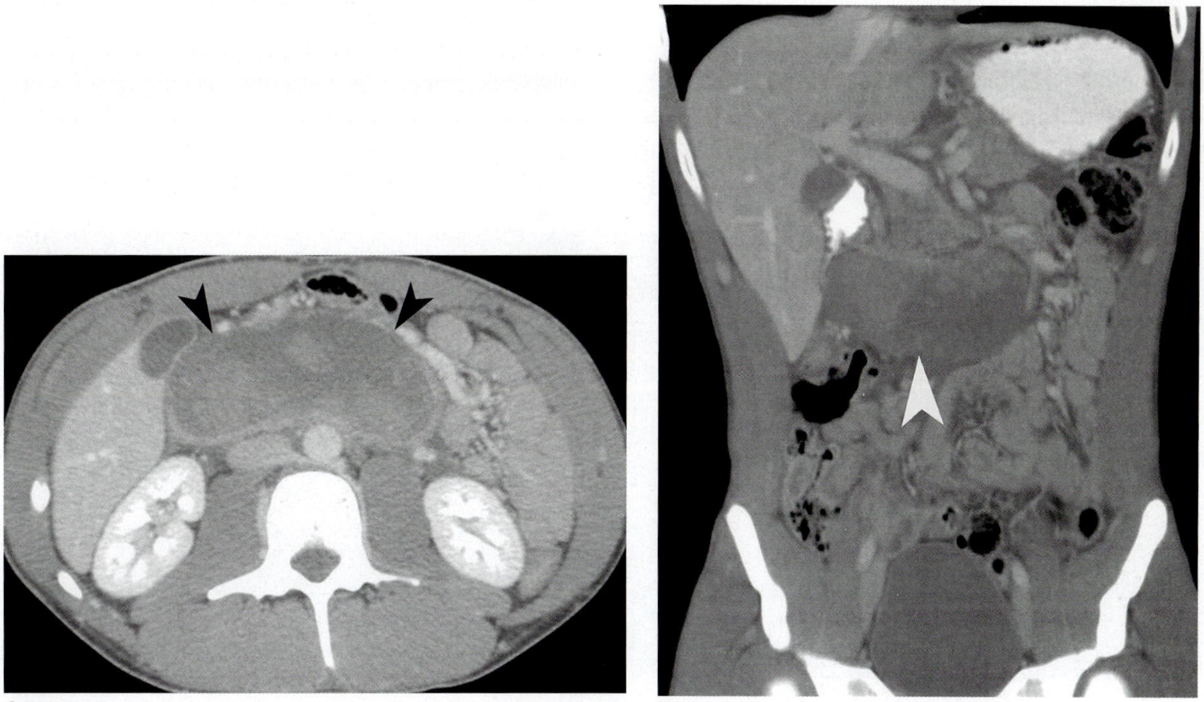

A B

**FIG. 4A.15 • Posttraumatic duodenal hematoma. A, B:** Axial and coronal contrast-enhanced CT demonstrates large submucosal hematoma (*arrowheads*) involving the third and fourth portion of the duodenum.

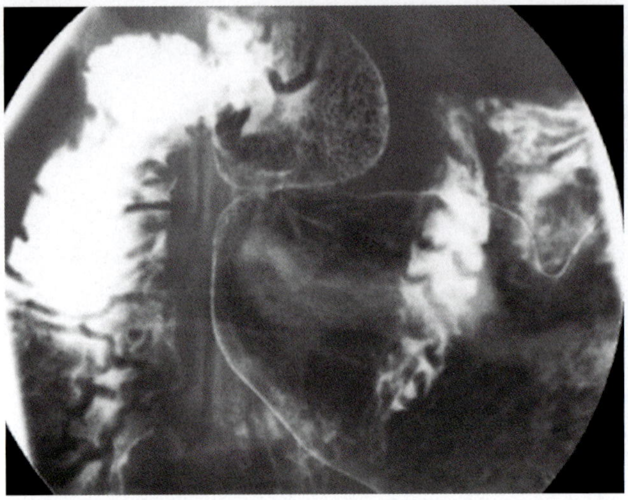

**FIG. 4A.16 • Brunner gland hyperplasia.** Double contrast upper GI study demonstrates multiple small nodular filling defects in the duodenal bulb due to hyperplasia of the Brunner glands.

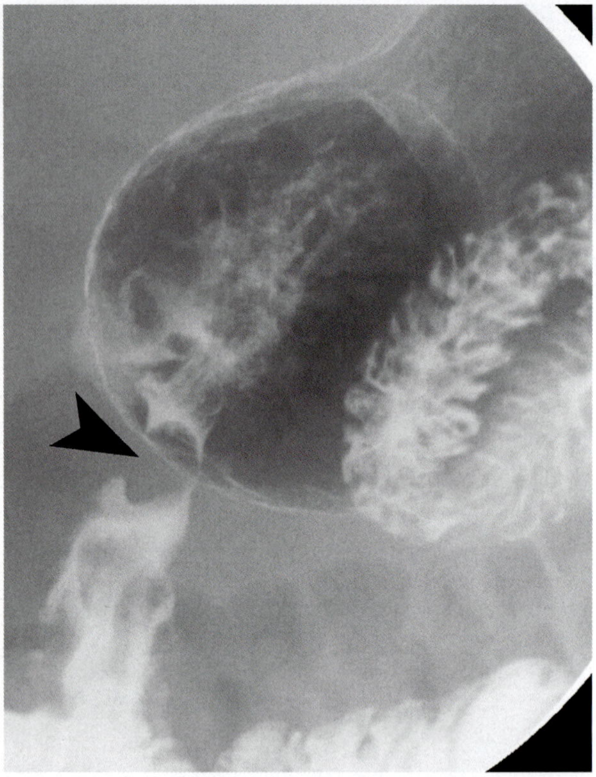

**FIG. 4A.17 • Duodenal polyp.** The upper GI series demonstrates a smooth well-defined nodular filling defect (*arrowhead*) in the proximal duodenum, which on biopsy was found to represent inflammatory polyp.

lymphoid hyperplasia, heterotopic gastric mucosa, polyposis syndromes, and duodenitis.

## BENIGN TUMORS

Unlike gastric polyps that are mostly hyperplastic polyps, duodenal polyps are mostly adenomatous polyps. They are seen on imaging as smooth, solitary, sessile filling defect measuring less than 2 cm in diameter in the first or second portion of the duodenum (Fig. 4A.17).

Benign duodenal tumors are more common than malignant duodenal tumors, and most commonly include lipoma and leiomyoma. The three types of duodenal adenomas include tubular, villous, and Brunner gland adenoma.

## MALIGNANT TUMORS

Duodenal carcinoma accounts for less than 1% of gastrointestinal neoplasm, most commonly located beyond the duodenal bulb. Adenocarcinomas are the most common malignancy of the duodenum. The frequency of duodenal carcinoma is increased in patients with celiac disease, familial adenomatous polyposis (FAP), Gardner syndrome, Crohn disease, and neurofibromatosis.[15,16]

On the upper GI study, they are most commonly seen as mass lesion distal to the ampulla of Vater, producing a polypoidal, annular, or ulcerative lesion. On CT scan study, duodenal carcinoma can be seen as a focal polypoidal or intramural mass, most often in second or third portion of the duodenum (Fig. 4A.18). In later stages, there is loss of fat

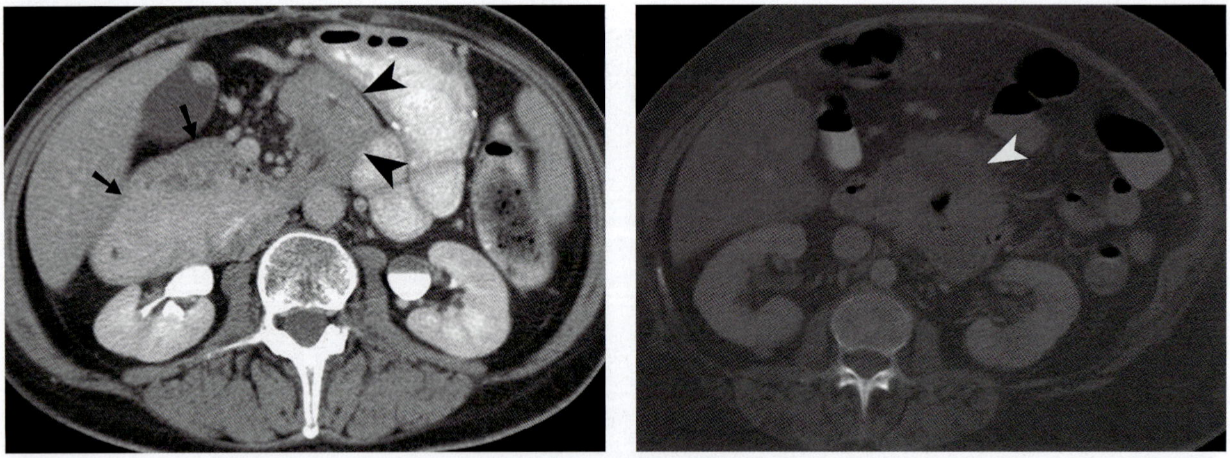

A B

**FIG. 4A.18 • Duodenal adenocarcinoma. A:** Axial contrast-enhanced CT scan study demonstrates dilatation of the second and third portion of the duodenum (*arrows*) secondary to adenocarcinoma involving the fourth portion of the duodenum (*arrowheads*). **B:** Axial contrast-enhanced CT demonstrates circumferential mass (*arrowhead*) surrounding the distal duodenum.

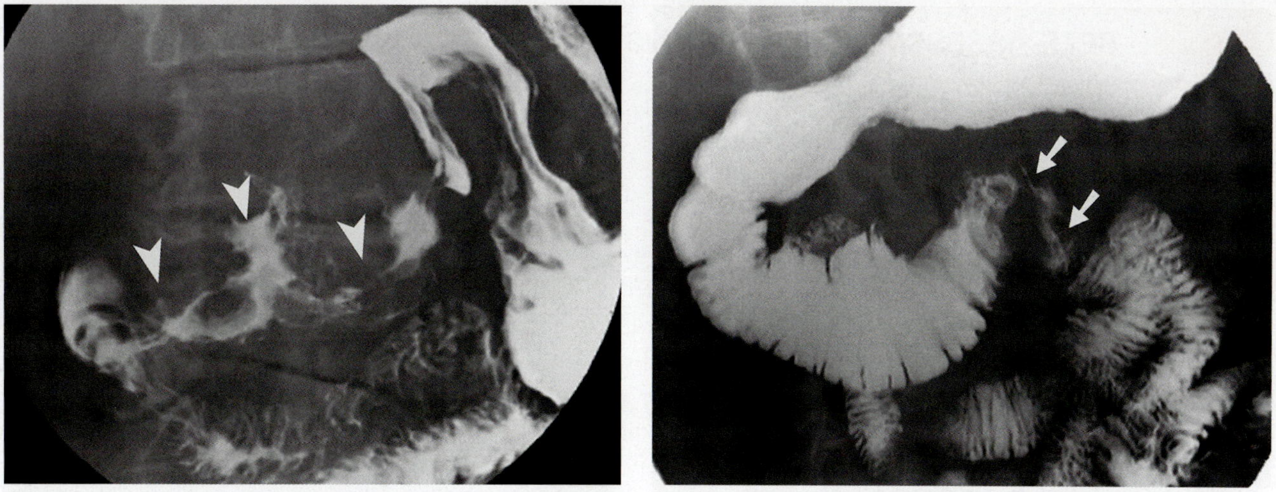

A B

**FIG. 4A.19 • Duodenal lymphoma. A:** The upper GI study demonstrates infiltrating mass lesion (*arrowheads*) involving the second portion of the duodenum with nodular filling defects and mucosal irregularity. There is no obstruction to flow of contrast seen on the upper GI study. **B:** The upper GI study series demonstrates neoplastic process at the duodenojejunal junction, indicated by multiple nodular filling defects and narrowing of the lumen (*arrows*) with dilatation of the more proximal duodenum.

planes around the mass, lymphadenopathy, pancreaticobiliary ductal obstruction, vascular encasement, and hematologic metastases.

Lymphoma of the duodenum can be primary or secondary, often seen as segmental nodular wall thickening or eccentric mass extending outside (Fig. 4A.19). Secondary invasion of the duodenum can occur with pancreatic or colonic neoplasm (Fig. 4A.20).

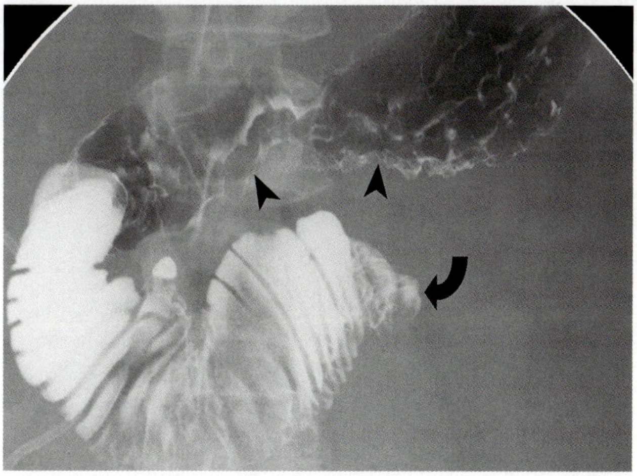

**FIG. 4A.20 • Distal duodenal obstruction due to gastric adenocarcinoma.** The upper GI study demonstrates dilatation of the duodenum due to focal narrowing (*curved arrow*) in the fourth portion of the duodenum due to direct spread of gastric adenocarcinoma. The gastric adenocarcinoma is indicated by the presence of extensive nodular filling defects in the distal gastric body and antrum (*arrowheads*). Incidental note is made of a small diverticulum arising from the second portion of the duodenum.

## References


1. Traubici J. The double bubble sign. *Radiology*. 2001;220(2):463–464.
2. Carbo AI, Sangster GP, Caraway J, et al. Acquired constricting and restricting lesions of the descending duodenum. *Radiographics*. 2014;34(5):1196–1217.
3. Jayaraman MV, Mayo-Smith WW, Movson JS, et al. CT of the duodenum: an overlooked segment gets its due. *Radiographics*. 2001;21(Spec No):S147–S160.
4. Sandrasegaran K, Patel A, Fogel EL, et al. Annular pancreas in adults. *AJR Am J Roentgenol*. 2009;193(2):455–460.
5. Chroeder TC, Hartman M, Heller M, et al. Duodenal diverticula: potential complications and common imaging pitfalls. *Clin Radiol*. 2014;69(10):1072–1076.
6. Bittle MM, Gunn ML, Gross JA, et al. Imaging of duodenal diverticula and their complications. *Curr Probl Diagn Radiol*. 2012;41(1):20–29.
7. Akhrass R, Yaffe MB, Fischer C, et al. Small-bowel diverticulosis: perceptions and reality. *J Am Coll Surg*. 1997;184(4):383–388.
8. Gelfand DW, Ott DJ, Chen MY. Radiologic evaluation of gastritis and duodenitis. *AJR Am J Roentgenol*. 1999;173(2):357–361.
9. Rakita D, Newatia A, Hines JJ, et al. Spectrum of CT findings in rupture and impending rupture of abdominal aortic aneurysms. *Radiographics*. 2007;27(2):497–507.
10. Bas A, Simsek O, Kandemirli SG, et al. Evolution of computed tomography findings in secondary aortoenteric fistula. *Iran J Radiol*. 2015;12(2):e22759.
11. Hernandorena González M, Domínguez MB, Muñoz RD, et al. CT findings for internal paraduodenal hernias. *Radiologia*. 2009;51(4):444–445.
12. Falk GA, Yurcisin BJ, Sell HS. Left paraduodenal hernia: case report and review of the literature. *BMJ Case Rep*. 2010 23;2010.
13. Prada-Arias M, Sanchís-Solera L, Pérez-Candela V, et al. Computed tomography diagnosis of symptomatic right paraduodenal hernia associated with enteric duplication cyst. *J Pediatr Surg*. 2007;42(11):1938–1941.
14. Takeyama N, Gokan T, Ohgiya Y, et al. CT of internal hernias. *Radiographics*. 2005;25(4):997–1015.
15. Carbo AI, Sangster GP, Caraway J, et al. Acquired constricting and restricting lesions of the descending duodenum. *Radiographics*. 2014;34(5):1196–1217.
16. Nikolaidis P, Hammond NA, Day K, et al. Imaging features of benign and malignant ampullary and periampullary lesions. *Radiographics*. 2014;34(3):624–641.

## SELF-ASSESSMENT QUESTIONS

1. What is the incidental imaging finding seen on the upper GI study?

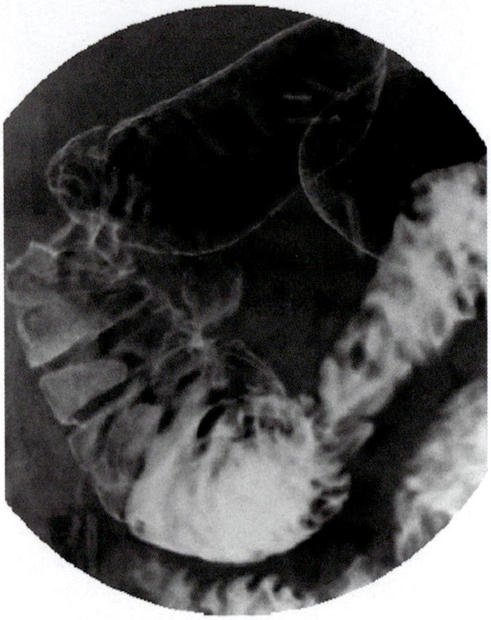

A. Adenocarcinoma
B. Polyp
C. Diverticulum
D. Ulcer

2. What is the congenital abnormality seen on the prenatal US?

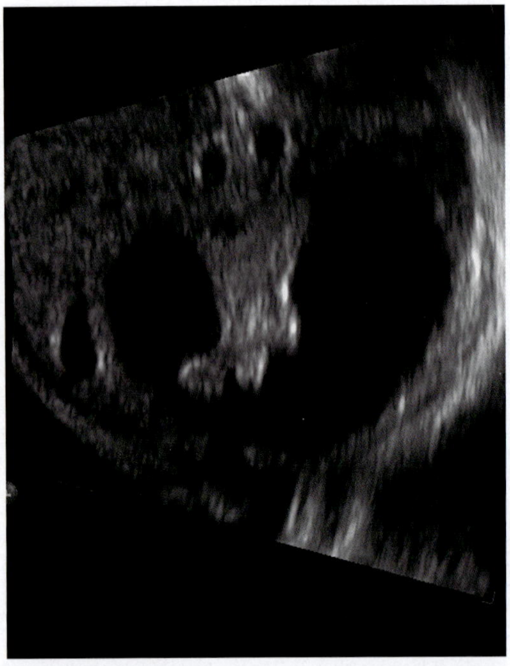

A. Duplication cyst
B. Duodenal atresia
C. Annular pancreas
D. Malrotation

3. What is the cause of bowel obstruction on the CT scan study?

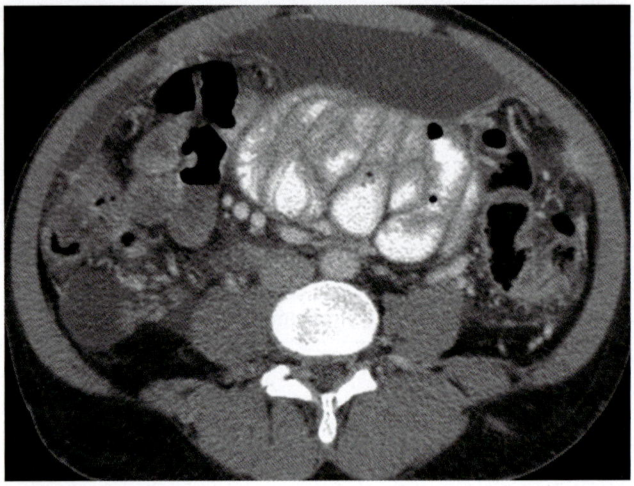

A. Malrotation
B. Volvulus
C. Paraduodenal hernia
D. Serosal metastasis

### Answers to Self-Assessment Questions

**1. C.** The upper GI series depicts a diverticulum arising from the medial aspect of the second portion of the duodenum. This location is the most common location of acquired duodenal diverticulum.

**2. B.** The US demonstrates distension of the stomach and duodenal bulb (double bubble sign) due to duodenal atresia. It can also be due to annular pancreas or volvulus.

**3. C.** The CT depicts encapsulated cluster of small bowel loops either located lateral to the ascending duodenum (left paraduodenal hernia).

# Small Bowel 4B

*Alexander Kessler, Akshya Gupta, and Refky Nicola*

## LEARNING OBJECTIVES

1. Review the normal anatomic features and characteristics of the small bowel.
2. Discuss the various imaging modalities used in the evaluation of the small bowel.
3. Discuss the imaging features of both neoplastic and non-neoplastic small bowel disorders.

The mesenteric small bowel represents the segment of the intestine which extends from the duodenojejunal flexure to the ileocecal valve. It lies entirely within the peritoneal cavity and is suspended from the posterior abdominal wall by a mesentery of connective tissue and vessels.

Jejunum:

- It constitutes the proximal two-fifths.
- It has a wide lumen, feathery mucosa, and prominent valvulae conniventes.
- Valvulae conniventes tends to be relatively thin (1 to 2 mm in thickness) and more in number (4 to 7 folds/inch).

Ileum:

- The ileum constitutes the distal three-fifths.
- It has more featureless mucosa, narrower lumen, and less prominent valvulae conniventes.
- The valvulae conniventes are thicker (2 to 3 mm in thickness) and less numerous (2 to 4 folds/inch) (Fig. 4B.1A).

## IMAGING OF THE SMALL INTESTINE

Since the mesenteric small bowel is literally beyond the scope of traditional endoscopy, imaging plays a central role in its assessment. Over the years, the tests of choice have been fluoroscopic techniques, namely the small bowel follow through (SBFT) and enteroclysis.

SBFT is often performed as part of an upper GI series and involves having the patient drink barium while multiple supine abdominal radiographs are obtained as the contrast transits through the small bowel. Once contrast reaches the terminal ileum, spot fluoroscopy images are obtained with or without peroral pneumocolon (insufflation of air into the rectum to cause reflux of air through the ileocecal valve) to better visualize terminal ileal pathology. Although easy to perform, overlap of small bowel loops, variable distension, and unpredictable transit time often limit diagnostic interpretation and sensitivity for detecting disease.[1]

Enteroclysis requires the insertion of a special nasal or oral catheter into the distal duodenum or proximal jejunum. Barium (or double contrast mixtures of barium) is then instilled through the catheter directly into the small bowel, and fluoroscopic images are obtained until contrast reaches the cecum. Unlike SBFT, enteroclysis provides greater detail of the mucosa as well as more uniform distension of the bowel lumen. The combination of enteroclysis with thin section CT or MRI (CT/MR enteroclysis) is also performed and provides the added advantage of depicting extraluminal extent of disease (Fig. 4B.1B). Although once standard techniques for diagnosis, the inherent invasiveness of enteroclysis has now led to the development of alternative enterography techniques to limit patient discomfort.

CT enterography protocols revolve around having the patient ingest a large volume of oral contrast (approximately 1.5 L) over a relative short period of time (45 to 60 minutes) to fully distend the bowel and coat the mucosa, followed by a contrast-enhanced CT scan. The most common oral contrast agents used are negative agents such as polyethylene glycol. However, positive contrast agents, such as dilute barium, can also be used. Although luminal distension is not as uniform as with CT enteroclysis, the lack of patient discomfort make this a good test of choice for most patients. Common diseases being evaluated with CT enterography are those with intraluminal pathology, including Crohn disease, small bowel tumors, and polyposis syndromes.[2,3]

Like CT enterography, MR enterography involves the use of similar amounts of oral contrast, following which high-resolution, ultra-fast sequences are acquired in the axial and coronal planes. Typically, these sequences consist of axial T2-SSFSE,

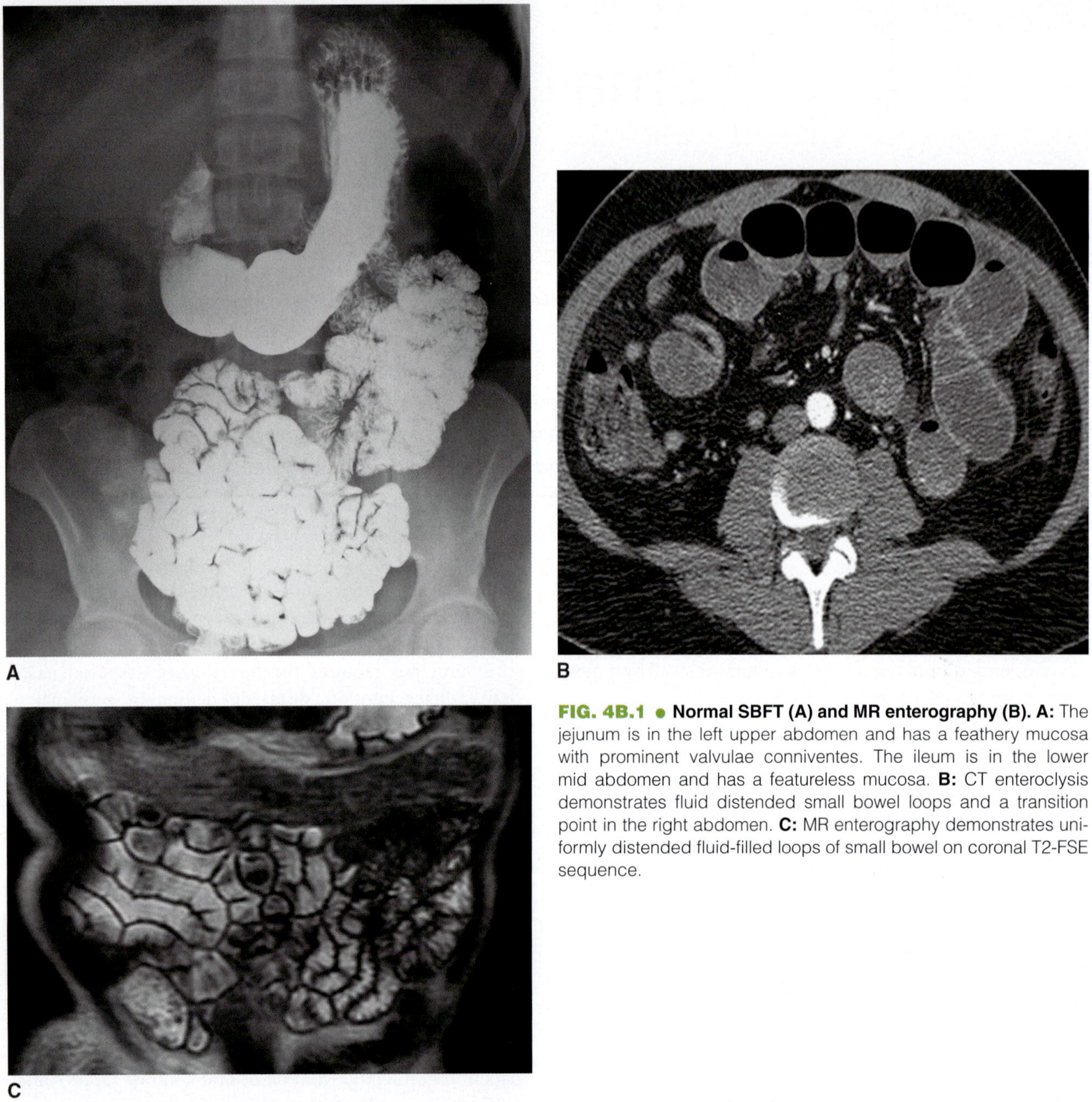

**FIG. 4B.1 • Normal SBFT (A) and MR enterography (B). A:** The jejunum is in the left upper abdomen and has a feathery mucosa with prominent valvulae conniventes. The ileum is in the lower mid abdomen and has a featureless mucosa. **B:** CT enteroclysis demonstrates fluid distended small bowel loops and a transition point in the right abdomen. **C:** MR enterography demonstrates uniformly distended fluid-filled loops of small bowel on coronal T2-FSE sequence.

coronal T2- SSFSE, coronal 2D/3D-SSFP, and axial/coronal T1+C dynamic images (Fig. 4B.1C). Unlike its CT counterpart, the inherent improvement in intraluminal contrast resolution and lack of radiation make this especially beneficial in pediatric patients with Crohn disease. However, patient motion can be a limiting factor.[4–6]

## SMALL BOWEL FOLDS

The most widely used approach on SBFT in differentiating diseases is based on identifying whether or not the bowel wall folds are thick or thin. The majority of small bowel diseases fall into one of these two categories, which allows us to make a helpful differential diagnosis.

## THINNED OR EFFACED FOLDS

Thinning or loss of small bowel folds is seen with a variety of processes that cause luminal dilatation of the small bowel. As the bowel dilates, the thickness of the bowel wall folds decrease (less than 2 to 3 mm) or become completely effaced, producing a featureless mucosa. Classically, this occurs due to either mechanical obstruction or smooth muscle dysfunction.

Smooth muscle dysfunction appears as abnormally dilated bowel with thinned folds that gradually taper to normal appearing bowel. The majority of cases are due to adynamic ileus, although other causes including malabsorption syndromes (celiac disease) and collagen vascular diseases (scleroderma) can be responsible.

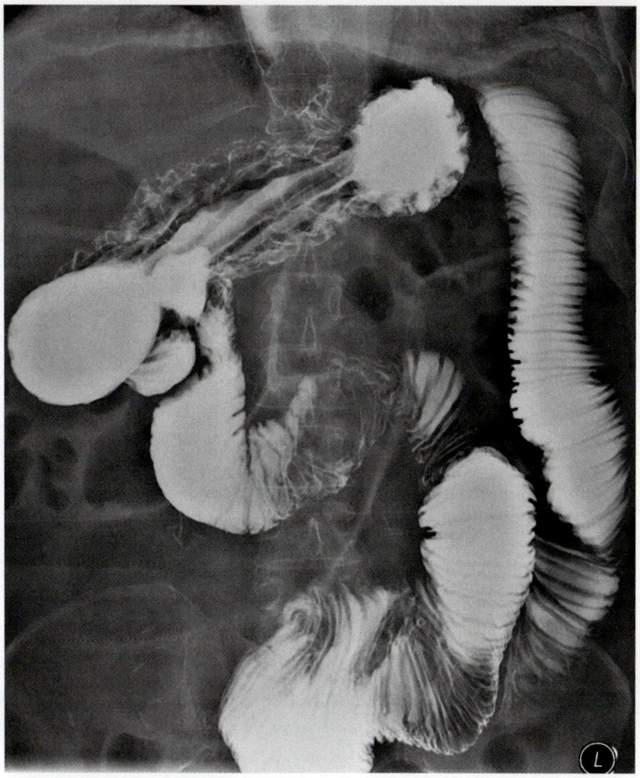

**FIG. 4B.2 • Scleroderma.** SBFT demonstrates jejunal dilatation and crowding of valvulae conneventes, producing a hidebound appearance.

In scleroderma, gastrointestinal involvement is clinically seen in 40% of cases and is the second most common organ system involved next to the skin. In the small bowel, the smooth muscle degenerates and is replaced by fibrosis, leading to severe dysmotility and classically causes prolonged transit times during fluoroscopy with retention of barium in the small bowel up to 24 hours after ingestion.

The imaging findings of scleroderma include the following:

- Prolonged transit time due to hypomotility on SBFT.
- Increased intraluminal fluid.
- Thinning and crowding of the valvulae conniventes produce a "hidebound" or "stack of coins" appearance in greater than 60% of cases (nearly pathognomonic) (Fig. 4B.2), due to fibrosis.
- Wide-mouthed sacculations along mesenteric border, due to asymmetric fibrosis.
- As the disease progresses, the affected bowel becomes aperistaltic and markedly dilated.
- Rarely, transient intussusception and pneumatosis intestinalis.
- On CT/MRI, there is pseudoobstruction in which there is dilated atonic small bowel juxtaposed with normal caliber, relatively uninvolved small bowel.

## THICKENED FOLDS

Thickening of small bowel folds is defined as a thickness greater than 3 mm. Histopathologically, this represents infiltration of the bowel wall submucosa by fluid or cells. To better manage the differential, it is helpful to further define the thickening as either uniform and straight or nodular and irregular.

Table 4B.1 **DIFFERENTIAL DIAGNOSIS OF UNIFORM OR STRAIGHT FOLD THICKENING**

| | |
|---|---|
| Edema | CHF<br>Portal hypertension<br>Hypoproteinemia<br>Lymphatic obstruction<br>Radiation enteritis<br>Mesenteric fibrosis |
| Hemorrhage | Trauma<br>Ischemia/infarction<br>Vasculitis<br>Coagulation disorders<br>Anticoagulation medications |

### Uniform and Straight (Table 4B.1)

Uniform fold thickening is seen with processes that cause infiltration with fluid. Most commonly, this is seen in cases of bowel wall edema (CHF and portal hypertension) or bowel wall hemorrhage (trauma and ischemia). On fluoroscopy, the thickened folds narrow the barium-filled spaces between them, creating a scalloped appearance known as thumbprinting (Fig. 4B.3). On CT, the bowel wall thickening is readily

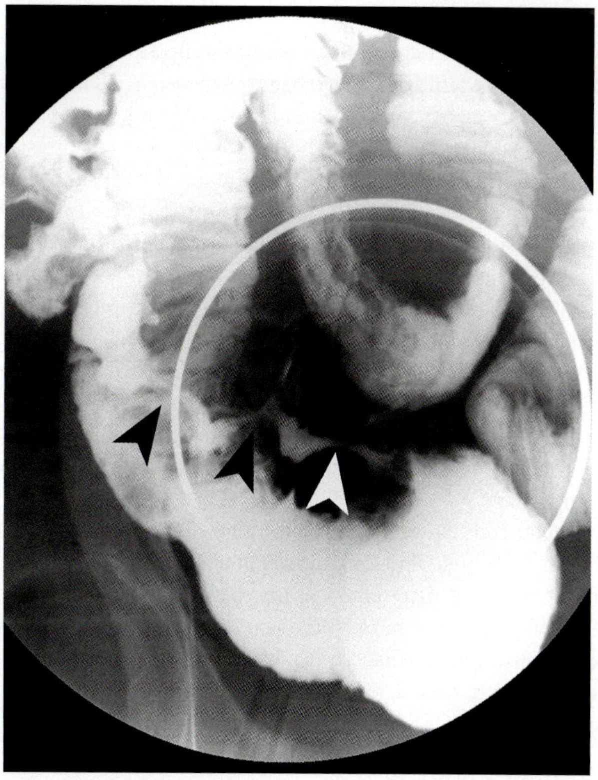

**FIG. 4B.3 • Thumbprinting.** Spot compression image of the terminal ileum demonstrates markedly thickened mucosal folds (*arrowheads*), producing a scalloped appearance known as thumbprinting.

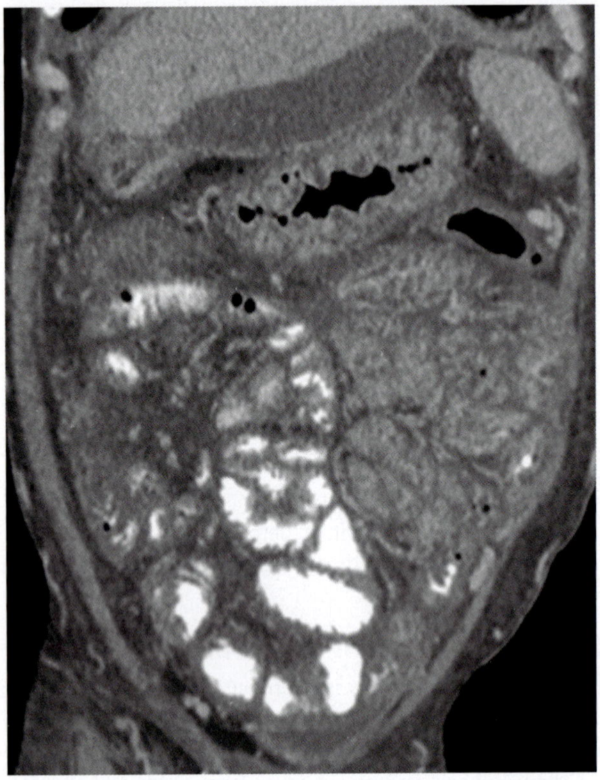

**FIG. 4B.4 • Bowel wall edema.** Coronal contrast-enhanced CT reformation demonstrates diffuse small bowel and gastric wall thickening from edema in a cirrhotic patient with long-standing portal hypertension.

apparent and the degree of attenuation reflects the presence of submucosal edema or hemorrhage.

Infiltration of the bowel wall with edema is typically a diffuse process seen throughout the entire small intestine. Cirrhosis and congestive heart failure are the most common syndromes responsible, although venous congestion, portal hypertension, or hypoproteinemia can also produce similar findings (Fig. 4B.4). Other less common causes of diffuse intestinal edema include lymphatic obstruction, radiation enteritis, mesenteric fibrosis, and the extremely uncommon angioneurotic edema. It is important to note that certain conditions (i.e., small bowel ischemia, Crohn disease, and eosinophilic enteritis) can produce intramural edema that is more focal in distribution, mimicking intramural hemorrhage.

Unlike bowel wall edema, intramural hemorrhage causes thicker folds and involves a focal segment of small bowel at the site of insult. In daily practice, trauma or mesenteric ischemia (Fig. 4B.5) are the most common etiologies. However, other conditions that predispose to bleeding including vasculitis, coagulation disorders, or anticoagulant medications can also be responsible.

### Nodular and Irregular

Irregular fold thickening represents infiltration of the bowel wall by cells or other nonfluid substances. It is seen with a wide variety of disorders including infectious, inflammatory, and

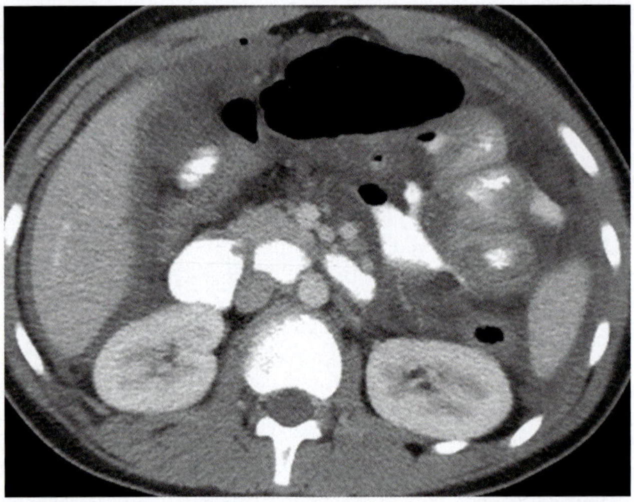

**FIG. 4B.5 • Bowel wall hemorrhage.** Contrast-enhanced CT demonstrates a small bowel wall thickening in the left upper abdomen from bowel wall hemorrhage.

neoplastic processes. On fluoroscopy, this appears as irregular folds causing distortion of the bowel lumen. On CT/MRI, stricturing or nodular soft tissue thickening of the bowel wall can be seen depending on the etiology. As with uniform thickening, distinguishing diffuse from focal involvement is helpful in creating a useful differential as many diseases have a propensity to affect only certain portions of the small intestine (Table 4B.2).

## COMMON SMALL BOWEL DISORDERS

### Small Bowel Obstruction

The overwhelming majority of cases of mechanical obstruction (approximately 75%) occur secondary to postsurgical adhesions that focally narrow the bowel lumen. Other causes include external hernias, luminal compression from extrinsic masses, and intraluminal obstruction from tumors, foreign bodies, or intussusception. Whatever the cause, the loops of

Table 4B.2 **DIFFERENTIAL DIAGNOSIS OF NODULAR OR IRREGULAR FOLD THICKENING**

| | |
|---|---|
| Jejunum | Giardiasis, Strongyloides, Whipple disease |
| | Eosinophilic enteritis |
| Ileum | Crohn disease |
| | Behcet disease |
| | Cystic fibrosis |
| Diffuse | *Campylobacter*, *Salmonella*, *Yersinia*<br>AIDS-related infections<br>Lymphoma, metastases<br>Polyposis syndromes<br>Amyloidosis<br>Histoplasmosis<br>Mastocytosis<br>Waldenstrom macroglobulinemia |

small bowel proximal to the site of obstruction dilate (greater than 3 cm) and patients develop abdominal pain, nausea, and vomiting.

On upright or decubitus radiographs, small bowel obstruction (SBO) classically appears as multiple dilated loops of small bowel with differential air–fluid levels in a stepwise pattern within the same loop of bowel (Fig. 4B.6A). In fact, a separation of greater than 1 cm in air–fluid levels almost always represents some degree of obstruction. When SBO is suspected on abdominal radiographs, a CT with oral contrast is the most appropriate imaging modality to evaluate for the source and site of obstruction. If high grade bowel obstruction is suspected, then oral contrast should not be used. On CT, SBO appears as multiple dilated loops of small bowel with a discrete transition to normal caliber bowel. As the obstruction progresses, the bowel folds are thinned and intraluminal contents proximal to the site of obstruction mix with gas producing the small bowel feces sign (Fig. 4B.6B). The small bowel distal to the site of obstruction decompresses and the site of obstruction can be more easily identified. Identifying the cause and site of obstruction is critical as incarcerated hernias or high grade obstructions often do not respond to medical management and require surgical treatment (Fig. 4B.6C).

Closed loop obstruction is a type of SBO where a segment of bowel gets obstructed at two places located at one point. It is most commonly caused by adhesions and hernia. The trapped loop progressively dilates and unlike traditional SBO, the loops of bowel proximal to the closed loop stay relatively decompressed. Typically, this occurs at sites of multiple adhesions or internal hernia. There is a high risk of strangulation (10% to 35%), and prompt CT is the diagnostic modality of choice for closed loop obstruction. SBFT and enteroclysis should not be performed in these patients.

The imaging findings of closed loop obstructions are as follows:

- Dilated loop in a U- or C-shaped configuration with tapered "beak signs" at the sites of transition (Fig. 4B.7).
- Small bowel mesentery gets stretched and may demonstrate a swirled appearance, as is seen with volvulus.
- Radial configuration of the mesenteric vessels points to the site of obstruction.
- Bowel wall edema and in late stage, pneumatosis or perforation.
- Variable bowel wall enhancement, with lack of enhancement indicating ischemia.
- Edema in small bowel mesentery, fluid and mesenteric vascular enlargement.

## Crohn Disease

Crohn disease is an inflammatory disorder of the GI tract that typically presents in young adults (peak age, 15 to 25 years), with a smaller peak in 50- to 80-year-old age group. Although

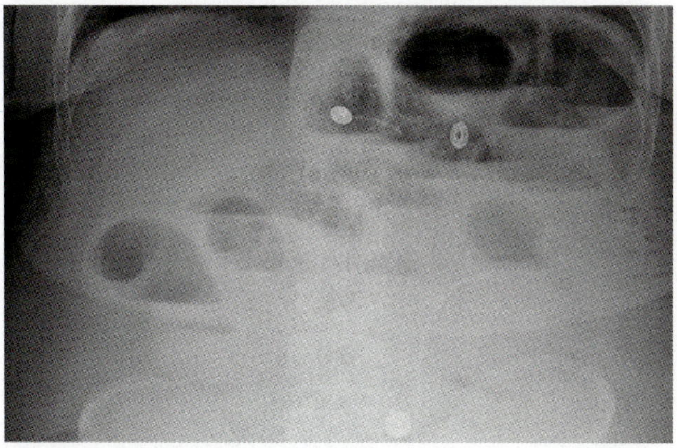

A

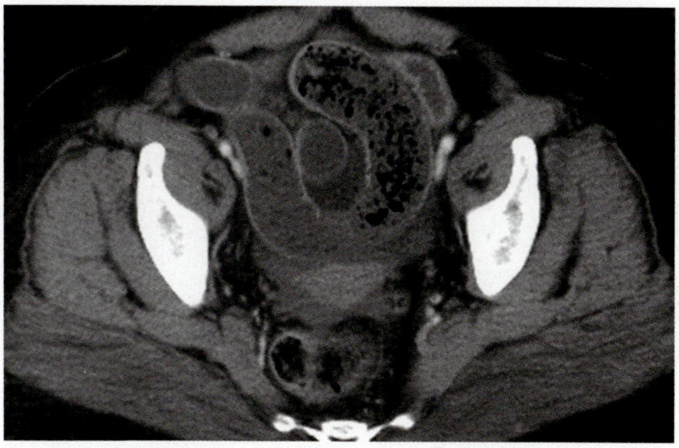

B

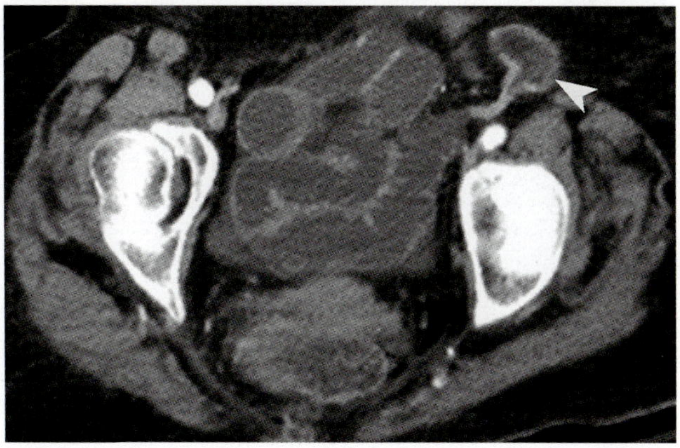

C

**FIG. 4B.6 • Small bowel obstruction. A:** Upright AP radiograph of the abdomen demonstrates dilated loops of small bowel with multiple air–fluid levels and differential air–fluid levels in step ladder pattern. **B:** Axial contrast-enhanced CT demonstrates small bowel feces sign in an ileal loop at the site of transition. **C:** Strangulated hernia: axial contrast-enhanced CT of the pelvis demonstrates multiple dilated loops of small bowel with a discrete transition point as bowel passes out of a left inguinal hernia (*arrowhead*).

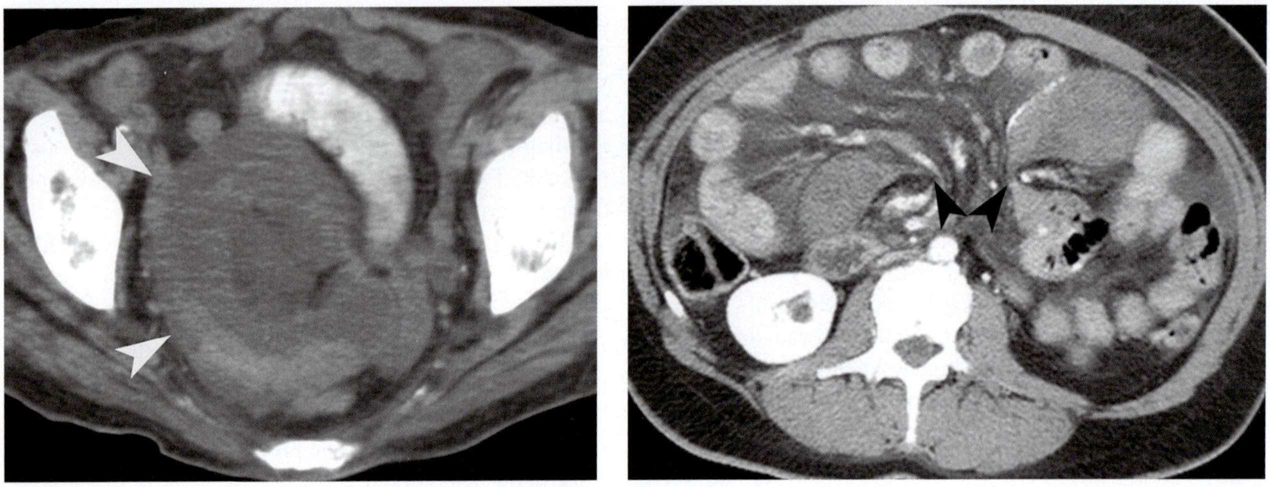

A B

**FIG. 4B.7 • Closed loop obstruction. A:** Axial contrast-enhanced CT shows a C-shaped small bowel loop (*arrowheads*) in the pelvis, representing the bowel loop with obstruction at two places. **B:** Axial contrast-enhanced CT images demonstrate a dilated central loop of small bowel with relatively decompressed small bowel proximally and distally. There is adjacent swirling of the mesentery and the two tapered beaks (*arrowheads*) of the closed loop are identified.

it may manifest anywhere from mouth to anus, terminal ileum involvement is nearly always seen (95%), and one-third of the patients have disease isolated to the small bowel. Pathologically, Crohn is characterized by aphthous ulcers, transmural inflammation, and noncaseating granulomas. During acute flares, Crohn's produces the classic pattern of skip lesions in which there are focal areas of inflamed bowel with unaffected bowel in between.

The imaging findings on barium studies include the following:

- Early stages: Aphthous ulcers (target lesions due to central pooling of barium surrounded by a ring of edema), lymphoid hyperplasia, and bowel wall edema.
- Ulcerations and fissures producing a "cobblestone pattern" due to barium collecting within the deep linear ulcers and fissures surrounding mounds of unaffected mucosa (Fig. 4B.8).
- Mesenteric border involvement is more severe than antimesenteric border involvement, leading to mesenteric border foreshortening and formation of the antimesenteric border pseudodiverticulosis (Fig. 4B.9).

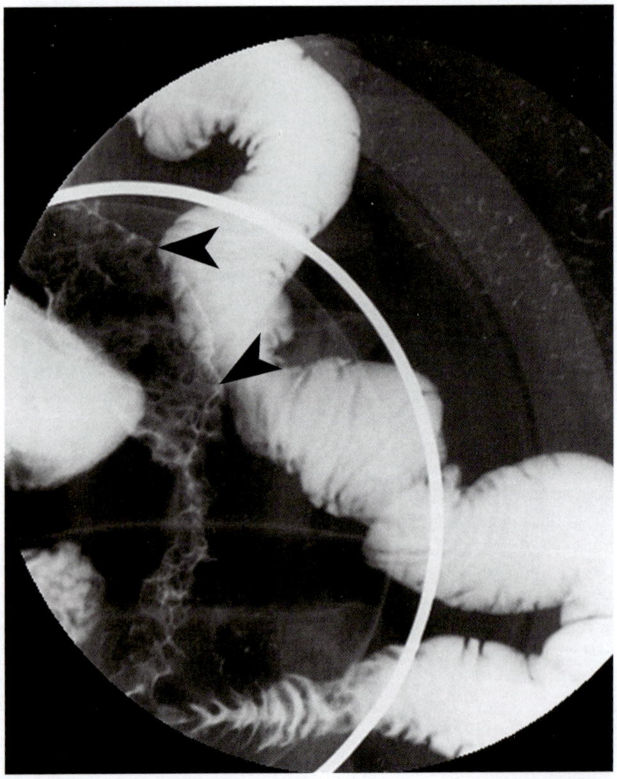

**FIG. 4B.8 • Crohn disease with cobblestoning of ileal mucosa.** SBFT study demonstrates pooling of contrast in fissures and ulcers, producing a cobblestone appearance (*arrowheads*) of the terminal ileum.

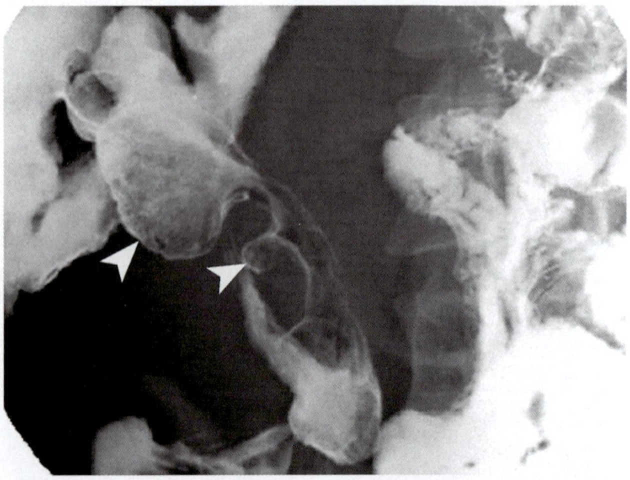

**FIG. 4B.9 • Crohn disease with pseudosacculations.** SBFT demonstrates multiple pseudosacculations (*arrowheads*) along the antimesenteric border, caused by foreshortening of the mesenteric border of ileum from fibrosis.

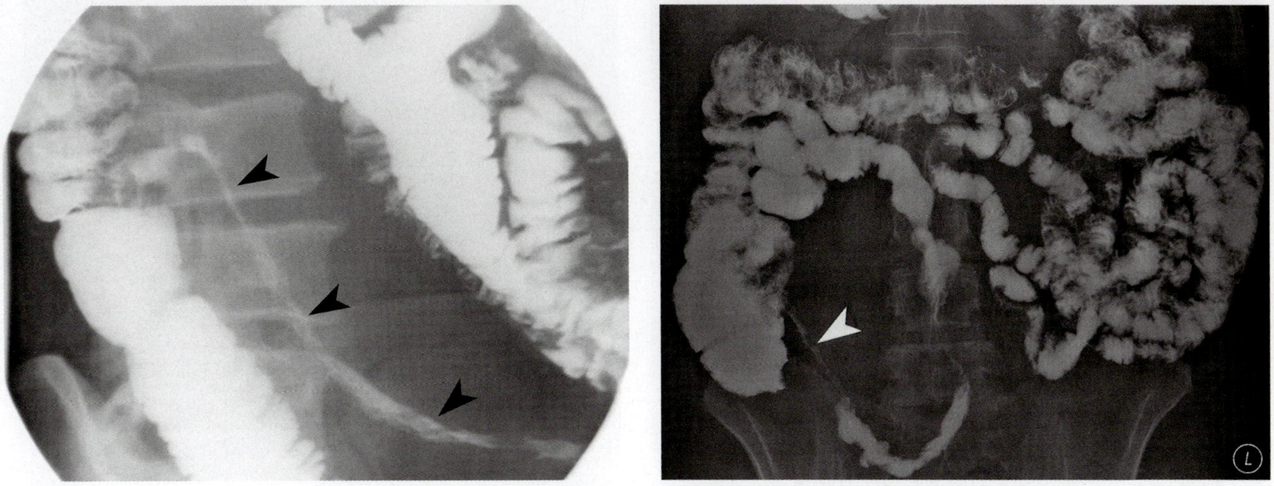


A B

**FIG. 4B.10 • String sign in Crohn disease. A, B:** SBFT study in two patients with long-standing Crohn disease demonstrates stricture of the terminal ileum (*arrowheads*), producing a classic string sign.

- Late stages: Fibrosis and stricturing of segments of the bowel wall produces the string sign that can be caused by bowel wall spasm or fibrosis (Fig. 4B.10).
- Focal bowel wall edema in the remaining mucosa can cause pseudopolyps.
- Deep fissures and fistulization is seen in advanced disease. Perianal fistulas are the most common (approximately 50% cases), followed by enteroenteric, rectovaginal, enterocutaneous, and enterovesical fistulas. One-fifth of the patients can develop abscess.

Although contrast-enhanced CT of the abdomen with intravenous contrast or CT enterography are considered the first-line imaging modality for acute initial presentation of Crohn disease in adult population, for nonacute presentations of Crohn disease in the adult population CT enterography and MR enterography are both considered front-line imaging modalities. In children MR, enterography is considered the imaging modality of choice for assessment of initial presentation as well as for follow-up of known Crohn disease.

On CT/MR enterography, bowel wall thickening (sometimes stratification), bowel wall hyperenhancement, and abscess formation are commonly seen with active flares. In active inflammation, the surrounding mesentery produces the comb sign, which is characterized by engorged mesenteric vessels surrounded by fibrofatty proliferation, otherwise known as creeping fat (Fig. 4B.11). In long-standing inflammation, CT and MR are particularly useful in identifying fistulae and sinus tracts (Fig. 4B.12). Of additional clinical importance is that Crohn patients are also at increased risk of developing intestinal small bowel adenocarcinomas (0.5%) and neuroendocrine tumors.

## Celiac Disease

Celiac disease is an autoimmune disorder in which the body mounts a T-cell mediated immune response toward ingested gluten. This immune response causes mucosal damage of the small bowel, resulting in villous atrophy, most severely in the proximal jejunum. Clinically, these patients typically present as young adults with symptoms of malabsorption, including steatorrhea, weight loss, and flatulence. As chronic mucosal injury occurs, patients develop an increased risk of developing small bowel adenocarcinoma, small bowel lymphoma, and pharyngoesophageal squamous cell carcinoma.

Despite the recent popularity of antibody tests and advanced endoscopic techniques, imaging can still play a role in helping to confirm a suspected diagnosis.

The imaging findings of celiac disease include dilatation of the small bowel with reversal of the normal jejunoileal fold pattern (number of mucosal folds in the jejunum decrease and the number of folds in the ileum increase). Majority of the patients with celiac disease have three or less number of folds per inch. Although commonly seen in celiac disease, this pattern may be seen with other causes of chronic malabsorption (Fig. 4B.13). On CT/MRI, in addition to the reversal of the small bowel fold pattern, the jejunum typically demonstrates circumferential wall thickening with submucosal edema producing a "halo sign." There may be reactive retroperitoneal and mesenteric lymphadenopathy.

## Small Bowel Ischemia

Acute ischemia of the small bowel most often occurs when there is compromised flow within the SMA or vein. Embolic occlusion is more common than thrombotic occlusion of celiac artery. It is most commonly seen in patients older than 50, and in overwhelming majority of cases is due to embolic or thrombotic arterial occlusion (60% to 90%). However, hypovolemia, shock, and sepsis can also produce acute ischemia without total vascular occlusion. Patients often present with acute onset abdominal pain out of proportion to physical exam findings and elevated lactate (greater than 2 mEq/L). The mortality is as high as 80% for acute arterial and much lower for venous occlusion.

On SBFT, edema and hemorrhage infiltrate the bowel wall causing uniform thickening of the bowel wall and is most evidenced by separation of bowel loops. The bowel wall folds also

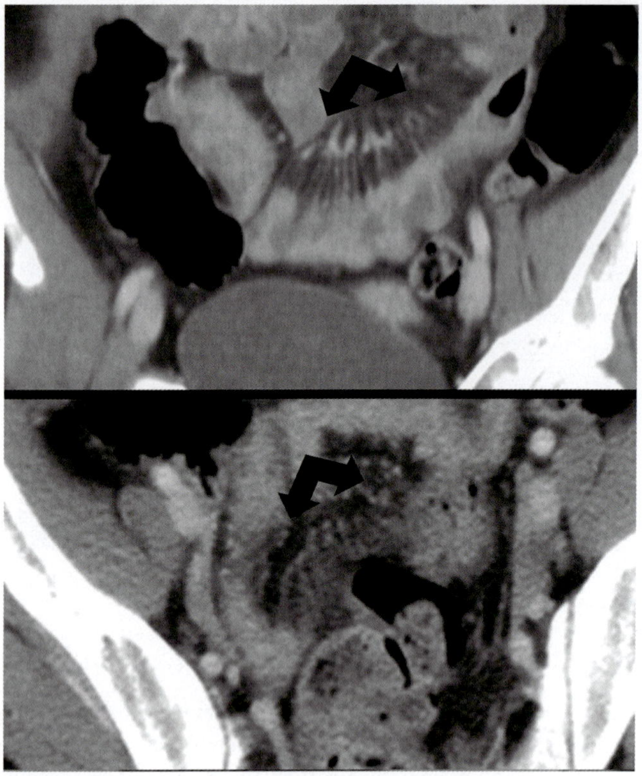

A

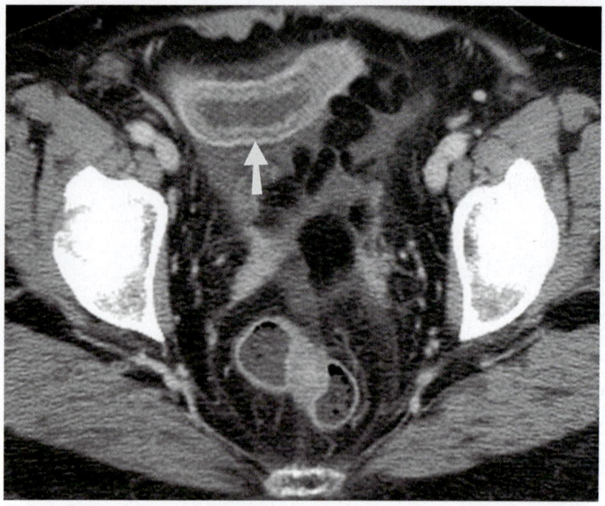

B

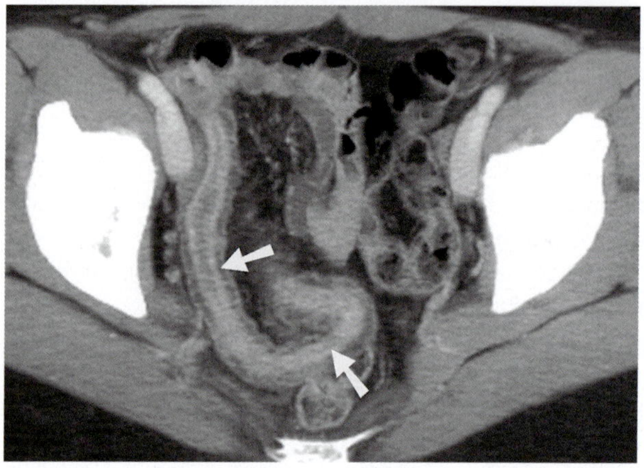

C

**FIG. 4B.11 • Crohn disease. A:** Comb sign: Axial and coronal contrast-enhanced CT of the pelvis. The distal ileum is thick walled. There are engorged mesenteric vessels and fibrofatty proliferation along the mesenteric border producing a comb sign (*bifid arrows*). **B, C:** Axial contrast-enhanced CT shows intense distal ileal mucosal enhancement with stratification of the wall (*arrows*).

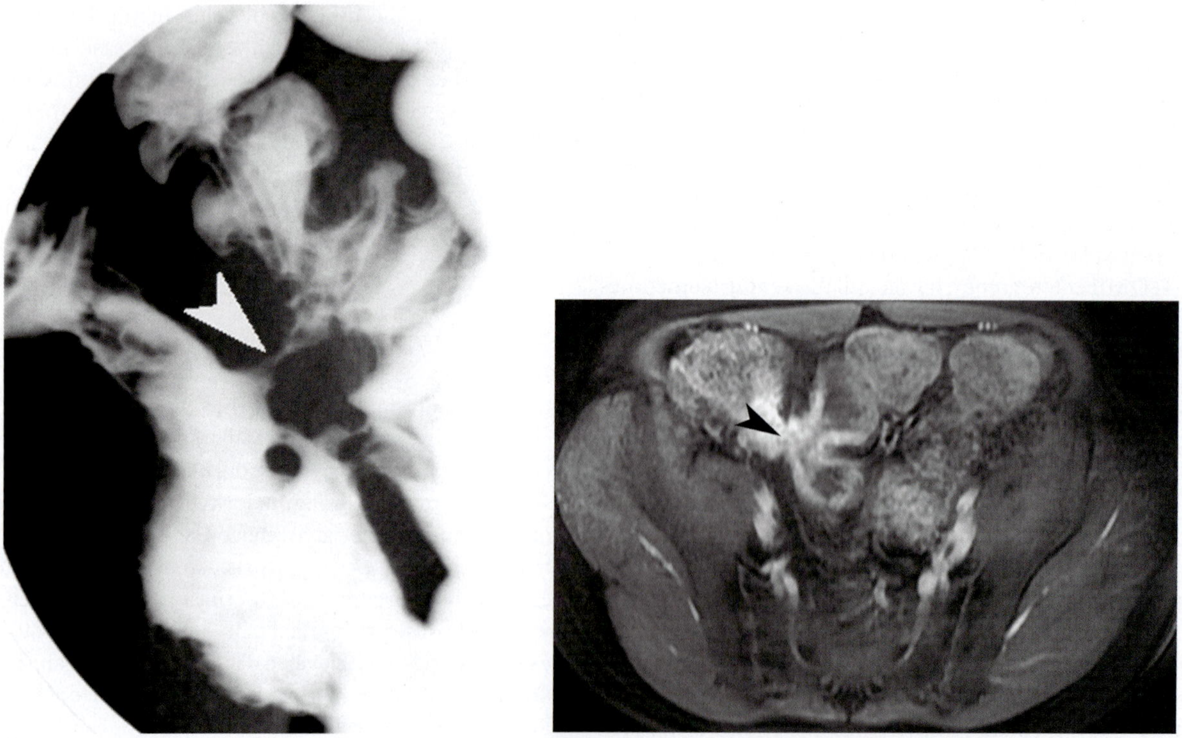

A B

**FIG 4B.12 • Crohn fistula. A:** SBFT spot fluoroscopic film demonstrates fistulous communication (*arrowhead*) between two ileal loops in the right lower quadrant. **B:** Axial Gadolinium-enhanced T1-WI during MR enterography demonstrates wall thickening and enhancement of the terminal ileum with loss of tissue plane with adjacent colon from an enterocolonic fistula (*arrowhead*).

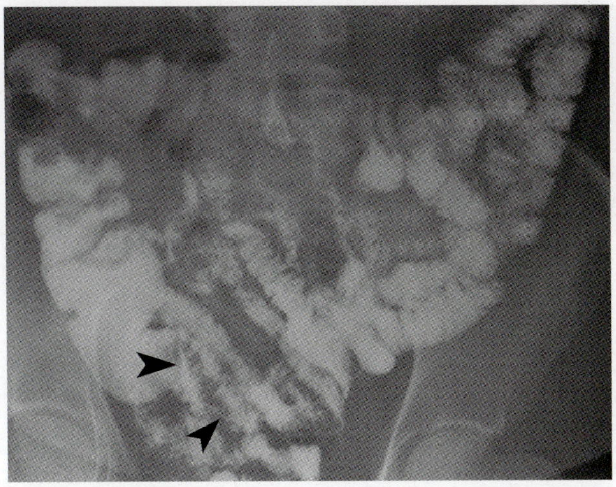

**FIG. 4B.13 • Celiac disease.** SBFT demonstrates increased number of mucosa folds in the ileum in a pattern referred to as jejunization (*arrowheads*). This appearance is consistent with chronic malabsorption.

become thickened, creating a scalloped appearance known as thumbprinting.[7]

The CT findings of small bowel ischemia include the following:

- Dilatation of small bowel due to paralytic ileus
- Bowel wall thickening (most common finding), more common after venous occlusion
- Decreased or absent enhancement of bowel wall
- Vascular occlusion or stenosis on arterial or venous phase (Fig. 4B.14A)
- Ascites and mesenteric edema
- Pneumatosis and portal venous gas, respectively (Fig. 4B.14B, C)

In patients with acute hypovolemia from trauma, there can be reversible ischemia of the small bowel mucosa, described as shock bowel syndrome (Fig. 4B.15). These patients have intense small bowel mucosal enhancement, flattened IVC, adrenal hyperenhancement, and peripancreatic edema.

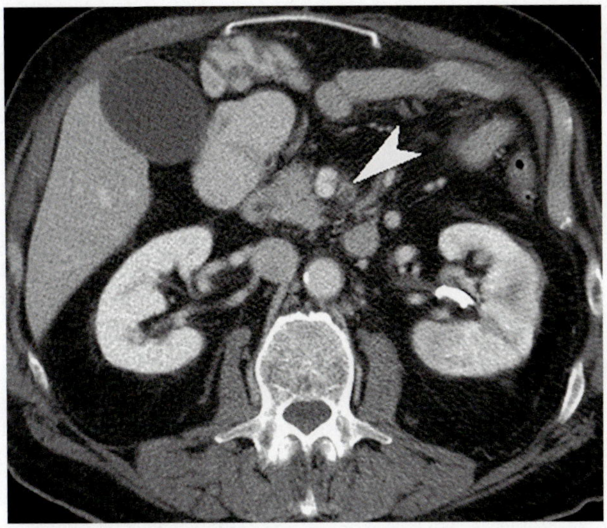

A

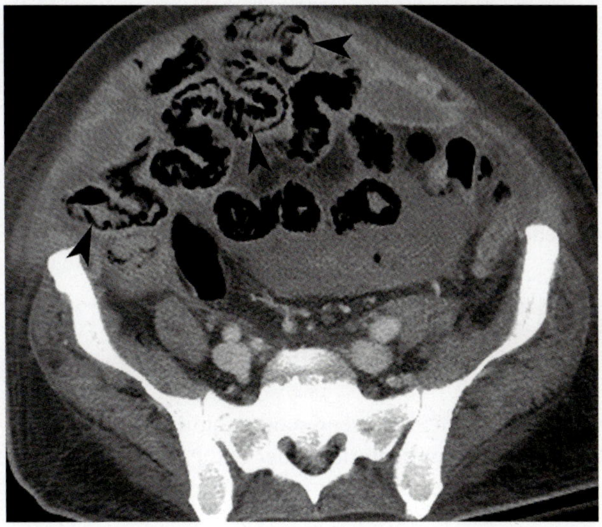

B

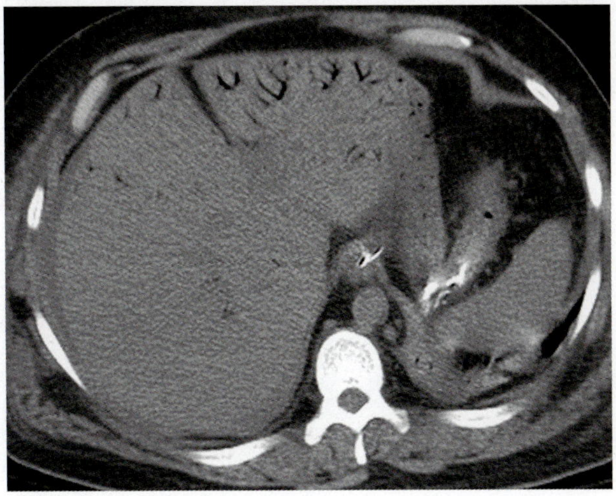

C

**FIG. 4B.14 • Small bowel ischemia findings: SMA occlusion (A), pneumatosis intestinalis (B), and portal vein gas (C). A:** Axial contrast-enhanced CT demonstrates thrombosis of the SMA (*arrowhead*), from thrombotic occlusion. The patient also had small bowel wall thickening of distal ileum (not pictured here), consistent with ongoing ischemia. **B:** Axial contrast-enhanced CT demonstrates pneumatosis (*arrowheads*) and decreased enhancement of multiple loops of distal small bowel. This patient had acute thrombosis of their superior mesenteric vein and extensive portal venous gas (not pictured here). **C:** Axial contrast-enhanced CT demonstrates extensive air in the portal veins, produced by strangulated hernia.

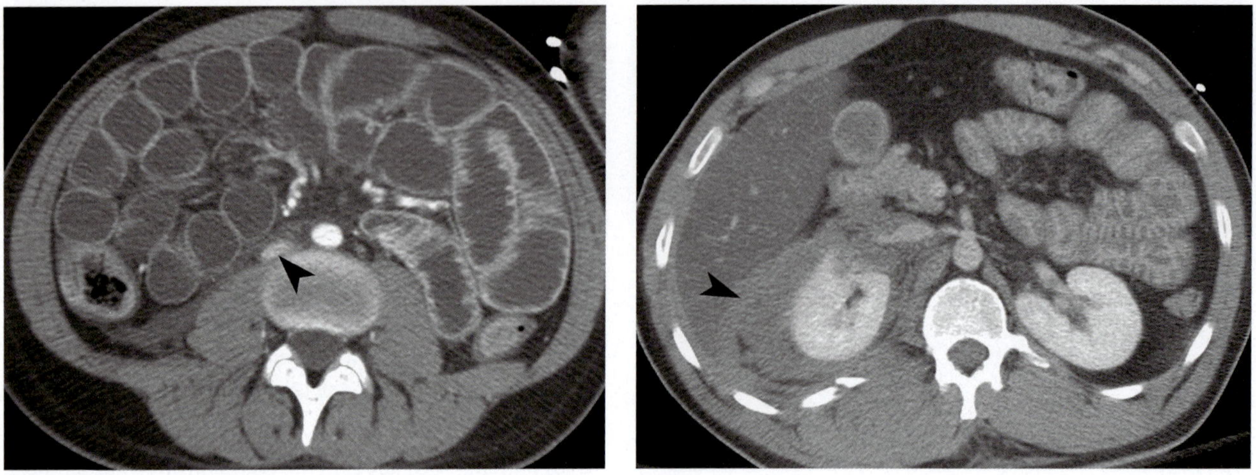

A B

**FIG. 4B.15 • Shock bowel syndrome. A:** Axial contrast-enhanced CT demonstrates paralytic ileus and intense small bowel wall enhancement. The IVC (*arrowhead*) is collapsed due to hypovolemia. **B:** Axial contrast enhanced CT demonstrates right perinephric hematoma (*arrowhead*) and intense small bowel mucosal enhancement.

Chronic mesenteric ischemia is most often seen on elderly women with smoking history. The patients typically complain of postprandial pain, fear of food, and weight loss. For mesenteric ischemia to develop, at least two out of three mesenteric arteries are compromised. For the diagnosis, US is often used as a screening test. A peak systolic velocity of more than 275 cm/s in SMA and more than 200 cm/s in celiac artery is considered abnormal in a fasting patient.

## OTHER SMALL BOWEL ABNORMALITIES

### Small Bowel Diverticulosis and Meckel Diverticulum

Small bowel diverticulosis represents acquired mucosal outpouching from the mesenteric border of the small bowel. The diverticula are more commonly present in the jejunum than ileum. They are mostly asymptomatic but can be associated with food stasis induced bacterial overgrowth, malabsorption, perforation, bleeding, and diverticulitis. On SBFT and CT, they can be seen as smooth outpouchings along the mesenteric border, present in 2% of the population (Fig. 4B.16). When inflamed, there is thickening of the wall of the diverticulum, and surrounding inflammation or free air (Fig. 4B.17).

Meckel diverticulum is a congenital anomaly in which there is a true diverticulum within the ileum as a result of persistence of the omphalomesenteric duct. At least 60% of cases contain heterotopic mucosa, of which gastric mucosa is the most common (50%). When ectopic gastric mucosa is present, secretion of gastric acid causes local inflammation and increases the risk of ulceration, bleeding, or perforation. Classically, these diverticula are present in 2% of the population, located within 2 feet of the ileocecal valve, and are symptomatic before the age

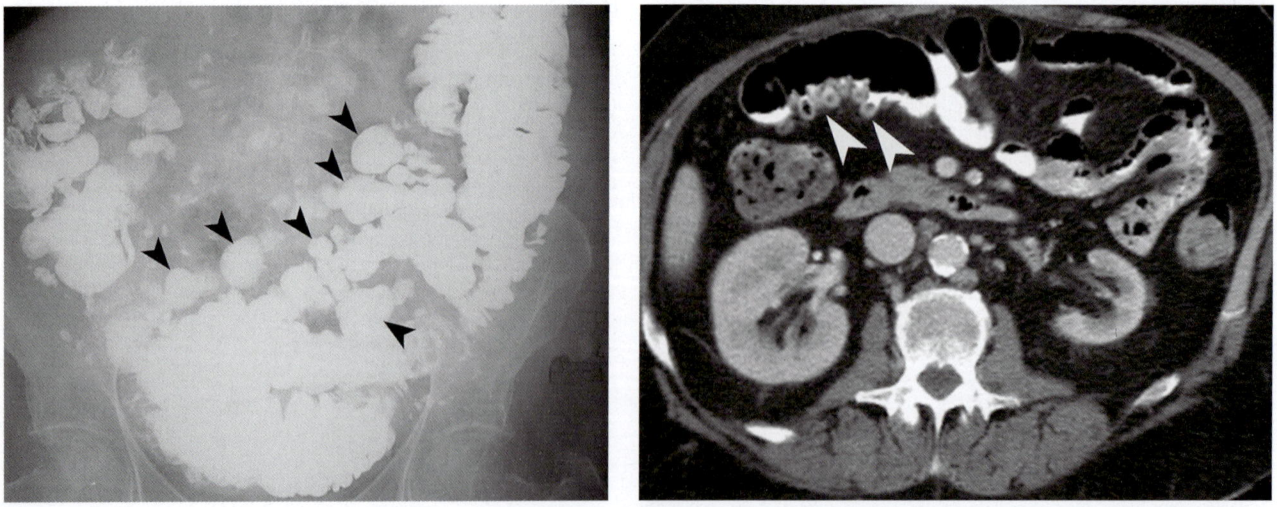

A B

**FIG. 4B.16 • Small bowel diverticulosis. A:** SBFT demonstrates multiple diverticula (*arrowheads*), represented by oval collections of barium throughout the abdomen and pelvis. **B:** Axial contrast-enhanced CT of the abdomen demonstrates multiple small bowel diverticula (*arrowheads*) along the mesenteric border of the ileum.

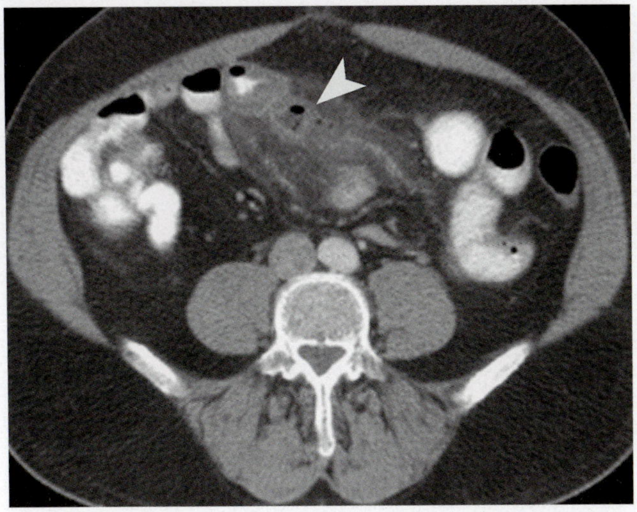

**FIG. 4B.17 • Small bowel diverticulitis.** Axial contrast-enhanced CT demonstrates an inflamed small bowel diverticulum (*arrowhead*) with surrounding edema.

of 2 (Rule of 2's). On CT, active Meckel diverticulitis appears as a blind ending ileal pouch with surrounding inflammatory changes (Fig. 4B.18A).[8] On technetium-99m pertechnetate scintigraphy (Meckel scan), diverticula that contain ectopic gastric mucosa classically demonstrate uptake of radiotracer by the mucin secreting gastric mucosa (Fig. 4B.18B). Because of this, Meckel scans have become the tests of choice for identifying gastric containing Meckel diverticula that would be otherwise occult on traditional CT.

Pseudodiverticula are sacculations along the antimesenteric border of the small intestine due to inflammatory or fibrosing small bowel disease. Crohn disease and scleroderma are the most common etiologies.

## Gallstone Ileus

Gallstone ileus is a rare condition where mechanical obstruction occurs secondary to impaction of a gallstone most commonly in the distal small bowel after it had eroded into the duodenum and migrated through the small intestine. Long-standing inflammation of the gall bladder wall, as is seen with chronic cholecystitis, is thought to be the major predisposing factor. Diagnosis is primarily made with CT and findings include Rigler triad of SBO, pneumobilia, and ectopic gallstone (Fig. 4B.19). Classically, obstruction occurs at the narrowest portions of the small bowel, namely the ligament of Treitz and ileocecal valve. If the gallstones are large enough, there can be proximal duodenal or distal gastric obstruction (Bouveret syndrome).[9]

## Intestinal Malrotation

Although adults with malrotation of bowel are usually asymptomatic, children with intestinal malrotation can present with small bowel obstruction due to midgut volvulus (due to short mesentery) or Ladd bands. Ninety percent of the symptomatic cases occur in infants.

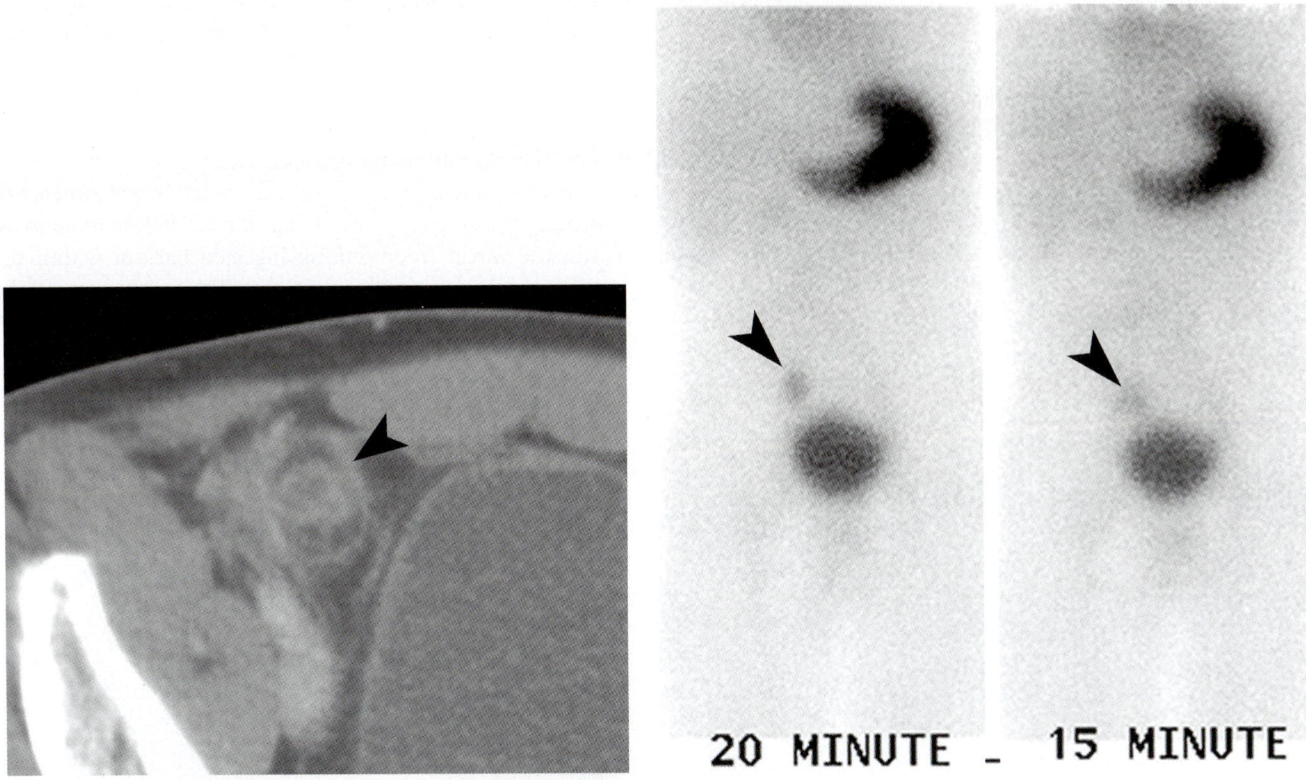


A B

**FIG. 4B.18 • Meckel diverticulum. A:** Contrast-enhanced CT demonstrates inflamed Meckel diverticulum (*arrowhead*) in the right lower quadrant. **B:** Tc-99m pertechnetate Meckel scan performed in a 3-year-old male with painless rectal bleeding demonstrates a focus of radiotracer activity (*arrowheads*) in the right lower quadrant compatible with ectopic gastric mucosa.

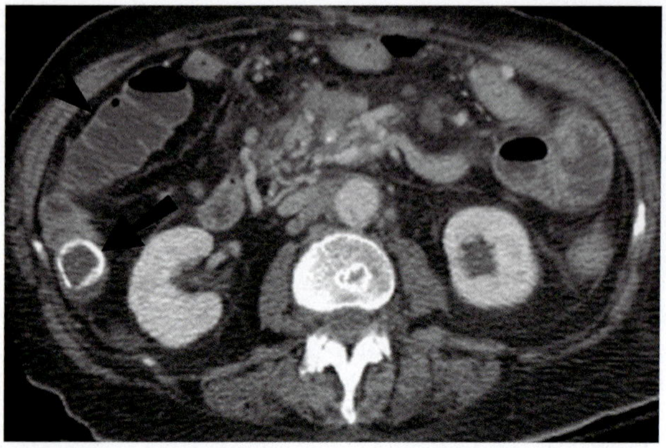

**FIG. 4B.19 • Gallstone ileus.** Axial contrast-enhanced CT shows a gallstone (*arrow*) in a small bowel loop, causing dilatation of more proximal bowel (*arrowhead*).

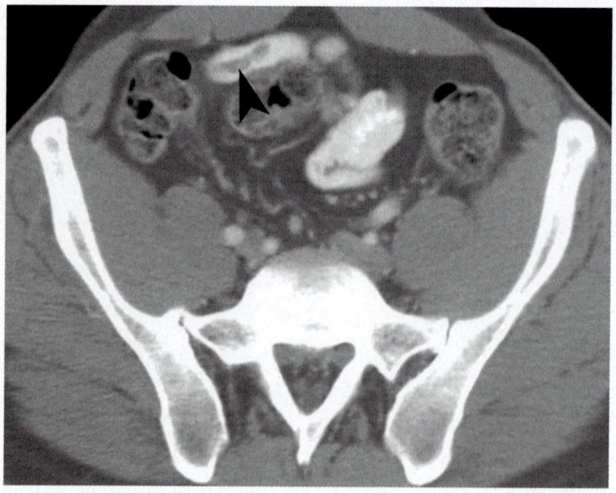

**FIG. 4B.21 • Ascariasis.** Axial contrast-enhanced CT demonstrates a tubular hypoattenuating filling defect within a contrast filled loop small bowel consistent with an ascaris worm (*arrowhead).*

The normal duodenojejunal junction is located to the left of the lumbar spine, and the duodenojejunal junction is located to the left of the spine, at the level of the duodenal bulb. The normal small bowel rotates a total of 270 degrees so that the cecum is in the right lower quadrant and duodenojejunal junction is to the left of midline. Any variation in the 270 degrees rotation results in one of the following: nonrotation, hyper rotation, malrotation, and reversed rotation. In patients with nonrotation of bowel, the cecum is located on the left side and the jejunum as well as ileum on the right side of the abdomen. In patients with malrotation, the duodenojejunal junction is located to the right of midline while the small bowel is located either on the right side or in the mid abdomen (Fig. 4B.20A). In patients with hyper rotation of the small bowel, the cecum is located in the left upper quadrant, while patient with reversed rotation the transverse colon is located in the right upper quadrant.

## Duplication Cyst

Enteric duplication cysts are cysts lined by all layers of the bowel, most commonly occur in the region of the ileum and duodenum. They are typically discovered in childhood and represent incomplete embryologic recanalization of the GI tract. They appear as round or tubular cystic lesions that may communicate (20% cases) with the lumen of adjacent small bowel (Fig. 4B.20B).[10]

## Ascariasis

Infestation with the roundworm *Ascaris lumbricoides* is the most common small bowel worm, affecting approximately 25% of the world population. These worms enter the GI system through ingestion of *Ascaris* eggs in contaminated food or water. After hatching, the larvae penetrate the small bowel wall and migrate to the lung via the vascular system. The larvae then migrate up the airways and are swallowed back into the GI tract where they mature in the small bowel. As the worms grow, a large cluster can become a nidus for small bowel obstruction. On all imaging modalities, these worms appear as round or tubular lesions within the small bowel lumen. On fluoroscopy, a characteristic string-like white line of contrast within the worm (representing ingested barium within the worm's intestine) is commonly seen.[11] The worms can also be seen in the bowel lumen on CT imaging (Fig. 4B.21).

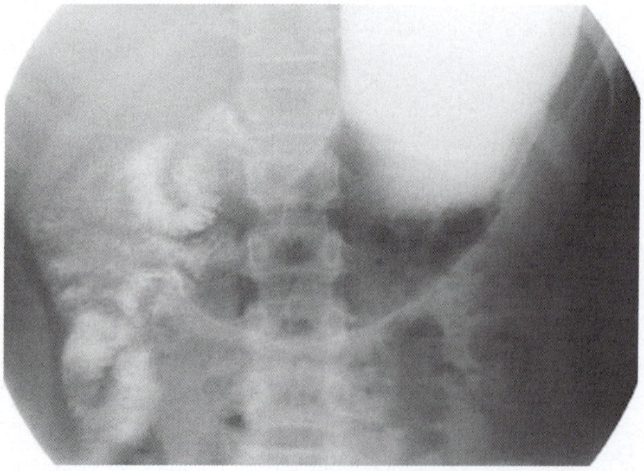

A

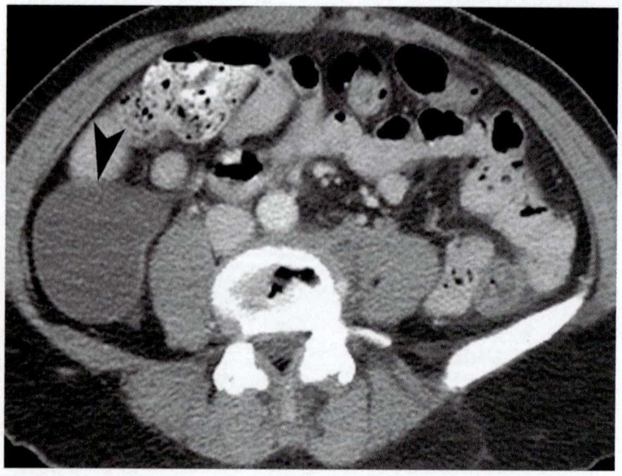

B

**FIG. 4B.20 • Malrotation (A) and duplication cyst (B). A:** SBFT demonstrates the duodenojejunal junction and jejunal loops located to the right of midline in this patient with malrotation. **B:** Axial contrast-enhanced CT of the abdomen demonstrates a round cystic lesion (*arrowhead*) with thin wall in the right lower quadrant.

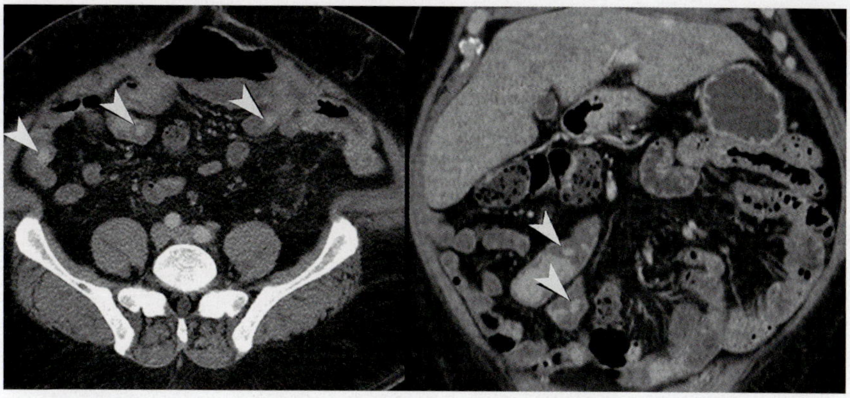

**FIG. 4B.22 • Peutz-Jeghers syndrome.** Axial and coronal contrast-enhanced CT enterography images demonstrate multiple enhancing intraluminal polyps (*arrowheads*) throughout the small bowel.

# BENIGN TUMORS

## Adenoma

Adenomas are mucosal tumors derived from glandular epithelium. As in the colon, these tumors appear as intraluminal polyps and carry the potential for malignant degeneration. Historically, adenomas are best seen with enteroclysis and SBFT studies. However, advanced endoscopic techniques (i.e., capsule endoscopy) and CT enterography have now become the diagnostic tests of choice.

## Polyposis Syndromes

Polyposis syndromes represent a group of conditions in which there are multiple small bowel polypoid masses associated with extra-intestinal manifestations. The majority of these polyps are characterized as adenomatous or hamartomatous.[12,13] Classically, adenomatous polyps carry the risk of neoplastic transformation, while hamartomatous polyps do not.

Peutz-Jeghers syndrome involves multiple hamartomatous polyps associated with hyperpigmentation of mucus membranes and the skin of the face, palms, and soles (Fig. 4B.22). Although the polyps are not premalignant, 13% of patients develop concomitant small bowel adenocarcinoma.

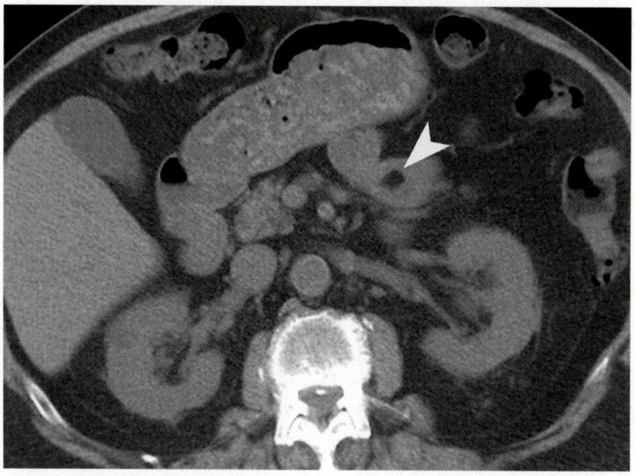

**FIG. 4B.23 • Lipoma.** Axial unenhanced CT image of the abdomen demonstrates a round fat density lesion (*arrowhead*) within a loop of proximal small bowel consistent with a lipoma.

Cronkhite-Canada syndrome involves multiple hamartomatous polyps associated with protein-losing enteropathy, alopecia, and nail atrophy.

Cowden syndrome involves multiple hamartomatous polyps associated with a predisposition for breast, thyroid, and skin cancers.

Juvenile polyposis, FAP, and Gardner syndrome predominantly have colonic adenomatous polyps, although associated small bowel polyps are occasionally seen.

## Lipoma

Lipomas are well-encapsulated tumors derived from submucosal fat. On fluoroscopy, these tumors appear as rounded intraluminal masses that are easily compressible due to their fat content. On CT, a well-circumscribed fat density mass is virtually diagnostic (Fig. 4B.23). Although typically asymptomatic, the pliability of these tumors may form pedunculated intraluminal masses that can become lead points for intussusception.

## Hemangioma

Hemangiomas are small submucosal masses caused by proliferation of vascular channels. When symptomatic, these tumors present with GI bleeding and are located predominantly in the jejunum. Fluoroscopy shows small intraluminal polyps and IV contrast-enhanced CT demonstrates small enhancing submucosal nodules. While this appearance is nonspecific, identification of a calcified phlebolith on CT is nearly diagnostic.

# MALIGNANT TUMORS

## Carcinoid Tumor

Carcinoid tumor is the most common small bowel malignancy representing one-third of all small bowel tumors. Histologically, it is a low grade neuroendocrine tumor arising from enterochromaffin cells within the bowel wall mucosa. Most of the carcinoid tumors occur in the appendix, rectum, and small bowel. Unlike adenocarcinoma, small bowel carcinoid tumor is predominantly found within the ileum (90%) rather than proximal small bowel.

On CT, carcinoid typically appears as a homogenous, intensely enhancing small bowel mass with a surrounding "sunburst pattern" of mesenteric fibrosis and infiltration

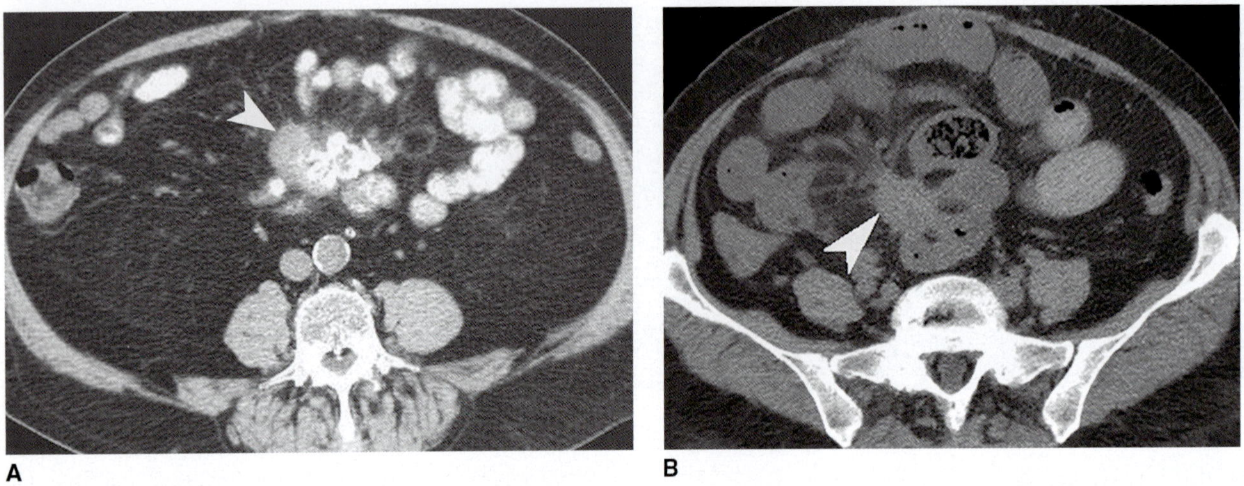


**FIG. 4B.24** • **Carcinoid tumor. A:** Axial contrast-enhanced CT demonstrates a mesenteric mass (*arrowhead*) with calcifications and surrounding desmoplastic scarring. **B:** Axial unenhanced CT image demonstrates a mesenteric mass (*arrowhead*) with a surrounding sunburst pattern of fibrosis consistent with desmoplastic reaction.

(Fig. 4B.24). Histologically, this represents local extension of tumor into the surrounding mesentery with release of serotonin causing a desmoplastic reaction with tethering and retraction of adjacent small bowel loops. Majority (70%) of the mesenteric speculated masses contain calcifications. Once carcinoid tumors reach 2 cm in size, metastases to the liver are seen in approximately 90% of cases.

CT is the most helpful modality to define the extent of disease with liver metastases appearing as hypoattenuating lesions that avidly enhance on postcontrast images.[14,15] Of note, it is with liver metastases that the classic carcinoid syndrome of cutaneous flushing, wheezing, and diarrhea can develop secondary to bypass of the normal hepatic degradation of serotonin into 5-hydroxyindoleacetic acid and resulting shunting of serotonin into the systemic circulation.

## Adenocarcinoma

Adenocarcinoma is the second most common malignant tumor of small bowel, representing approximately 25% of small bowel malignancies. More than 50% occur in the duodenum, while the rest occur in jejunum and ileum. Many disorders are associated with an increased relative risk of developing small bowel adenocarcinoma, including celiac disease (60-80 fold), Crohn disease (60 fold), and polyposis syndromes such as familial adenomatous polyposis (330 fold). Most patients are symptomatic at the time of diagnosis presenting with abdominal pain, GI bleeding, intussusception, or small bowel obstruction. If discovered early, adenocarcinoma may appear as a polypoid sessile mass producing an intraluminal filling defect on barium studies. More commonly, however, adenocarcinoma has an infiltrating morphology showing the characteristic "apple core" or annular constricting lesion on fluoroscopy (Fig. 4B.25). On CT, this has the appearance of an abrupt transition from thin walled normal caliber bowel to mass-like circumferential wall thickening with marked intraluminal narrowing (Fig. 4B.26).

## Gastrointestinal Stromal Tumor

Gastrointestinal stromal tumors (GISTs) are smooth muscle mesenchymal tumors that arise from the interstitial cells of Cajal. They are most commonly located in the stomach (70%), followed by small bowel (20%). On fluoroscopy, these tumors produce rounded, submucosal filling defects with or without ulceration.

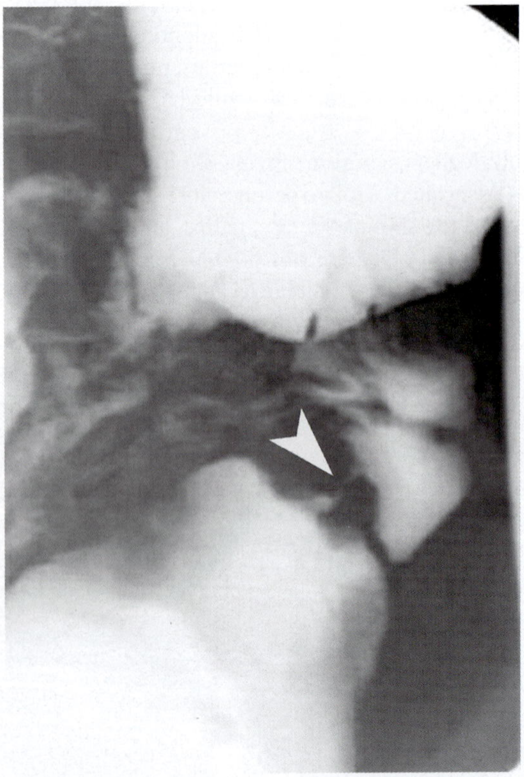

**FIG. 4B.25** • **Ileal adenocarcinoma.** Spot fluoroscopic image demonstrates an annular constricting lesion in a distal small bowel loop with an abrupt transition from normal caliber lumen to markedly narrowed lumen producing the characteristic apple core stricture (*arrowhead*).

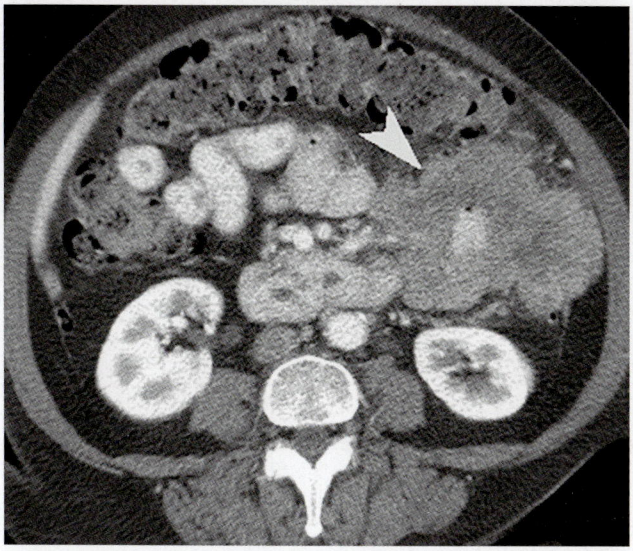

**FIG. 4B.26 • Jejunal adenocarcinoma.** Axial contrast-enhanced CT of the abdomen demonstrates large mass lesion (*arrowhead*) involving a jejunal loop with extension in to the surrounding mesenteric fat.

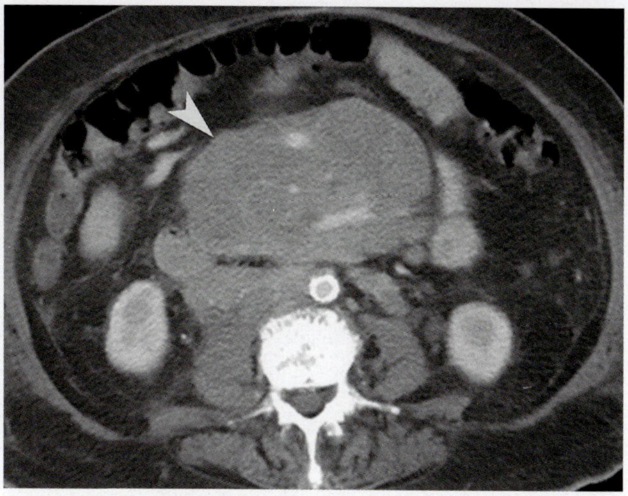

**FIG. 4B.28 • Mesenteric lymphoma.** Axial contrast-enhanced CT image demonstrates large conglomerate lymph nodal mass (*arrowhead*) encasing mesenteric vessels, producing the sandwich sign.

On CT, GISTs classically appear as well circumscribed masses with exoenteric growth pattern when they are more than 3 cm in diameter. When less than 2 cm in diameter these tumors demonstrate homogeneous enhancement with no metastases. However, as they enlarge, enhancement becomes patchy owing to various degrees of internal necrosis (Fig. 4B.27). Distinguishing benign from malignant GISTs can be difficult although necrotic tumors larger than 5 cm should raise the suspicion for malignancy.[16,17]

## Lymphoma

Small bowel lymphoma accounts for 20% of all primary malignant small bowel tumors and represents the second most common site of gastrointestinal tract lymphoma, after stomach. It is typically non-Hodgkin B-cell lymphoma and arises predominantly in the distal ileum, the region where the majority of small bowel lymphoid tissue resides. Traditionally, small bowel lymphoma is classified as being primary (arising from the small bowel) or mesenteric (from mesenteric lymph nodes). In the primary form, lymphoma destroys the muscularis and autonomic plexus of the small bowel wall, causing luminal dilatation. Therefore, unlike most other mass lesions within the small bowel, it rarely causes obstruction.

It is well recognized that immunocompromised patients and celiac patients are at increased risk of developing small bowel lymphoma. Unlike most other cases of small bowel lymphoma, celiac patients tend to develop a T-cell lymphoma which occurs predominantly in the proximal small bowel at the site of greatest villous injury. Lymphoma in immunocompromised

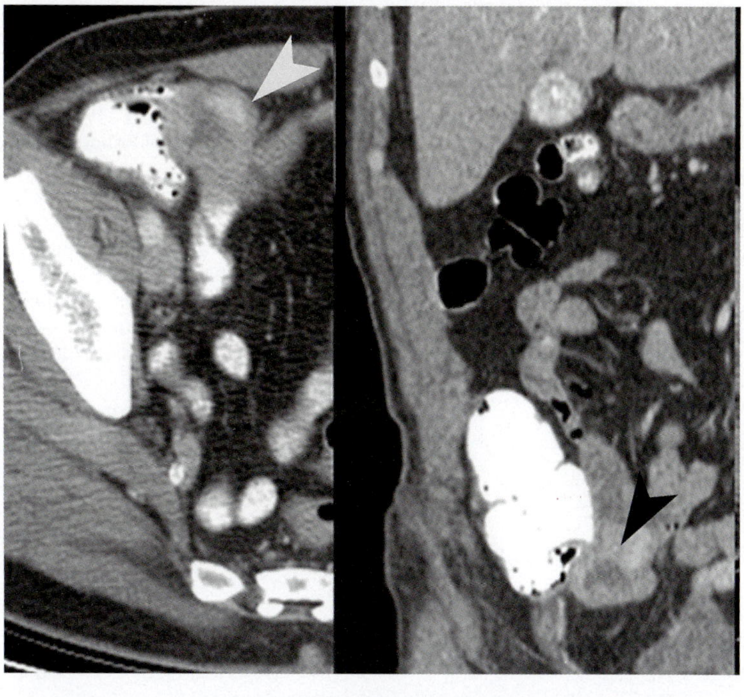

**FIG. 4B.27 • Gastrointestinal stromal tumor of ileum.** Coronal contrast-enhanced CT demonstrates an exophytic heterogeneously enhancing mass (*black arrowhead*) arising from distal ileum (*white arrowhead*). There is central hypoattenuation consistent with necrosis.

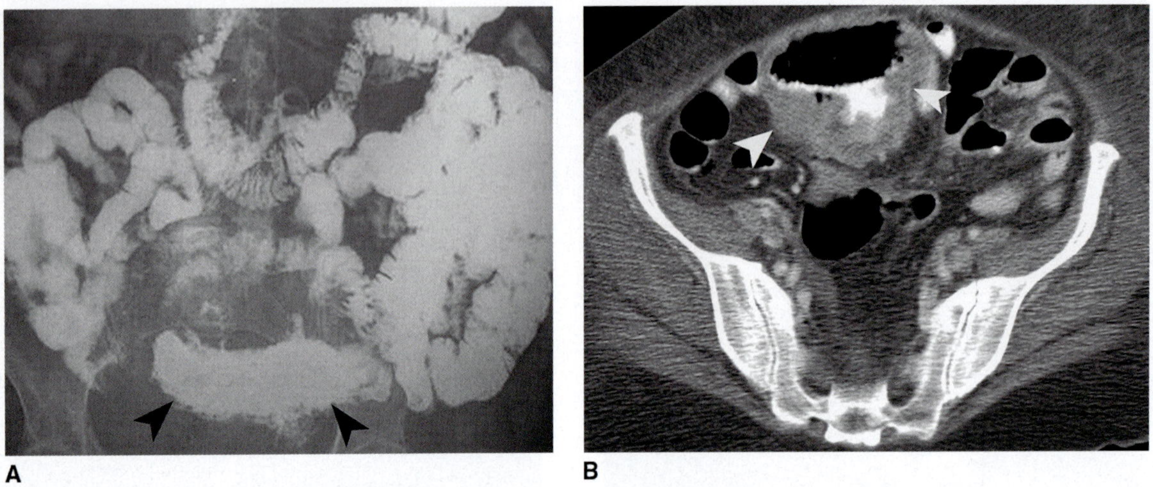


**FIG. 4B.29 • Ileal lymphoma. A:** SBFT demonstrates aneurysmal dilatation of an ileal (*arrowheads*) loop, caused by lymphomatous infiltration of myenteric plexus. **B:** Axial contrast-enhanced CT shows an aneurysmally dilated (*arrowheads*) small bowel loop with wall thickening in the pelvis.

patients was traditionally described with AIDS patients but is now more commonly seen with transplant or rheumatologic patients on high dose immunosuppressive medications.

Most commonly, primary small bowel lymphoma is infiltrative in morphology and involves a longer segment of bowel than other small bowel tumors. It appears as eccentric, circumferential wall thickening on CT and irregular thickened folds on SBFT. Less common morphologic patterns of primary small bowel lymphoma include mural nodules, polypoid masses, or exophytic masses. In the mesenteric form, confluent adenopathy produces solid soft tissue masses that can encase mesenteric fat and vessels producing the classic "sandwich sign" on CT (Fig. 4B.28). Dilatation of the bowel lumen due to myenteric plexus neoplastic destruction may occur and is described as aneurysmal dilatation of bowel (Fig. 4B.29).[18,19]

## References

1. Hara AK, Leighton JA, Sharma VK, et al. Imaging of small bowel disease: comparison of capsule endoscopy, standard endoscopy, barium examination, and CT. *Radiographics.* 2005;25:697–718.
2. Wittenberg J, Harisinghani MG, Jhaveri K, et al. Algorithmic approach to CT diagnosis of the abnormal bowel wall. *Radiographics.* 2002;22:1093–1109.
3. Balthazar EJ. CT of the gastrointestinal tract: principles and interpretation. *AJR Am J Roentgenol.* 1991;156:23–32.
4. Lee SS, Kim AY, Yang SK, et al. Crohn disease of the small bowel: comparison of CT enterography, MR enterography, and small-bowel follow-through as diagnostic techniques. *Radiology.* 2009; 251(3):751–761.
5. Amzallag-Bellenger E, Oudjit A, Ruiz A, et al. Effectiveness of MR enterography for the assessment of small-bowel diseases beyond Crohn disease. *Radiographics.* 2012; 32(5):1423–1444.
6. Grand DJ, Harris A, Loftus EV. Imaging for luminal disease and complications: CT enterography, MR enterography, small-bowel follow-through, and ultrasound. *Gastroenterol Clin North Am.* 2012; 41(2): 497–512.
7. Gore RM, Yaghmai V, Thakrar KH, et al. Imaging in intestinal ischemic disorders. *Radiol Clin North Am.* 2008;46(5):845–875.
8. Thurley PD, Halliday KE, Somers JM, et al. Radiological features of Meckel's diverticulum and its complications. *Clin Radiol.* 2009;64(2):109–118.
9. Lassandro F, Romano S, Ragozzino A, et al. Role of helical CT in diagnosis of gallstone ileus and related conditions. *AJR Am J Roentgenol.* 2005;185(5):1159–1165.
10. Macpherson RI. Gastrointestinal tract duplications: clinical, pathologic, etiologic, and radiologic considerations. *Radiographics.* 1993;13(5):1063–1080.
11. Suzuki A, Yabushita Y, Takahashi H, et al. Education and imaging. Gastrointestinal: ascariasis. *J Gastroenterol Hepatol.* 2008;23(11):1770.
12. Cho GJ, Bergquist K, Shwartz AM. Peutz-Jeghers syndrome and the hamartomatous polyposis syndromes: radiologic-pathologic correlation. *Radiographics.* 1997;17(3):785–791.
13. Hamed RK, Buck JL, Sobin LH. The hamartomatous polyposis syndromes: clinical and radiologic features. *AJR Am J Roentgenol.* 1995;164(3):565–571.
14. Buckley JA, Fishman EK. CT evaluation of small bowel neoplasms: spectrum of disease. *Radiographics.* 1998;18(2):379–392.
15. Laurent F, Drouillard J, Lecesne R, et al. CT of small-bowel neoplasms. *Semin Ultrasound CT MR.* 1995;16(2):102–111.
16. King DM. The radiology of gastrointestinal stromal tumors (GIST). *Cancer Imaging.* 2005;15(5):150–156.
17. Ulusan S, Koc Z, Kayaselcuk F. Gastrointestinal stromal tumors: CT findings. *Br J Radiol.* 2008;81(968):618–623.
18. Rubesin SE, Gilchrist AM, Bronner M, et al. Non-Hodgkin lymphoma of the small intestine. *Radiographics.* 1990;10(6):985–998.
19. Balthazar EJ, Noordhoorn M, Megibow AJ, et al. CT of small-bowel lymphoma in immunocompetent patients and patients with AIDS: Comparison of findings. *AJR Am J Roentgenol.* 1997;168(3):675–680.

## SELF-ASSESSMENT QUESTIONS

1. Based on the barium enema examination, what is the cause of the patient's chronic diarrhea?

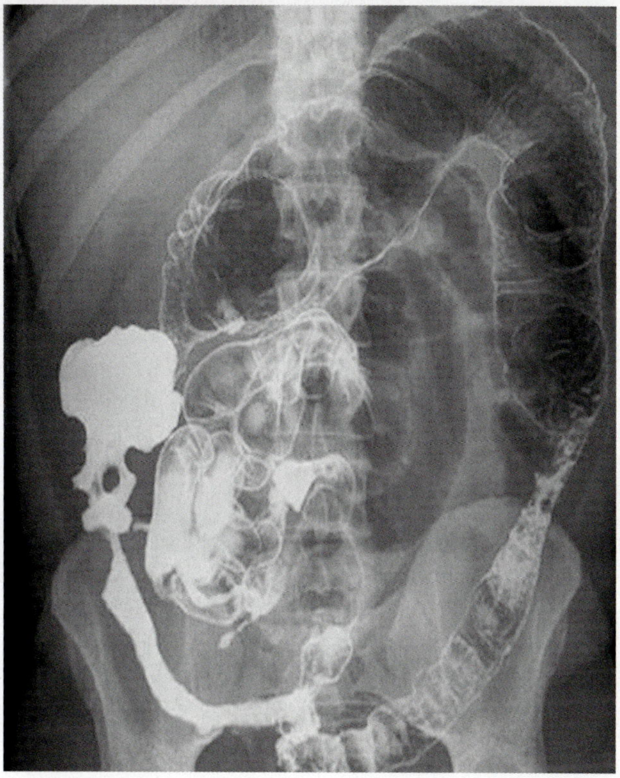

   A. Ulcerative colitis
   B. Intussusception
   C. Crohn disease
   D. Sarcoidosis

2. What is a likely cause of the pathology (arrowhead) shown on the CT of a patient with abdominal pain out of proportion to physical exam findings?

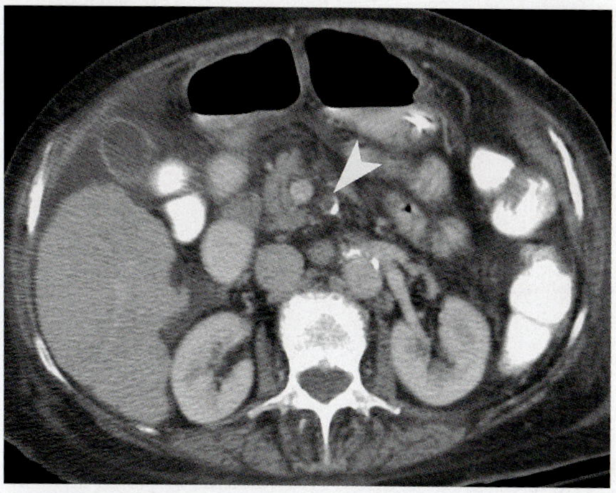

   A. Septicemia
   B. Trauma
   C. Atrial fibrillation
   D. Jejunitis

### *Answers to Self-Assessment Questions*

**1. C.** Crohn disease. The barium enema demonstrates strictures in the transverse and descending colon. There is a long segment stricture also seen in the ileum, consistent with late stage of Crohn disease.

**2. C.** Atrial fibrillation. The contrast-enhanced CT shows thrombus in the SMA, which is often due to embolism from cardiac source (atrial fibrillation, endocarditis, myocarditis, etc.).

# Large Bowel: Non-neoplastic Lesions

# 5A

*Vijetha Vinod Maller, Randall L. Scott, and Sridhar Shankar*

## LEARNING OBJECTIVE

**1.** Review the imaging features of the congenital, infectious, and inflammatory pathologies of the colon.

Plain film radiography and fluoroscopy still play an important but diminishing role in the imaging of nonneoplastic diseases of the colon. Advances in multidetector CT and newer, faster sequences in MRI have revolutionized diagnostic imaging and have opened the door to noninvasive characterization of lesions.

## DIVERTICULOSIS AND DIVERTICULITIS

Diverticulosis is one of the most common large bowel disorders in Western countries with approximately 30% of the population being affected over the age of 60 years and 80% of the population affected over the age of 85.[1,2] Colonic diverticula occur due to the herniation of the mucosa through a defect in the muscularis and are common on the mesenteric side of the colon where the nutrient arteries enter. Although the sigmoid colon is affected most commonly, the entire colon may be involved.[1] Diverticulitis occurs as a consequence of obstruction of the neck of the diverticula causing perforation, inflammation, and infection.

On double-contrast barium enema, diverticula appear as air filled, lined with a thin layer of barium projecting extraluminally on tangential views (Fig. 5A.1A). On single-contrast study, the diverticula appear to be completely filled with barium. On en face views, the double-contrast barium study demonstrates a ring shadow or double-ring shadow with the neck of the diverticulum projecting in the center. Partly filled diverticula demonstrate the meniscus sign with the meniscus fading centrally.[3] Although most colonic diverticula are less than 2 cm in diameter, giant sigmoid diverticulum measures more than 4 cm in diameter (Fig. 5A.1B). Barium enema is not used to make the diagnosis of diverticulitis but can be used to evaluate the fistula and surgical planning (Fig. 5A.2).

Diverticulosis is seen on CT as air- or contrast-filled outpouchings with sizes ranging from few millimeters to few centimeters. The Hinchey classification of acute diverticulitis addresses the surgical significance of the various manifestations (Table 5A.1).[4] The CT findings of diverticulitis include the following:

- Segmental colonic wall thickening, hyperemia, and enhancement with higher inner and outer attenuation with a middle layer of lower attenuation are seen.
- Pericolonic fat stranding is disproportionately prominent compared to the degree of bowel wall thickening (Figs. 5A.3 and 5A.4A, B).
- Diverticular perforation causes extravasation of air and fluid into the pelvis and peritoneal cavity resulting in the abscess formation (Figs. 5A.4C and 5A.5).
- Fistula formation with the adjacent viscera (bladder, vagina, colon, small bowel, or skin) can occur as a complication.[5]

CT features of acute diverticulitis can also be present in carcinoma of the colon, although the two can coexist. While there are limited data about follow-up colonoscopy after a CT diagnosis of acute diverticulitis, professional societies such as the American Society of Colon and Rectal Surgeons and the American College of Gastroenterology recommend that patients undergo colonoscopy to exclude colon cancer after an episode of acute diverticulitis.[6]

Features distinguishing diverticulitis from colon cancer:

- Fluid in the sigmoid mesocolon, engorged mesenteric vessels, and pericolonic edema have high predictive value for the diagnosis of acute diverticulitis.
- Demonstration of pericolonic lymph nodes, luminal mass, and abrupt zone of transition favors the diagnosis of colonic neoplasm.
- Demonstration of segmental colonic wall thickening with pericolonic inflammation, in the absence of pericolonic lymph nodes, strongly favors the diagnosis of diverticulitis.

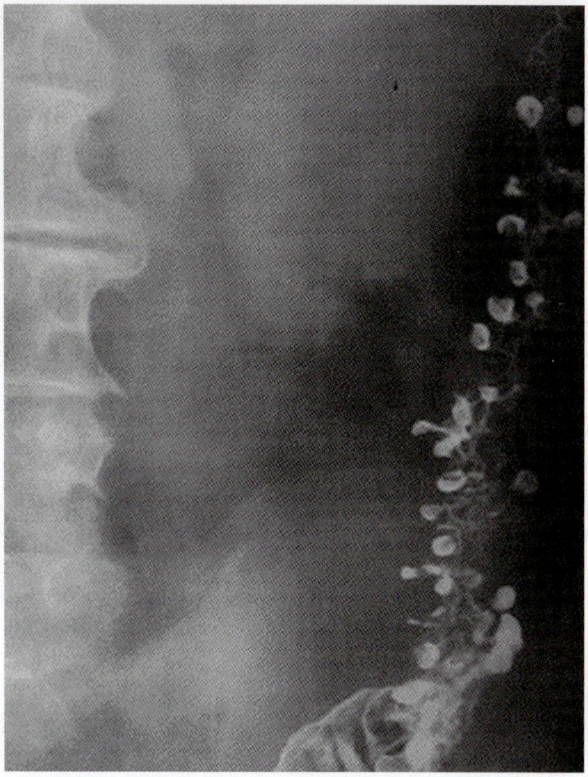

A

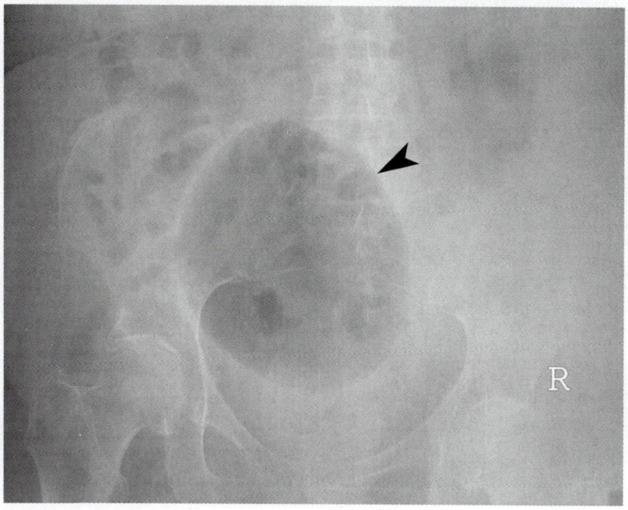


B

**FIG. 5A.1 ● Colonic diverticulosis. A:** Postevacuation film after barium enema shows multiple outpouchings lined with barium pointing away from the lumen of descending colon. **B:** Plain radiograph shows an 8-cm diameter air-containing viscous, consistent with giant sigmoid diverticulum (*arrowhead*). The differential diagnosis of the radiographic finding could also include an abscess.

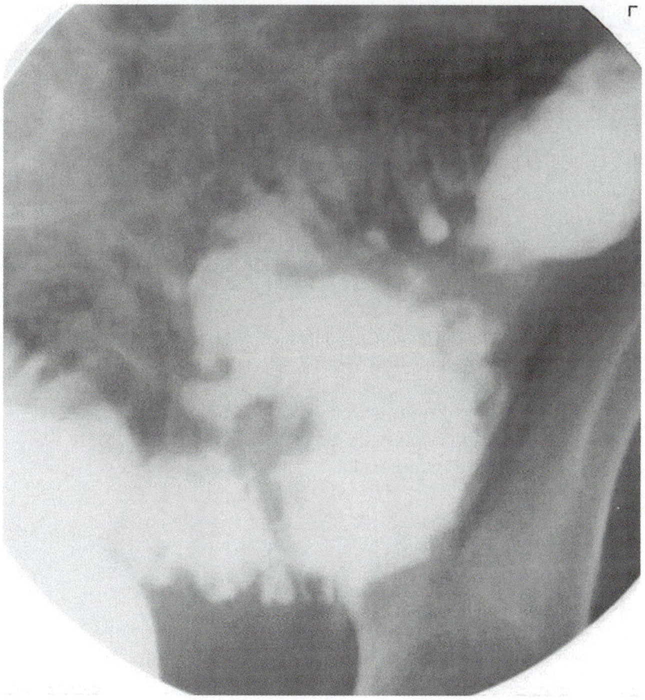

**FIG. 5A.2 ● Acute diverticulitis.** Single-contrast barium enema shows multiple colonic diverticula with mucosal thickening and irregularity of the sigmoid colonic wall.

## ACUTE EPIPLOIC APPENDAGITIS

Epiploic appendages are grape-like fatty peritoneal outpouchings that arise from the serosal surface of the colon, containing adipose tissue and vessels, which can measure up to 5 cm in length. Epiploic appendagitis is a rare self-limiting inflammatory process involving the epiploic appendages, which can be due to torsion or vascular occlusion. Although any part of the colon may be involved, the sigmoid junction and descending colon are the most common.

The imaging features of acute epiploic appendagitis include the following:

- On US, rounded, noncompressible, hyperechoic mass, without internal vascularity and surrounded by hypoechoic line.

Table 5A.1 **HINCHEY CLASSIFICATION OF ACUTE DIVERTICULITIS**

| | |
|---|---|
| Stage 1a | Phlegmon |
| Stage 1b | Diverticulitis with pericolic or mesenteric abscess |
| Stage 2 | Diverticulitis with walled off pelvic abscess |
| Stage 3 | Diverticulitis with generalized purulent peritonitis |
| Stage 4 | Diverticulitis with generalized fecal peritonitis |

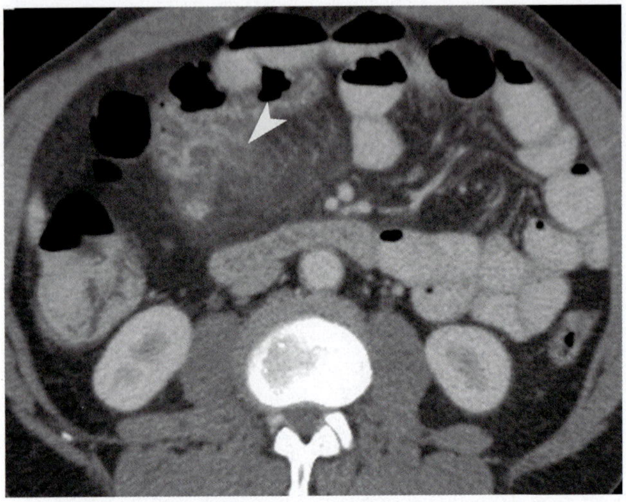

**FIG. 5A.3 • Acute diverticulitis.** Axial contrast-enhanced CT of the abdomen demonstrates an inflamed transverse colonic diverticulum (*arrowhead*) with wall thickening and pericolic fat stranding.

- On CT, 1.5- to 3.5-cm, fat density ovoid structure abutting the colon with thin high-density rim (Fig. 5A.6). Surrounding inflammatory fat stranding and thickening of the adjacent peritoneum can be seen. Central hyperdense dot due to the thrombosed vascular pedicle is present and is approximately half the cases.[7]

## INFLAMMATORY BOWEL DISEASE

Inflammatory bowel disease is a group of disorders with intestinal inflammation, extraintestinal manifestations and a relapsing course. This group of disorder includes ulcerative colitis and Crohn disease.

## ULCERATIVE COLITIS

Patients with ulcerative colitis usually present with persistent diarrhea, urgency of defecation, and tenesmus, often associated with fever, pain, and weight loss. Males are more commonly affected than females (1.3:1) with most individuals between the age group of 14 to 40 years.[8] Unlike Crohn disease, which is characteristically a transmural disease, ulcerative colitis is usually limited to the mucosa and submucosa (Table 5A.2). The rectum is most commonly affected, accounting for 95% of involvement.[9] The colon is involved to a varying extent with continuous involvement unlike skip lesions in Crohn disease. The entire colon may be involved with edema of the terminal ileum termed backwash ileitis. Extraintestinal manifestations include primary sclerosing cholangitis, seronegative spondyloarthropathy,

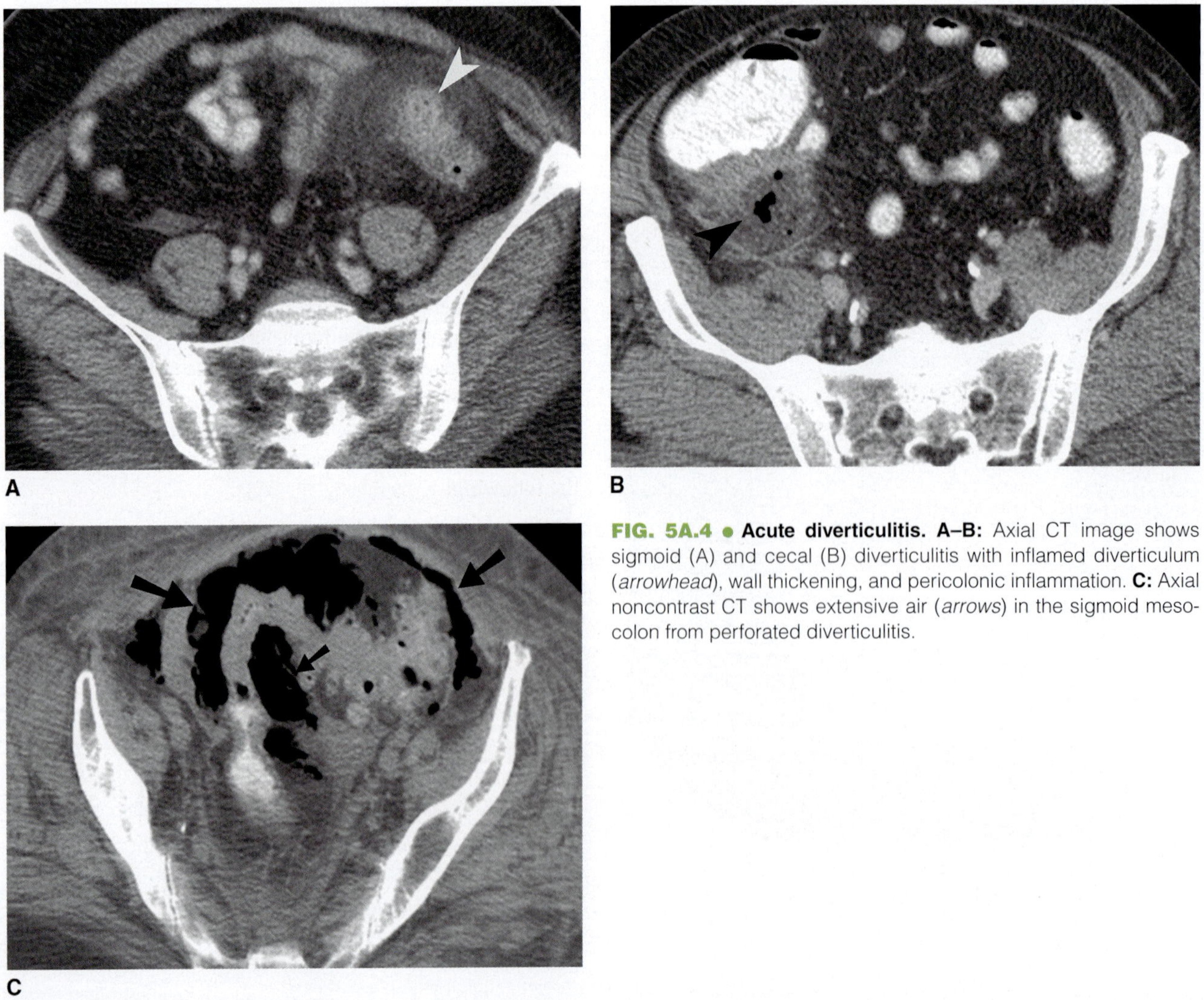

**FIG. 5A.4 • Acute diverticulitis. A–B:** Axial CT image shows sigmoid (A) and cecal (B) diverticulitis with inflamed diverticulum (*arrowhead*), wall thickening, and pericolonic inflammation. **C:** Axial noncontrast CT shows extensive air (*arrows*) in the sigmoid mesocolon from perforated diverticulitis.

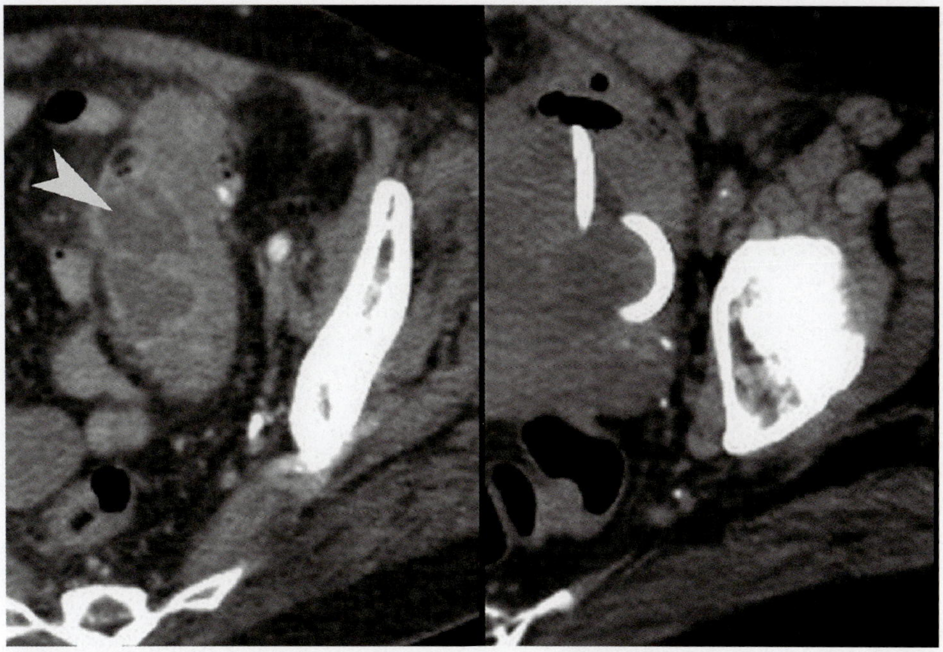

A

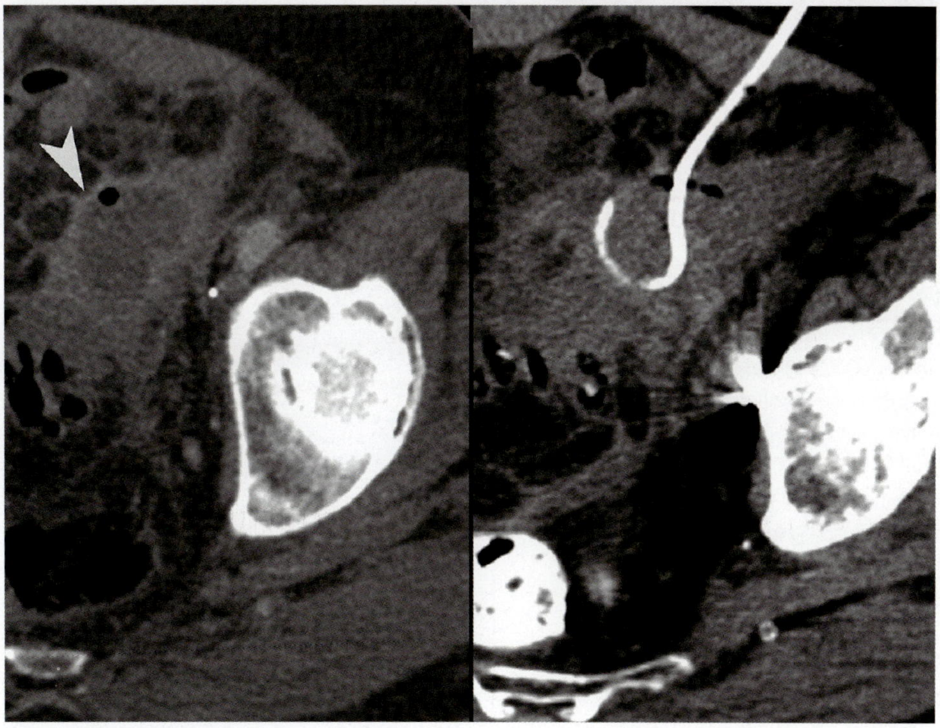

B

**FIG. 5A.5 • A, B: Diverticular abscess.** Axial contrast-enhanced CT of two patients demonstrates sigmoid colon diverticulitis with pericolic abscess (*arrowhead*) before and after pigtail catheter drainage.

uveitis, iritis, erythema nodosum, pyoderma gangrenosum, thrombotic complications, and fatty liver.

Radiographic findings are nonspecific and vary with severity of inflammation (Fig. 5A.7). With severe inflammation, thumbprinting (mucosal edema) may be seen. Double-contrast barium enema allows detailed evaluation of the colonic mucosa; however, it is contraindicated in acute severe colitis due to the risk of perforation.

The imaging findings of ulcerative colitis include the following:

- Granular mucosal appearance with thickening of the haustra (Figs. 5A.8 and 5A.9).
- Mucosal ulcer margins are undermined and result in a collar button appearance.
- With destruction of most of the mucosa, the remaining islands of ragged mucosa can have a pseudopolyp appearance.

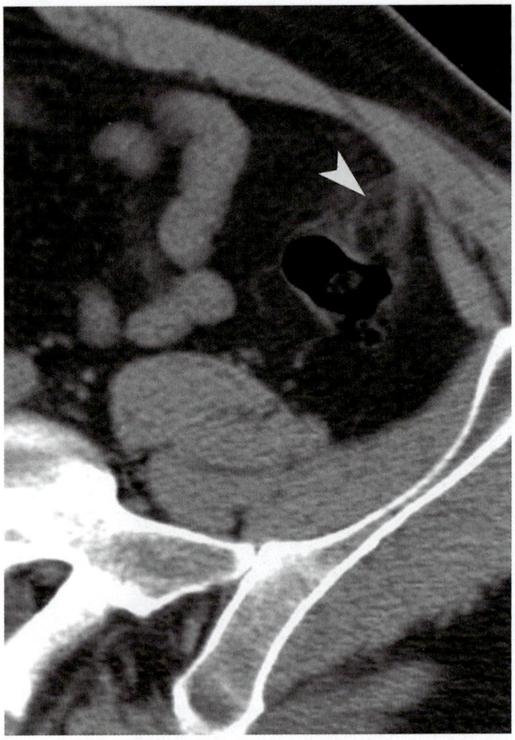

**FIG. 5A.6 • Acute epiploic appendagitis.** Axial contrast-enhanced CT abdomen images show fat density ovoid structure (*arrowhead*) with thin high-density rim, central high-density dot, and surrounding inflammatory fat stranding.

Table 5A.2 **DIFFERENCE BETWEEN ULCERATIVE COLITIS AND CROHN DISEASE**

| Ulcerative Colitis | Crohn Disease |
|---|---|
| Rectal involvement is seen in 95% of the cases with the terminal ileum involved in pancolitis causing backwash ileitis. | Small bowel is involved in 70%–80% with colon being involved in 20% of the cases. |
| Male predominance | No gender predominance |
| Continuous involvement from the rectum to varying proximal extent | Skip lesions are seen. |
| Button-shaped superficial ulcers | Aphthous ulcers |
| Fat halo sign is more common. | Less common |
| Lead pipe appearance in chronic cases | Cobblestone appearance |
| Mesenteric creeping fat not seen | Mesenteric creeping fat seen in chronic cases |
| Abscess formation is uncommon | Abscess formation is common |
| Perianal complications are less common. Colon carcinomas are more common | Ischiorectal fat stranding, sinuses, and fistulas are more common. Colon carcinomas are less common |

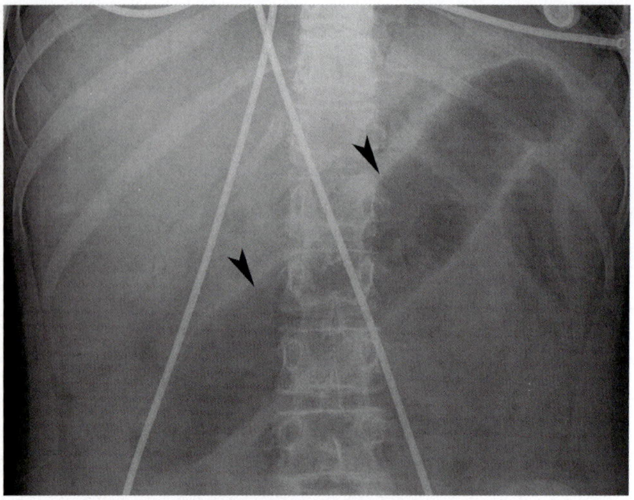

**FIG. 5A.7 • Ulcerative colitis.** Plain radiograph of the abdomen demonstrates loss of haustral folds, resulting in featureless loop of the transverse colon (*arrowheads*).

- Toxic megacolon is seen in less than 5% of patients and is characterized by dilatation of the colon to at least 6 cm and evidence of systemic toxicity.[10]
- In chronic cases, the bowel becomes featureless with loss of normal haustral markings, luminal narrowing, and bowel shortening giving it a lead pipe appearance. Colorectal carcinoma (CRC), which may occur as a complication of ulcerative colitis, is frequently sessile and may appear as a simple stricture.

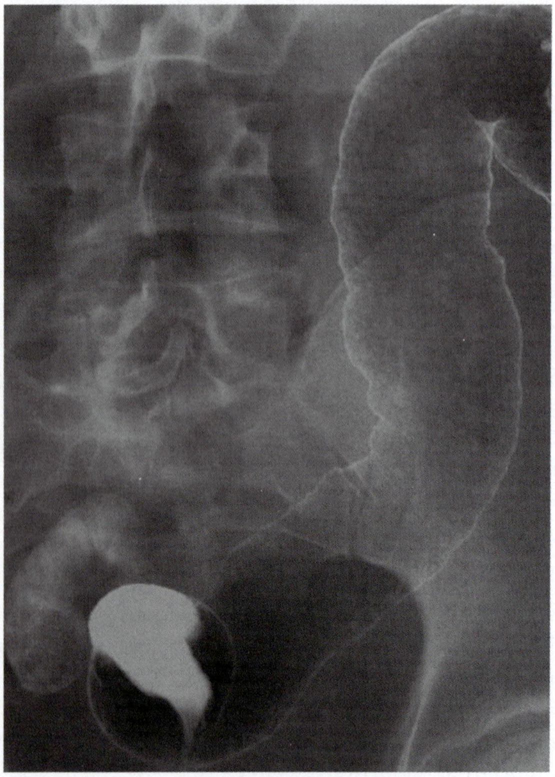

**FIG. 5A.8 • Ulcerative colitis.** Double-contrast barium enema demonstrates a granular mucosal appearance of the rectum and sigmoid colon.

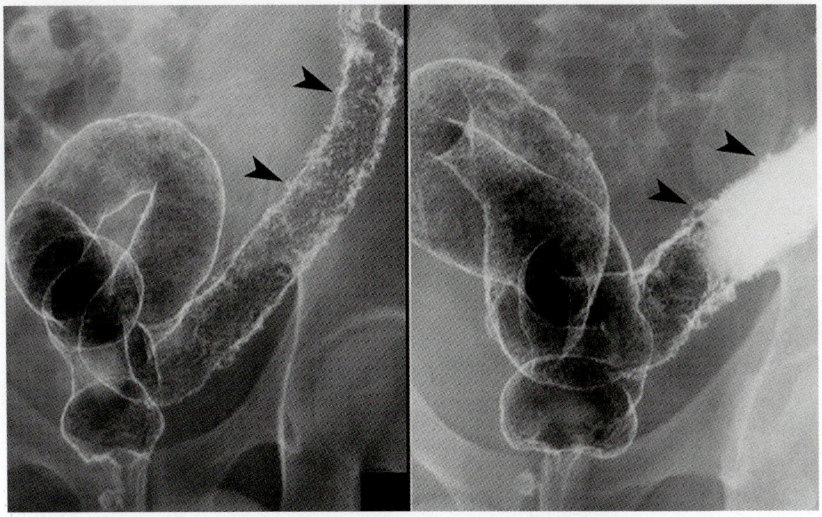

**FIG. 5A.9 • Ulcerative colitis.** Double-contrast barium enema demonstrates granular mucosal appearance of the rectum, sigmoid, and descending colon. There are mucosal ulcers (*arrowheads*) and loss of normal haustra in the descending colon.

CT has emerged as a valuable tool of evaluation of intraperitoneal complications, including abscess, fistula, and perforation. The thickened bowel may show halo sign due to mural stratification and concentric rings of varying attenuation (Fig. 5A.10A). In chronic cases, submucosal fat deposition is seen particularly in the rectum giving a fat halo sign (Fig. 5A.10B). Extramural deposition of fat in this region may lead to thickening of the perirectal fat and widening of the presacral space. Muscularis mucosa hypertrophy may cause loss of normal haustral pattern giving the bowel a lead pipe appearance similar to that seen on barium enema. Strictures are also common as the muscularis mucosa hypertrophies. Focal loss of mural stratification or excessive mural thickness should arouse suspicion for CRC, which often appears as a sessile polyp and should prompt endoscopic evaluation.[11] CT colonography can be used as an alternative technique to colonoscopy in the follow-up evaluation of patients with ulcerative colitis. CT colonography is performed by distending the colon with air or carbon dioxide with prior patient preparation. However, CT colonography is contraindicated in severe acute colitis.

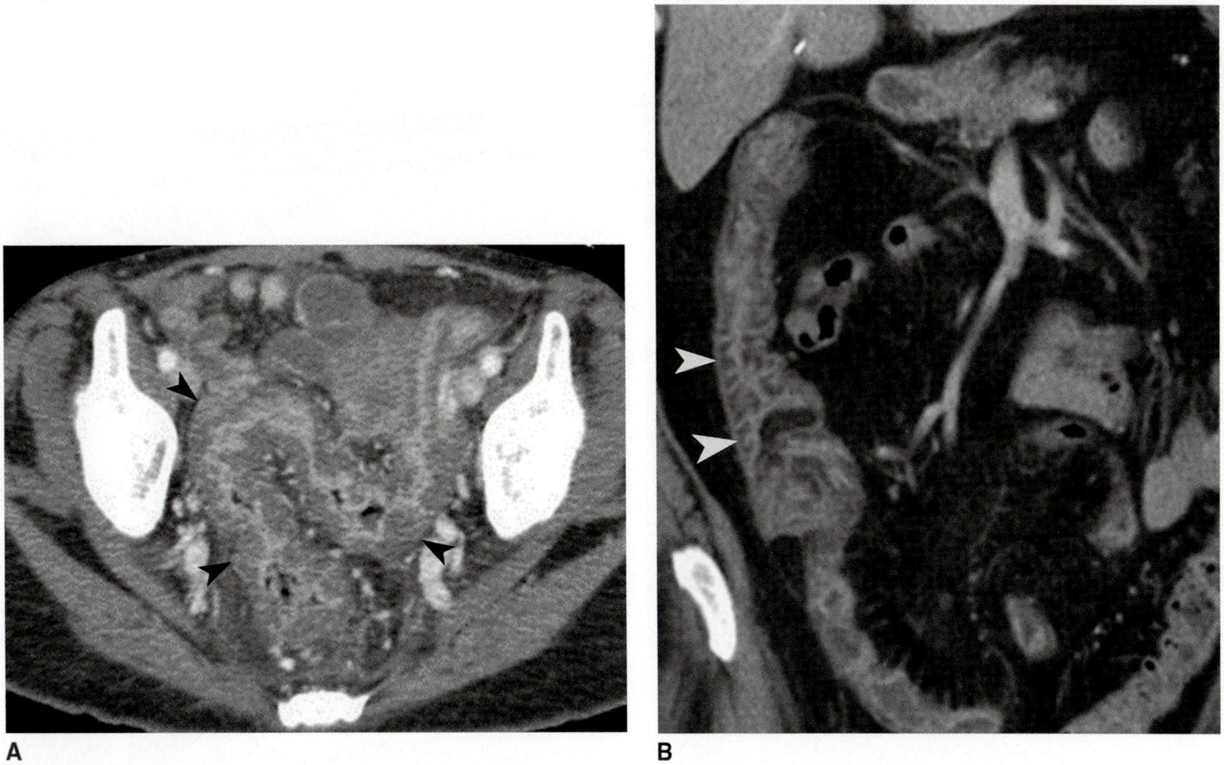


**FIG. 5A.10 • Ulcerative colitis. A:** Axial contrast-enhanced CT image shows wall thickening and mural stratification of the rectum and sigmoid colon (*arrowheads*) with enhancement of the mucosa, producing water halo sign. **B:** Coronal CT reformation of another patient with chronic ulcerative colitis demonstrates submucosal fat infiltration of the ascending colon (*arrowheads*) and ileum, resulting in fat halo sign.

MR colonography can be used as a useful imaging modality in the evaluation of ulcerative colitis. Bowel cleansing is started with low-fiber diet, which is started 2 days prior to the procedure. The patient is overnight fasting and drinks 3 to 3.5 L of polyethylene glycol electrolyte solution. For optimal bowel distention, 1.5 to 2.5 L of warm water enema solution may be performed. Intravenous contrast material can be used in combination. Just prior to the rectal instillation of water, an antiperistaltic agent such as 20-mg scopolamine and 1 mg of glucagon is administered. The patient position may be supine or prone. A comprehensive imaging protocol should include both T2- and T1-weighted sequences to help detect and characterize all lesions. True fast imaging with steady-state precession (FISP) is performed in the coronal plane to ensure sufficient and homogeneous filling of the entire colon and rectum. In early disease with mild activity, MR colonography often cannot help detect alterations because the disease is limited to the mucosa and only superficial changes such us edema and hyperemia are present. In severe disease, a granular mucosa with ulcers and inflammatory pseudopolyps may be visualized. Mural thickening, loss of haustra, and luminal narrowing are seen in chronic situations. Submucosal fatty infiltration may also be demonstrated with fat halo sign.[12]

## CROHN DISEASE

Crohn disease is a chronic granulomatous inflammatory disease of the gastrointestinal tract, which can affect any part of the gastrointestinal tract from the mouth to the anus, the hallmarks being multiple discontinuous sites of involvement and a tendency toward remission and relapse. Crohn disease is most often seen in 15- to 25-year age group, with a second smaller peak in the 50- to 80-year age group.[13,14] Involvement of the colon with small bowel occurs in 50% of the cases, while large bowel involvement without small bowel involvement occurs in approximately 20%.[15]

Aphthous ulcer is an early finding, while cobblestone appearance is seen in severe cases (Fig. 5A.11). The other findings include string sign due to spasm or stricture, prestenotic dilatation, pseudodiverticula, skip lesion, fistula, sinus, abscess, increased vascularity of the vasa recta (comb sign), and mesenteric adenopathy (Figs. 5A.12 to 5A.14).[16,17]

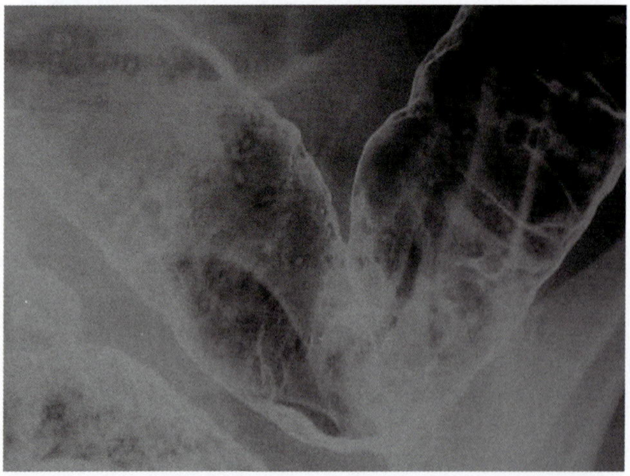

**FIG. 5A.11 • Crohn disease.** Double-contrast barium enema shows multiple superficial aphthous ulcers in the sigmoid colon and distal descending colon.

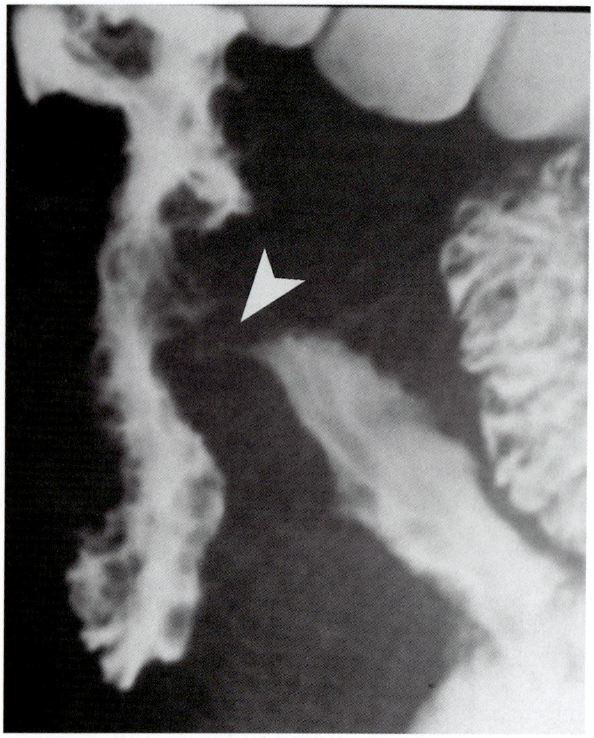

**FIG. 5A.12 • Crohn disease.** Barium meal follow-through images demonstrate stricture of the terminal ileum (*arrowhead*) at the ileocecal junction and cecum.

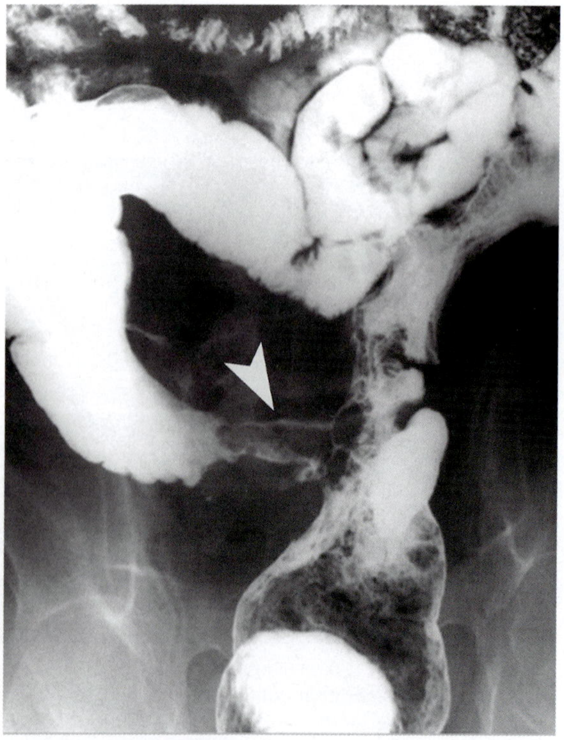

**FIG. 5A.13 • Crohn disease.** SBFT shows enterocolic fistula (*arrowhead*) between the ileum and sigmoid colon.

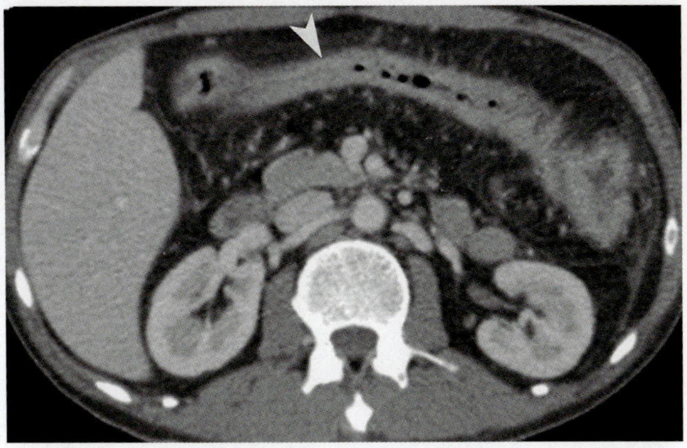

**FIG. 5A.14 • Crohn disease.** Axial contrast-enhanced CT of the abdomen demonstrates the comb sign, which is the hypervascularity in transverse mesocolon. There is transverse colonic wall thickening (*arrowhead*) and pericolonic inflammatory infiltration.

## INFECTIOUS COLITIS

Infectious colitis the is inflammation of the colon due to infective causes, which could be bacterial, viral, fungal, or parasitic. There is overlap of imaging features of infective colitis caused by various organisms; however, different organisms have affinity to particular segments of the colon. Ameba, shigella, and salmonella usually affect the right side of the colon; while gonorrhea, chlamydia, and herpes involve the rectosigmoid, schistosomiasis involves the left colon. Diffuse colonic involvement occurs in cytomegalovirus (Fig. 5A.15) and *Escherichia coli*. Imaging features include colon wall thickening and edema, air–fluid level in the colon, and pericolonic fat stranding.[18] Deep mucosal ulcerations occur in amebic colitis.

## PSEUDOMEMBRANOUS COLITIS

It is caused by *Clostridium difficile* in patients on antibiotics or chemotherapy. On plain radiographs, bowel dilatation, mural thickening, and thumbprinting may be seen (Fig. 5A.16). In patients who are untreated or in those with fulminant disease, toxic megacolon and subsequently perforation and pneumoperitoneum may occur. Barium studies demonstrate findings similar to plain radiography. A pseudomembrane, which is sloughed-off mucosa comprising of fibrin, white cells, and cellular debris, may be visible on double-contrast studies. CT shows bowel wall thickening, shaggy mucosal outline, pericolic stranding, and peritoneal free fluid. An accordion sign may be seen when rectal contrast is given as a result of contrast trapped between edematous haustral folds and pseudomembranes (Fig. 5A.17).[19]

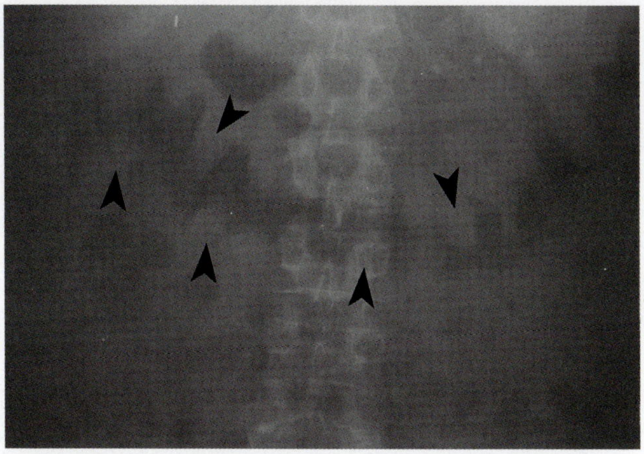

**FIG. 5A.16 • Pseudomembranous colitis.** Plain radiograph of the abdomen shows thumbprinting (*arrowheads*) of the transverse colon (thumb-like indentations on the air-filled lumen).

## ILEOCECAL TUBERCULOSIS

Although tuberculosis (TB) can affect any part of the gastrointestinal tract, ileocecal region is the most common site to be affected. Computed tomography can detect these changes as well as extraluminal changes, abscesses, and complications. The findings on barium study include the following:

- Thickening of the ileocecal valve, gaping of the valve, and narrowing of the terminal ileum are called inverted umbrella signs of Fleischner.
- Gooseneck deformity is caused by loss of normal ileocecal angle and dilated terminal ileum, appearing suspended from a retracted fibrosed cecum (Fig. 5A.18).

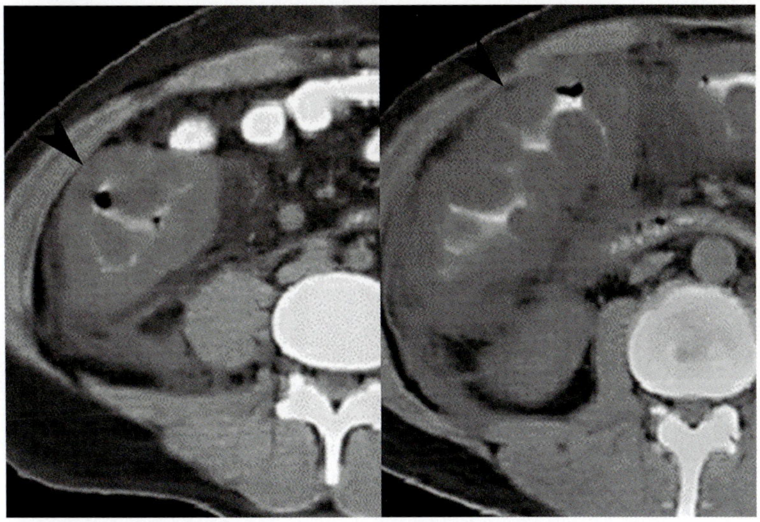

**FIG. 5A.15 • CMV colitis.** In an HIV-infected patient, axial contrast-enhanced CT of the abdomen shows extensive colonic wall (*arrowheads*) and haustral fold thickening.

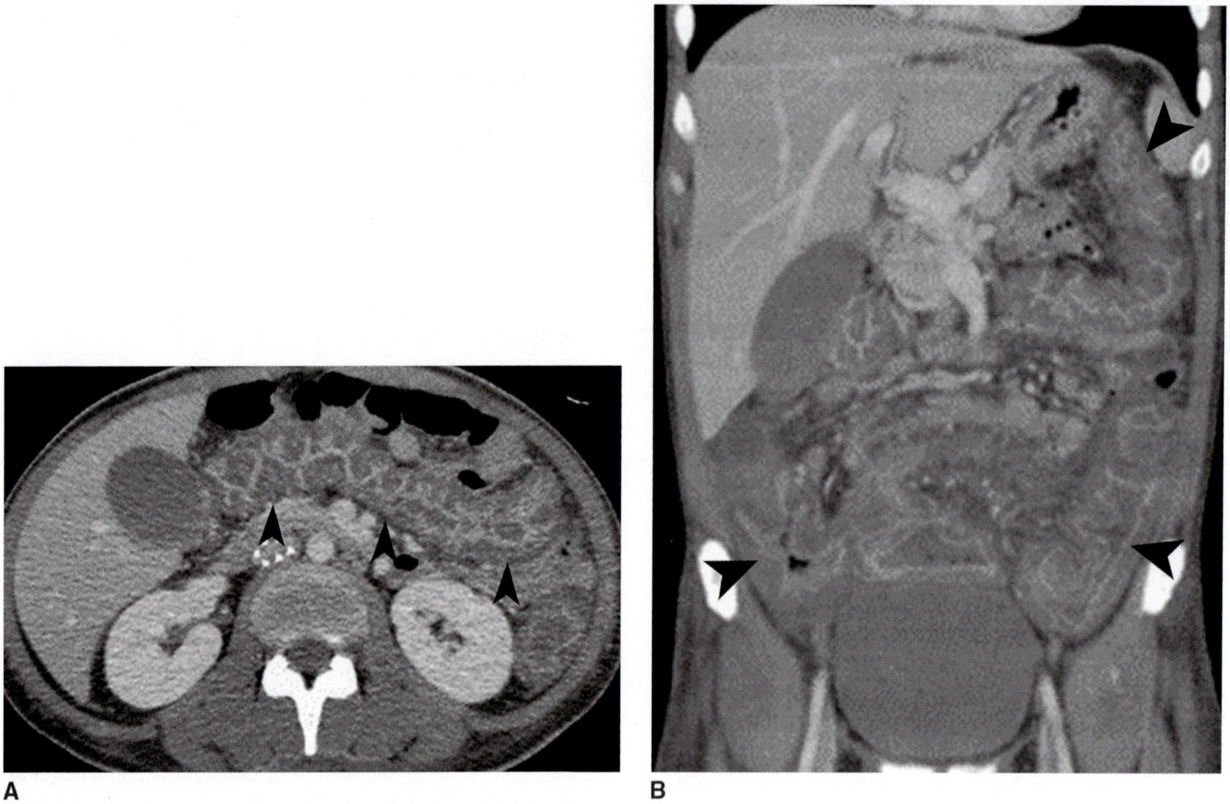

FIG. 5A.17 • **Pseudomembranous colitis. A, B:** Axial contrast-enhanced CT images show extensive submucosal edema in the colonic wall (*arrowheads*), simulating accordion sign.

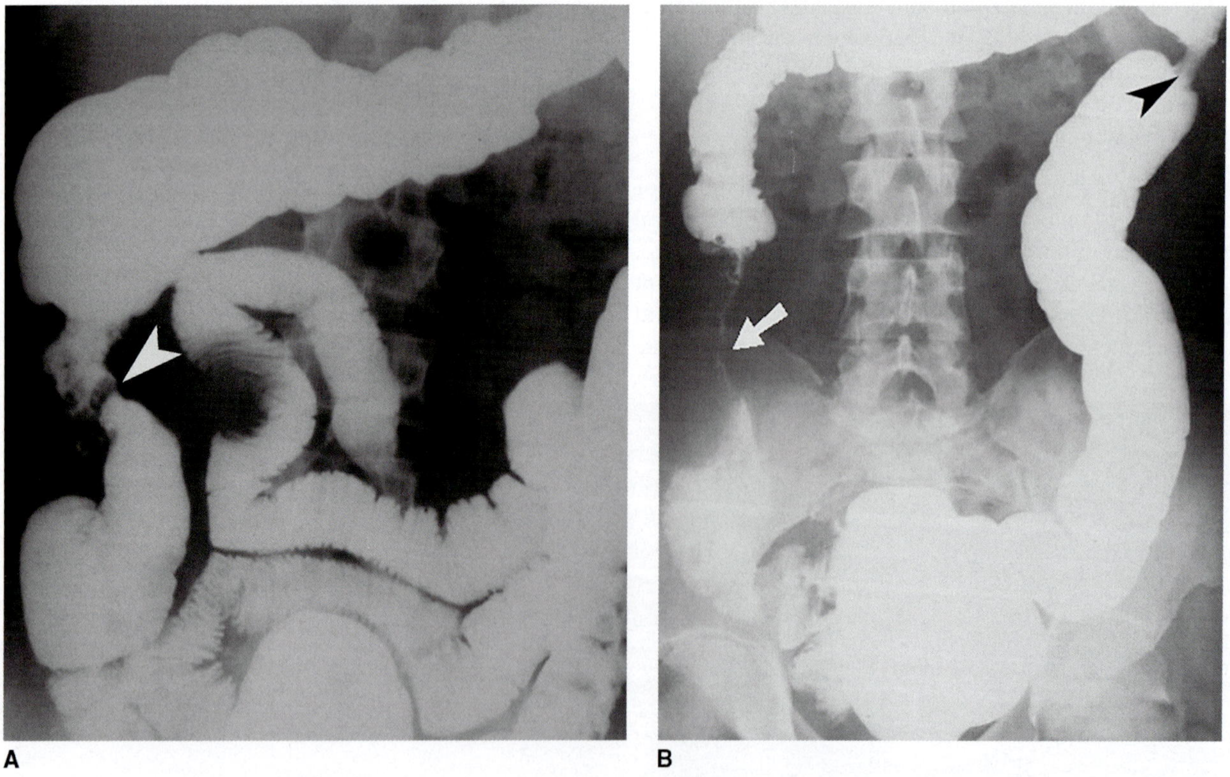

FIG. 5A.18 • **Ileocecal tuberculosis. A:** SBFT shows gooseneck deformity caused by loss of normal ileocecal angle and dilated terminal ileum, appearing suspended from a retracted fibrosed cecum (*arrowhead*). **B:** SBFT shows stricture of the terminal ileum (*arrow*) with proximal dilatation of the ileum. The cecum is extensively fibrosed and retracted upward. There is a second stricture seen in the proximal descending colon (*arrowhead*).

- Conical cecum is shrunken in size and pulled out of the iliac fossa due to contraction and fibrosis of the mesocolon.
- Purse string stenosis is due to localized stenosis opposite the ileocecal valve with a rounded off smooth cecum and a dilated terminal ileum.
- Stierlin sign is due to the lack of barium retention in the inflamed segments of the ileum, cecum, and variable length of the ascending colon with a normal configured column of barium on either side.
- String sign is a persistent narrow stream of barium indicating stenosis.[20]

## ISCHEMIC COLITIS

Ischemic colitis is one of the common vascular disorders of the colon in the elderly and usually occurs in the seventh decade of life.[21] Ischemic colitis can be classified as occlusive and nonocclusive arterial and venous etiology.[22] Nonocclusive ischemic colitis can be caused by low-flow states like hypotension, congestive heart failure, and cardiac arrhythmias. Bowel overdistention can cause ischemia as a result of compromised local microcirculation due to the elevation of intraluminal pressure (e.g., Ogilvie syndrome).[23] The splenic flexure and rectosigmoid junction are watershed areas that are susceptible to ischemia.

Plain radiographs may demonstrate thumbprinting and ileus. Pneumatosis coli may occur due to necrosis and localized intramural air. With peritonitis, generalized ileus may be seen. Similar to the plain film, barium enema may show thumbprinting on single-contrast study, local spasm, and serrated mucosa (Fig. 5A.19).

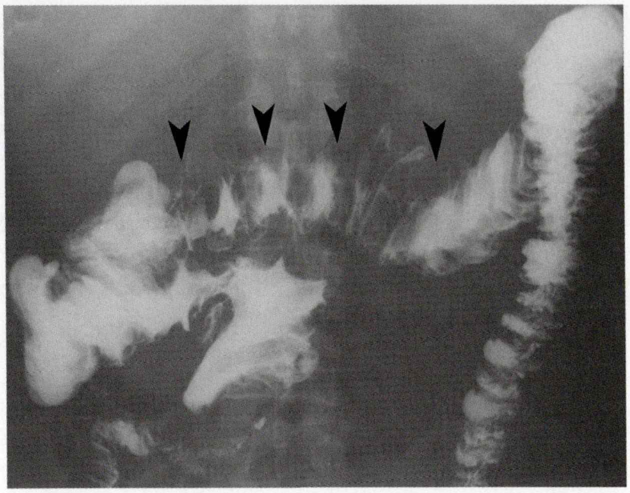

**FIG. 5A.19 • Ischemic colitis.** Single-contrast barium shows submucosal edema, resulting in thumbprinting (*arrowheads*) of the transverse colon.

Initial acquisition of unenhanced CT scans will delineate vascular calcifications, hyperdense intravascular clot, and acute submucosal or intramural hemorrhage. Intravenous administration of contrast material is necessary to demonstrate the presence of thrombi in the mesenteric arteries or veins (Fig. 5A.20). CT demonstrates a gray attenuation sign with thickened, hypoenhancing or nonenhancing bowel wall.[24] A water halo sign may also be seen, which is thickened bowel wall consisting of either two or three symmetrically thickened layers. Double halo sign is composed of either a higher-attenuation outer annular ring of muscularis propria surrounding a second luminally oriented annular ring of gray attenuation or a higher-attenuation inner layer of mucosa with outer ring of gray attenuation. The target sign is composed of three rings consisting of outer high-attenuation muscularis propria, a middle ring of gray attenuation submucosa, and a luminally oriented ring of high-attenuation mucosa.[24] Other features of ischemic colitis include dilatation, absent wall enhancement, mesenteric stranding, vascular engorgement, ascites, pneumatosis, perforation, and portal venous gas. Paper-thin colonic wall may be found in conditions where ischemia is not followed by effective reperfusion.[25]

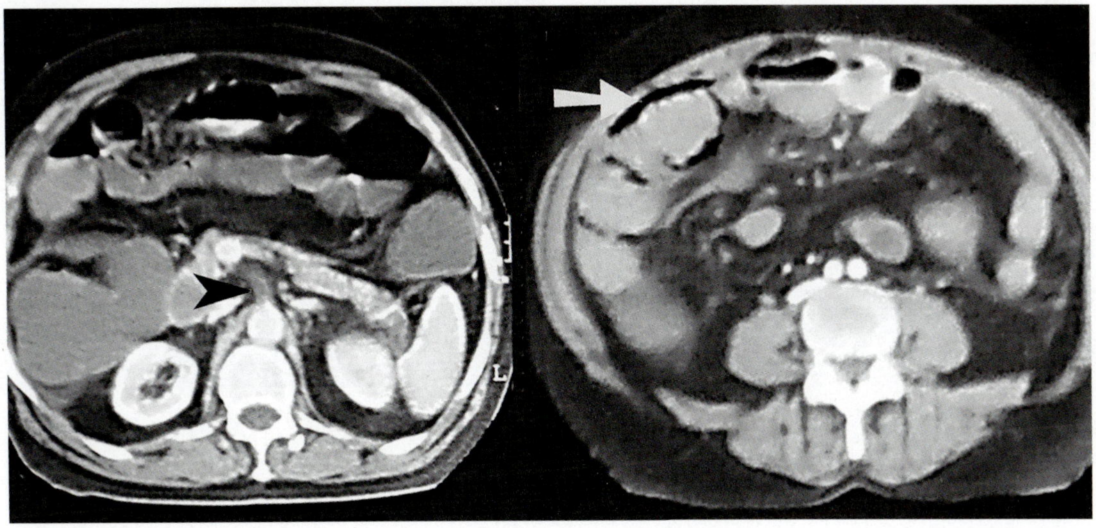

**FIG. 5A.20 • Ischemic colitis.** Axial contrast-enhanced CT of the abdomen in a 70-year-old patient with lower gastrointestinal bleeding demonstrates SMA thrombus (*arrowhead*) and pneumatosis coli (*arrow*).

## RADIATION COLITIS

Greater than half of all patients receiving more than 3,000 cGy of radiation to the pelvis will experience acute proctitis.[26] Radiation colitis, which is usually self-limiting, occurs during the first few weeks of radiation exposure, and imaging typically is not necessary for the diagnosis. CT demonstrates nonspecific inflammatory stranding of the affected segment of the colon with water halo sign, similar to that seen in ischemic colitis.[24] Chronic radiation injury of the colon and rectum can lead to nonspecific wall thickening, increased pelvic fat, thickening of the perirectal fibrous tissue, strictures, and fistulas.[4,26]

## LARGE BOWEL OBSTRUCTION

Colorectal cancers are the most common cause of the large bowel obstruction in the Western world. Other causes of large bowel obstruction are diverticulitis, inflammatory bowel disease, volvulus, ischemic strictures, hernias, pelvic malignancy, and fecal impaction.

On plain radiograph, the large bowel dilates proximal to the site of obstruction with a cutoff value of 9 cm for the cecum and 6 cm for the rest of the colon. Multiple air–fluid levels within the large bowel are seen. If the ileocecal valve is patent, the small bowel loops also dilate. In advanced cases, pneumatosis coli and pneumoperitoneum may be seen. Ultrasound can play an important role in differentiating obstruction from paralytic ileus. In obstruction, there will be an initial increase in peristalsis; however, with the progression of obstruction, there will be a decrease in peristalsis. In paralytic ileus, there will be absence of peristalsis, which can be detected by the presence of akinesis of more than 5 minutes.[1] Computed tomography plays an important modality in identifying the site and cause of obstruction. It allows early diagnosis of complications such as ischemia, incarceration, and perforation.

## VOLVULUS

Volvulus is the twisting around of the bowel around its mesentery. Redundant mesentery and chronic constipation are some of the risk factors. Sigmoid volvulus (50% to 75%) is the most common type of large bowel volvulus, cecal volvulus (25% to 40%) being the second most common. Other parts of the colon that may undergo volvulus include the transverse colon, splenic flexure, and compound volvulus or ileosigmoid knot. Unlike cecal volvulus, which occurs in 20- to 40-year age group, sigmoid volvulus is most common in older population.

On plain radiography, sigmoid volvulus is seen as a dilated ahaustral air-filled sigmoid colonic loop with inverted U appearance giving a coffee bean appearance arising from the pelvis. Frimann-Dahl sign is the presence of three dense lines converging toward the site of obstruction (Fig. 5A.21A). There is an absence of rectal gas with complete obstruction.[27]

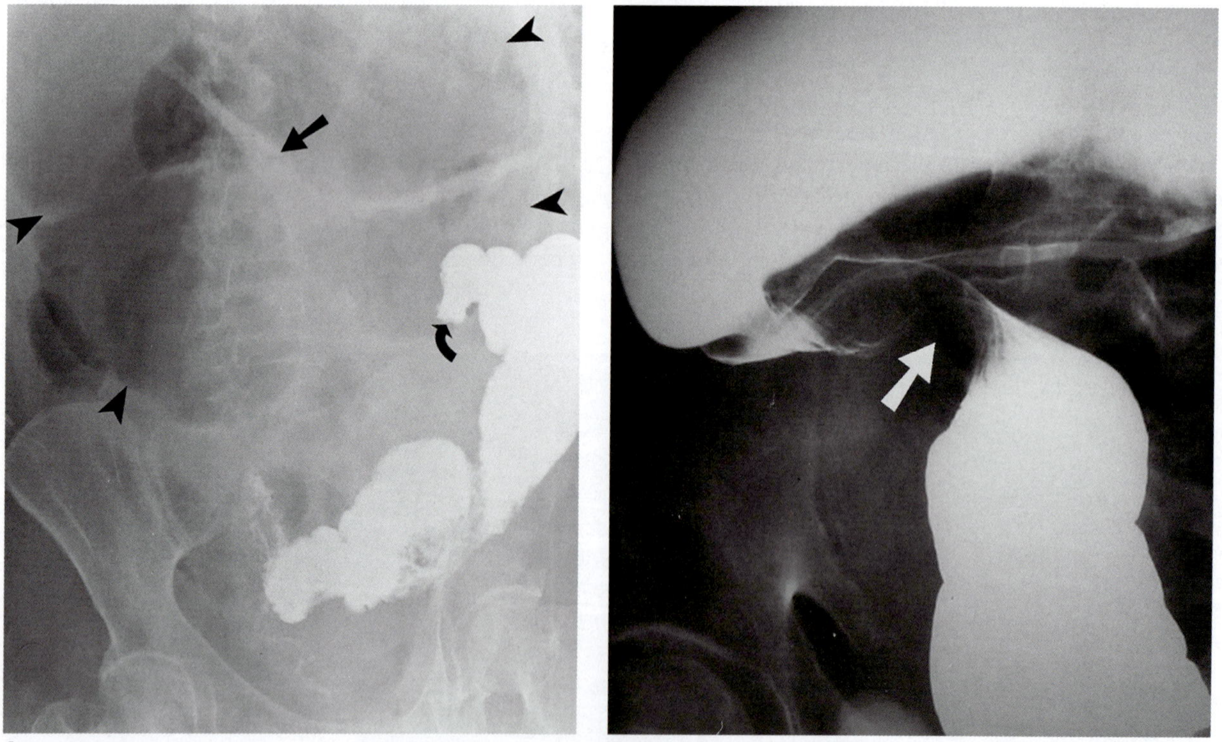

A B

**FIG. 5A.21 • Colonic volvulus. A:** Single-contrast barium enema shows inverted U appearance of the dilated sigmoid colon (*arrowheads*), giving a coffee bean appearance. There are three dense lines consisting of two lines caused by lateral walls of the sigmoid loop and one line caused by opposed medial walls (*straight arrow*) of the sigmoid loop. These three lines converging toward the site of obstruction is called Frimann-Dahl sign and suggests sigmoid volvulus. There is obstruction to the flow of contrast in the distal sigmoid colon (*curved arrow*). **B:** Single-contrast barium enema shows smooth tapering (*arrow*) toward the point of torsion at rectosigmoid junction, consistent with bird-of-prey sign.

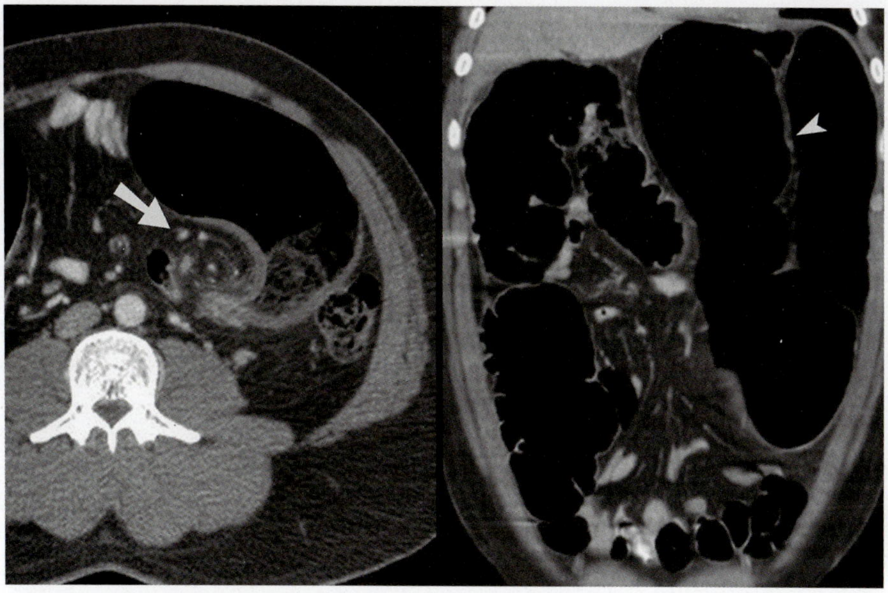

**FIG. 5A.22 • Sigmoid volvulus.** Axial contrast-enhanced CT of the abdomen shows whirl sign (*arrow*) at the site of the torsion. Coronal CT reformation demonstrates dilated sigmoid colonic loop extending up to the left upper quadrant, with two walls opposed together (*arrowhead*).

Cecal volvulus is often seen as a round air-filled dilated loop with haustral markings in the left upper abdomen. Depending upon the length and mobility of the colon, the distended twisted cecum can be found anywhere from the right lower quadrant to the epigastrium or left upper quadrant.[28]

Water-soluble contrast is preferred over the barium with avoidance of air insufflation to minimize the risk of perforation. There is smooth tapering toward the point of torsion, giving a "bird-beak" appearance or "bird-of-prey sign" (Fig. 5A.21B).

On CT, the two limbs of the sigmoid colonic loop taper to converge at the site of the torsion. Bird-beak sign although originally applied to the appearance of sigmoid volvulus on conventional radiographs can also be appreciated on CT images (best seen on coronal or sagittal reformations). The whirl sign is a CT-specific sign for volvulus, which is composed of spiraled loops of collapsed cecum, low-attenuating fatty mesentery with enhancing engorged vessels radiating from the twisted bowel (Fig. 5A.22). Tapering of the afferent limb and efferent limb toward the point of torsion can be seen.[27,28]

## LARGE BOWEL TRAUMA

Bowel and mesentery injuries are more likely with gunshot and stab injuries than with blunt abdominal trauma. The mechanism of injury is crush or compression type, shearing type (from fixed point of mesentery) or burst type (from increased intraluminal pressure).[29] The types of injury include perforation, mural hematoma, edema, serosal tear, and active hemorrhage (Fig. 5A.23). Mesenteric injuries include laceration with active bleeding or hematoma.[29] Moderate or large volume of free fluid without solid organ injury is suspicious for bowel or mesenteric injury. Bowel wall hyperenhancement may be seen due to vascular permeability secondary to hypoperfusion. Shock bowel may occur due to posttraumatic hypovolemic

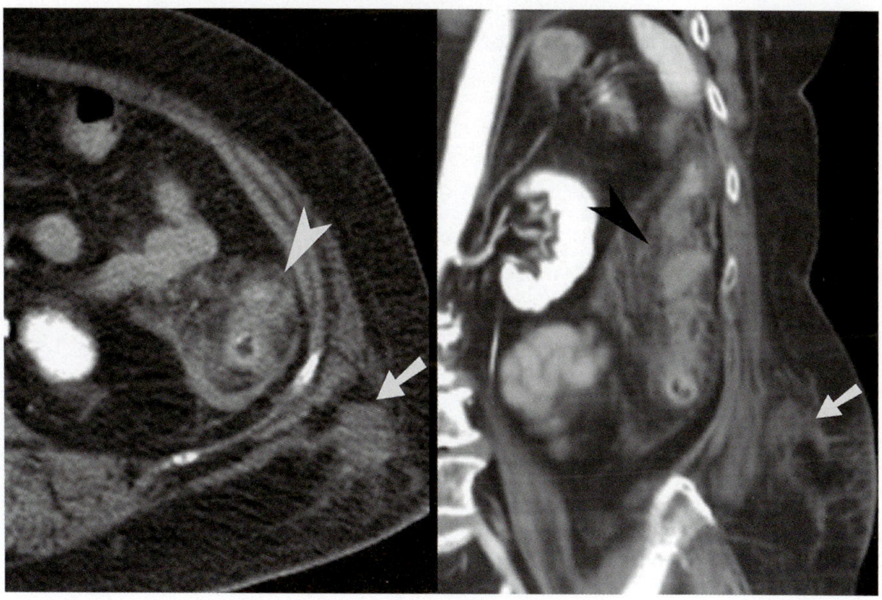

**FIG. 5A.23 • Colonic trauma.** Axial and coronal contrast-enhanced CT of the abdomen in a patient with history of blunt trauma shows descending colon wall thickening and pericolonic fat stranding suggesting colonic wall contusion (*arrowhead*) with associated mesenteric injury. Subcutaneous tissue injury (*arrow*) is seen in the left lateral abdominal wall.

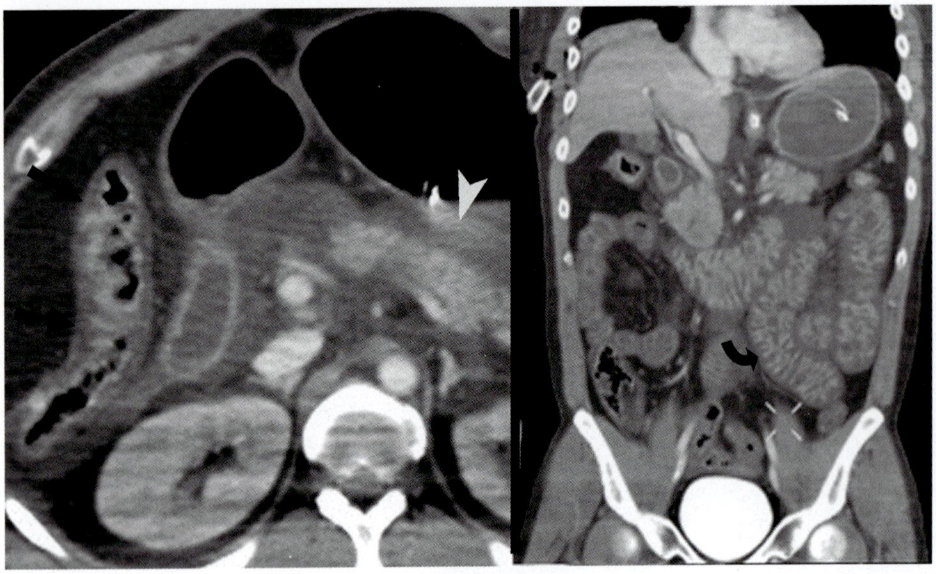

**FIG. 5A.24 • Hypoperfusion complex.** Axial and coronal contrast-enhanced CT images show thickened small bowel (*curved arrow*) and large bowel loops (*arrows*) with enhancing mucosa, small caliber abdominal aorta, and peripancreatic fluid (*arrowhead*).

shock (Fig. 5A.24) (thickened bowel loops with enhancing walls with white attenuation pattern of bowel wall, together with other visceral manifestations).[30]

## LOWER GASTROINTESTINAL TRACT BLEEDING

Lower gastrointestinal bleeding is defined as bleeding distal to the ligament of Treitz. On the arterial phase of CT imaging, active bleeding will demonstrate intraluminal extravasation of contrast material, which helps in identifying the origin of the bleeding. The change from noncontrast CT, which shows no intraluminal hyperattenuation to the appearance of a blush on arterial phase imaging, which blooms on portal venous phase, confirms the presence of active bleeding.[31] One of the more common causes of lower GI bleeding is diverticulosis (Fig. 5A.25). Nodular hypertrophied submucosal vessels in angiodysplasia and nodular vessels extending through the mucosa and submucosa into the muscular layer of the bowel in arteriovenous malformation (AVM)

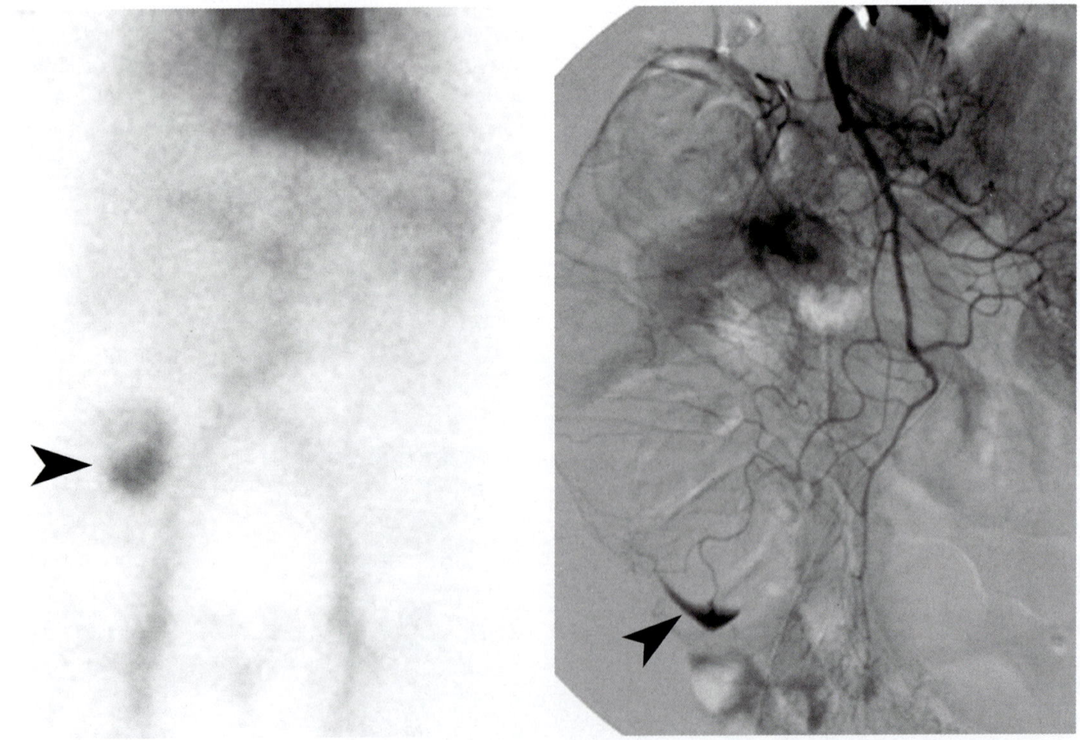

A B

**FIG. 5A.25 • Active diverticular bleeding. A–B:** Tc-99 RBC scan and digital subtraction angiography demonstrates active bleeding (*arrowhead*) in the right lower quadrant. **C:** Arterial phase, coronal MIP-reformatted image demonstrates active extravasation of contrast (*arrow*) in the descending colon.

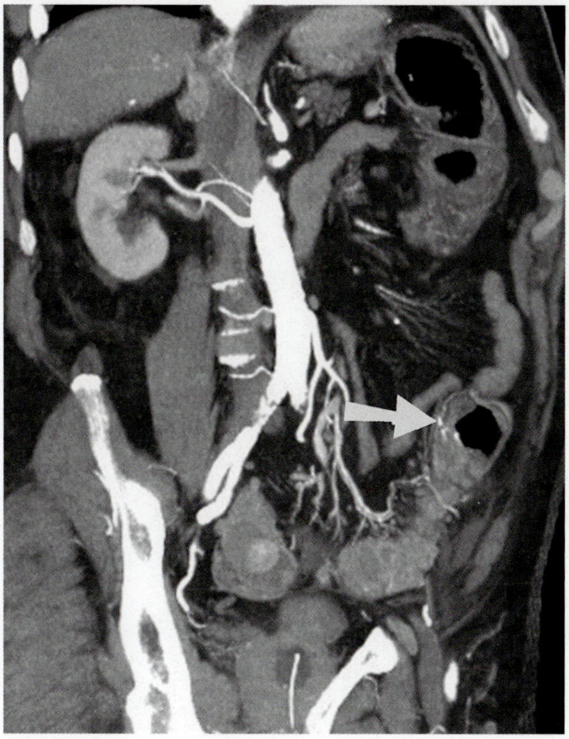

C

**FIG. 5A.25** • (*Continued*)

can be seen on the arterial phase images with an early draining vein (Fig. 5A.26). Other causes for lower GI bleeding include ischemic colitis, inflammatory bowel disease, infective colitis, chronic radiation proctopathy, and CRC. CT angiography detects active bleeding that exceeds 0.3 to 0.5 mL/min, a rate that is slightly higher than the threshold assigned to catheter angiography (0.5 mL/min), and a rate that is lower than that of scintigraphy with 99mTc-labeled red blood cells.[31]

## INTUSSUSCEPTION

Intussusception is characterized by telescoping of the intussusceptum into a distal bowel segment called intussuscipiens. In children, majority of the patients with intussusception do not have a pathologic lead point. Peak incidence of intussusception is seen in infants less than 10 months of age. In adult population, 90% of the intussusceptions have an underlying cause, which most commonly includes neoplastic process and less likely other causes such as venous malformation, Meckel diverticulum, and inflammation. In adults, small bowel intussusception without a lead point is more common than one with a lead point. In adults, large bowel intussusception is mostly due to a lead point, which is most often malignant neoplasm. Colonic adenocarcinoma is the commonest malignant neoplasm, and lipoma the commonest benign tumor causing colonic intussusception.

On barium enema, barium between the intussusceptum and intussuscipiens produces a coiled spring appearance. On ultrasound imaging, a target or doughnut sign is seen, characterized by hypoechoic intussuscipiens wall, surrounding hyperechoic central intussusceptum, and mesenteric fat (Fig. 5A.27A). On CT scan study, intussusception is seen on transverse imaging of the bowel loop as target sign, characterized by concentric bowel wall rings, with fat in between (Fig. 5A.27B).

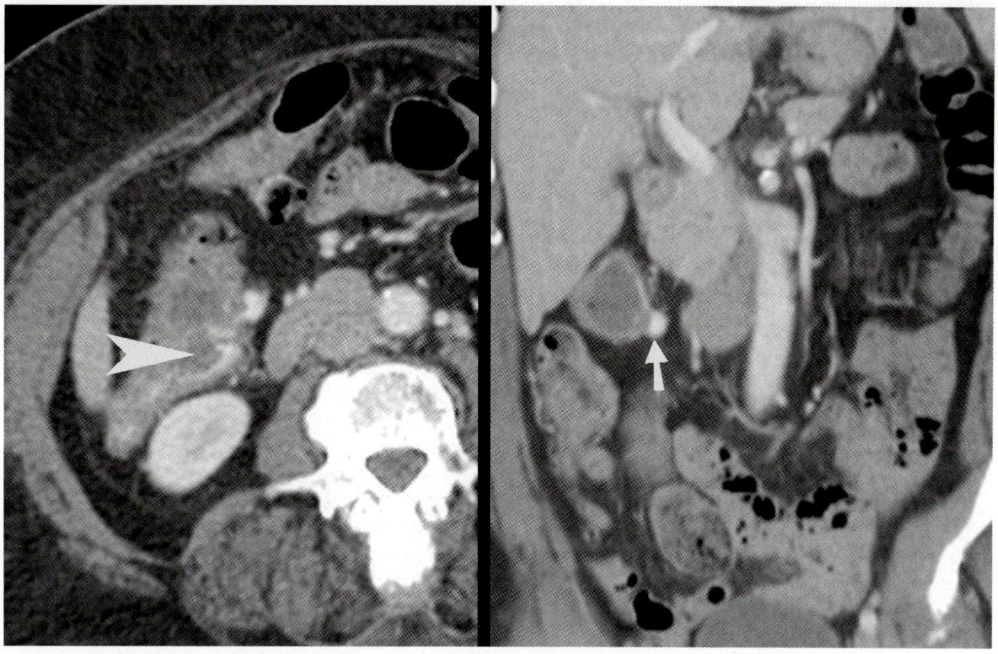

**FIG. 5A.26** • **Arteriovenous malformation of hepatic flexure.** Axial and coronal contrast-enhanced CT of the abdomen demonstrates distinct vascular nidus (*arrow*) within the hepatic flexure wall with early filling of veins. The intraluminal extravagated contrast due to active bleeding (*arrowhead*) is evident.

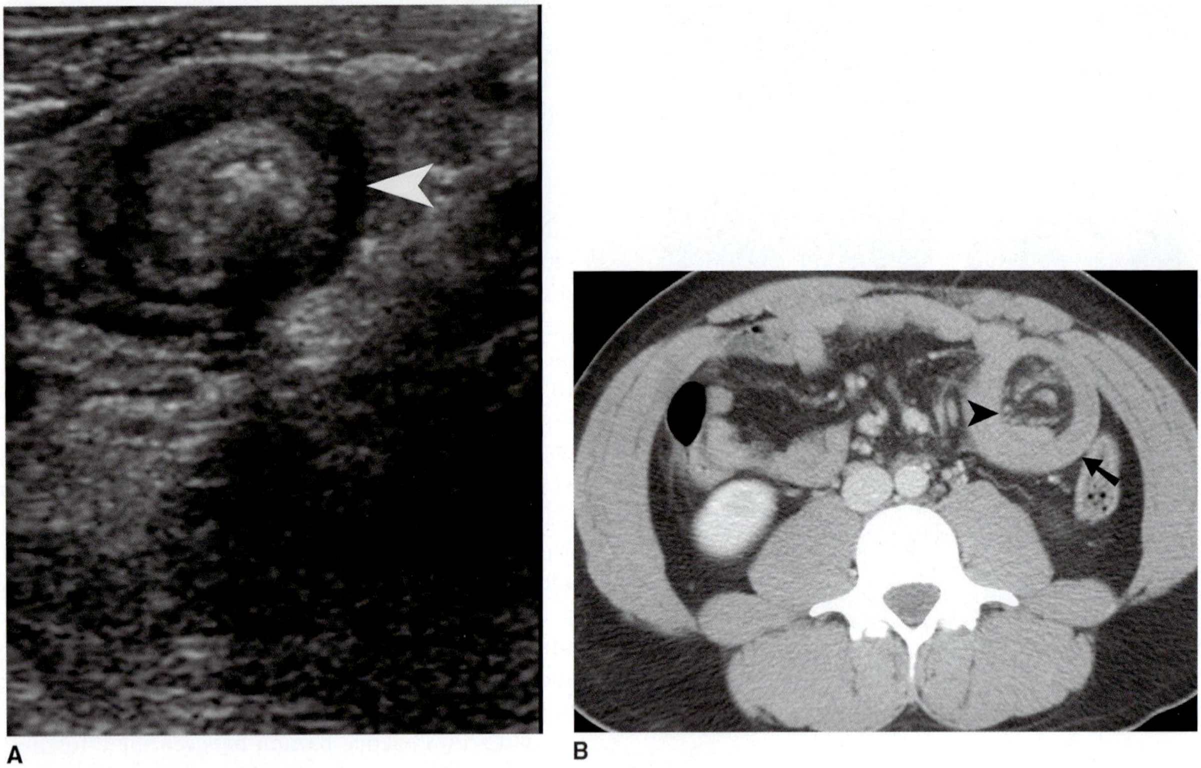

**FIG. 5A.27 • Intussusception. A:** US demonstrates central hyperechoic intussusceptum and outer hypoechoic intussuscipiens (*arrowhead*). **B:** Axial contrast-enhanced CT shows outer intussuscipiens (*arrow*) and central fat density from mesenteric fat (*arrowhead*).

## References


1. Avunduk C. *Manual of Gastroenterology, Diagnosis and Therapy*. Philadelphia, PA: Lippincott Williams & Wilkins; 2008.
2. Ferzoco LB, Raptopoulos V, Silen W. Acute diverticulitis. *N Engl J Med*. 1998;338:1521–1526.
3. Keller CE, Halpert RD, Feczko PJ, et al. Radiologic recognition of colonic diverticula simulating polyps. *AJR Am J Roentgenol*. 1984;143(1):93–97.
4. Hinchey EJ, Schaal PG, Richards GK. Treatment of perforated diverticular disease of the colon. *Adv Surg*. 1979;12:85–109.
5. Horton KM, Corl FM, Fishman EK. CT evaluation of the colon: inflammatory disease. *Radiographics*. 2000;20(2).
6. Sai VF, Velayos F, Neuhaus J, et al. Colonoscopy after CT diagnosis of diverticulitis to exclude colon cancer: a systematic literature review. *Radiology*. 2012;263(2):383–390. doi: 10.1148/radiol.12111869.
7. Singh AK, Gervais DA, Hahn PF, et al. CT appearance of acute appendagitis. *AJR Am J Roentgenol*. 2004;183(5):1303–1307.
8. Loftus EV Jr. Clinical epidemiology of inflammatory bowel disease: incidence, prevalence, and environmental influences. *Gastroenterology*. 2004;126:1504–1517.
9. Kornbluth A, Sachar DB. Ulcerative colitis practice guidelines in adults (update): American College of Gastroenterology, Practice Parameters Committee. *Am J Gastroenterol*. 2004;99:1371–1385.
10. Jalan KN, Sircus W, Card WI, et al. An experience of ulcerative colitis. I. Toxic dilation in 55 cases. *Gastroenterology*. 1969;57:68–82.
11. Gore RM, Marn CS, Kirby DF, et al. CT findings in ulcerative, granulomatous, and indeterminate colitis. *AJR Am J Roentgenol*. 1984;143(2):279–284.
12. Rimola J, Orlando SR, Bosch OG, et al. Role of 3.0-T MR colonography in the evaluation of inflammatory Bowel disease. *Radiographics*. 2009;29(3):701–719.
13. Fleischer DE, Grimm IS, Friedman LS. Inflammatory bowel disease in older patients. *Med Clin North Am* 1994;78:1303–1319.
14. Przemioslo RT, Ciclitira PJ. Pathogenesis of Crohn's disease. *QJM*. 1995;88:525–527.
15. Herlinger H, Caroline DF. Crohn's disease of the small bowel. In: Gore RM, Lenine MS, eds. *Textbook of Gastrointestinal Radiology*. 2nd ed. Philadelphia, PA: Saunders; 2000;726–745.
16. Del Campo L, Arribas I, Valbuena M, et al. Spiral CT findings in active and remission phases in patients with Crohn disease. *J Comput Assist Tomogr*. 2001;25:792–797.
17. Holzknecht N, Helmberger T, von Ritter C, et al. Breathhold MRI of the small bowel in Crohn's disease after enteroclysis with oral magnetic particles. *Radiologe*. 1998;38:29–36.
18. Thoeni RF, Cello JP. CT imaging of colitis. *Radiology*. 2006; 240(3):623–638.
19. Kirkpatrick ID, Greenberg HM. Evaluating the CT diagnosis of *Clostridium difficile* colitis: should CT guide therapy? *AJR Am J Roentgenol*. 2001;176(3):635–639.
20. Bandyopadhyay S. Tuberculosis in gastroenterology practice: clinical challenges. *Medicin Update*. 2011. apiindia.org.
21. Sotiriadis J, Brandt LJ, Behin DS, et al. Ischemic colitis has a worse prognosis when isolated to the right side of the colon. *Am J Gastroenterol*. 2007;102:(10):2247–2252.
22. Brandt L, Boley S, Goldberg L, et al. Colitis in the elderly. *Am J Gastroenterol*. 1981;76:239–245.
23. Saegesser F, Sandblom P. Ischemic lesions of the distended colon: a complication of obstructive colorectal cancer. *Am J Surg*. 1975;129:309–315.
24. Wittenberg J, Harisinghani MG, Jhaveri JK, et al. Algorithmic approach to CT diagnosis of the abnormal bowel wall. *Educ Exhib—CME*. 2002;22(5).
25. Mazzei MA, Mazzei FG, Marrelli D. Computed tomographic evaluation of mesentery: diagnostic value in acute mesenteric ischemia. *J Comput Assist Tomogr*. 2012;36(1):1–7.
26. Otchy DP, Nelson H. Radiation injuries of the colon and rectum. *Surg Clin North Am*. 1993;73:1017–1035.

27. Levsky JM, Den EI, Dubrow RA, et al. CT findings of sigmoid volvulus. *AJR Am J Roentgenol.* 2010;194(1):136–143. doi: 10.2214/AJR.09.2580.
28. Frank AJ, Goffner LB, Fruauff AA, et al. Cecal volvulus: the CT whirl sign. *Abdom Imaging.* 1993;18(3):288–289.
29. Butela ST, Federle MP, Chang PJ, et al. Performance of CT in detection of bowel injury. *AJR Am J Roentgenol.* 2001;176(1):129–135.
30. Tarrant AM, Ryan MF, Hamilton PA, et al. A pictorial review of hypovolaemic shock in adults. *Br J Radiol.* 2008;81(963): 252–257.
31. Artigas JM, Martí M, Soto JA, et al. Multidetector CT angiography for acute gastrointestinal bleeding: technique and findings. *Radiographics.* 2013;33(5):1453–1470.

## SELF-ASSESSMENT QUESTIONS

1. What is the most common cause of colocolic intussusception?
   A. Lipoma
   B. Duplication cyst
   C. Lymphoma
   D. Adenocarcinoma

2. Which segment of the bowel is dilated on the plain film?

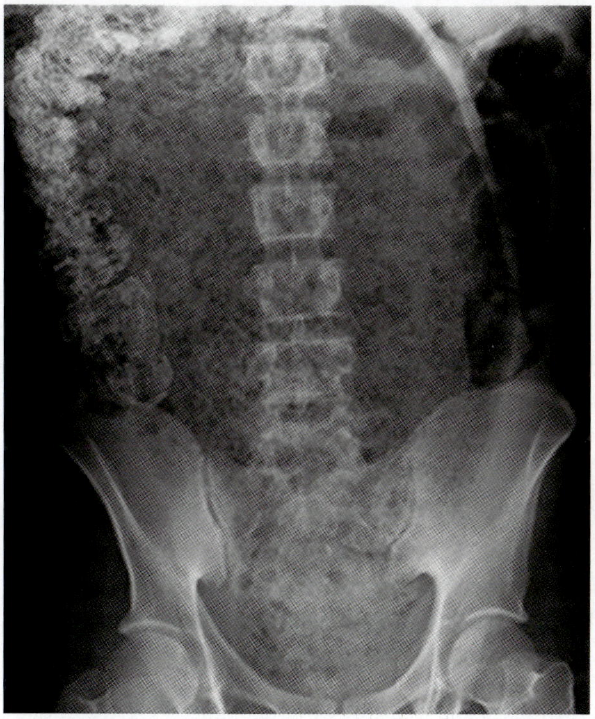

   A. Cecum
   B. Sigmoid colon
   C. Stomach
   D. Small bowel

3. What is the classical sign shown on the CT?

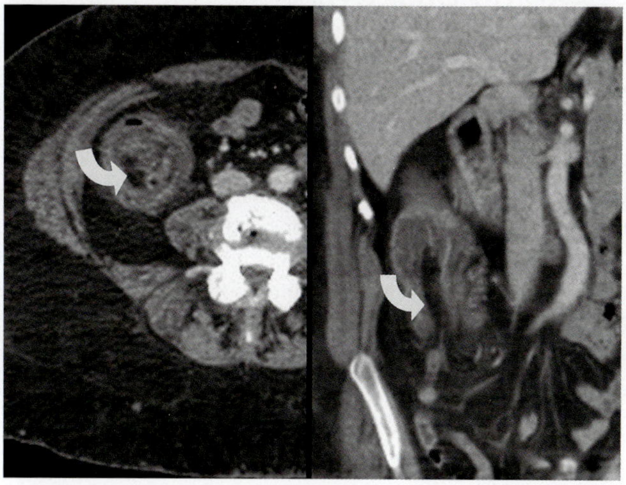

   A. Target sign
   B. Whirl sign
   C. Accordion sign
   D. Comb sign

### Answers to Self-Assessment Questions

**1. D.** Adenocarcinoma. In adults, large bowel intussusception is mostly due to a lead point, which is most often malignant neoplasm. Colonic adenocarcinoma is the most common malignant, and lipoma is the most common benign neoplasm causing colocolic intussusception.

**2. B.** The plain radiograph demonstrates large amount of fecal matter in the sigmoid colon and rectum. The cecum and ascending colon are opacified with intraluminal contrast.

**3. A.** Target sign. On CT, the target sign is seen as concentric bowel wall rings, with fat in between.

# Large Bowel: Neoplastic Lesions

# 5B

*Vijetha Vinod Maller, Vijay S. Pande, Randall L. Scott, and Sridhar Shankar*

## LEARNING OBJECTIVE

**1.** Review the imaging features of the benign and malignant neoplastic pathologies of the colon.

Colorectal cancer is the third most common cancer and the third leading cause of cancer death in the United States. Although screening for colon cancer includes several different tests, the CDC recommends occult blood and sigmoidoscopy/colonoscopy only. While advances in CT colonography and MR colonography rival optical colonoscopy in terms of accuracy for the detection of lesions, widespread adoption has been slow because of the lack of support from third-party payers.

## COLONIC POLYPS

Colonic polyps are seen in 10% of the population, most commonly in the left colon. Colonic polyps are sessile or pedunculated lesions protruding from the colonic mucosa and can be nonneoplastic or neoplastic. Nonneoplastic polyps can be hyperplastic, hamartomatous, or inflammatory in nature. Neoplastic polyps are adenomatous and are further classified as tubular, tubulovillous, or villous. Villous polyps have an increased risk of adenocarcinoma. Adenomatous polyps less than 1 cm have 1% risk of adenocarcinoma, polyps 1 to 2 cm have 10% to 20% risk, and polyps greater than 2 cm have a nearly 50% risk.[1] Any polyp more than 0.5 cm in diameter is typically resected.

Polyps can be syndromic or acquired, and polyposis syndromes may be familial inherited (autosomal dominant) or nonfamilial. Inherited polyposis syndromes can further be subdivided depending on whether or not the polyps are adenomas or hamartomas. Adenomatous polyposis syndromes include the classic familial adenomatous polyposis (FAP) (Fig. 5B.1), Gardner syndrome (Fig. 5B.2), and Turcot syndrome, all of which have extremely high risk for the development of colorectal cancers. Hamartomatous familial polyposis syndromes include Peutz-Jeghers syndrome, juvenile polyposis syndrome, Cowden disease, and Ruvalcaba-Myhre-Smith syndrome. Noninherited polyposis syndromes include the Cronkhite-Canada syndrome among others.

Acquired causes include sporadic adenomatous polyps, hyperplastic polyps, and inflammatory polyps. Hyperplastic polyps are found frequently at colonoscopy and represent a large fraction of polyps smaller than 1 cm.

On barium enema, sessile polyps on the dependent wall appear as a radiolucent filling defect, while those on the nondependent wall show a ring shadow with barium-coated white rim on en face view.

**Bowler-hat sign:** It is seen with both polyps and diverticulum. It is seen on oblique views of polyp, due to the projection of the rim of barium adjacent to the base of the polyp surrounding a layer of barium coating the surface of the polyp (Fig. 5B.3A).

**Mexican hat sign:** It is seen with pedunculated polyps where the meniscus of barium around the stalk is surrounded by second ring of barium around the dome of polyp.

Villous sessile adenomatous polyps are larger in size than hyperplastic polyps (Fig. 5B.3B, C). There is barium trapped within the indentations of the irregular surface giving it a frond-like appearance. Carpet lesions (flat/sessile) may be noted with elevation of the mucosal surface with little or no protrusion into the lumen. Tiny coalescent plaques appear as a fine nodular and reticular pattern on en face views.

CT colonography is a minimally invasive examination of the colon to evaluate colorectal polyps. Screening studies are performed using a low-dose, nonenhanced CT technique on a multidetector CT in prone and supine position after colonic distention by rectal air/$CO_2$ insufflation. Bowel preparation and tagging can be performed prior to the procedure.[2] The use of water-soluble contrast alone or in combination with low-volume barium is the preferred tagging method. The goal of tagging is to incorporate contrast into any residual fluid and stool, which helps to differentiate these from polyps. The acquired image data set is then displayed on a workstation with image analysis software that renders images simulating those obtained at conventional colonoscopy. These software programs display the images for analysis by the radiologist in two-dimensional (2D) and three-dimensional (3D) display formats (Fig. 5B.4). 3D fly-through technique and virtual dissection help in the detection of polyps.

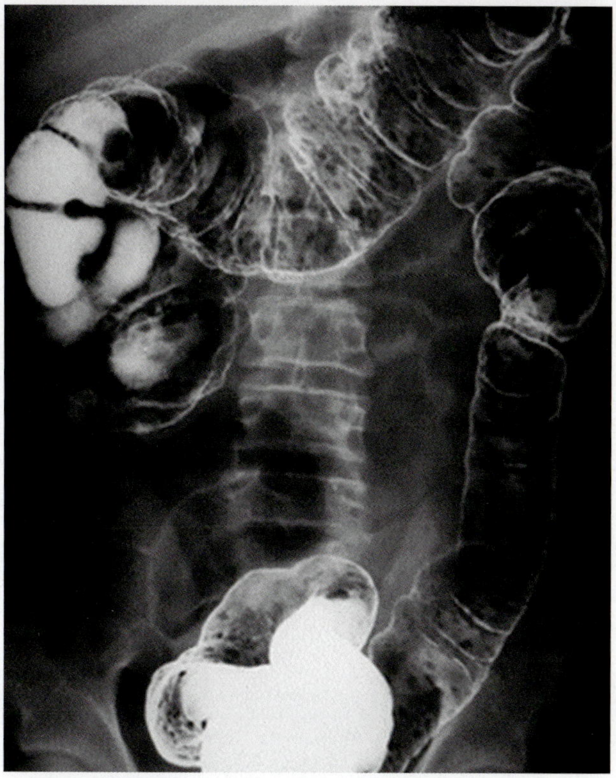

**FIG. 5B.1 • Familial adenomatous polyposis.** Double-contrast barium enema shows numerous radiolucent filling defects and ring shadows etched with barium, consistent with polyps.

Diagnostic CTC may require intravenous contrast to characterize intracolonic and extracolonic structures. Typically, sessile and flat polyps appear flame or pea shaped, while pedunculated polyps are more varied and may be flame, club, or bizarre shaped (Fig. 5B.5).[3] Diagnostic contrast-enhanced CT colonography should include an initial low-dose noncontrast prone series followed by a supine series with intravenous contrast and normal dose. It is important to note that there is some consensus among practitioners that polyps less than 4 mm in diameter are not clinically significant and may not be reported.

MR colonography involves bowel preparation and stool tagging methods similar to CT colonography. The use of an antispasmodic agent such as butyl scopolamine or glucagon is recommended to minimize peristalsis-related artifacts at MR colonography. There are two methods of colonic distention for MR colonography: bright-lumen and dark-lumen techniques. Bright-lumen MR colonography involves administration of a gadolinium chelate-spiked enema, whereas the dark-lumen approach involves the administration of water, carbon dioxide, or room air. Supine prone or dual positioning may be done. 3D T1-weighted spoiled GRE sequences are used for bright lumen and a combination of 3D T1-weighted spoiled GRE and T2-weighted short-echo HASTE sequences are utilized for the dark-lumen method. In dark-lumen colonography, intravenous administration of a gadolinium chelate allows visualization of the colonic wall against the dark lumen. Pre- and postcontrast T1-weighted spoiled GRE fat suppression sequences are used.[4] When a mass or polyp is seen to protrude into the lumen on postcontrast T1-weighted images, the same part of the colon should be re-examined on precontrast images. True colorectal lesions typically enhance, whereas residual stool particles do not. Polyps are seen as sessile broad based without a stalk or pedunculated with a stalk. Flat polyps are sessile lesions with only minimal elevation and therefore can be difficult to identify.[4]

## COLON CARCINOMA

CRC is the third most commonly diagnosed cancer in males and second in females with a median age at diagnosis of 60 to 80 years.[5] Low-fiber, high-fat, and animal protein diet, smoking, and inflammatory bowel disease are risk factors. FAP and its variants (Gardner syndrome, Turcot syndrome, and attenuated adenomatous polyposis coli) account for less than 1% of colorectal cancers.[6] Lynch syndrome or hereditary nonpolyposis colorectal cancer is an autosomal

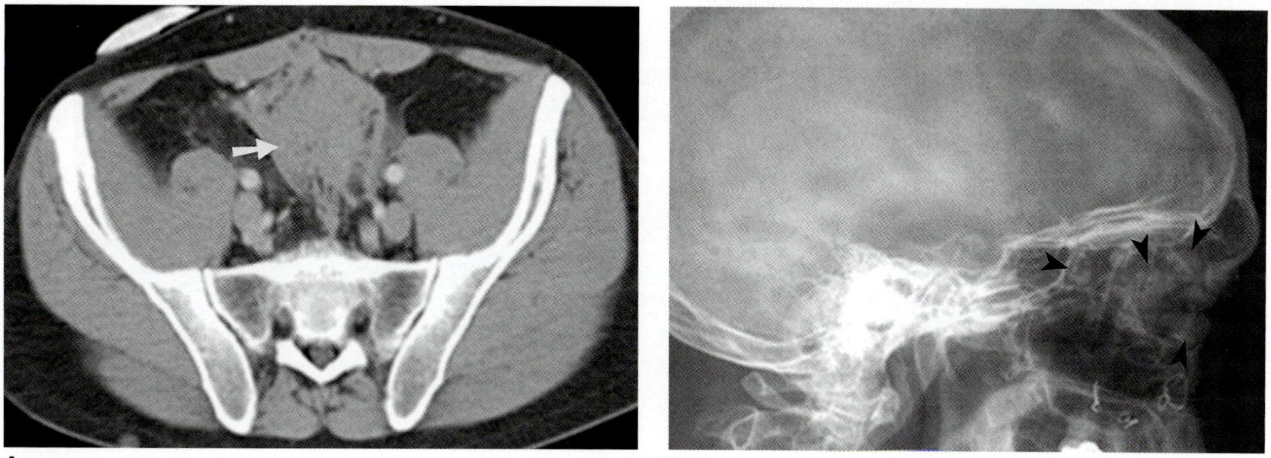

A B

**FIG. 5B.2 • Gardner syndrome. A:** Axial contrast-enhanced CT of the abdomen shows mesenteric desmoid (*arrow*). **B:** Skull radiograph of the same patient shows multiple osteomas (*arrowheads*).

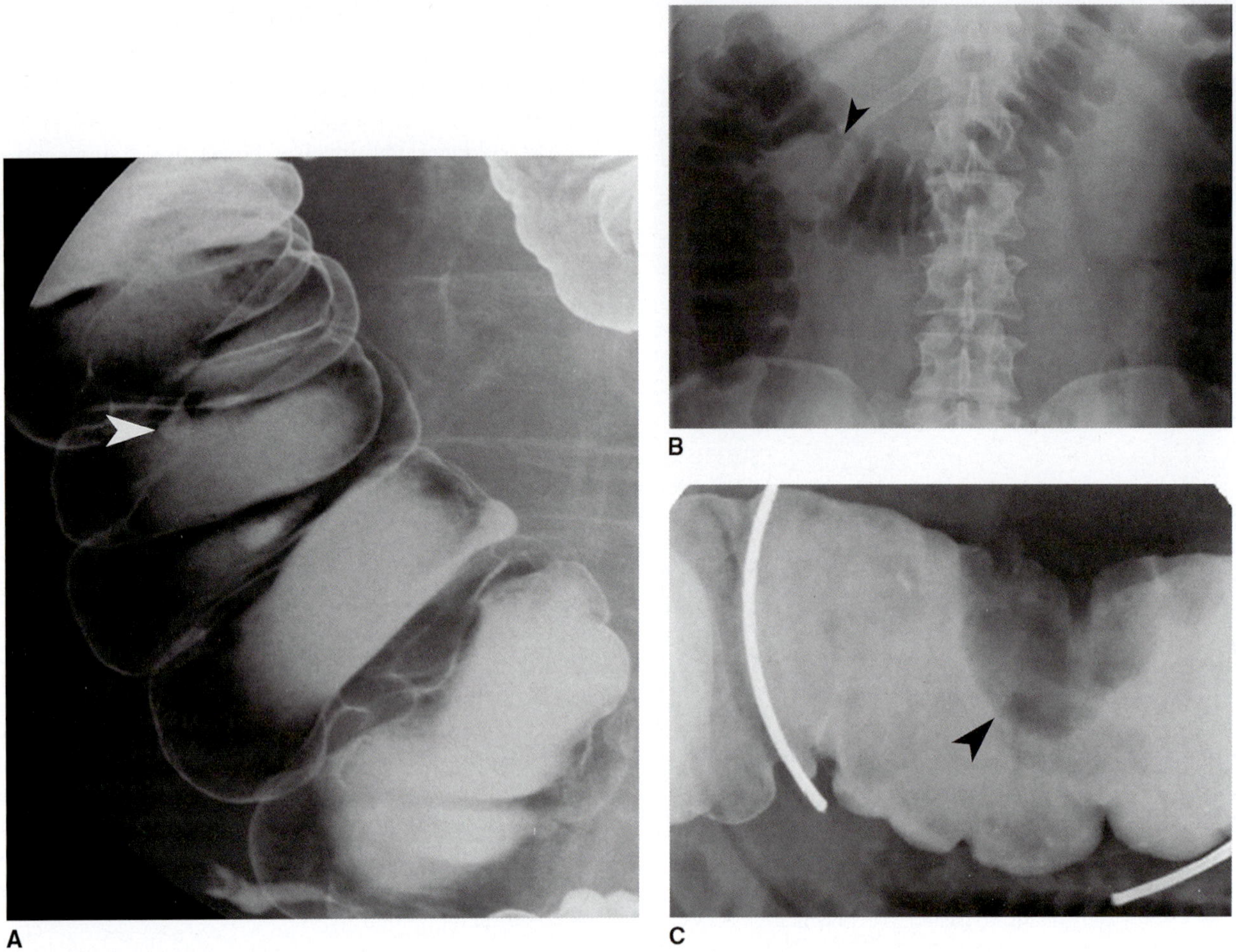


**FIG. 5B.3 • Colonic polyp. A:** Double-contrast barium enema shows a sessile polyp in the cecum with the characteristic bowler-hat sign (*arrowhead*). **B:** Plain radiograph shows a large soft tissue mass (*arrowhead*) within the proximal transverse colon, outlined by air. Given the large size, this polyp has high malignant potential. **C:** Double-contrast barium enema shows a large lobulated villous adenoma in the transverse colon (*arrowhead*).

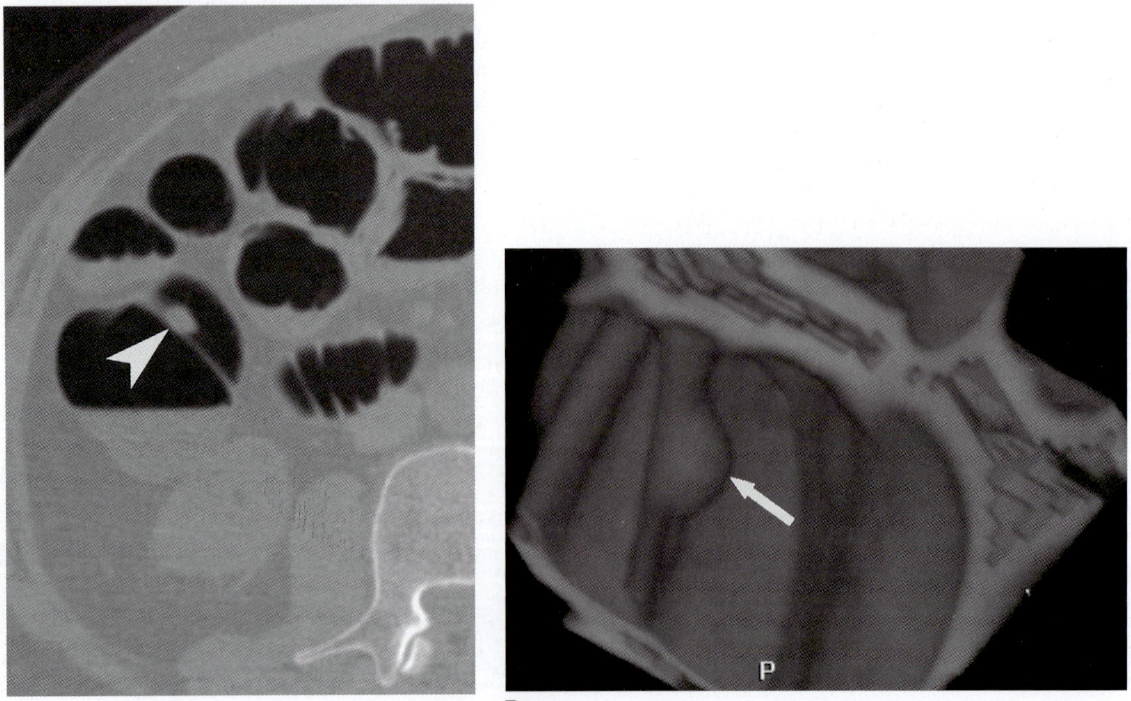


**FIG. 5B.4 • Colonic polyp. A:** Axial CT colonography demonstrates a subcentimeter polyp (*arrowhead*) located on a mucosal fold. **B:** 3D reformation clearly demonstrates the sessile polyp (*arrow*) in the ascending colon.

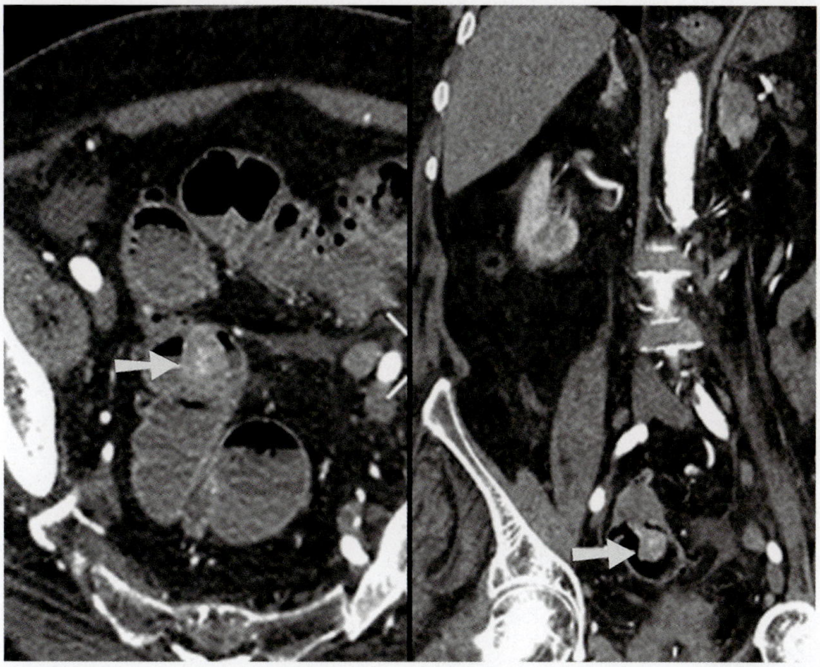

**FIG. 5B.5 • Pedunculated polyp.** Axial and coronal contrast-enhanced CT abdomen images demonstrate enhancement of pedunculated polyp (*arrows*).

dominant syndrome that accounts for approximately 3% to 5% of all colonic adenocarcinomas being more common than FAP.[7]

Approximately 55% of colorectal cancers occur in the rectosigmoid region, 22% in the cecum and ascending colon, 11% in the transverse colon, and 6% in the descending colon.[5] Morphologically, colon carcinomas can be sessile, exophytic, circumferential (apple core), ulcerated, and desmoplastic.

Barium enema is useful in the detection of polyps and carcinoma, although it is decreasing in popularity as a primary study. The diagnosis of colorectal cancer requires a careful examination of the entire colon since 5% of patients have a synchronous colon cancer, and more than one-third have additional adenomatous polyps.[8]

Early carcinoma of the colon is often sessile and flat lesion, more than 1 cm in diameter. Advanced carcinomas will appear as irregular filling defect in the barium on the dependent wall, while on the nondependent wall, it will appear to be etched with barium (Fig. 5B.6). Semiannular or saddle-shaped appearance may be appreciated. In further advanced colonic cancers, apple core lesions with proximal shouldering, mucosal destruction, and overhanging borders will be demonstrated (Fig. 5B.7).

CT performed with positive (barium/iodinated media) or negative (low concentration barium 0.1%, whole milk) intraluminal contrast agent use, in addition to IV contrast, significantly enhances the lesion detectability. These can be administered the night before the study as well as 30 to 90 minutes prior to the study to ensure that adequate contrast material reaches the colon. Neutral agents (water) or negative agents (air) can also be easily administered via a rectal tube and provide excellent contrast for colonic imaging.[9,10] Intravenous contrast material is essential for complete staging of known colorectal cancer and for evaluation of recurrent or metastatic disease. CT virtual colonoscopy is also a potential method for screening patients for polyps and colon cancers (Fig. 5B.8).

Typically, primary colonic malignancy is demonstrated on CT as a focal colonic wall thickening with narrowing of the

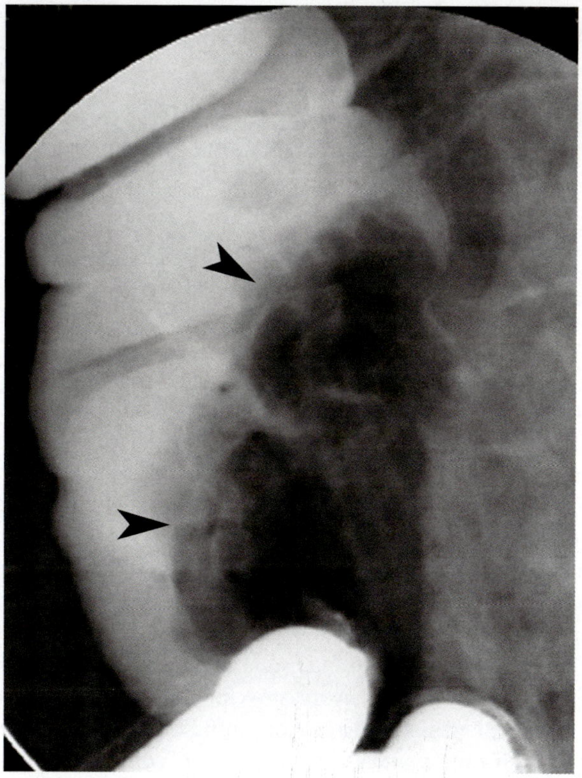

**FIG. 5B.6 • Cecal adenocarcinoma.** Barium enema exam demonstrates a large lobulated mass (*arrowheads*) lesion in the cecum.

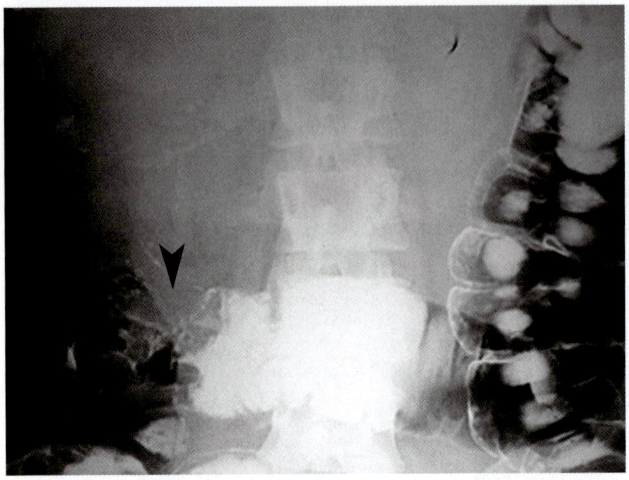

A

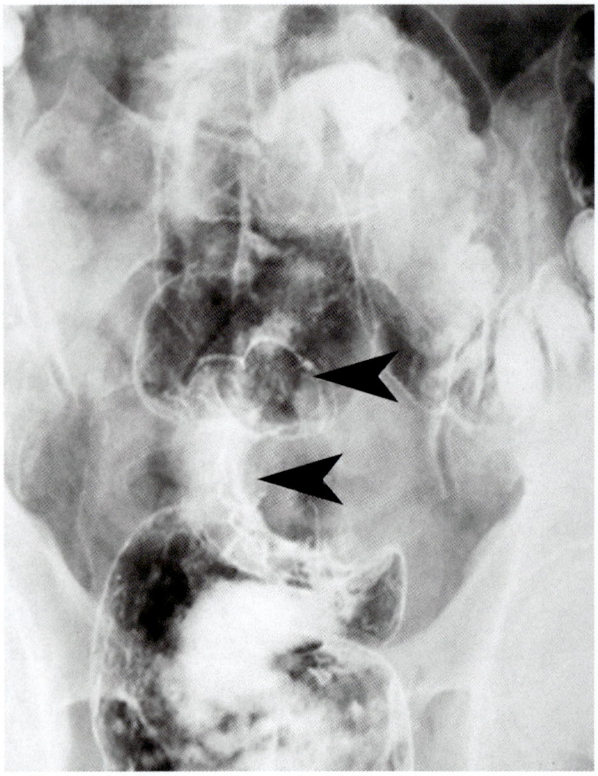

B

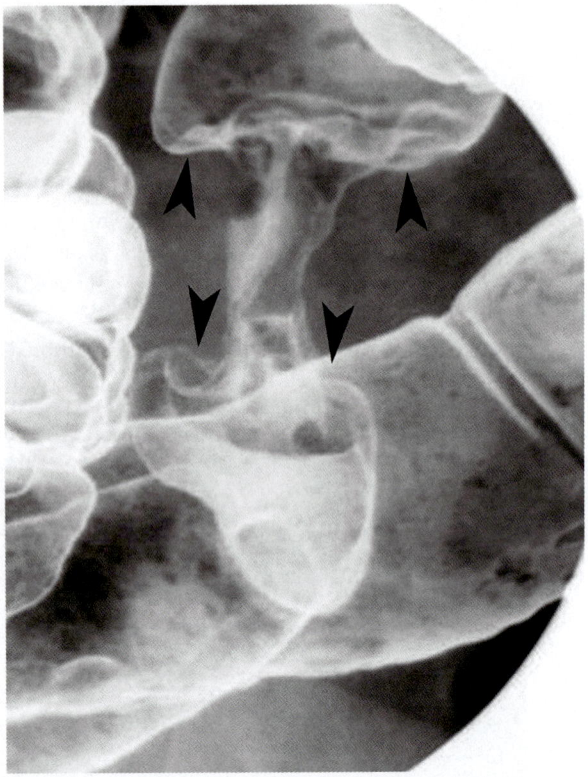

C

**FIG. 5B.7 • Colonic adenocarcinoma. A:** Barium enema shows short-segment stenosis, mucosal irregularity, and distal shouldering caused by malignant mass in the hepatic flexure (*arrowhead*). **B:** Double-contrast barium enema shows a polypoidal mass (*arrowheads*) at the rectosigmoid junction, causing luminal narrowing and apple core appearance. **C:** Double-contrast study demonstrates an apple core lesion with proximal and distal shouldering (*arrowheads*).

lumen (Figs. 5B.9 and 5B.10). Polypoidal lesions project into the lumen and are seen as a discrete soft mass that narrows the lumen. Larger mass lesion can undergo central necrosis with central hypodensity and may contain air, which may give it the appearance of an abscess. It is usually difficult to differentiate short-segment malignant and benign strictures as seen with diverticulitis on CT alone. Primary colonic malignancies may initially present with complications such as obstruction (Fig. 5B.11), perforation, and fistula, and these are readily visualized with CT. Colonic neoplasms can present as intussusception with or without obstruction. Intussusceptions appear as a target-like mass with alternating rings of soft tissue and fat.

The greatest utility of CT is in the assessment of local extension and distant metastasis of colonic malignancies (staging) and evaluation of treatment response (restaging). Local extension of tumor appears as an extracolic mass or as thickening and infiltration of pericolic fat (Figs. 5B.12 and 5B.13). Pericolic spread of tumor is also suggested by loss of fat planes between the colon and adjacent organs. It is important to identify the involvement of adjacent organs, such as the bladder, vagina, and abdominal or pelvic musculature. Lymph node enlargement of more than 1 to 1.5 cm in short-axis diameter is considered pathologic.[11] Hepatic metastases, a common site for blood-borne spread, usually appear as hypoattenuating masses and are best visualized during the portal venous phase of liver enhancement (Fig. 5B.14). Mucinous colorectal cancer can produce cystic or calcified hepatic metastases. Other common sites of metastases from colon cancer include the lungs, adrenal

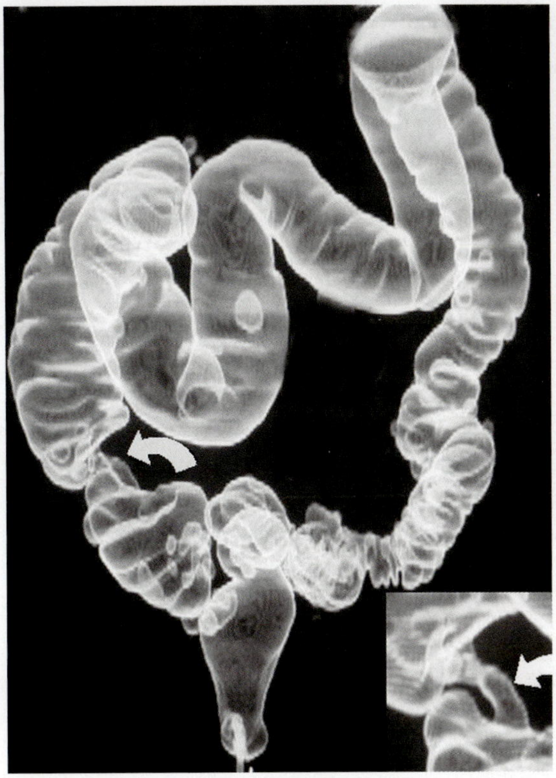

**FIG. 5B.8 • Colonic adenocarcinoma on CT colonography.** 3D-rendered image from CT colonography demonstrates an apple core stricture (*curved arrow*) in the ascending colon with proximal and distal shouldering.

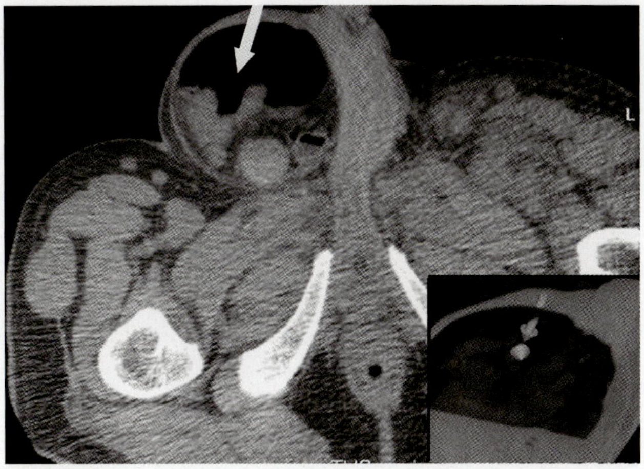

**FIG. 5B.10 • Cecal carcinoma.** CT colonography demonstrates a right inguinal hernia sac, containing a cecal mass (*arrow*) with central ulceration.

glands, bones, and peritoneum (peritoneal carcinomatosis and pseudomyxoma peritonei with mucinous adenocarcinoma).

Recent developments in the technique, increased availability, and widespread introduction of integrated FDG PET/CT imaging have made it a valuable tool for the differentiation of posttreatment changes from recurrent colorectal malignancy, to differentiate benign from malignant metastatic lesions (indeterminate lymph nodes, hepatic, and pulmonary lesions), and in evaluation of patients with rising tumor markers.[12]

MRI is utilized in the evaluation of the rectosigmoid malignancies, especially in preoperative staging for total mesorectal excision (Tables 5B.1 and 5B.2). T1 and T2 tumors are limited to the bowel wall and can be accurately identified with MR, because the rectal wall will have an intact black line. A T3 tumor grows through all layers and extends into the perirectal fat tissue. Perirectal fat stranding does not necessarily indicate tumor spread and may represent desmoplastic reaction or inflammatory stranding. Since there is no accurate way of differentiation, perirectal fat stranding should be labeled as T3. The perirectal fat is bounded by the mesorectal fascia, which is seen as a fine line of low signal intensity. The shortest distance from the tumor or lymph nodes to the mesorectal fascia is called the circumferential

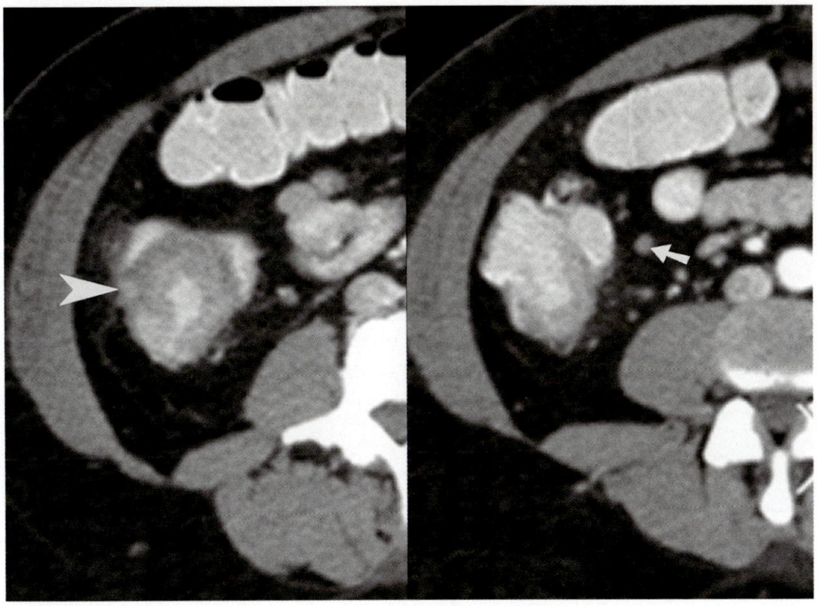

**FIG. 5B.9 • Carcinoma ascending colon.** Axial contrast-enhanced CT of the abdomen shows circumferential wall thickening (*arrowhead*) of the ascending colon segment with luminal narrowing. Pericolonic lymph node (*arrow*) is seen in the ascending mesocolon.

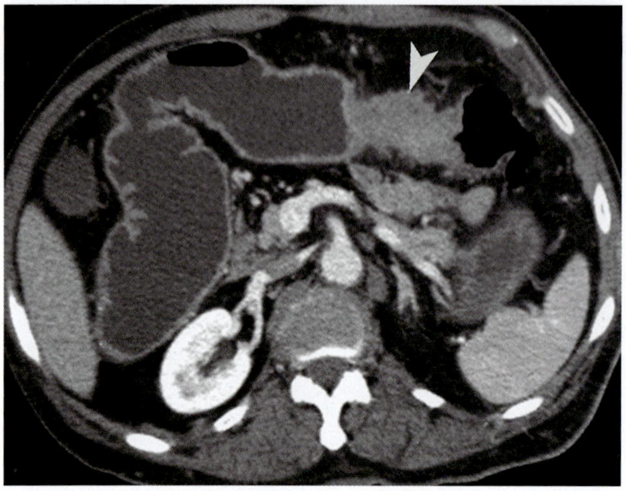

**FIG. 5B.11 • Adenocarcinoma transverse colon.** Axial contrast-enhanced CT of the abdomen shows distal transverse colon mass (*arrowhead*), causing large bowel obstruction.

resection margin (CRM), which is the most powerful predictor for local recurrence (Fig. 5B.15). The mesorectal fascia is involved if the distance between the tumor and the fascia is less than or equal to 1 mm.[13,14]

## COLONIC LYMPHOMA

Primary colorectal lymphoma comprises large cell lymphoma, low-grade B-cell lymphoma arising from MALT, mantle cell lymphoma, and T-cell lymphoma.

Double-contrast barium enema examination and CT may demonstrate polypoid masses (Fig. 5B.16A), circumferential infiltration, a cavitary mass excavating into the mesentery, endo-exo-enteric tumors, mucosal nodularity, and fold thickening (Fig. 5B.16B). Aneurysmal dilatation (Fig. 5B.17), focal strictures, or ulcerative forms with fistula formation may also be seen. Intussusception may occur with cecal involvement.

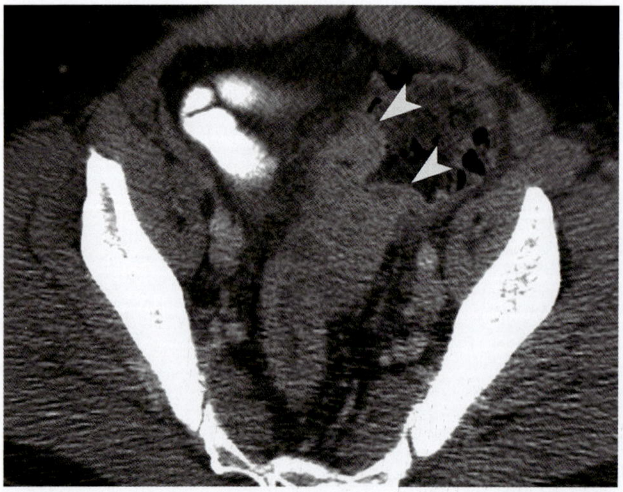

**FIG. 5B.12 • Sigmoid colonic adenocarcinoma.** Axial contrast-enhanced CT shows infiltrating sigmoid colonic mass, causing luminal narrowing and proximal shouldering (*arrowheads*).

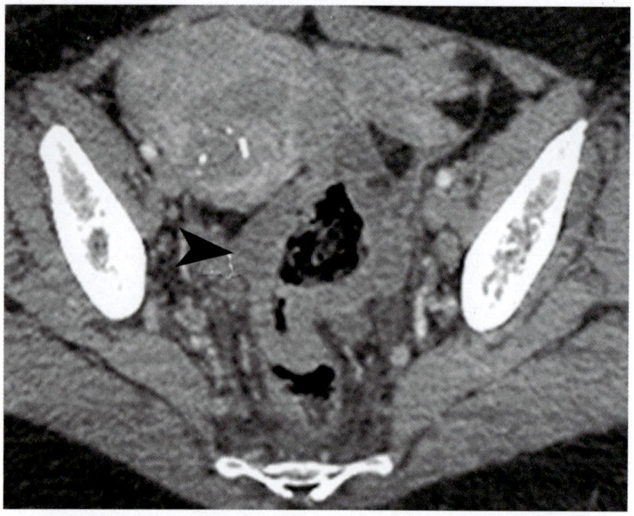

**FIG. 5B.13 • Rectosigmoid carcinoma.** Axial contrast-enhanced CT of the abdomen shows segmental rectosigmoid wall thickening (*arrowhead*) with abrupt distal transition. Incidental note is made of calcified uterine myomas in the right lower quadrant.

Features that can differentiate lymphoma from adenocarcinoma are:

1. Extension into the terminal ileum
2. Well-defined margins with preservation of fat planes
3. Less likely to cause obstruction because it does not elicit a desmoplastic response and submucosal lymphoid infiltration weakens the muscularis propria of the wall[15]
4. Aneurysmal dilatation

## MESENCHYMAL TUMORS OF COLON

A wide variety of benign and malignant mesenchymal tumors arise from the large bowel. Lipomas are tumors of mature adipose tissue with a fibrotic capsule, which usually arise from the submucosa of the cecum or sigmoid colon.[16] On barium, the submucosal mass present as well-defined, smooth hemispherical filling defect with right angle or obtuse margins with the colonic lumen (Fig. 5B.18).

Neurofibromas, schwannomas, and leiomyomas are other mesenchymal tumors occurring in the colorectum. Vascular tumors are classified into benign tumors like hemangiomas, lymphangiomas, and angiomatosis: malignant tumors such as hemangioendotheliomas and angiosarcomas. These mesenchymal tumors may present with intussusception (Fig. 5B.19).

Kaposi sarcoma is a mesenchymal tumor involving the lymphovascular system, usually seen in HIV/AIDS patients. Double-contrast barium studies may detect colorectal masses with or without central ulceration, demonstrating bull's-eye or target lesions. Polypoid submucosal masses with irregular fold thickening may be detected in CT.[17]

## GASTROINTESTINAL STROMAL TUMOR

Gastrointestinal stromal tumors were classified as smooth muscle tumors (leiomyosarcomas) until 1983 when electron microscopy and immunohistochemistry findings demonstrated

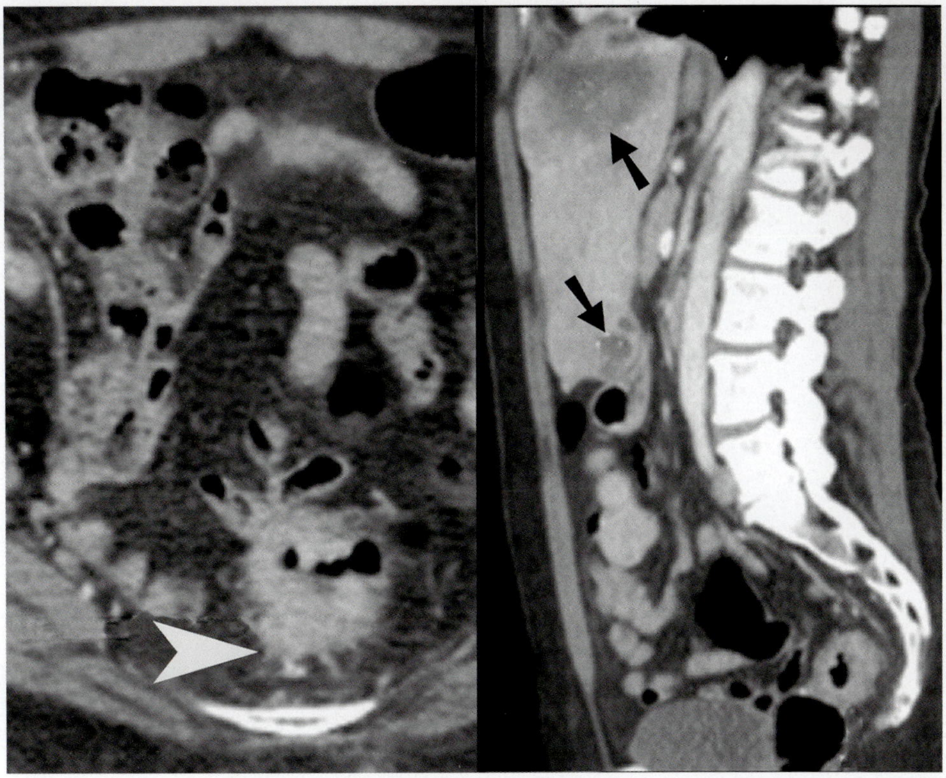

**FIG. 5B.14 • Carcinoma at rectosigmoid junction with hepatic metastasis.** Axial and coronal CT abdomen images show distal sigmoid colon wall thickening with pericolonic fat stranding (*arrowhead*). Multiple hepatic metastases are also seen (*arrows*).

a lack of smooth muscle and Schwann cells. They are mesenchymal tumors arising from the interstitial cells of Cajal and are most commonly benign (75%).[18] Tumors of small bowel origin tend to have more aggressive behavior and thus a worse prognosis than that of tumors originating in other gastrointestinal sites. These tumors arise from the muscularis propria with the bulk of the mass growing exophytically rather than intraluminally or intramurally.[19] Since most of these tumors are submucosal in location, they can attain a large size without causing bowel obstruction by the time of diagnosis (Fig. 5B.20). The enhancement pattern varies from homogenously enhancing to heterogeneously enhancing, with or without ulceration.

## ENDOCRINE TUMORS OF THE COLON

Most colorectal carcinoids arise in the rectum followed by the cecum. While metastatic disease from rectal carcinoids is not associated with carcinoid syndrome, metastatic disease from colonic carcinoids may produce carcinoid syndrome. Carcinoids of the proximal colon are polypoid intraluminal masses and are difficult to distinguish from polypoid

Table 5B.1 **STAGING OF COLORECTAL CANCER WITH TNM AND DUKES SYSTEM**

| | | |
|---|---|---|
| T0—no evidence of primary tumor | N0—no regional lymph node metastases | M0—no distant metastases |
| Tis—carcinoma in situ: intraepithelial or invasion of the lamina propria | N1—metastases in 1–3 regional lymph nodes | M1—distant metastases |
| T1—tumor invades submucosa | N2—metastases in ≥4 regional lymph nodes | |
| T2—tumor invades muscularis propria | | |
| T3—tumor invades through the muscularis propria into the subserosa or into the pericolic tissues | | |
| T4—tumor directly invades other organs or structures and/or perforates the visceral peritoneum | | |

Table 5B.2 **STAGING OF COLORECTAL CANCER WITH TNM AND DUKES SYSTEM**

| TNM | Dukes | |
|---|---|---|
| Stage 0—TisN0M0 | | Carcinoma in situ |
| Stage I—T1–2, N0M0 | Stage A | Limited to the bowel wall. No extrarectal spread or lymph node metastasis |
| Stage IIA—T3 N0 M0<br>Stage IIB—T4 N0 M0 | Stage B | Cancer extends through the bowel wall into perirectal tissue. No lymph node metastasis. |
| IIIA—T1–2, N1, M0<br>III B—T3–4, N1 M0<br>IIIC—any T N2 M0 | Stage C | Lymph node metastasis |
| Stage IV any T, any N, M1 | Stage C | Distant metastasis |

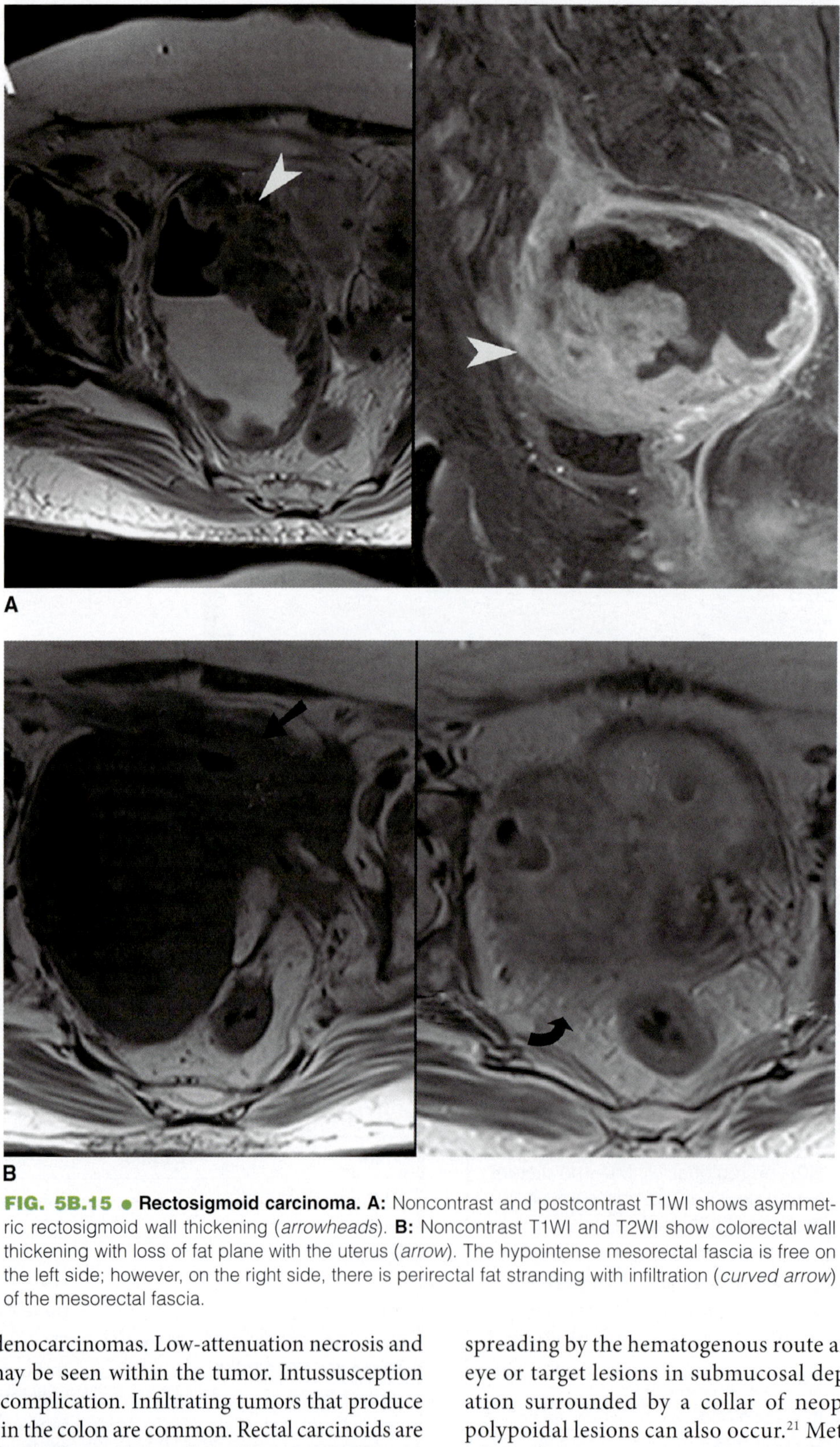

**FIG. 5B.15 ● Rectosigmoid carcinoma. A:** Noncontrast and postcontrast T1WI shows asymmetric rectosigmoid wall thickening (*arrowheads*). **B:** Noncontrast T1WI and T2WI show colorectal wall thickening with loss of fat plane with the uterus (*arrow*). The hypointense mesorectal fascia is free on the left side; however, on the right side, there is perirectal fat stranding with infiltration (*curved arrow*) of the mesorectal fascia.

adenomas or adenocarcinomas. Low-attenuation necrosis and degeneration may be seen within the tumor. Intussusception may occur as a complication. Infiltrating tumors that produce annular lesions in the colon are common. Rectal carcinoids are most commonly small mural or polypoid masses. Malignant rectal carcinoids may invade adjacent pelvic structures.[20]

## COLONIC METASTASES

Malignant melanoma is one of the more common malignancies to metastasize to the gastrointestinal tract spreading by the hematogenous route and presents as bull's-eye or target lesions in submucosal deposits (central ulceration surrounded by a collar of neoplastic tissue). Large polypoidal lesions can also occur.[21] Metastatic colonic serosal implants can cause colonic wall retraction due to the intense desmoplastic reaction, thickened separated mucosal folds traversing only part of the bowel lumen without extending across the entire colonic lumen giving striped colon appearance on double-contrast barium enema examinations (Fig. 5B.21).

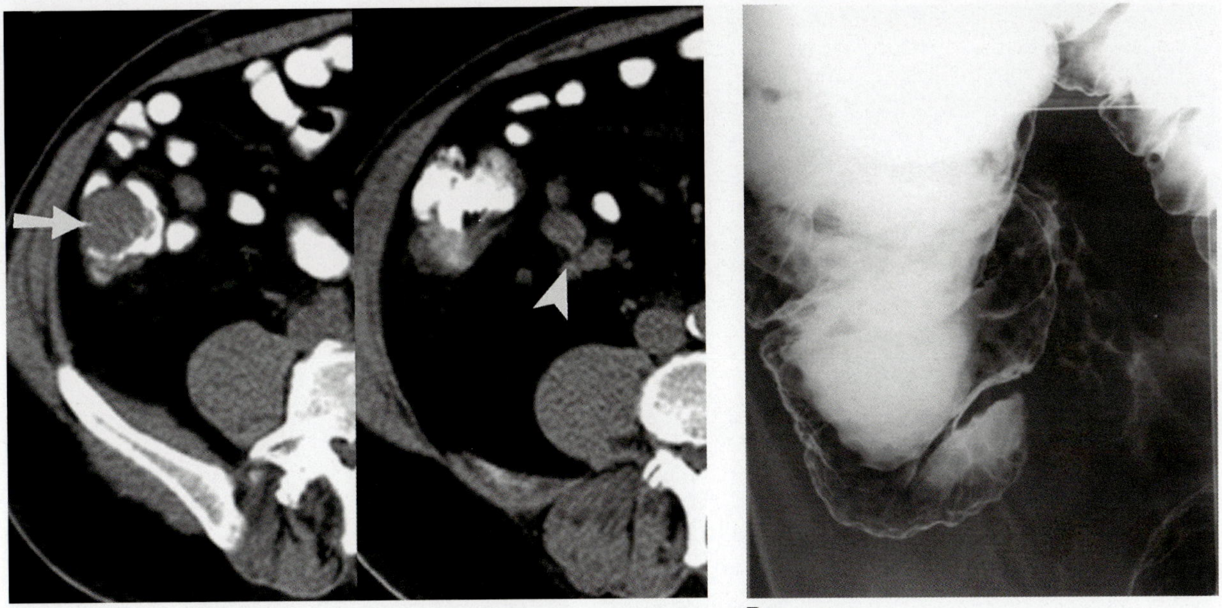

A B

**FIG. 5B.16 • Colonic lymphoma. A:** Axial CT of the abdomen shows a polypoidal mass (*arrow*) in the cecum. Multiple enlarged lymph nodes are also demonstrated (*arrowhead*). **B:** Barium enema demonstrates numerous mucosal nodules in the cecum, with fold thickening and nodularity of the terminal ileum.

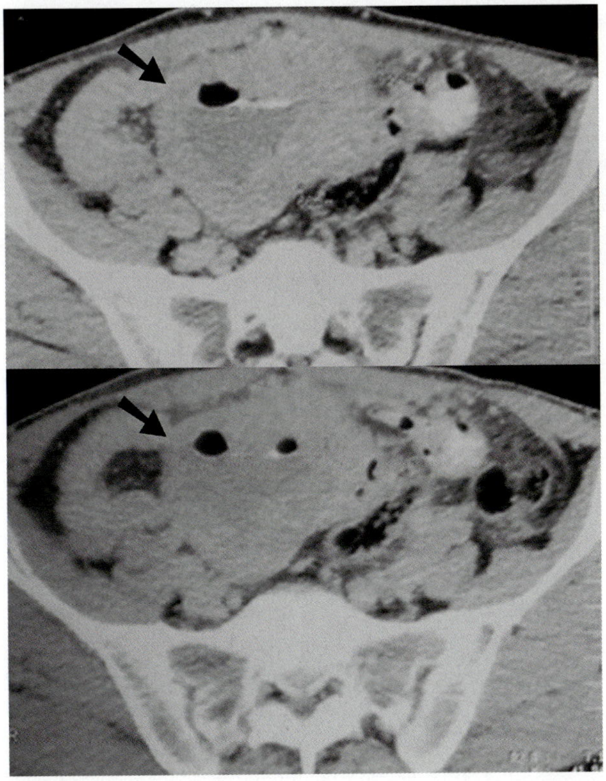

**FIG. 5B.17 • Colonic lymphoma.** Axial CT shows circumferential wall thickening and luminal dilatation of the sigmoid colon with intraluminal air–fluid level (*arrows*).

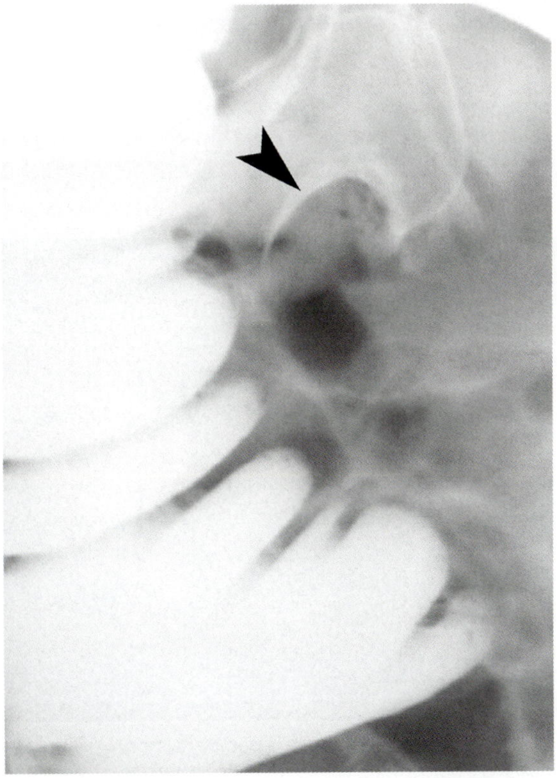

**FIG. 5B.18 • Colonic lipoma.** Double-contrast barium demonstrates smooth hemispherical submucosal mass (*arrowhead*) in the transverse colon.

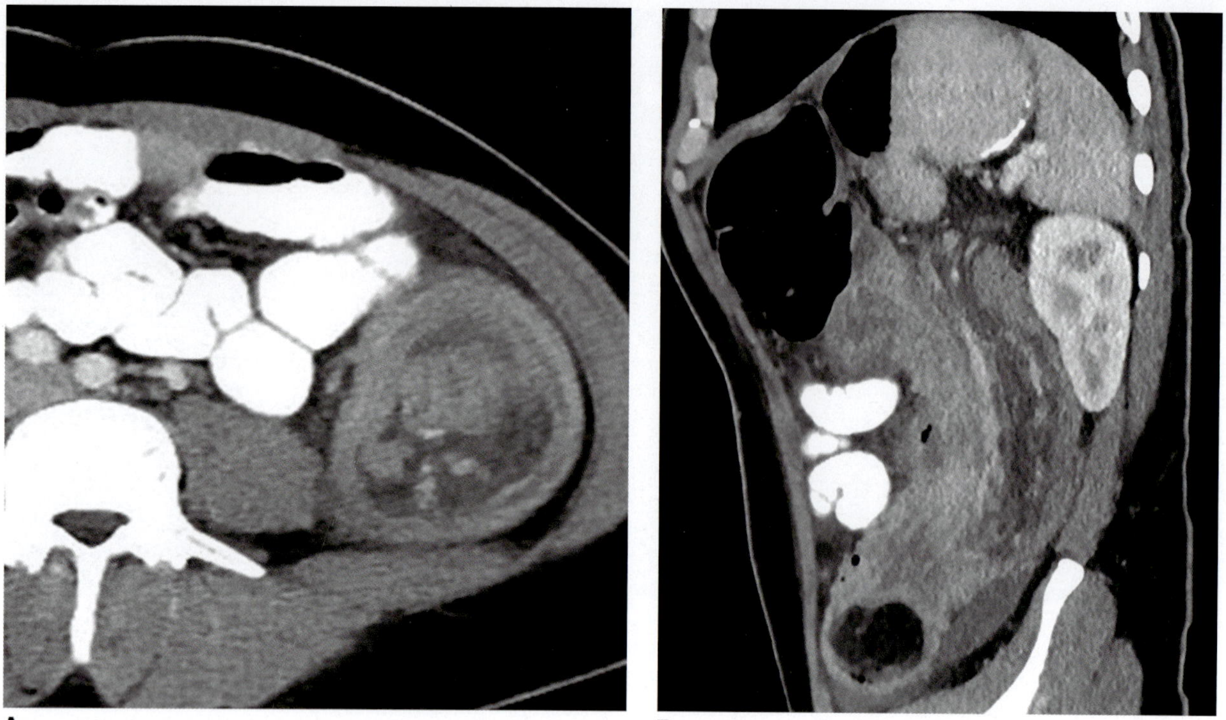

A B

**FIG. 5B.19 • Colocolic intussusception due to lipoma. A:** Axial contrast-enhanced CT of the inner intussusceptum separated from the intussuscipiens (*arrow*) by transverse mesocolonic fat. **B:** Sagittal CT image demonstrates a lipoma as the lead point.

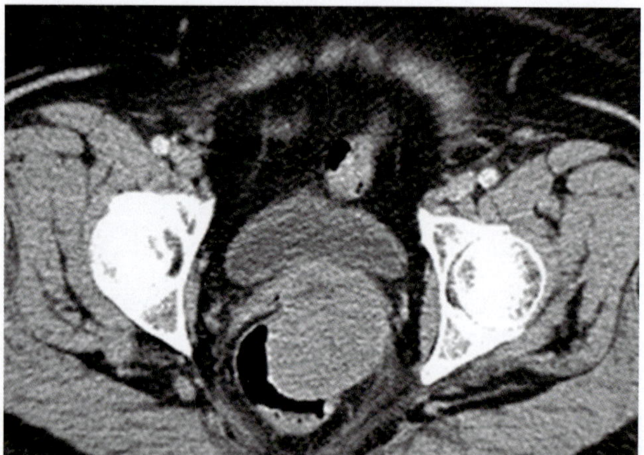

**FIG. 5B.20 • Gastrointestinal stromal tumor.** Axial contrast-enhanced CT pelvis image shows enhancing mass arising from the rectum projecting into the lumen and also with anterior exophytic extension. (Image courtesy of N. Ramaiya, MD, Dana Farber Cancer Institute.)

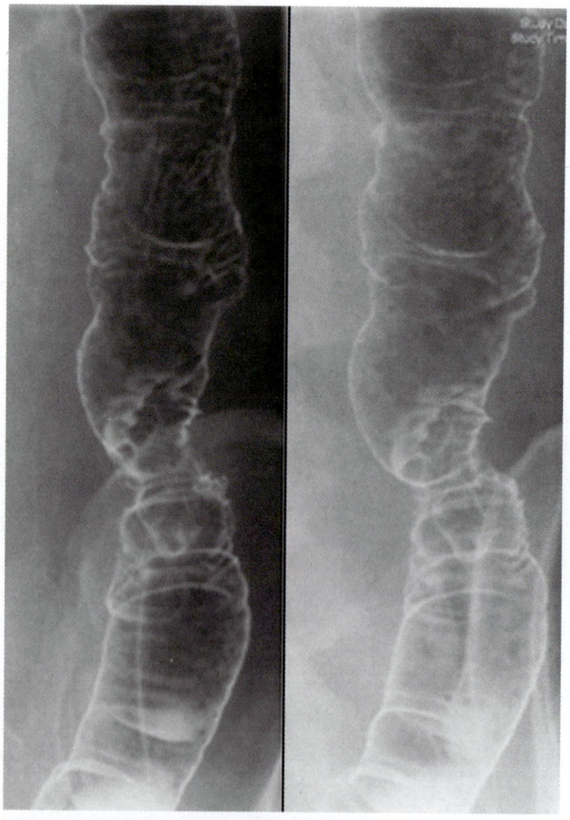

**FIG. 5B.21 • Colonic serosal implants.** Barium enema shows serosal spiculation adjacent to nodular tumor implantation. Also present are numerous transverse folds of the descending colon giving the characteristic striped colon appearance.

## References


1. Muto T, Bussey HJ, Morson BC. The evolution of cancer of the colon and rectum. *Cancer*. 1975;36(6):2251–2270.
2. Yee J, Kim DH, Rosen MP, et al. ACR appropriateness criteria colorectal cancer screening. *J Am Coll Radiol*. 2014;11(6):543–551.
3. Silva AC, Wellnitz CV, Hara AK. Three-dimensional virtual dissection at CT colonography: unraveling the colon to search for lesions. *Radiographics*. 2006;26:1669–1686.
4. Thornton E, Morrin MM, Yee J. Current status of MR colonography. *Radiographics*. 2010;30(1):201–218.
5. Kumar V, Abbas AK, Fausto N, et al. *Robbins and Cotran Pathologic Basis of Disease*. Philadelphia, PA: WB Saunders Co.; 2005. ISBN: 0721601871.
6. Burt RW, DiSario JA, Cannon-Albright L. Genetics of colon cancer: impact of inheritance on colon cancer risk. *Annu Rev Med*. 1995;46:371.
7. Chan TL, Yuen ST, Kong CK, et al. Heritable germline epimutation of MSH2 in a family with hereditary nonpolyposis colorectal cancer. *Nat Genet*. 2006;38:1178.
8. Cunliffe WJ, Hasleton PS, Tweedle DE, et al. Incidence of synchronous and metachronous colorectal carcinoma. *Br J Surg*. 1984;71(12):941–943.
9. Angelelli G, Macarini L, Lupo L, et al. Rectal carcinoma: CT staging with water as contrast medium. *Radiology*. 1990;177:511–514.
10. Gossios KJ, Tsianos EV, Kontogiannis DS, et al. Water as contrast medium for computed tomography study of colonic wall lesions. *Gastrointest Radiol*. 1992;17:125–128.
11. Freeny PC, Marks WM, Ryan JA, et al. Colorectal carcinoma evaluation with CT: preoperative staging and detection of postoperative recurrence. *Radiology*. 1986;158:347–353.
12. Delbeke DI, Martin WH. FDG PET and PET/CT for colorectal cancer. *Methods Mol Biol*. 2011;727:77–103.
13. Brown G, Richards CJ, Newcombe RG, et al. Rectal carcinoma: thin section MR imaging for staging in 28 patients. *Radiology*. 1999;211:215–222.
14. MERCURY. Study group: extramural depth of tumor invasion at thin section MR in patients with rectal cancer: results of the MERCURY study. *Radiology*. 2007;243:132–139.
15. Lee HJ, Han JK, Kim TK, et al. Primary colorectal lymphoma: a spectrum of imaging findings with pathologic correlation. *Eur Radiol*. 2002;12:2242–2249.
16. Nallamothu G, Adler DG. Large colonic lipomas. *Gastroenterol Hepatol (NY)*. 2011;7(7):490–492.
17. Pantongrag-Brown L, Nelson AM, Brown AE, et al. Gastrointestinal manifestations of acquired immunodeficiency syndrome: radiologic-pathologic correlation. *Radiographics*. 1995;15:1155–1178.
18. Burkill GJ, Badran M, Al-Muderis O, et al. Malignant gastrointestinal stromal tumor: distribution, imaging features, and pattern of metastatic spread. *Radiology*. 2003;226(2):527–532.
19. Hersh MR, Choi J, Garsett C, et al. Imaging gastrointestinal stromal tumours. *Cancer Control*. 2005;12:111–115.
20. Levy AD, Sobin LH. From the archives of the AFIP: gastrointestinal carcinoids: imaging features with clinicopathologic comparison. *Radiographics*. 2007;27(1):237–257.
21. Reintgen DS, Thompson W, Garbutt J, et al. Radiologic, endoscopic, and surgical considerations of melanoma metastatic to the gastrointestinal tract. *Surgery*. 1984;95(6):635–639.


## SELF-ASSESSMENT QUESTIONS

1. A 52-year-old man presenting with anemia, pain on the abdomen, and weight loss. What is the most likely diagnosis on the barium enema?

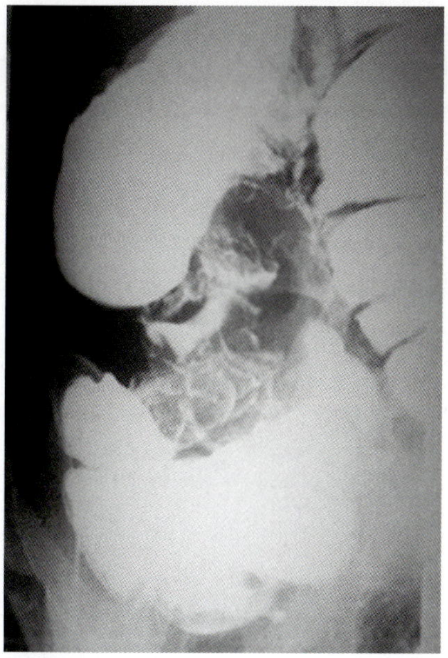

A. Diverticulitis
B. Carcinoma
C. Polyp
D. Tuberculosis

2. A 57-year-old man presents with weight loss and diarrhea. What is the imaging finding of lymphoma on the barium enema?

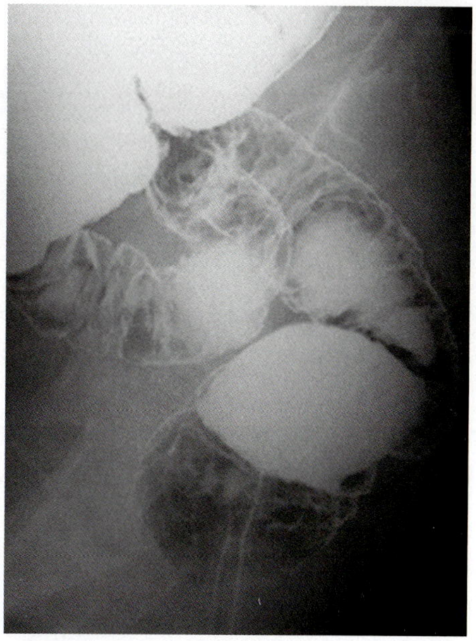

A. Nodularity
B. Ulcerations
C. Diverticulosis
D. Pseudopolyps

## Answers to Self-Assessment Questions

**1. B.** Carcinoma. The barium enema demonstrates a malignant apple core lesion with proximal as well as distal shouldering.

**2. A.** Nodularity. The barium enema demonstrates innumerable polypoidal filling defects in the distal sigmoid colon and rectum.

# Appendix 6

*Ajay K. Singh*

## LEARNING OBJECTIVES

1. Describe the imaging features of acute appendicitis.
2. Describe noninflammatory pathologies of the appendix.

The normal appendix is a blind-ending tubular structure measuring on average 8 cm in length. It is most often located posteromedial to the cecum, most commonly located at 2:00 to 6:00 o'clock position (Fig. 6.1). The appendix is supplied by the ileocolic artery, which is a branch of the superior mesenteric artery. The appendicular artery, which supplies the appendix, is a terminal artery, thereby making the appendix more prone to ischemia. While the normal appendix can be seen on CT scan study in more than 90% of the population, it can be seen on US in less than 10% of the population.[1–7] The appendix can be visualized on MR in 70% to 100% of patients. Clinically, the appendix is an important organ, especially because acute appendicitis is the most common cause of surgical abdomen in emergency room patients.

## ACUTE APPENDICITIS

There are more than 250,000 acute appendicitis surgeries performed in the United States every year, representing the most common surgical cause of the acute abdomen. Acute appendicitis is most commonly seen in the second decade, slightly more common in males than in females. The lifetime risk of developing acute appendicitis is approximately 9% in males and 7% in females. Approximately 20% of patients with acute appendicitis have perforation, most commonly in infants and elderly population.

Acute appendicitis is due to obstruction caused most commonly by appendicolith and less commonly by other pathologies, such as lymphoid hyperplasia, foreign bodies, tumors, etc. Appendicolith results in stasis of secretions in the appendiceal lumen, causing increased intraluminal pressure, finally leading to ischemia and gangrenous changes.

Based on the clinical examination alone, there is approximately 20% false positivity rate for the diagnosis of acute appendicitis. This is the reason why cross-sectional imaging, especially CT, is considered the most appropriate imaging modality for the assessment of the appendicitis in adult population. CT in patients with suspected appendicitis is most optimally performed using intravenous contrast and either oral or rectal contrast. In general, CT is believed to be more sensitive than US for diagnosing acute appendicitis. According to the American College of Radiology appropriateness criteria, US is the most appropriate imaging modality for the evaluation of suspected appendicitis in pediatric patients (less than 14-year-old) and pregnant population.

Plain radiograph has very limited sensitivity and demonstrates appendicolith in 10% of the population. Appendicoliths are typically solitary, less than 2 cm in diameter, rounded densities in the right lower quadrant, which may be laminated (Fig. 6.2). The other findings include localized paralytic ileus, ill definition of the psoas outline, free air, and gasless cecum (due to spasm).

Graded compression US findings include noncompressible blind-ending tubular structure measuring more than 6 mm in diameter, sometimes containing appendicolith (Fig. 6.3A, B). Color Doppler US can demonstrate increased vascularity in the wall of the appendix, which is decreased in patients with gangrenous appendicitis (Fig. 6.3C).

The CT findings of acute appendicitis include the dilated appendix measuring more than 7 mm in diameter with periappendiceal inflammatory changes (Figs. 6.4 to 6.7). The dilated appendix alone should not be taken as definite criteria to make the diagnosis of acute appendicitis because appendiceal caliber of up to 10 mm can be seen in minority of normal population. The other findings of acute appendicitis are appendicolith (in 20%), reactive lymphadenopathy, phlegmonous changes, distal small bowel obstruction, paralytic ileus, wall thickening (greater than 3 mm), and stratification of the appendiceal wall. The arrowhead sign refers to funneling of contrast into the base of the cecum in an arrowhead configuration, due to spasticity of the cecum (Fig. 6.8A). Cecal bar sign refers to thickening of

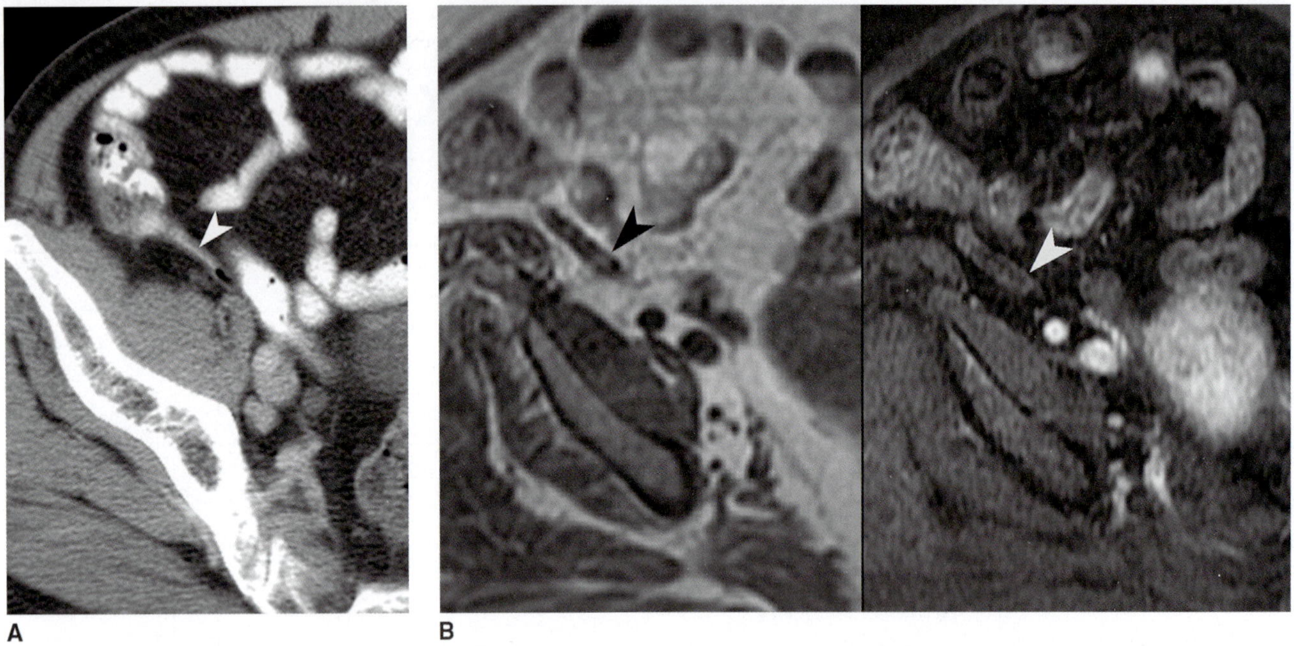

**FIG. 6.1 • Normal appendix. A:** Axial contrast-enhanced CT demonstrates the normal-caliber appendix (*arrowhead*), filling with oral contrast. **B:** T2WI and postgadolinium T1WI demonstrates the normal appendix (*arrowheads*) located posteromedial to the cecum.

the base of the cecum at the site of insertion of the appendix, due to inflammatory changes (Fig. 6.8B).

The diagnosis of appendiceal perforation has important clinical implications as these patients have higher morbidity and mortality. These patients are often initially managed with catheter drainage and antibiotics. CT has a sensitivity of 62% to 94% and specificity of 81% to 100% in diagnosing perforation.[8,9] The imaging findings of appendiceal perforation include (Fig. 6.9):

1. Extraluminal appendicolith
2. Discontinuous enhancement of the wall
3. Periappendiceal abscess
4. Periappendiceal air

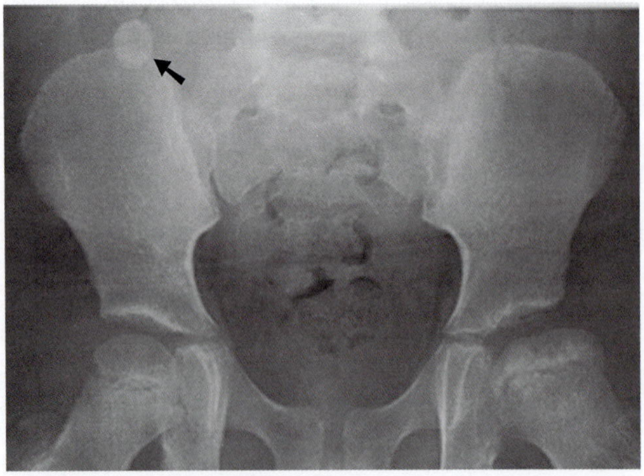

**FIG. 6.2 • Appendicolith.** Plain x-ray of the abdomen demonstrates calcified appendicolith (*arrow*) in the right lower quadrant.

MR is the most appropriate imaging modality in pregnant patients with nondiagnostic US.[10–13] It should use phased array body coil due to higher signal-to-noise ratio (SNR) associated with it. Eight channel or higher surface coils allow imaging of the abdomen and pelvis with excellent SNR. Oral Gastromark (Mallinckrodt Medical, St. Louis, Missouri), which was used in the past, is no longer available as contrast agent for gastrointestinal tract. Gadolinium (0.1 mmol/kg or approximately 20 mL) is routinely used intravenously except in pregnant patients. The contrast-enhanced T1-weighted sequence used is a fat-saturated 3D volumetric isotropic acquisition (VIBE/THRIVE/FAME/LAVA). The cornerstone of MR protocol in pregnant patients is T2-weighted sequence (SSFSE and T2-FSE) because of their ability to provide excellent evaluation of ascites, inflammation, wall edema, and dilated bowel loops.[7]

On MR, the inflamed appendix is 7 mm or more in diameter and demonstrates periappendiceal T2 hyperintense inflammation and thickened T2 hyperintense appendiceal wall (Figs. 6.10 and 6.11). Abscess, free fluid, bowel dilatation, and inflammatory phlegmon are the other findings seen on MR (Fig. 6.12). MR has high sensitivity (97%), specificity (92%), accuracy (92%), negative predictive value (96%), and positive predictive value (94%) for diagnosing acute appendicitis.[10]

The differential diagnoses of the right lower quadrant pain include segmental omental infarction, acute epiploic appendicitis, infectious enterocolitis (*Salmonella*, tuberculosis, *Campylobacter*, *Yersinia*), diverticulitis, typhlitis, inflammatory bowel disease, and Meckel diverticulitis.

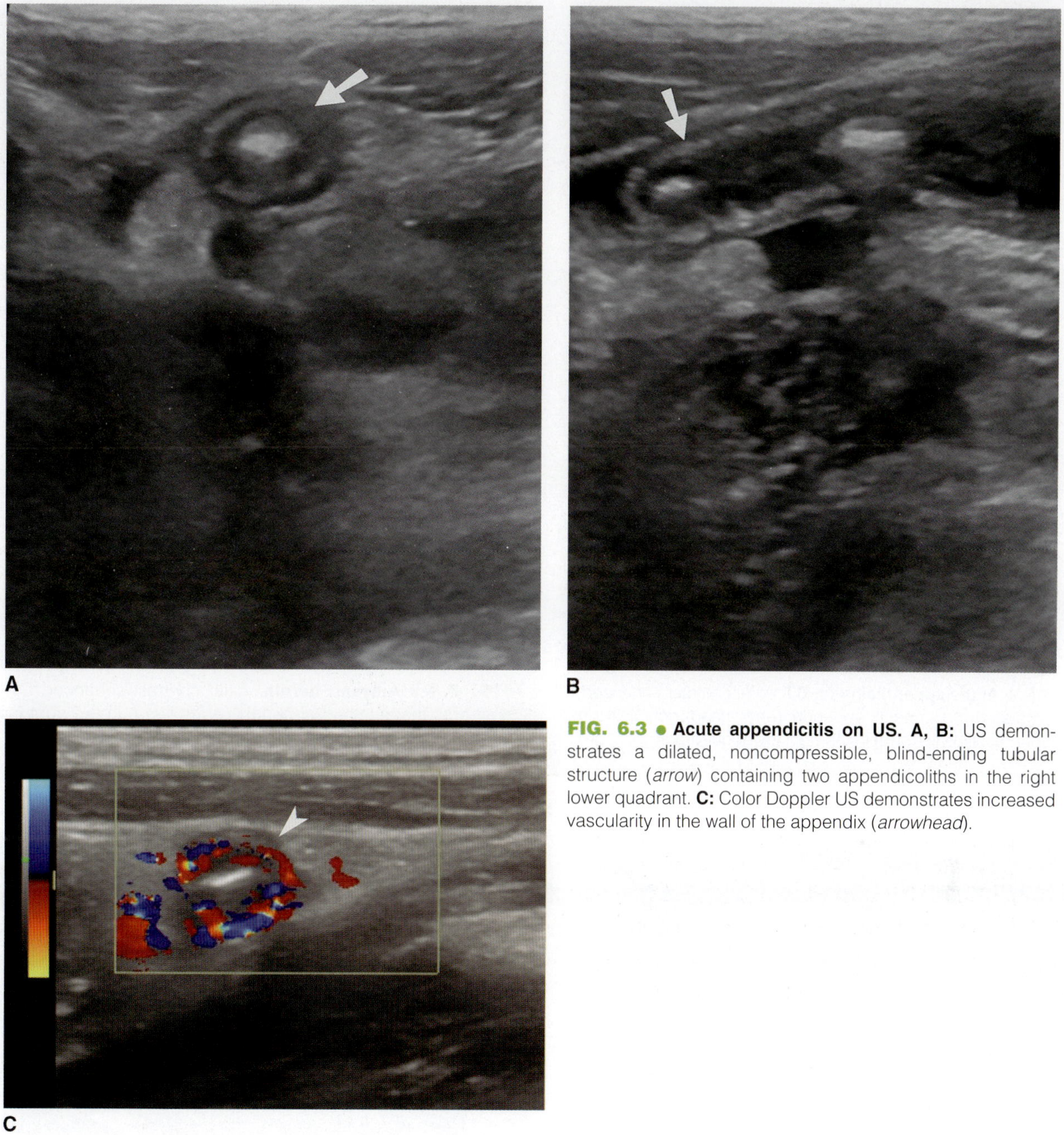

**FIG. 6.3 • Acute appendicitis on US. A, B:** US demonstrates a dilated, noncompressible, blind-ending tubular structure (*arrow*) containing two appendicoliths in the right lower quadrant. **C:** Color Doppler US demonstrates increased vascularity in the wall of the appendix (*arrowhead*).

## Inflammatory Bowel Disease

Appendiceal involvement by Crohn disease is seen in approximately one-third of the cases. It is also seen in two-thirds of the patient with ulcerative colitis and pancolitis. Crohn disease involvement of the appendix is characterized by the presence of transmural granulomatous inflammation. The presence of imaging finding of terminal ileitis on imaging is helpful in making the diagnosis and differentiating from acute appendicitis (Figs. 6.13 and 6.14).

## Mesenteric Lymphadenitis

Mesenteric lymphadenitis is the most common nonsurgical cause of the right lower quadrant pain. The CT finding of primary mesenteric lymphadenitis is the demonstration of cluster of lymph nodes in the right lower quadrant, which are at least 5 mm in short-axis diameter, with the normal appendix (Fig. 6.15).[14] Sometimes, this is associated with distal ileal wall thickening. Secondary mesenteric lymphadenitis is characterized by enlargement of the mesenteric lymph nodes due to an underlying cause, such as appendicitis, diverticulitis, inflammatory bowel disease, etc.

## Appendiceal Diverticulitis

Similar to colonic diverticulum, appendiceal diverticulum is also pseudodiverticulum, typically measuring less than 1 cm

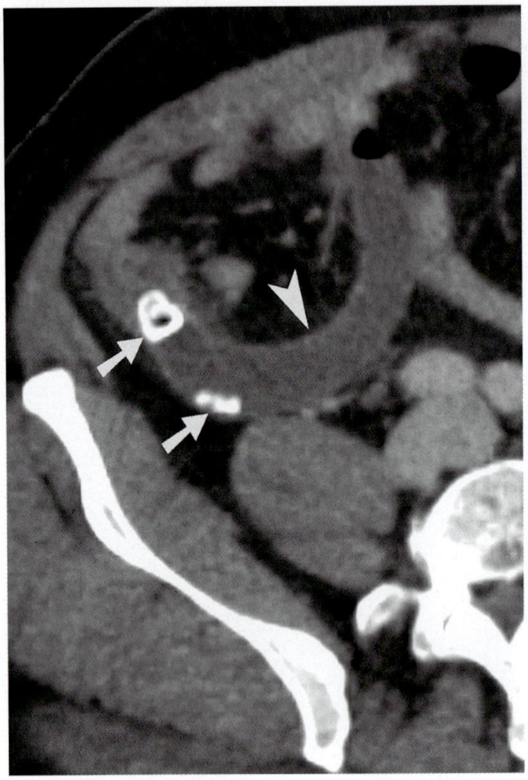

**FIG. 6.4 • Acute appendicitis on CT.** Axial contrast-enhanced CT demonstrates the distended appendix (*arrowhead*) containing multiple appendicoliths (*arrows*) in the right lower quadrant.

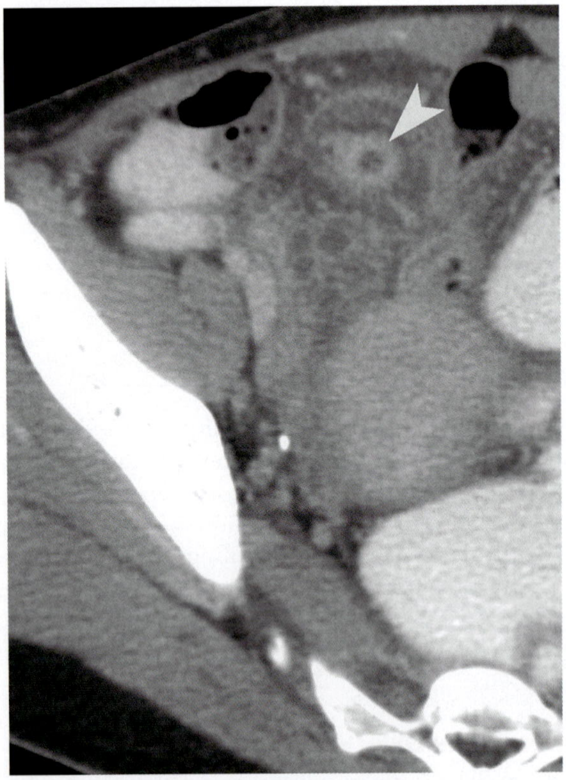

**FIG. 6.5 • Acute appendicitis on CT.** Axial contrast-enhanced CT demonstrates the dilated appendix with thickened enhancing wall (*arrowhead*) and extensive periappendiceal inflammatory changes.

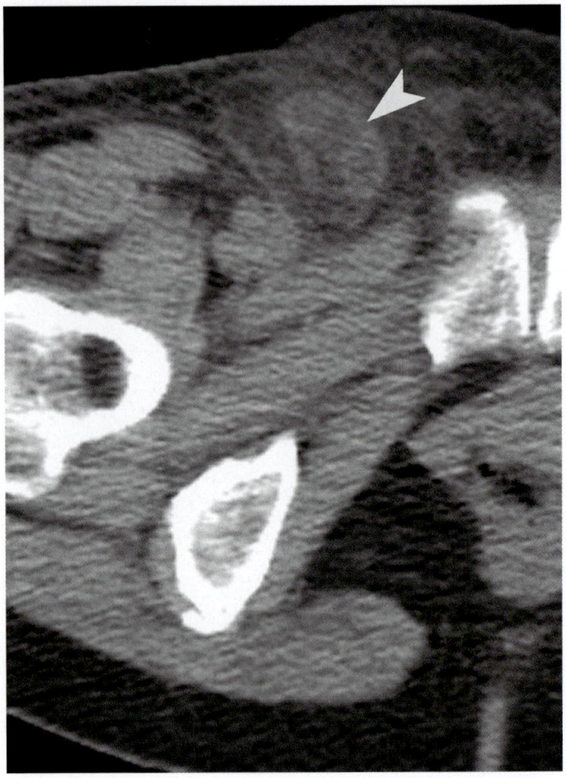

**FIG. 6.6 • Amyand hernia.** Axial contrast-enhanced CT demonstrates the inflamed appendix (*arrowhead*) in the right inguinal canal.

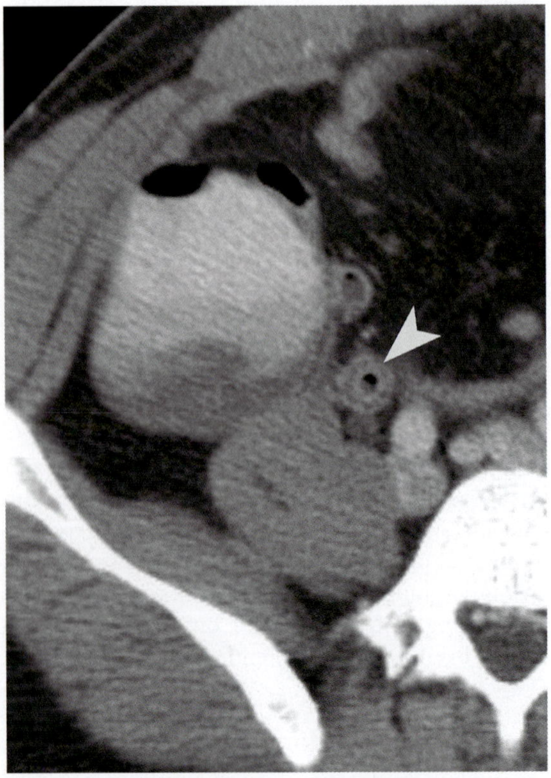

**FIG. 6.7 • Acute appendicitis with stratified wall.** Contrast-enhanced CT with rectal contrast demonstrates laminated appearance of the thickened appendiceal wall (*arrowhead*).

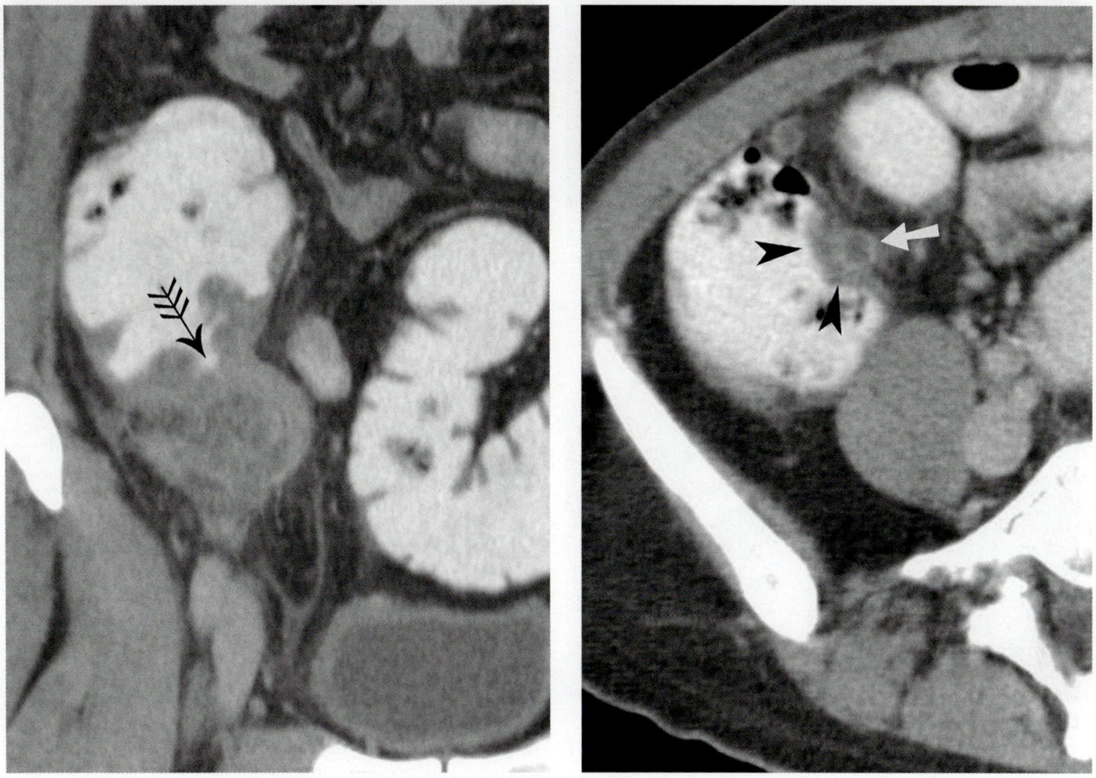

A B

**FIG. 6.8 • Arrowhead and cecal bar sign. A:** Arrowhead sign—coronal CT reformation demonstrates arrowhead appearance of the gastrointestinal contrast (*arrow*), funneling into the base of the cecum in a patient with acute appendicitis. **B:** Cecal bar sign—a bar of thickened cecal wall (*arrowheads*) is seen adjacent to the inflamed appendix (*arrow*).

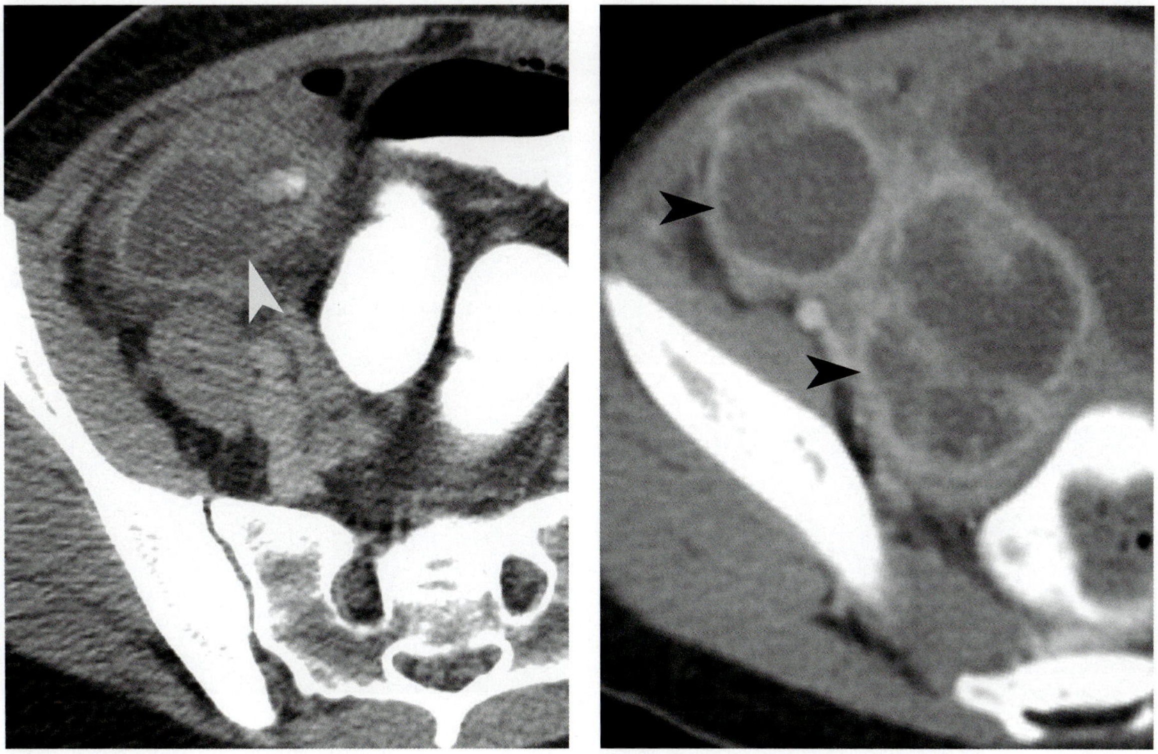

A B

**FIG. 6.9 • Perforated appendicitis. A:** Axial contrast-enhanced CT demonstrates abscess (*arrowhead*) containing an appendicolith in the right lower quadrant. **B:** Axial contrast-enhanced CT of a pediatric patient demonstrates multiple abscesses (*arrowheads*) in the right lower quadrant.

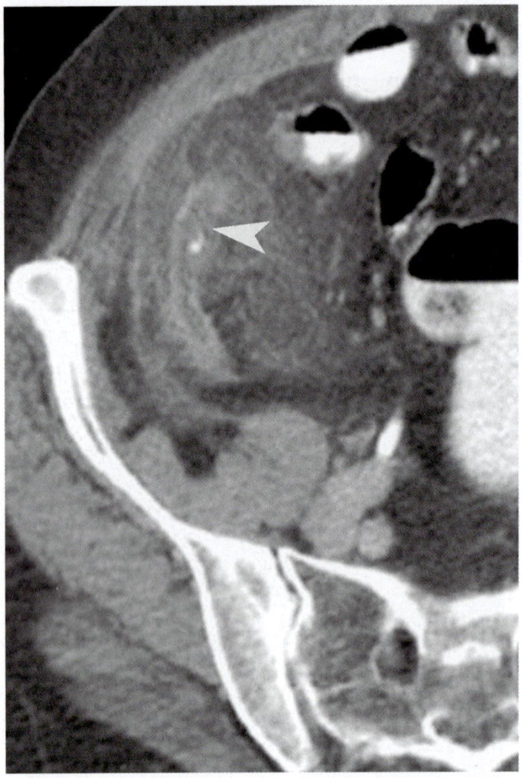

C

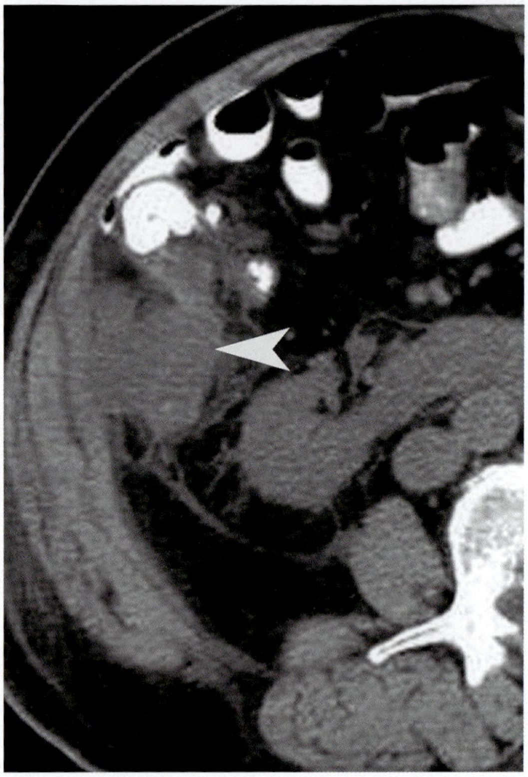

D

**FIG. 1.9** • (*Continued*) **C:** Axial contrast-enhanced CT shows discontinuity (*arrowhead*) in the appendiceal wall on the medial aspect arrowhead in a patient with perforated appendicitis. Note that the appendix is not dilated but there are extensive periappendiceal inflammatory changes. **D:** Axial noncontrast CT demonstrates inflammatory phlegmon (*arrowhead*) in the right lower quadrant, in the expected location of the appendix.

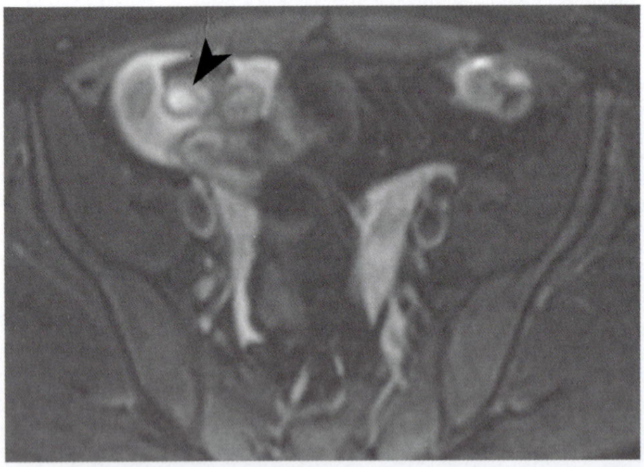

A

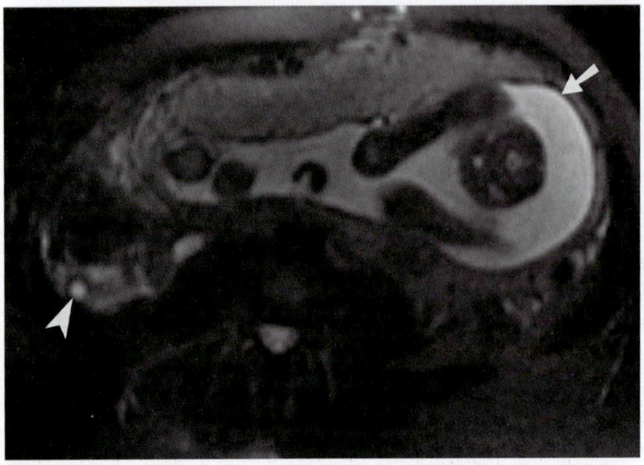

B

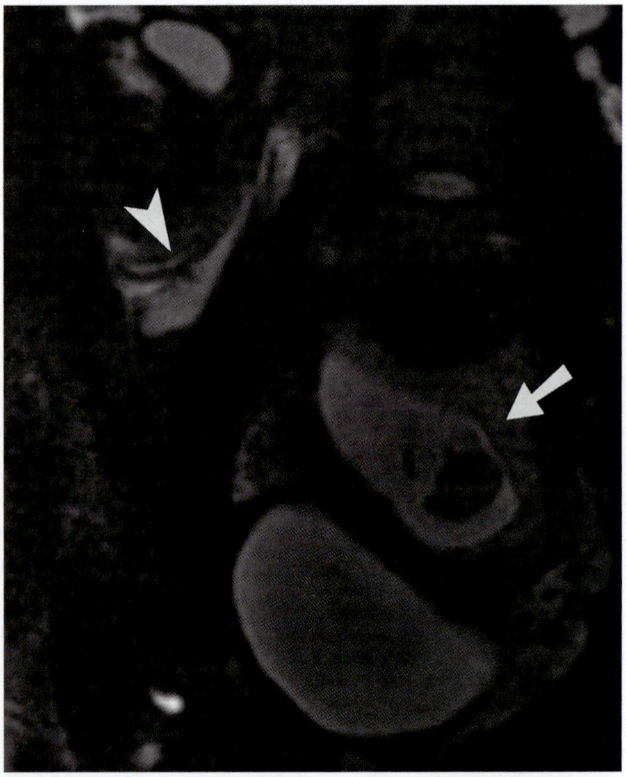

C

**FIG. 6.10** • **Acute appendicitis on T2-weighted sequence. A–C:** Axial (**A–B**) and coronal (**C**) T2-SSFSE with fat saturation in three different patients with acute appendicitis demonstrates the dilated appendix (*arrowheads*) in the right lower quadrant with surrounding free fluid. A gestational sac (*arrow*) (**B–C**) is seen in the uterus.

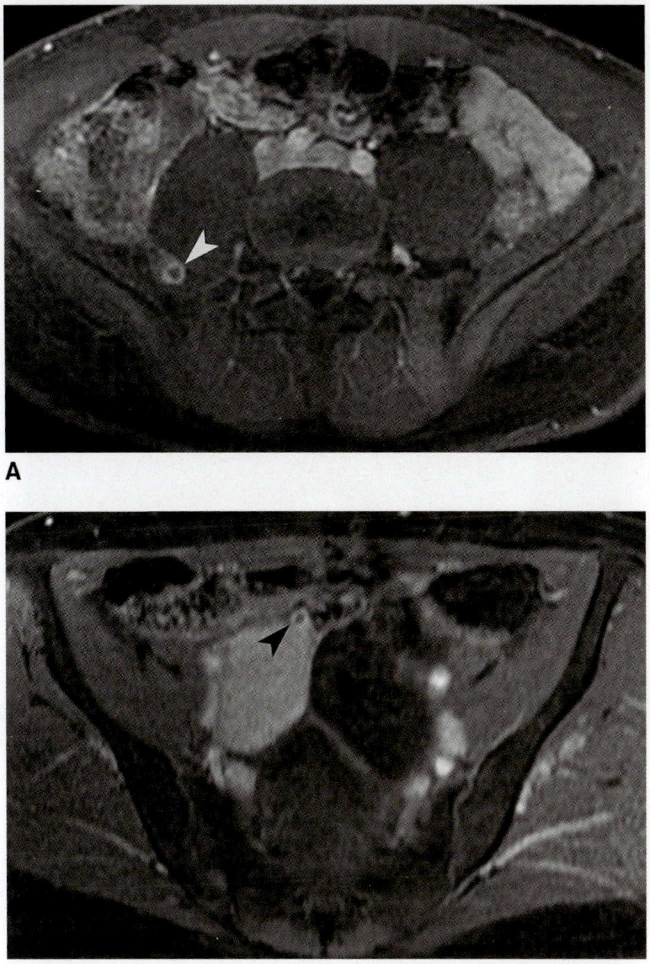

**FIG. 6.11 • Acute appendicitis on postgadolinium MR. A, B:** Axial contrast-enhanced T1WI demonstrates intensely enhancing appendiceal wall (*arrowheads*), consistent with acute appendicitis.

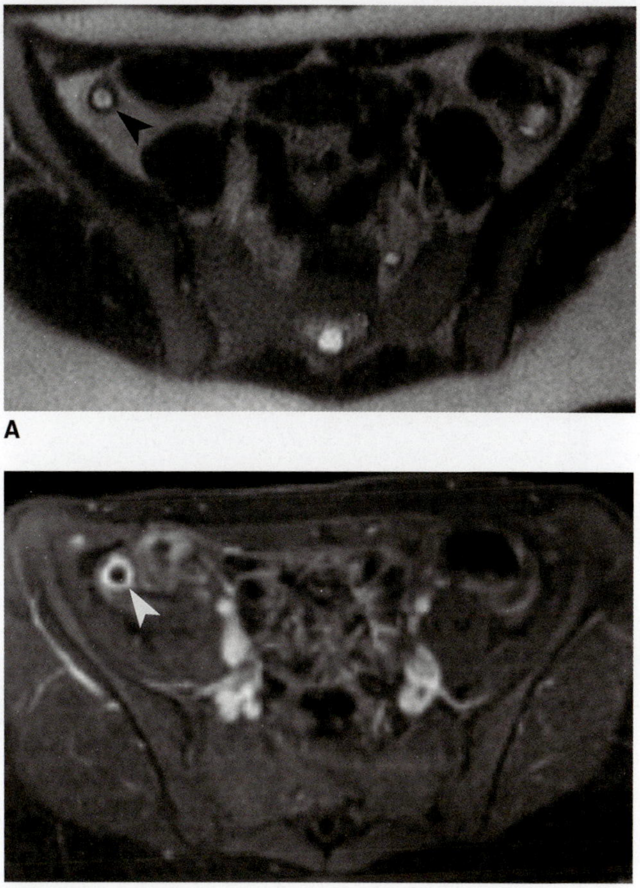

**FIG. 6.13 • Crohn disease involving the appendix. A, B:** Axial T2 and postcontrast T1WI in a patient with Crohn disease demonstrates the chronically dilated appendix (*arrowheads*) with thickened wall.

in diameter (Fig. 6.16). The appendiceal diverticulum can get inflamed, clinically mimicking acute appendicitis. Inflamed appendiceal diverticulum has four times higher risk for perforation compared to acute appendicitis.

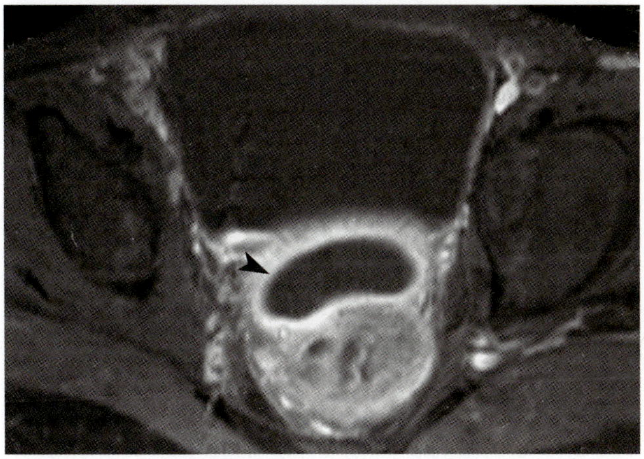

**FIG. 6.12 • Perforated appendicitis on MR.** Axial contrast-enhanced T1WI demonstrates a well-defined abscess (*arrowhead*) with intensely enhancing wall in the pelvis.

## APPENDICEAL NEOPLASM

Appendiceal tumors are most commonly seen in middle-aged or older patients with the exception of carcinoid tumors, which are often seen in young adult patients.[6] Carcinoid tumor of the appendix is the most common appendiceal tumor, accounting for up to 80% of the appendiceal neoplasm. The appendix is the second most common location of carcinoid tumor, accounting for approximately 20% of gastrointestinal carcinoids. Two-thirds of the appendiceal carcinoid are present in the distal third of the appendix and are typically less than 1 cm in size. Unlike other GI carcinoids, carcinoid tumors of the appendix are less likely to metastasize and cause carcinoid syndrome, thereby accounting for more than 90% 5-year survival rate. The imaging findings are sparse and include demonstration of a small primary tumor, which usually is not associated with metastatic disease process (Fig. 6.17).

The epithelial neoplasm of the appendix includes adenoma and adenocarcinoma. These are more likely to be detected because of their larger size at the time of diagnosis and higher metastasis rate, compared to carcinoid tumor. Mucinous tumors are primarily detected because of the presence of

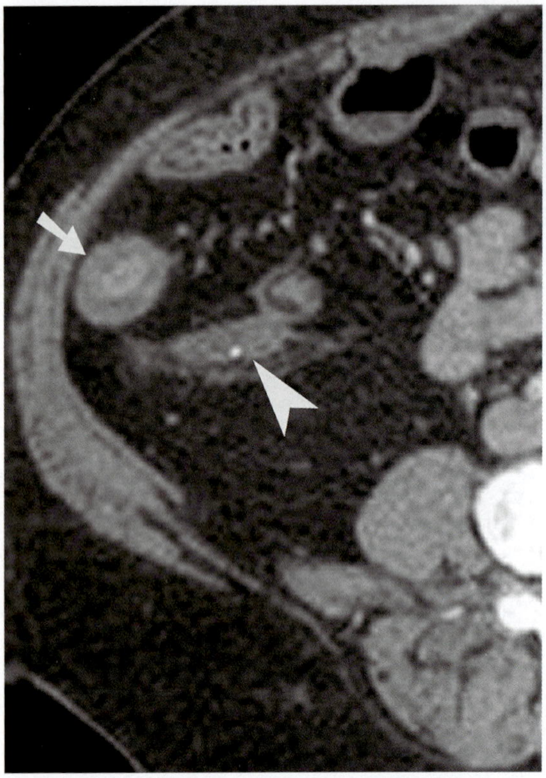

**FIG. 6.14 • Crohn disease with acute appendicitis.** Axial contrast-enhanced CT demonstrates thickened appendiceal wall (*arrowhead*) with mild periappendiceal inflammatory changes in the patient with acute appendicitis. The patient also has findings of terminal ileitis (*arrow*) from the patient's known Crohn disease.

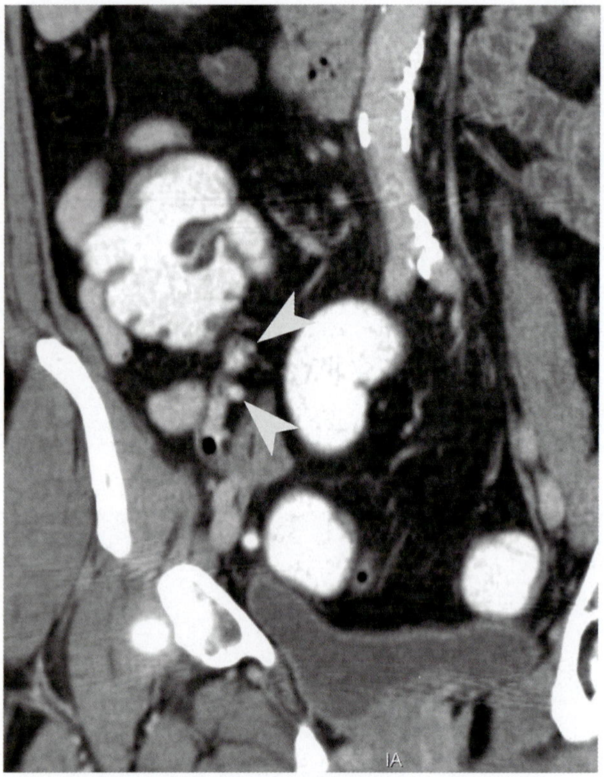

**FIG. 6.16 • Appendiceal diverticulosis.** Coronal CT reformation demonstrates multiple diverticulum (*arrowheads*) arising from the appendix.

associated mucocele. The CT findings include demonstration of a fluid density, cystic mass lesion arising from the base of the cecum, often associated with curvilinear wall calcification (Figs. 6.18 to 6.20). Nonmucinous epithelial neoplasms are rare in the appendix and demonstrate soft tissue mass without any associated mucocele formation (Fig. 6.21).

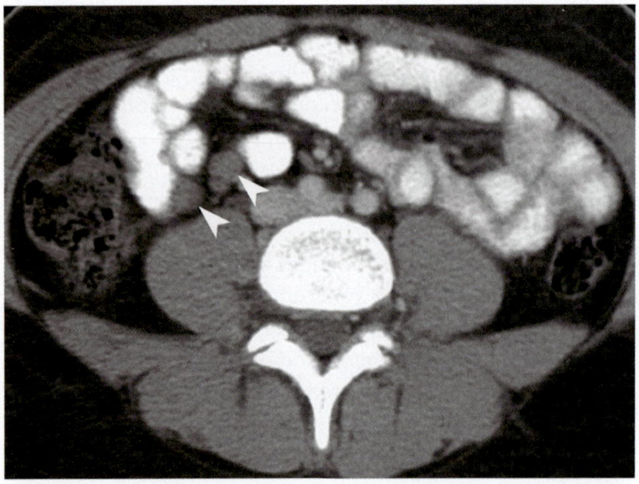

**FIG. 6.15 • Acute mesenteric lymphadenitis.** Axial contrast-enhanced CT demonstrates multiple prominent lymph nodes (*arrowheads*) in the right lower quadrant.

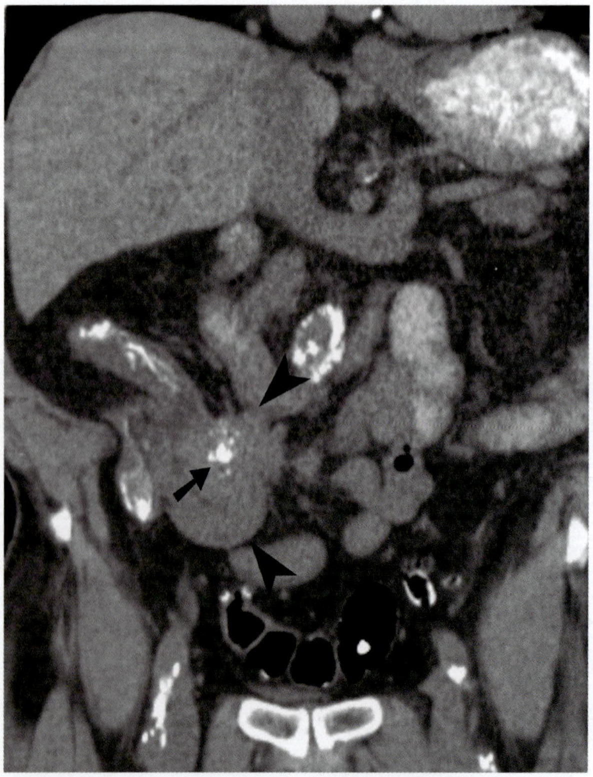

**FIG. 6.17 • Carcinoid tumor of the appendix.** Coronal CT reformation demonstrates an irregular soft tissue density mass (*arrowheads*) with central calcification (*arrow*) in the right lower quadrant.

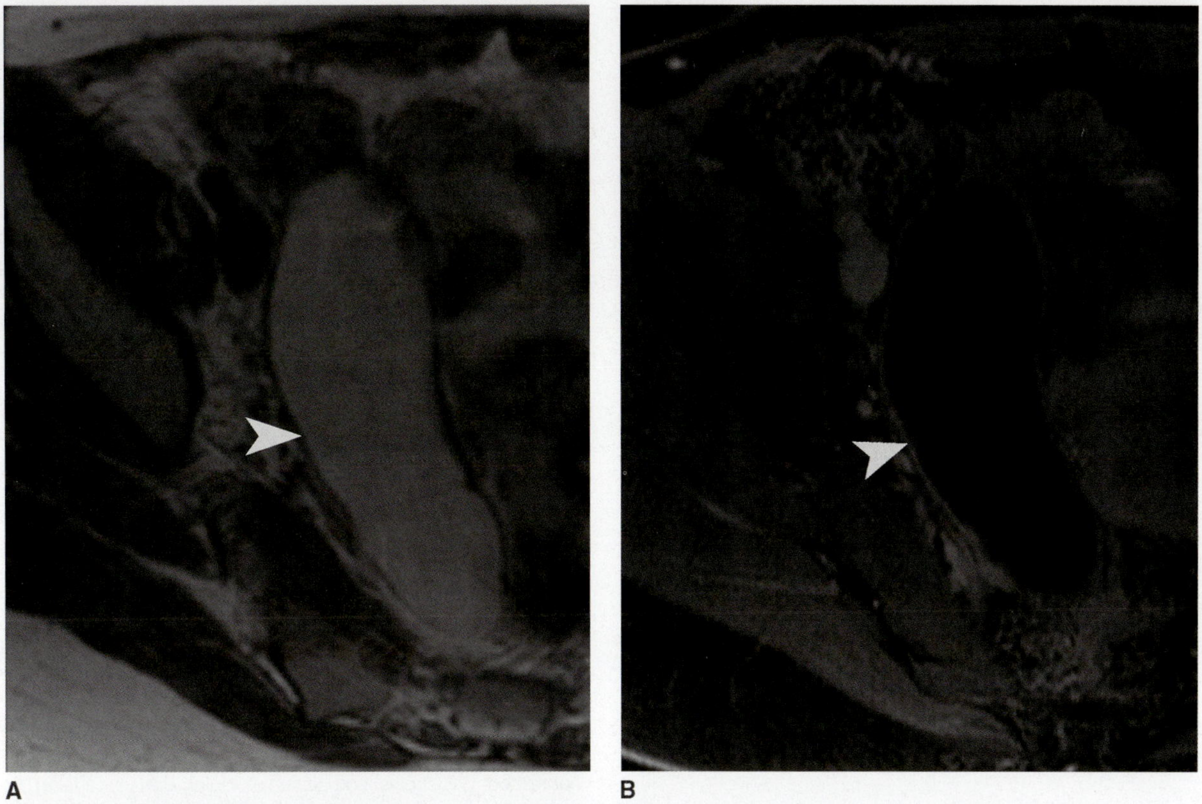

FIG. 6.18 • **Mucocele of the appendix. A, B:** T2 and postgadolinium T1WI demonstrates a cystic, sausage-shaped dilated appendix (*arrows*) in the right lower quadrant in a patient with mucinous low-grade cystadenocarcinoma.

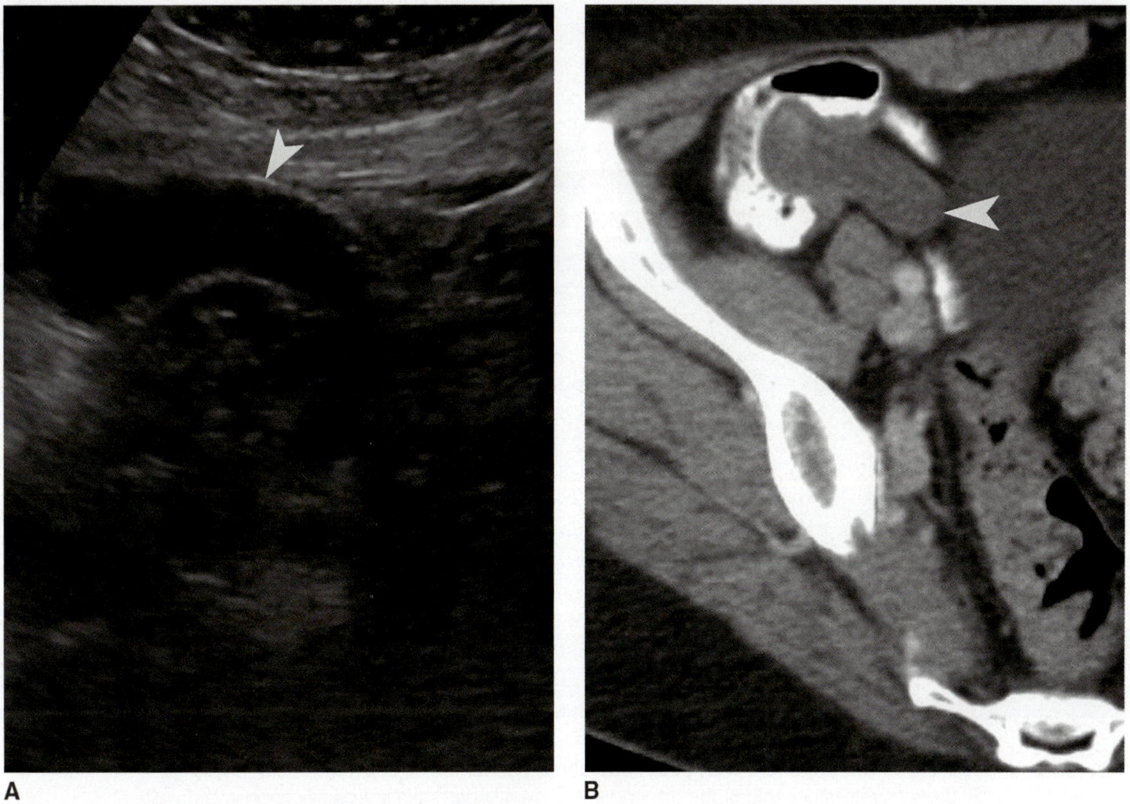

FIG. 6.19 • **Mucocele of the appendix.** US **(A)**, CT **(B)**, and coronal T2WI **(C)** demonstrate the chronically dilated appendix (*arrowheads*) without surrounding inflammation.

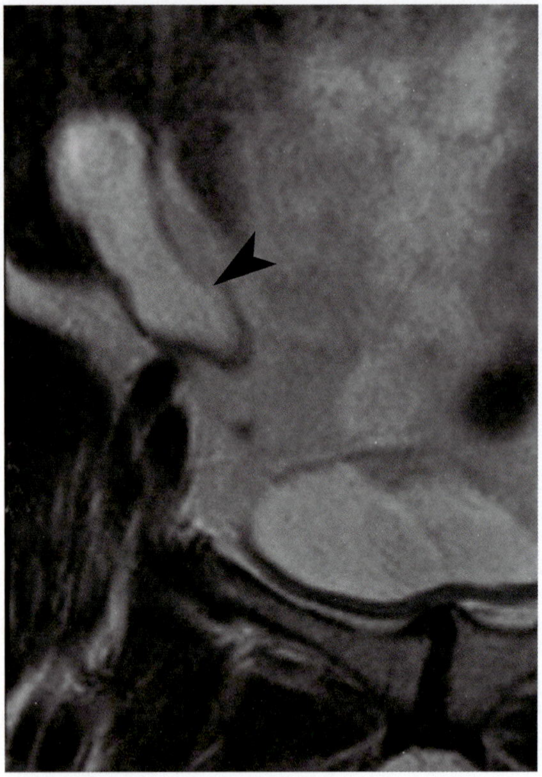

C

**FIG. 6.19** • (*Continued*)

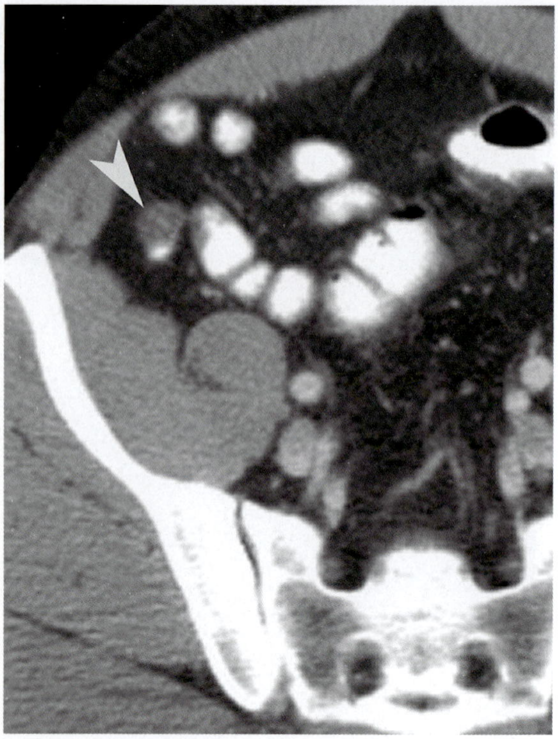

**FIG. 6.21** • **Adenocarcinoma of the appendix.** Axial contrast-enhanced CT shows soft tissue nodular density arising from the appendiceal wall (*arrowhead*) in a patient with metastatic adenocarcinoma without mucocele formation.

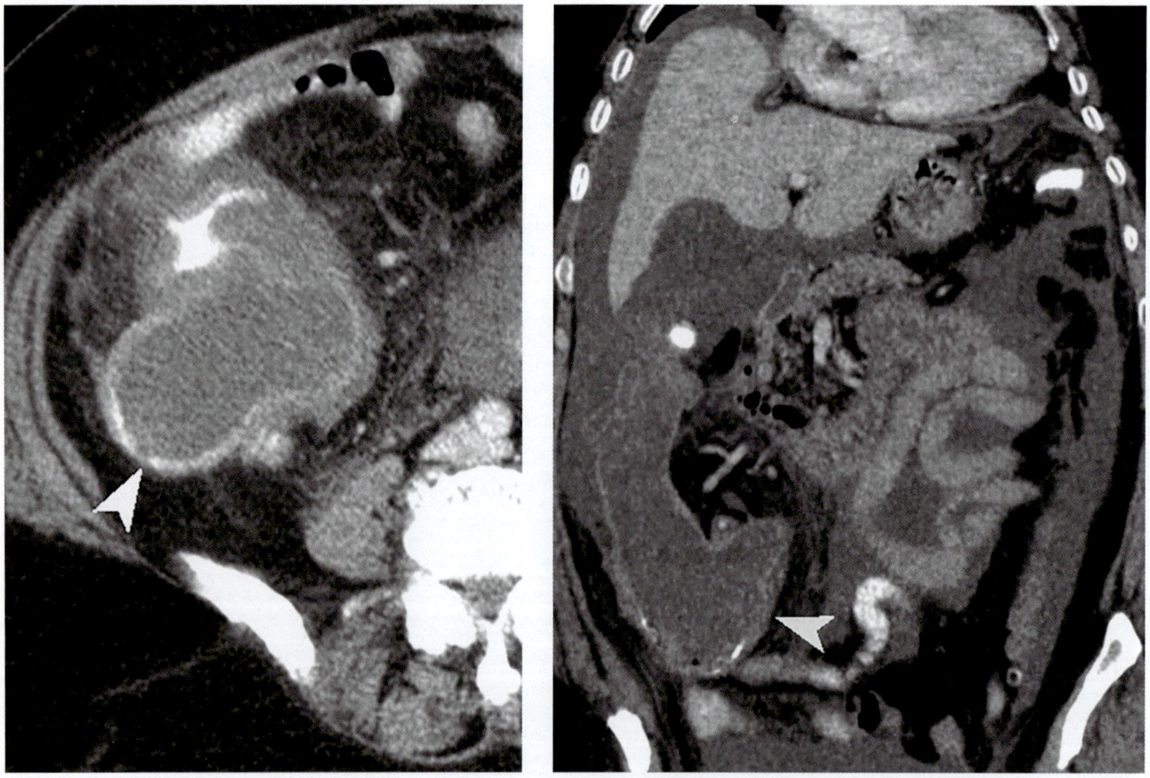

A B

**FIG. 6.20** • **Mucocele of the appendix with pseudomyxoma peritonei.** Axial **(A)** and coronal **(B)** contrast-enhanced CT demonstrate mucocele of the appendix with curvilinear calcified calcification in the wall (*arrowheads*). Fluid density in the peritoneal cavity is seen to cause scalloping of the liver outline and represents pseudomyxoma peritonei.

## MUCOCELE OF THE APPENDIX

Appendiceal mucocele can be classified into mucinous cystadenoma, mucosal hyperplasia, retention cyst, and mucinous cystadenocarcinoma. It is most commonly seen in the females in the sixth decade of life and is characterized by appendiceal distention due to retained mucus, often associated with mucinous cystadenoma or cystadenocarcinoma. Other causes of mucocele of the appendix include stricture, appendicolith, endometriosis, polyp, and other neoplasms (such as carcinoid and cecal cancer).

On imaging, appendiceal mucocele is most commonly 3- to 6-cm well-defined cystic mass, with curvilinear calcification in the wall (in less than 50%) (Fig. 6.20). On MR imaging, mucocele with high mucous content appears low signal intensity on T2-WI; however, if water content is high, then it appears high signal intensity on T2WI (Fig. 6.18). High mucous content also appears hyperintense on T1-WI. Mucocele rupture can lead to pseudomyxoma peritonei, which is characterized by loculated ascites, calcifications, and scalloping of the liver or spleen margin.

### *References*

1. Tkacz JN, Anderson SA, Soto J. MR imaging in gastrointestinal emergencies. *Radiographics*. 2009;29(6):1767–1780.
2. Pedrosa I, Zeikus EA, Levine D, et al. MR imaging of acute right lower quadrant pain in pregnant and nonpregnant patients. *Radiographics*. 2007;27(3):721–743.
3. Pickhardt PJ, Levy AD, Rohrmann CA Jr, et al. Primary neoplasms of the appendix: radiologic spectrum of disease with pathologic correlation. *Radiographics*. 2003;23(3):645–662.
4. O'Malley ME, Wilson SR. US of gastrointestinal tract abnormalities with CT correlation. *Radiographics*. 2003;23(1):59–72.
5. Sivit CJ, Siegel MJ, Applegate KE, et al. When appendicitis is suspected in children. *Radiographics*. 2001;21(1):247–262.
6. Gore RM, Levine MS. *Textbook of Gastrointestinal Radiology*. 3rd ed. 2007.
7. Singh A, Danrad R, Hahn PF, et al. MR imaging of the acute abdomen and pelvis: acute appendicitis and beyond. *Radiographics*. 2007;27(5):1419–1431.
8. Fraser JD, Aguayo P, Sharp SW, et al. Accuracy of computed tomography in predicting appendiceal perforation. *J Pediatr Surg*. 2010;45(1):231–234.
9. Kim MS, Park HW, Park JY, et al. Differentiation of early perforated from nonperforated appendicitis: MDCT findings, MDCT diagnostic performance, and clinical outcome. *Abdom Imaging*. 2014;39(3):459–466.
10. Incesu L, Coskun A, Selcuk MB, et al. Acute appendicitis: MR imaging and sonographic correlation. *AJR Am J Roentgenol*. 1997;168(3):669–674.
11. Pedrosa I, Lafornara M, Pandharipande PV, et al. Pregnant patients suspected of having acute appendicitis: effect of MR imaging on negative laparotomy rate and appendiceal perforation rate. *Radiology*. 2009;250(3):749–757.
12. Pedrosa I, Levine D, Eyvazzadeh AD, et al. MR imaging evaluation of acute appendicitis in pregnancy. *Radiology*. 2006;238(3):891–899.
13. Singh AK, Desai H, Novelline RA. Emergency MRI of acute pelvic pain: MR protocol with no oral contrast. *Emerg Radiol*. 2009;16(2):133–141.
14. Rao PM, Rhea JT, Novelline RA. CT diagnosis of mesenteric adenitis. *Radiology*. 1997;202(1):145–149.

## SELF-ASSESSMENT QUESTIONS

1. What is the pathology identified on the CT of a 71-year-old female with the right lower quadrant pain?

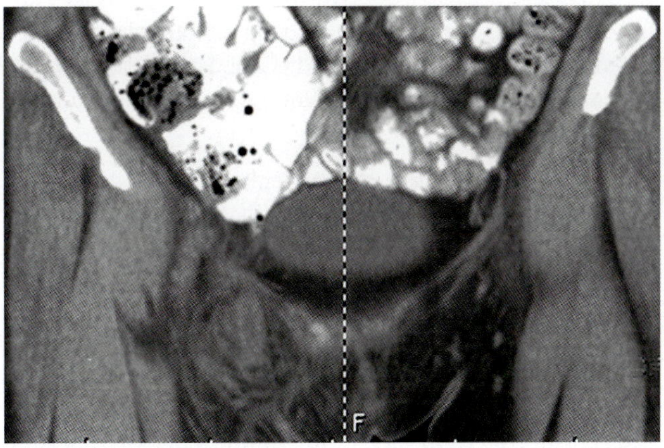

A. Amyand hernia
B. De Garengeot hernia
C. Carcinoid tumor
D. No pathology

2. What is the likely cause of the right lower quadrant pain in a patient who underwent a contrast-enhanced CT?

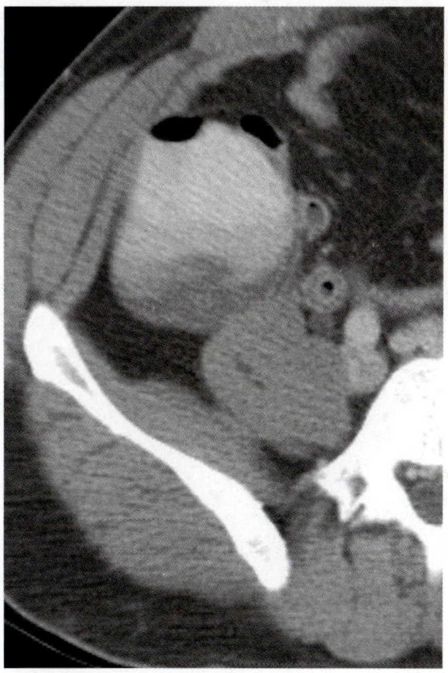

A. Crohn disease
B. Tuberculosis
C. Appendicitis
D. Typhlitis

3. A young adult patient presents with chronic right lower quadrant pain. What is the pathology (arrowhead) detected on the CT?

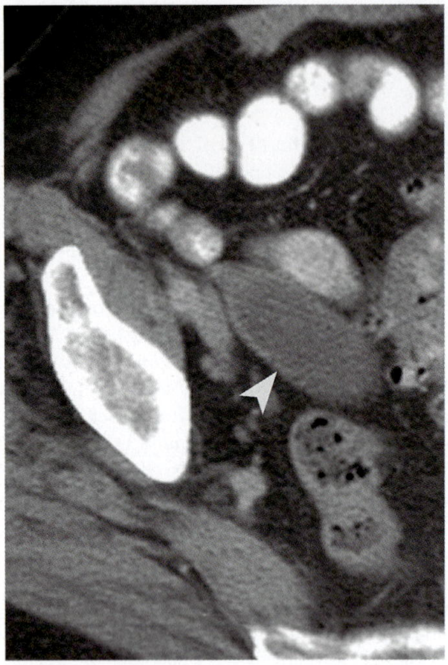

A. Acute appendicitis
B. Chronic appendicitis
C. Mucocele
D. Carcinoid

4. A patient presents with fever and right lower quadrant pain. What is the pathology depicted on the CT?

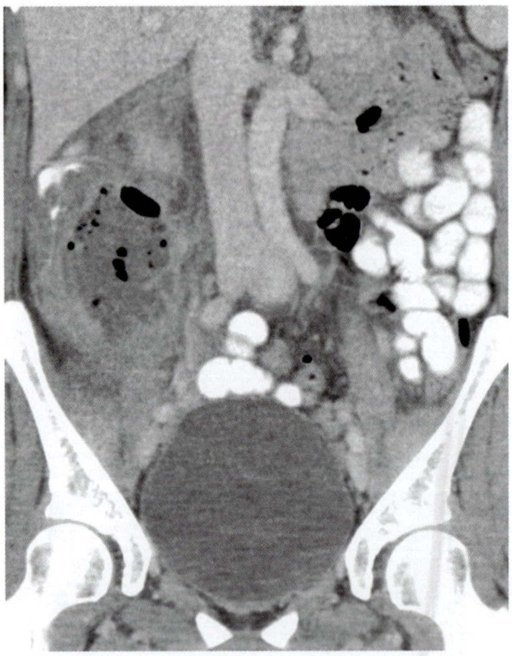

A. Typhlitis
B. Abscess
C. Crohn disease
D. Free fluid

5. What is the cause of acute appendicitis in a patient whose coronal CT reformation is shown?

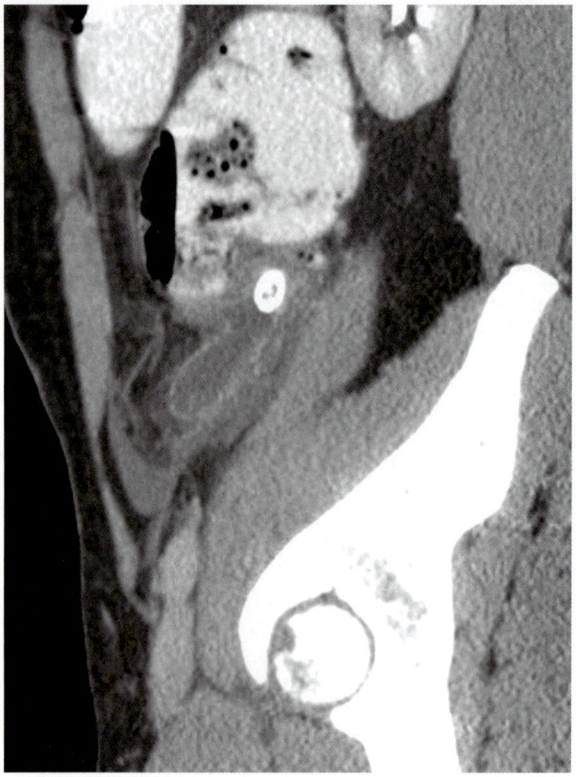

A. Lymphoid hyperplasia
B. Foreign body
C. Parasite
D. Appendicolith

## Answers to Self-Assessment Questions

**1. A.** Amyand hernia. The CT demonstrates the inflamed appendix in the right inguinal hernia, known as Amyand hernia. De Garengeot hernia is femoral hernia containing the appendix.

**2. C.** Appendicitis. The contrast-enhanced CT depicts the dilated appendix with thickened stratified wall and surrounding inflammation, consistent with appendicitis.

**3. C.** Mucocele. Contrast-enhanced CT shows a markedly dilated, fluid-filled appendix (arrowhead) without surrounding inflammation.

**4. B.** Coronal CT reformation shows fluid and air-containing abscess in the right lower quadrant with surrounding inflammation.

**5. D.** Sagittal CT reformation demonstrates a radiopaque appendicolith located at the base of the inflamed appendix.

# 7 Peritoneum

*Travis McKenzie, Amisha Khicha, and Kamran Ali*

## LEARNING OBJECTIVES

1. Review the anatomy of the peritoneal cavity with emphasis on pathology of disease spread.
2. Discuss the imaging of common intra-abdominal fluid collections and pathologies of the peritoneum.

The peritoneal anatomy consists of the peritoneal cavity, peritoneal ligaments, mesentery, and omentum. The peritoneum is subdivided into the parietal peritoneum, which lines the abdominal wall, and the visceral peritoneum, which covers the abdominal organs. Understanding the anatomic relationship of these structures is critical in identifying the pathology and establishing a diagnosis.

## PERITONEAL CAVITY

The peritoneal cavity consists of multiple potential spaces that are in partial communication with each other. The two major compartments of the peritoneal cavity are the greater sac and the lesser sac.

The greater sac can be divided into subspaces. The transverse mesocolon (Fig. 7.1) divides the supramesocolic and inframesocolic spaces. The left supramesocolic spaces consist of the perihepatic, left subphrenic, and perisplenic spaces. The right supramesocolic spaces consist of the hepatorenal space (Morrison pouch) and right subphrenic space (subdiaphragmatic space). The falciform ligament separates the left perihepatic space from the right subphrenic space (Fig. 7.2). The right supramesocolic spaces have a communication with the lesser sac via the foramen of Winslow. The lesser sac has boundaries formed by the posterior wall of the stomach, quadrate lobe of the liver, gastrocolic ligament, and lesser omentum.

The paracolic gutters are lateral to the peritoneal reflections of the ascending and descending colon. The right paracolic gutter freely communicates with the perihepatic space and pelvic cavity. The left paracolic gutter also freely communicates with the pelvis; however, the phrenicocolic ligament acts as a partial barrier to the perisplenic space.[1]

## PERITONEAL LIGAMENTS

The peritoneal ligaments act as barriers and guide flow of intra-abdominal fluid. The bare area of the liver is attached to the diaphragm and outlined by triangular ligaments (coronary ligaments). The falciform ligament is a longitudinally oriented ligament consisting of a peritoneal fold containing the remnant umbilical vein. Fluid or disease spread along the falciform ligament may be mistakenly diagnosed as a hepatic mass.[2]

The lesser omentum is a peritoneal fold that extends from the lesser curvature of the stomach to the duodenum and liver. The gastrohepatic and hepatoduodenal ligaments are contiguous with the lesser omentum. The gastrohepatic ligament contains the coronary vein and left gastric artery. The hepatoduodenal ligament contains the portal vein, hepatic artery, and biliary ducts. The hepatoduodenal ligament is a common site of spread from pancreatic diseases, biliary carcinoma, and gall bladder carcinoma.[3]

The greater omentum is a fat containing double-layered fold extending from the greater curvature of the stomach, draping over the abdomen. Given the lack of vital structures in the region, the omentum is an often overlooked site of disease spread.[4]

The mesentery is a fold of peritoneum that envelopes segments of the intestinal tract and connects to the posterior abdominal wall. The base of the small bowel mesentery extends obliquely from the ligament of Treitz to the cecum. The transverse mesocolon attaches the transverse colon to the posterior abdominal wall and contains the middle colic vessels. The sigmoid colon is invested in the sigmoid mesocolon, which can be an isolated source of disease spread.[3]

## ASCITES AND FLUID COLLECTIONS

The imaging characteristics and location of intra-abdominal fluid aids in determining the composition and etiology.

### Transudative Ascites (Simple Ascites)

The differential diagnosis for transudative ascites is extensive. The majority of cases of significant ascites are related to portal hypertension from cirrhosis, hypoproteinemia from liver/renal disease, or congestive heart failure. The characteristic CT

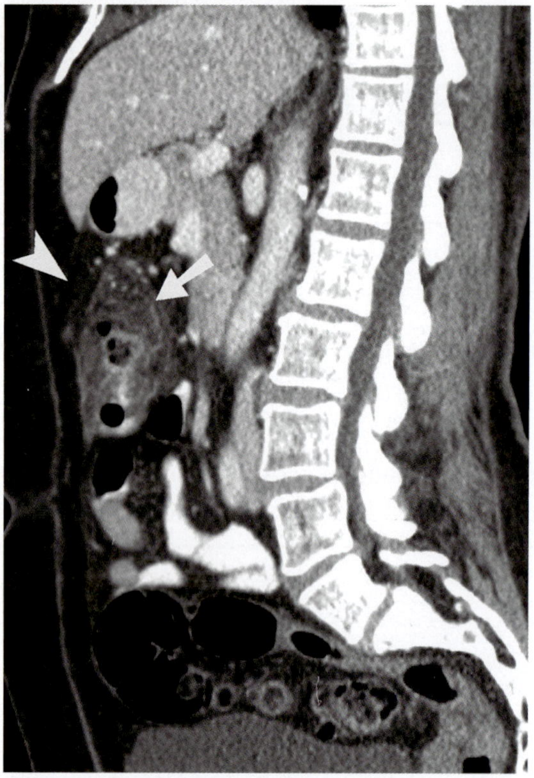

A

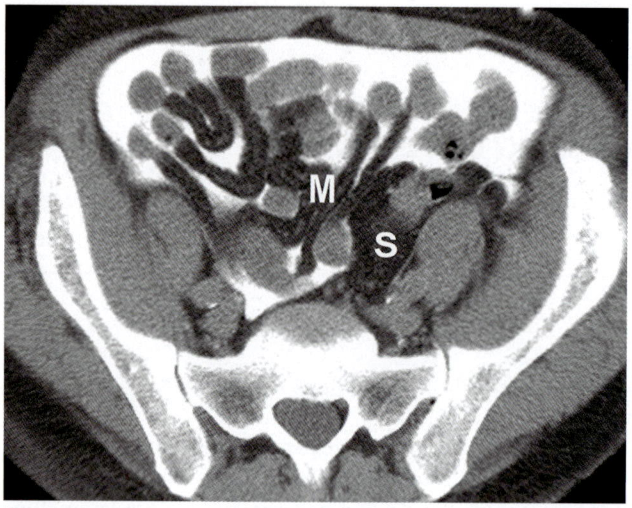


B

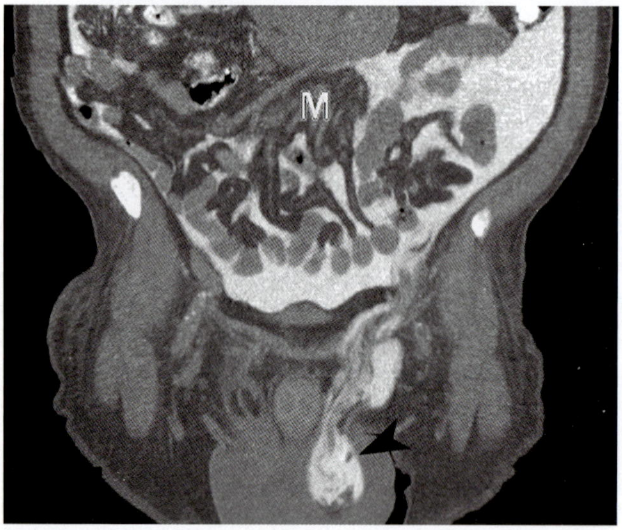


C

**FIG. 7.1 • CT anatomy of transverse mesocolon and mesentery. A:** Sagittal postcontrast abdominal CT reformation demonstrates inflammation in the transverse mesocolon from transverse colonic diverticulitis (*arrow*). The greater omentum (*arrowhead*) is arising from the greater curvature of the stomach and is located anterior to the transverse colon. **B, C:** Axial and coronal CT images demonstrate the fat containing small bowel mesentery (M), outlined by contrast injected into the peritoneal cavity. The sigmoid mesocolon (S) is located in the left lower quadrant. The contrast also extends into the left scrotum via patent processus vaginalis (*arrowhead*).

appearance is low-attenuating fluid, usually less than 10 HU. US demonstrates anechoic fluid. On MR, simple ascites is high signal on T2 and low signal on T1WI.

## Exudative Ascites

Exudative fluid has higher protein content than simple ascites. The etiology of exudative ascites includes metastatic peritoneal infiltration, infection, pancreatitis, and tuberculosis. On CT, the attenuation of fluid increases with the protein content and usually measures 10 to 30 HU. US demonstrates anechoic to hypoechoic fluid containing echogenic debris.[5] On MR, the high protein content results in variable signal on T1WI and high signal on T2WI.

## Acute Intraperitoneal Hemorrhage

FAST (focused assessment with sonography for trauma) is a useful screening modality in the emergency setting that can detect as little as 100 mL of free intraperitoneal fluid.[6] CT is the primary modality for identifying acute intraperitoneal hemorrhage, which appears as high-attenuating fluid measuring 30 to 60 HU (Fig. 7.3).[7] Sentinel clots are relatively high-attenuating regions (approximately 60 HU) representing coagulated blood. These are crucial to identify as they indicate the source of bleeding and are areas that are likely to rebleed. CT is performed with contrast to identify active contrast extravasation, a sign indicative of active hemorrhage.

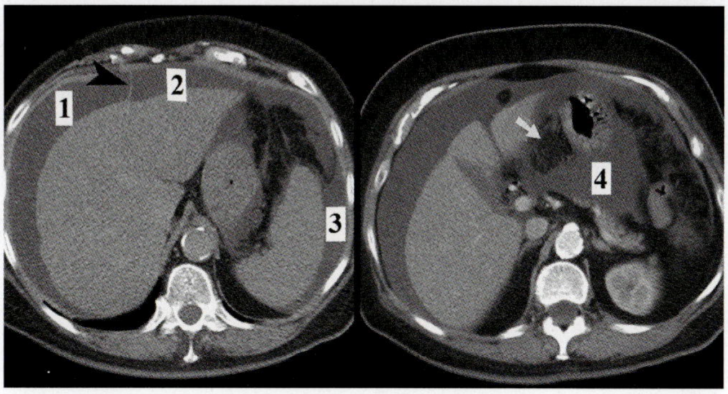


**FIG. 7.2 • Potential spaces in the abdomen.** Axial CT image demonstrates the falciform ligament (*arrowhead*) outlined by ascites, separating the right subphrenic space (*1*) from the left perihepatic space (*2*). Fluid is also visualized in the perisplenic space (*3*). There is fluid in the lesser sac (*4*), posterior to the stomach. There is fat attenuation of the lesser omentum (*arrow*) extending from the lesser curvature of the stomach to the liver.

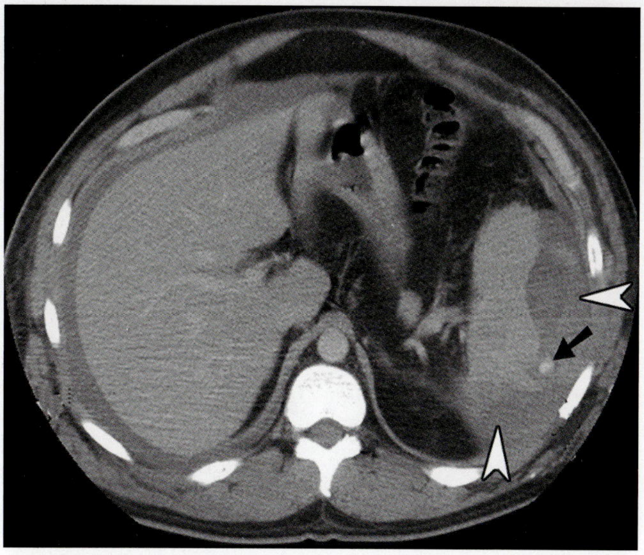

**FIG. 7.3 • Hemoperitoneum with splenic laceration.** Axial contrast-enhanced CT shows hyperdense fluid representing hemorrhage in the perisplenic area (*arrowheads*). A splenic laceration is present with a focal contrast blush representing active extravasation (*arrow*).

MR is infrequently performed for acute intraperitoneal hemorrhage and demonstrates variable signal intensity on T1WI and T2WI.

## Pseudomyxoma Peritonei

Thick gelatinous ascites associated with mucin-producing cells from ruptured appendiceal mucocele, mucinous ovarian cyst, or mucinous colorectal adenocarcinoma has been termed pseudomyxoma peritonei. Common sites of accumulation are in the right subdiaphragmatic space, along the omentum, in the left paracolic gutter, and in the pelvis. Pseudomyxoma peritonei is distinguished from simple ascites by the scalloped appearance on the adjacent organs, most commonly the liver and spleen (Fig. 7.4).[8]

On US, pseudomyxoma peritonei may show echogenic ascites and echogenic septations. The small bowel is usually displaced centrally by pseudomyxoma peritonei, sometime resulting in starburst appearance due to central, echogenic bowel in star-like configuration with surrounding hypoechoic fluid. Unlike mucinous carcinomatosis, pseudomyxoma peritonei typically does not extend into the chest.

## Chylous Ascites

Chylous ascites occurs from injury or obstruction of lymphatic flow. Chylous fluid has a milky appearance and can be confirmed with a triglyceride count of greater than 110 mg/dL.[9] The fluid measures fat attenuation on CT (−100 to 0 HU). Intra-abdominal malignancy, lymphoma, trauma, left subclavian vein thrombosis, and TB lymphadenitis represent potential causes for chylous ascites.

Cerebrospinal fluid from ventriculoperitoneal shunt placement (CSFoma) (Fig. 7.5), bile from bile duct injury, and urine

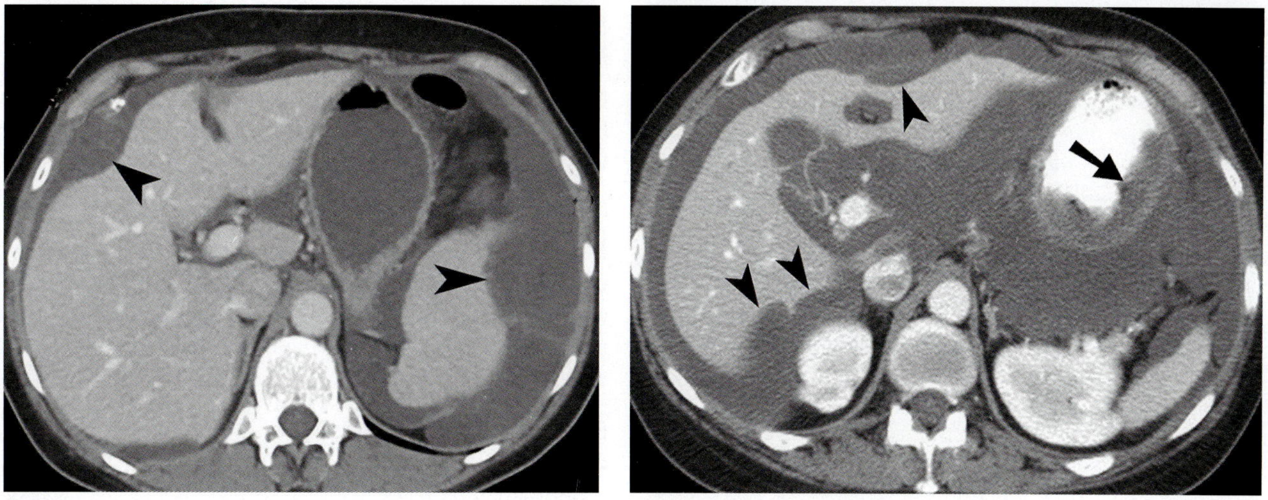

A B

**FIG. 7.4 • Pseudomyxoma peritonei. A, B:** Axial contrast-enhanced CT demonstrates septated fluid density in the upper abdomen with scalloping (*arrowheads*) of the solid viscera. The gastric adenocarcinoma is represented by gastric wall thickening (*arrow*).

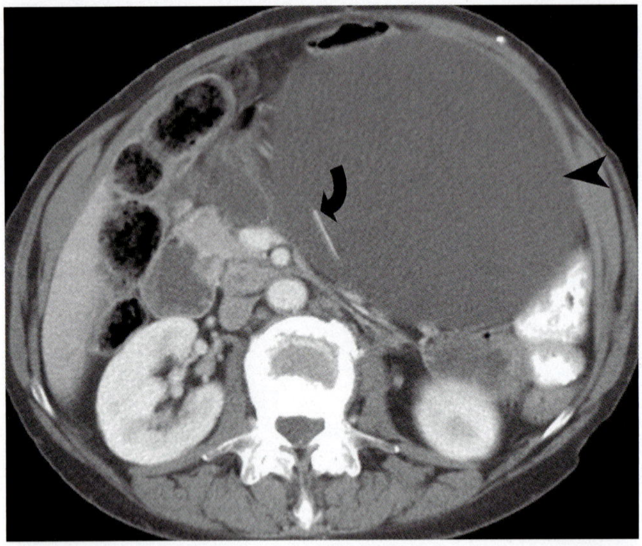

**FIG. 7.5 • CSFoma.** Contrast-enhanced CT shows a well-defined fluid density collection (*arrowhead*) around the tip of the VP shunt catheter (*arrow*).

from injury to the collecting system are other less common causes of ascites.

## Encapsulated Fluid Collections

### *Abscess*

Small postoperative seromas and hematomas are common and usually not a cause for concern unless there is worsening abdominal pain or signs of infection. Abscess formation is high on the differential in the late postoperative period (i.e., more than 5 days postoperative) with clinical signs of infection (e.g., fever, abdominal pain, leukocytosis). Common nonsurgical etiologies for abscess include complications of diverticulitis, inflammatory bowel disease, and perforated malignancy.

The classic appearance on CT is a rim-enhancing fluid collection (Fig. 7.6). Identifying air within the collection helps to solidify the diagnosis. US demonstrates a heterogeneous hypoechoic collection with echogenic debris. Droplets of air on ultrasound can appear as echogenic foci, whereas larger collections of air may demonstrate "dirty" acoustic shadowing. Abscesses are more difficult to diagnose on MR where fluid may have variable signal characteristics and small amounts of air are less conspicuous than on CT. Rim enhancement is the key finding.

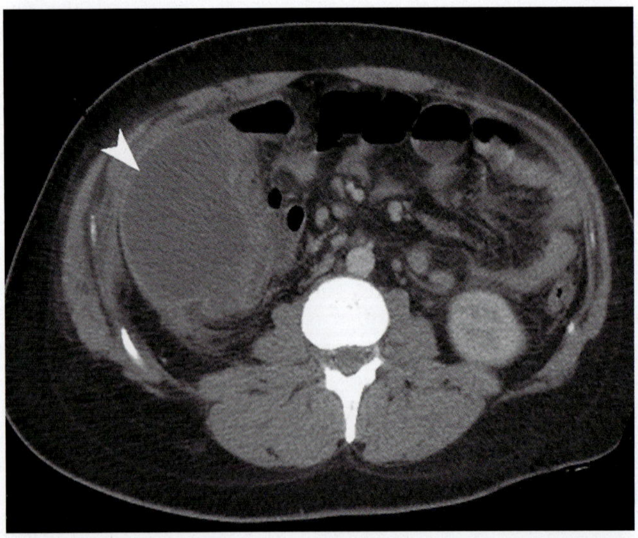

**FIG. 7.6 • Intra-abdominal abscess.** Axial contrast-enhanced CT of the abdomen demonstrates loculated abscess with rim (*arrowhead*) enhancement and surrounding inflammation.

### *Lymphangioma*

Lymphangiomas are located in the neck or axilla in 95% cases. Approximately 5% cases are seen in the abdomen or chest (excluding axilla). Abdominal lymphangiomas most frequently occur in the mesentery and less commonly in the retroperitoneum, omentum, and mesocolon. These are uncommon benign lymphatic malformations and may occur at any age. They tend to be large, thin-walled, and multiloculated collections (Fig. 7.7). The collections are typically water attenuation (less than 10 HU) and may have small peripheral calcifications. The classic appearance may be complicated by infection or hemorrhage.[10]

### *Peritoneal Inclusion Cyst*

Peritoneal inclusion cysts almost exclusively occur in premenopausal women with a history of prior abdominal surgery. Postoperative adhesions alter the physiologic ability of the peritoneum to absorb exudative fluid from the ovary. This causes a benign loculated fluid collection to form in the adnexal region of the pelvis (Fig. 7.8). The size varies from a few millimeters to larger lesions, which encompass the pelvis. US evaluation demonstrates a multicystic fluid collection in the pelvis that is separate from the ovary.

On CT, a peritoneal inclusion cyst is a contained fluid collection in the pelvis that conforms to the contour of the peritoneum with no peripheral enhancement. MR signal follows simple fluid characteristics.[11]

# MESENTERIC PATHOLOGY

## Misty Mesentery

Misty mesentery refers to non–mass-like increased attenuation of mesenteric fat. This may be due to fluid, inflammation, fibrosis, or tumor (Table 7.1).

## Mesenteric Inflammation

Mesenteric edema with engorged lymphatics (i.e., fat stranding) can often be the most salient feature of localized inflammation. The most common inflammatory diseases causing mesenteric edema are diverticulitis, appendicitis, Crohn disease, and pancreatitis.[12]

### *Sclerosing Mesenteritis*

Sclerosing mesenteritis refers to chronic mesenteric inflammation usually involving the root of the small bowel mesentery. It is associated with prior abdominal surgery, retroperitoneal fibrosis, orbital pseudotumor, Riedel thyroiditis, malignancy, infection, and sclerosing cholangitis.[13]

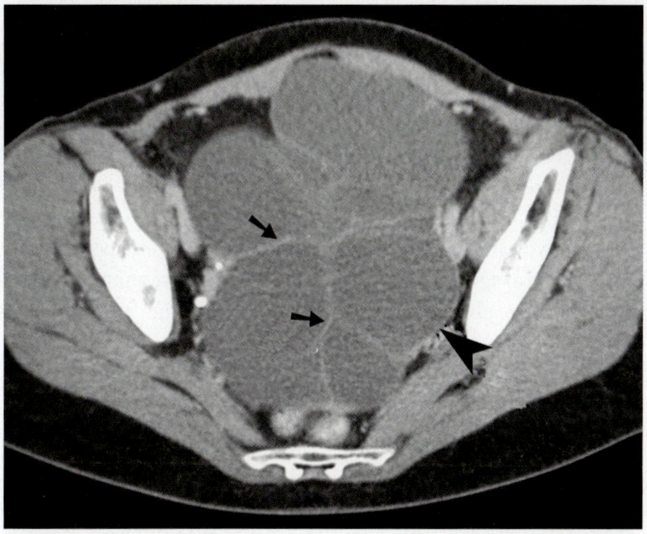

A

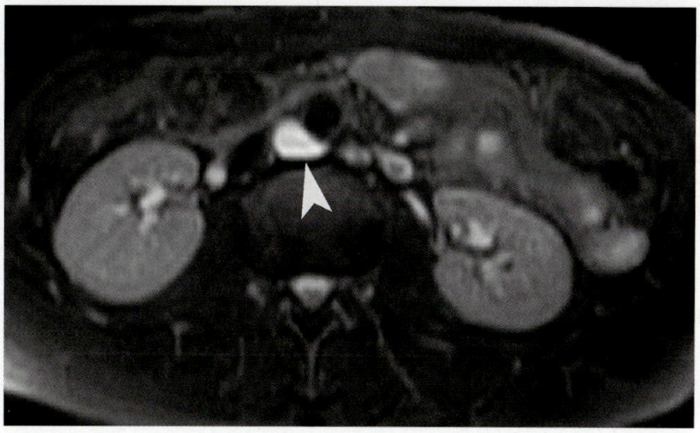

B

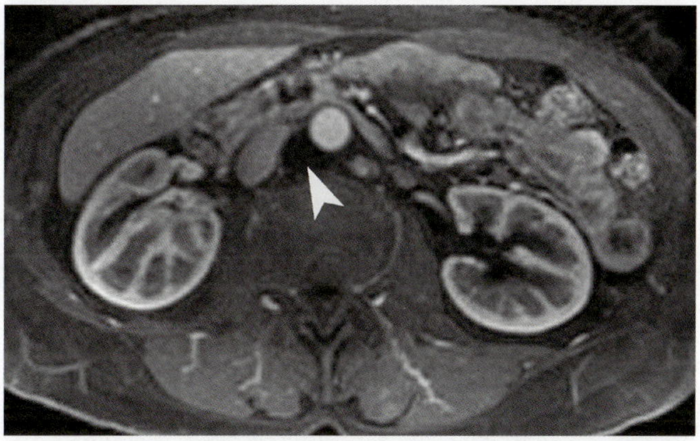

C

**FIG. 7.7 • Lymphangioma. A:** Axial contrast-enhanced abdominal CT shows a nonenhancing, septated (*arrows*) multicystic, low-attenuating lesion filling the pelvis (*arrowhead*). T2-FSE **(B)** and post-contrast T1WI **(C)** show a nonenhancing cystic lesion (*arrowhead*) in the retroperitoneum, which was stable over 3 years on cross-sectional imaging.

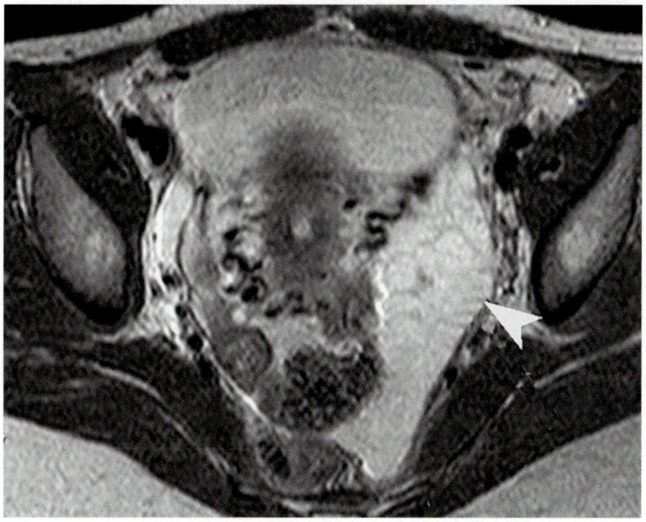

**FIG. 7.8 • Peritoneal inclusion cyst.** Axial MR T2WI in a patient with history of prior endometrial ablation demonstrates a multiseptated cystic lesion (*arrowhead*) in the left adnexa, which was separate from the left ovary.

Table 7.1 **MISTY MESENTERY DIFFERENTIAL DIAGNOSIS**

| | |
|---|---|
| Inflammation | Mesenteric panniculitis<br>Inflammatory bowel disease<br>Diverticulitis<br>Pancreatitis<br>Amyloidosis<br>Tuberculosis |
| Mesenteric edema | Lymphatic congestion<br>Portal hypertension<br>Heart failure<br>Nephrotic syndrome<br>Thrombosis of portal vein or mesenteric vessels<br>Hypoalbuminemia<br>Vasculitis |
| Hemorrhage | Trauma<br>Bowel ischemia |
| Neoplasm | Non-Hodgkin lymphoma<br>Carcinoid<br>Mesothelioma<br>Metastatic carcinoma<br>Melanoma |

Sclerosing mesenteritis is characterized by the presence of fibrosis, chronic inflammation, and fat necrosis. It is synonymous with retractile mesenteritis and is subdivided into three groups based on the histopathologic tissue type:

1. Mesenteric panniculitis
2. Mesenteric lipodystrophy
3. Retractile mesenteritis

Mesenteric panniculitis may have a misty mesentery appearance (Fig. 7.9) and classically demonstrates fat sparing surrounding the mesenteric vessels (fat ring sign), which helps distinguish it from other mesenteric pathologies. Subcentimeter lymph nodes can be seen with mesenteric panniculitis. In the absence of additional sites of significant adenopathy, the appearance is consistent with a benign etiology, and no further workup is necessary.[14]

Retractile mesenteritis typically presents as a mass-like lesion, consisting of mostly fibrotic with little inflammatory change. It can be difficult to differentiate retractile mesenteritis from carcinoid tumors. Additional imaging modalities such as octreotide scan can aid in the diagnosis. Sclerosing mesenteritis is favored when there is an absence of desmoplastic reaction on CT and absent radiotracer uptake on octreotide scan.[13]

## Desmoid Tumor

Primary tumors arising from the mesentery are rare benign tumors, which can be locally aggressive. The majority of primary mesenteric tumors are mesenchymal in origin and can occur most commonly in the abdominal wall, mesentery, or retroperitoneum.[8] Mesenteric desmoids, also known as aggressive fibromatosis, are associated with familial adenomatous polyposis (Gardner syndrome). The other associations include young women during or after pregnancy, estrogen therapy, abdominal surgery, and familial adenomatous polyposis.

CT is the imaging modality of choice and used for surgical planning as well as prognostication. These lesions present as mass with well-defined or infiltrating margin in the mesentery that are isoattenuating to muscle (Fig. 7.10A). Poor prognostic indicators include large size (greater than 10 cm), multiple lesions, and infiltrative or invasive features. On MR, the fibrotic nature results in low signal on T1WI. Aggressive lesions demonstrate high signal on T2WI.[8]

## Metastatic Mesenteric Tumors

Metastatic spread of lymphoma to the mesentery presents as multiple rounded nonenhancing soft tissue nodules.

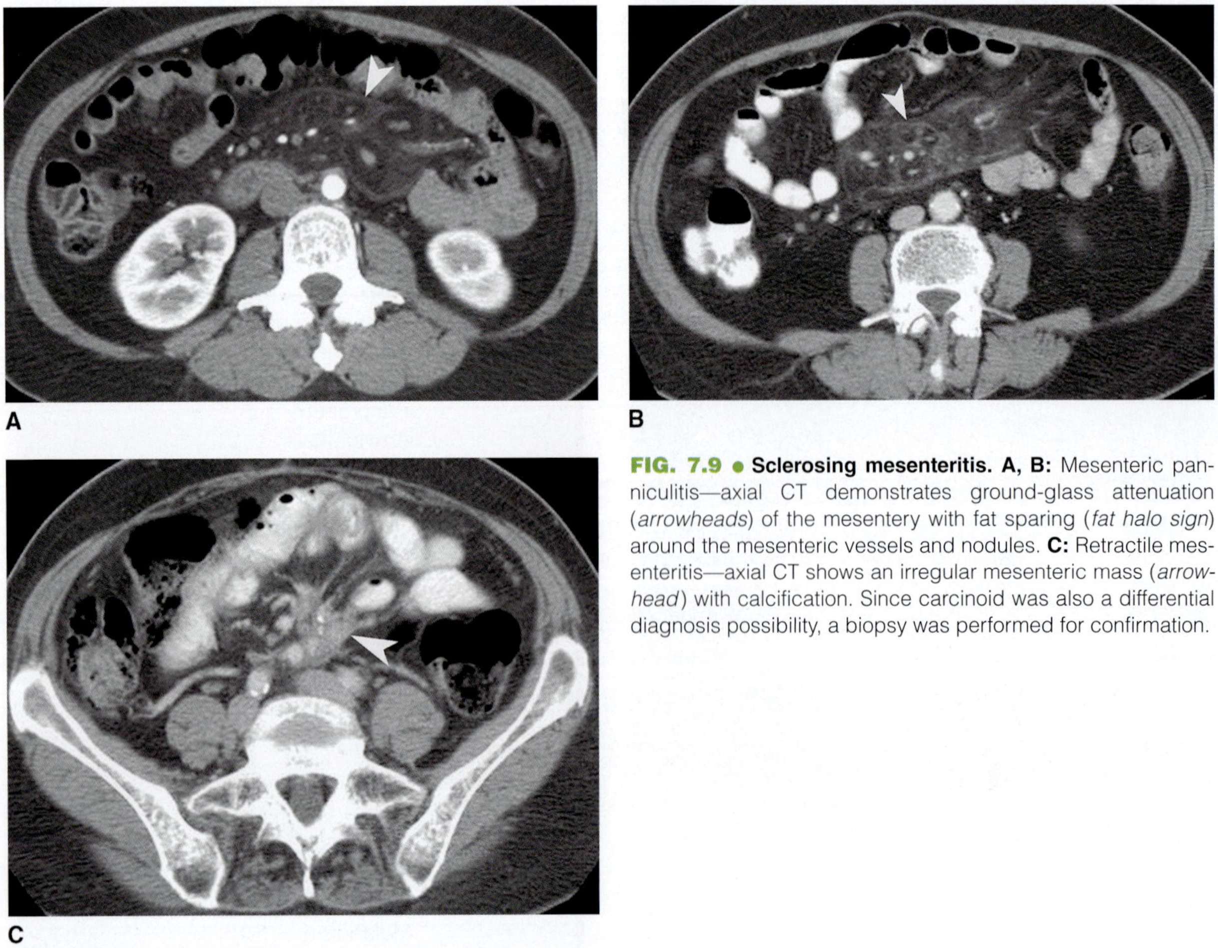

**FIG. 7.9 • Sclerosing mesenteritis. A, B:** Mesenteric panniculitis—axial CT demonstrates ground-glass attenuation (*arrowheads*) of the mesentery with fat sparing (*fat halo sign*) around the mesenteric vessels and nodules. **C:** Retractile mesenteritis—axial CT shows an irregular mesenteric mass (*arrowhead*) with calcification. Since carcinoid was also a differential diagnosis possibility, a biopsy was performed for confirmation.

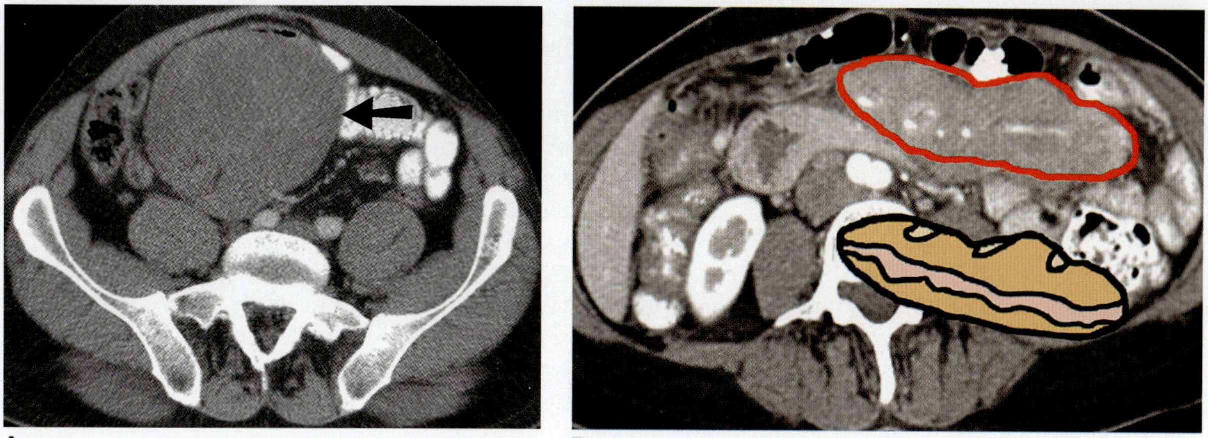

A B

**FIG. 7.10 • Desmoid (A) and lymphoma (B). A:** Axial contrast-enhanced CT demonstrates large well-defined soft tissue density desmoid (*arrow*) in the right pelvis. **B:** Axial contrast-enhanced CT demonstrates confluent mesenteric lymphnodal mass encasing the mesenteric vessels, described as sandwich sign.

Conglomerated lymph nodes can surround mesenteric vessels, giving the classic "sandwich" sign (Fig. 7.10B).

Metastatic carcinoid tumors to the mesentery are common and often more striking than the primary tumor, which usually arises in the ileum or jejunum. This typically presents as a mesenteric soft tissue mass with spiculations (Fig. 7.11). On MR, these lesions demonstrate low signal on T1WI and T2WI with minimal enhancement.[8]

There are four pathways of metastatic spread to the mesentery:[8]

1. Direct spread along the mesentery (e.g., gastrointestinal and pancreatic tumors)
2. Intraperitoneal seeding (ovarian carcinoma)
3. Lymphatic extension (lymphoma)
4. Hematogenous dissemination (melanoma, breast cancer, lung cancer)

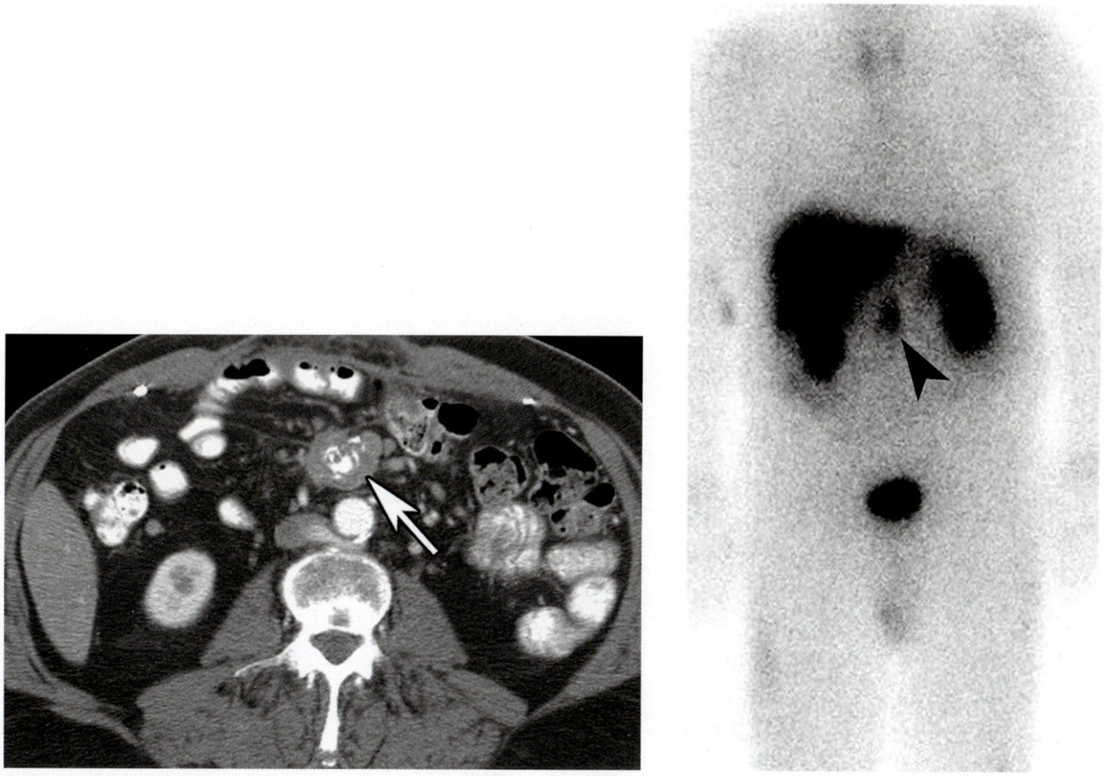

A B

**FIG. 7.11 • Mesenteric carcinoid. A:** Contrast-enhanced axial CT demonstrates an irregular mass in the mesentery with central coarse calcifications (*arrow*). Linear array of increased attenuation adjacent to the lesion represents desmoplastic reaction. **B:** Pentetreotide scan in a patient demonstrates radiotracer in the upper abdomen (*arrowhead*) from a known carcinoid.

### Infiltrative Mesenteric Lesions

Other less common diseases that have been shown to infiltrate the mesentery include tuberculosis, AIDS, Whipple disease, and amyloidosis.

## PERITONEAL AND OMENTAL PATHOLOGY

### Malignant Peritoneal Mesothelioma

Malignant peritoneal and pleural mesothelioma share similar imaging findings, characteristics, and risk factors. There is strong association with previous asbestos exposure, however, less so than with the pleural form. Plaque-like thickening and nodularity of the peritoneal lining are common features (Fig. 7.12). Calcified plaques may also be present. The appearance is described as dry or wet, depending on the presence of ascites. PET imaging aids in preoperative staging of the disease.[15] Imaging features of malignant peritoneal mesothelioma overlap with primary peritoneal serous carcinoma.

### Primary Peritoneal Serous Carcinoma

In contrast to malignant peritoneal mesothelioma, which predominately affects males, primary peritoneal serous carcinoma is more common in postmenopausal women. Plaque-like peritoneal thickening and intralesional calcifications are characteristic imaging findings (Fig. 7.13). The appearance can mimic findings associated with epithelial ovarian carcinoma. Management is surgical, consisting of total hysterectomy, oopherectomy, and tumor debulking.[15,16]

### Peritoneal Carcinomatosis

Many malignancies may spread to involve the peritoneum, including gastrointestinal and ovarian cancer (Fig. 7.14). Imaging findings include tumor studding of the peritoneum with development of malignant ascites as well as invasion of the omental fat producing omental caking.

The peritoneum and omentum should be searched extensively if there is ascites of unknown origin. Peritoneal studding may appear as hypoechoic nodules on US. While MR is not the primary modality, it can provide excellent visualization of the peritoneum. Gradual delayed enhancement (5 to 10 minutes) is common with carcinomatosis. FDG PET/CT has been reported as effective in the detection of peritoneal carcinomatosis (sensitivities 78% to 100%), but has limitation in spatial resolution to detect smaller nodules.[17] Metastatic spread of lymphoma or sarcoma to the peritoneum may be difficult to distinguish from peritoneal carcinomatosis.[18]

### Segmental Omental Infarct

Segmental omental infarction results from torsion of the vascular pedicle. This most commonly presents with acute onset of abdominal pain. It may be idiopathic or secondary to abdominal surgery. Unlike acute epiploic appendagitis, they are more commonly located on the right side and often mimic appendicitis. The right side predilection could be related to more tenuous vascular supply. Unlike acute epiploic appendagitis, which is most commonly seen in fifth decade of life, segmental omental infarction can occur in adult (85%) as well as pediatric (15%) patients. Predisposing factors for segmental omental infarction include strenuous exercise, congestive heart failure, recent abdominal surgery, obesity, and digitalis administration.

The characteristic imaging feature on CT is a heterogeneous fatty lesion measuring more than 5 cm in diameter and centered in the greater omentum (Fig. 7.15). Distinguishing segmental omental infarction from acute epiploic appendagitis is not necessary as the treatment of both conditions involves conservative management with pain medications. Recognition of these two pathologies is critical as they may mimic surgical abdomen.[19]

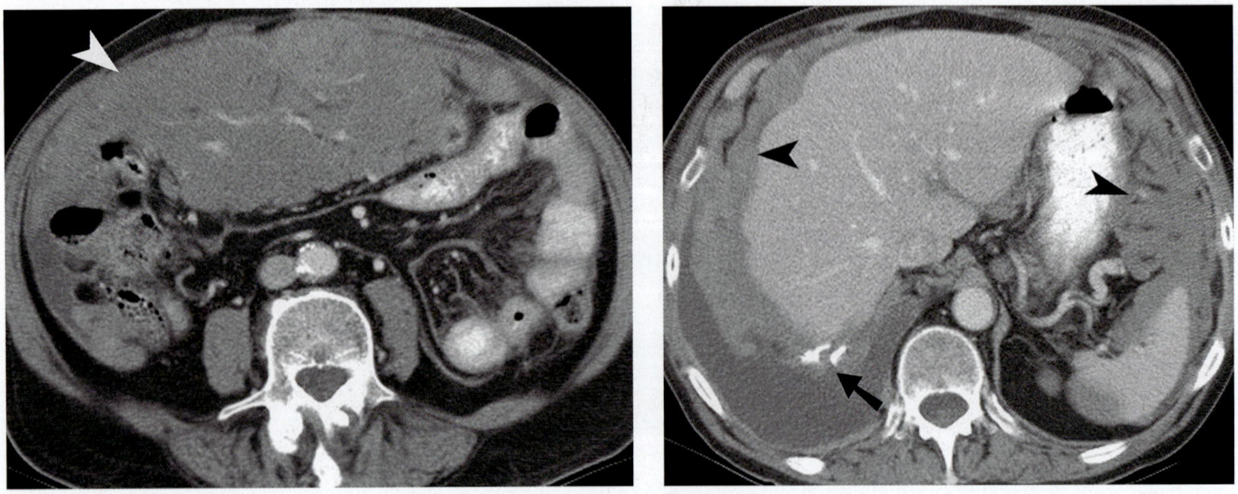

**FIG. 7.12 • Malignant peritoneal mesothelioma. A, B:** Axial contrast-enhanced abdominal CT demonstrates extensive peritoneal-based masses in the abdomen (*arrowheads*). There is calcified pleural plaque (*arrow*) also seen in the right hemithorax.

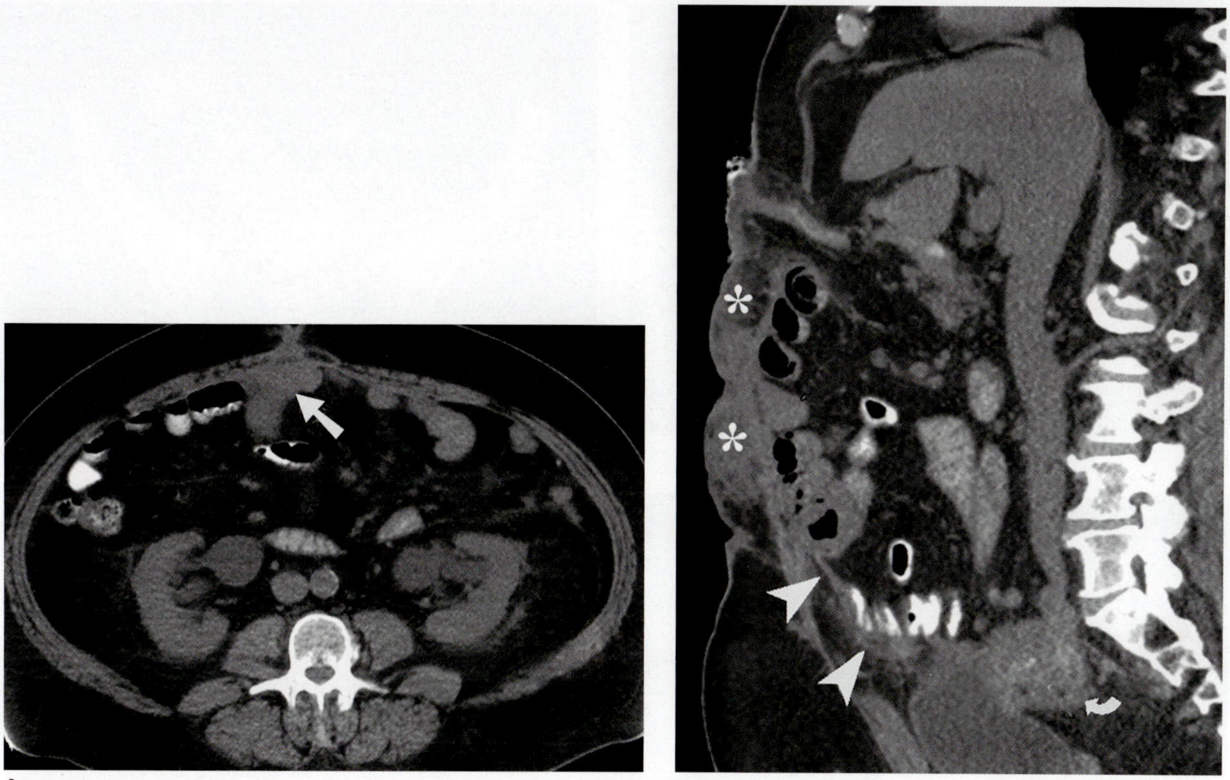

A B

**FIG. 7.13 • Primary peritoneal serous carcinoma.** Axial **(A)** and sagittal **(B)** CT images demonstrate plaque-like thickening (*arrow*) and nodularity (*arrowheads*) of the omentum with extension into the anterior abdominal wall (*asterisk*). A peritoneal soft tissue mass is seen in the pelvis with intralesional calcifications (*curved arrow*) and mild associated ascites (Courtesy: Mendy Smith, MD, West Virginia University.)

## Granulomatous Peritonitis

Granulomatous infection and inflammatory processes can result in caseating nodules along the peritoneum. Tuberculosis is a common cause. However, a myriad of other diseases and agents can incite a similar reaction (Table 7.2). Tuberculous ascites may be loculated and ranges in attenuation from fluid density to hyperdense. There is often peritoneal nodularity and calcifications. Other imaging findings may include miliary microabscesses in the liver or spleen, calcified lymph nodes, low-attenuating lymphadenopathy, and thickening of the cecum.[17]

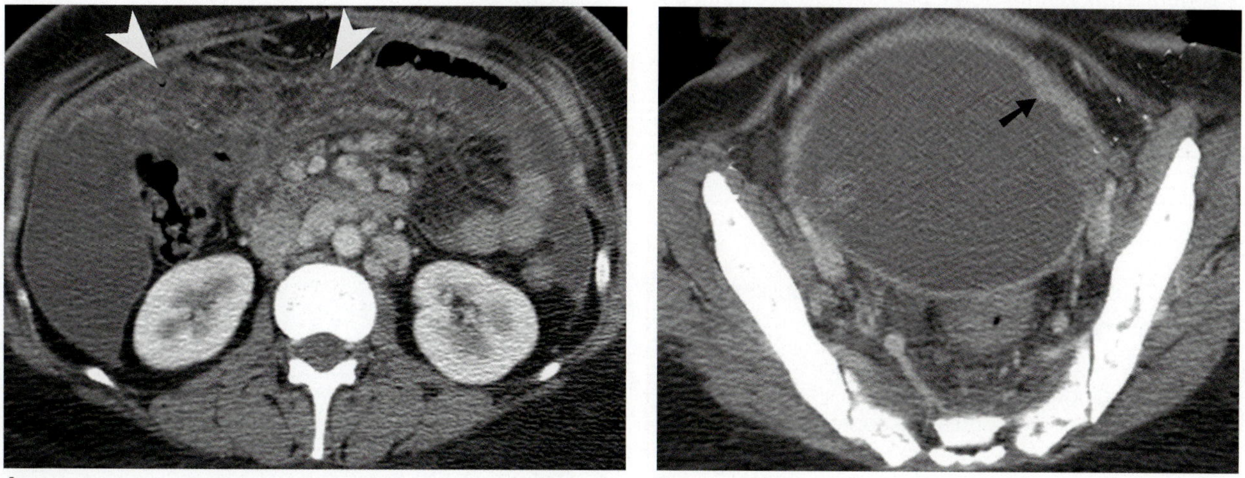

A B

**FIG. 7.14 • Peritoneal carcinomatosis. A:** Contrast-enhanced CT of a patient with history of gastric adenocarcinoma demonstrates soft tissue nodularity in the greater omentum representing omental caking (*arrowheads*). **B:** Contrast-enhanced pelvic CT of the same patient demonstrates ascites and enhancing nodular peritoneal thickening, representing metastatic implants (*arrow*).

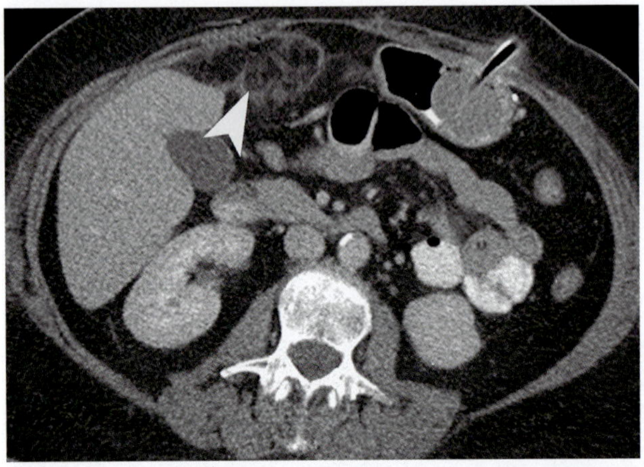

A

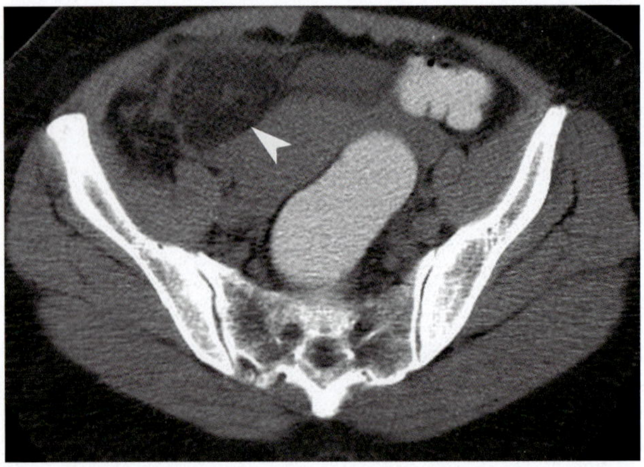

B

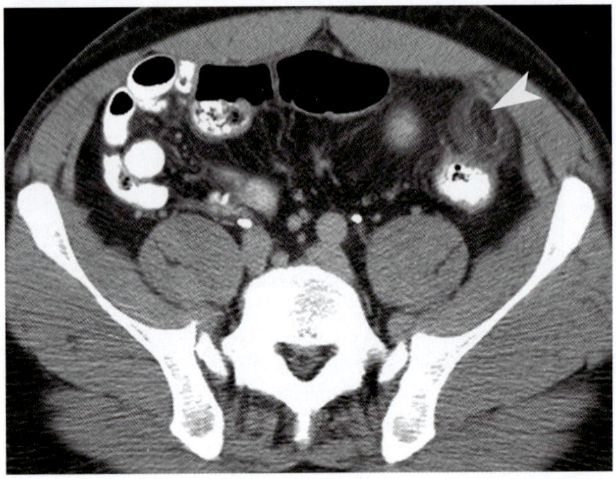

C

**FIG. 7.15 • Segmental omental infarct (A, B) and acute epiploic appendagitis (C). A, B:** Segmental omental infarct—axial contrast-enhanced CT in two patients with acute right-sided abdominal pain demonstrates a heterogeneous fatty lesion with a hyperdense rim in the greater omentum (*arrowhead*), consistent with omental infarct. **C:** Acute epiploic appendagitis—axial contrast-enhanced CT in a patient with acute left lower quadrant pain demonstrates an oval inflammatory fatty lesion arising from sigmoid colon with a hyperdense rim (*arrowhead*).

## Sclerosing Encapsulating Peritonitis

It is a chronic inflammatory process involving the peritoneum, seen in patients who undergo peritoneal dialysis. There is thickening of the peritoneum due to progressive collagen deposition from multiple episodes of peritonitis. On CT, there is diffuse thickening of the peritoneum, free fluid, and linear calcifications, often described as abdominal cocoon (Fig. 7.16).

Table 7.2 **GRANULOMATOUS PERITONITIS**

| | |
|---|---|
| Infection | Tuberculosis<br>Histoplasmosis<br>Pneumocystis organisms |
| Foreign material | Talc<br>Barium |
| Adjacent pathology | Meconium<br>Intestinal contents<br>Bile<br>Ruptured ovarian cysts |
| Systemic disease | Crohn disease<br>Sarcoidosis<br>Whipple disease |

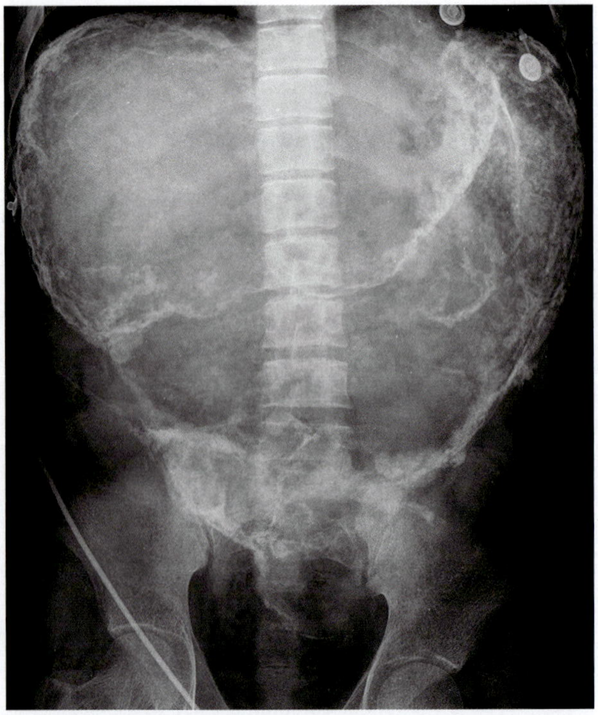

**FIG. 7.16 • Sclerosing encapsulating peritonitis.** Plain radiograph shows extensive calcifications along the peritoneum in a patient with multiple episodes of peritonitis from peritoneal dialysis.

## References


1. Tirkes T, Sandrasegaran K, Patel AA, et al. Peritoneal and retroperitoneal anatomy and its relevance for cross-sectional imaging. *Radiographics.* 2012;32(2):437–451.
2. Healy JC, Reznek RH. The peritoneum, mesenteries and omenta: normal anatomy and pathological processes. *Eur Radiol.* 1998;8(6):886–900.
3. DeMeo JH, Fulcher AS, Austin RF Jr. Anatomic CT demonstration of the peritoneal spaces, ligaments, and mesenteries: normal and pathologic processes. *Radiographics.* 1995;15(4):755–770.
4. Yoo E, Kim JH, Kim MJ, et al. Greater and lesser omenta: normal anatomy and pathologic processes. *Radiographics.* 2007;27(3):707–720.
5. Malde HM, Gandhi RD. Exudative v/s transudative ascites: differentiation based on fluid echogenicity on high resolution sonography. *J Postgrad Med.* 1993;39(3):132–133.
6. Von Kuenssberg Jehle D, Stiller G, Wagner D. Sensitivity in detecting free intraperitoneal fluid with the pelvic views of the FAST exam. *Am J Emerg Med.* 2003;21(6):476–478.
7. Federle MP, Jeffrey RB Jr. Hemoperitoneum studied by computed tomography. *Radiology.* 1983;148(1):187–192.
8. Sheth S, Horton KM, Garland MR, et al. Mesenteric neoplasms: CT appearances of primary and secondary tumors and differential diagnosis. *Radiographics.* 2003;23(2):457–473.
9. Press OW, Press NO, Kaufman, SD. Evaluation and management of chylous ascites. *Ann Intern Med.* 1982;96(3):358–364.
10. Sohn JH, Byun JH, Park SH. Abdominal cavernous lymphangiomas: CT findings. *Abdom Imaging.* 2005;30(6):689–693.
11. Jain KA. Imaging of peritoneal inclusion cysts. *AJR Am J Roentgenol.* 2000;174(6):1559–1563.
12. Thornton E, Mendiratta-Lala M, Siewert B, et al. Patterns of fat stranding. *AJR Am J Roentgenol.* 2011;197(1):W1–W14.
13. Horton KM, Lawler LP, Fishman EK. CT findings in sclerosing mesenteritis (panniculitis): spectrum of disease. *Radiographics.* 2003;23(6):1561–1567.
14. Corwin MT, Smith AJ, Karam AR, et al. Incidentally detected misty mesentery on CT: risk of malignancy correlates with mesenteric lymph node size. *J Comput Assist Tomogr.* 2012;36(1):26–29.
15. Cao S, Jin S, Cao J, et al. Advances in malignant peritoneal mesothelioma. *Int J Colorectal Dis.* 2014. doi:10.1007/s00384-014-2029-1.
16. Lubner MG, Hinshaw JL, Pickhardt PJ. Primary malignant tumors of peritoneal and retroperitoneal origin: clinical and imaging features. *Surg Oncol Clin N Am.* 2014;23(4):821–845.
17. Levy AD, Shaw JC, Sobin LH. Secondary tumors and tumorlike lesions of the peritoneal cavity: imaging features with pathologic correlation. *Radiographics.* 2009;29(2):347–373.
18. Cabral FC, Krajewski KM, Kim KW, et al. Peritoneal lymphomatosis: CT and PET/CT findings and how to differentiate between carcinomatosis and sarcomatosis. *Cancer Imaging.* 2013;13:162–170.
19. Singh AK, Gervais DA, Lee P, et al. Omental infarct: CT imaging features. *Abdom Imaging.* 2006;31(5):549–554.


## SELF-ASSESSMENT QUESTIONS

1. In a patient with pseudomyxoma peritonei, what is the most likely source of primary pathology?

   A. Rectum
   B. Pancreas
   C. Stomach
   D. Appendix

2. In four patients with misty mesentery, which CT image is best associated with mesenteric panniculitis?

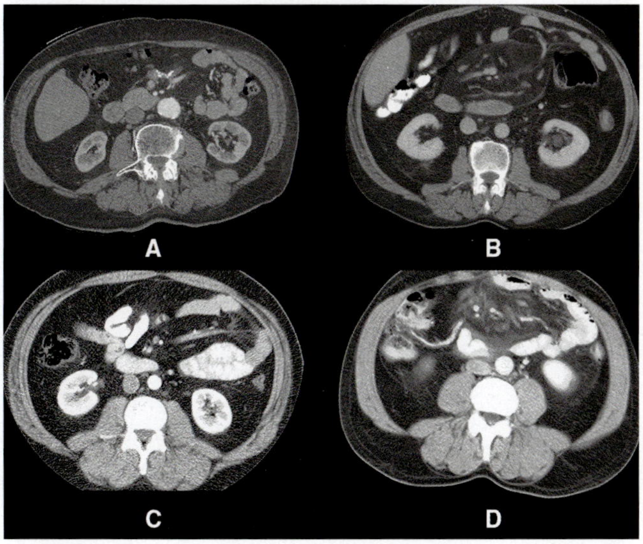


3. What is the likely diagnosis in a patient presenting with fever of unknown origin?

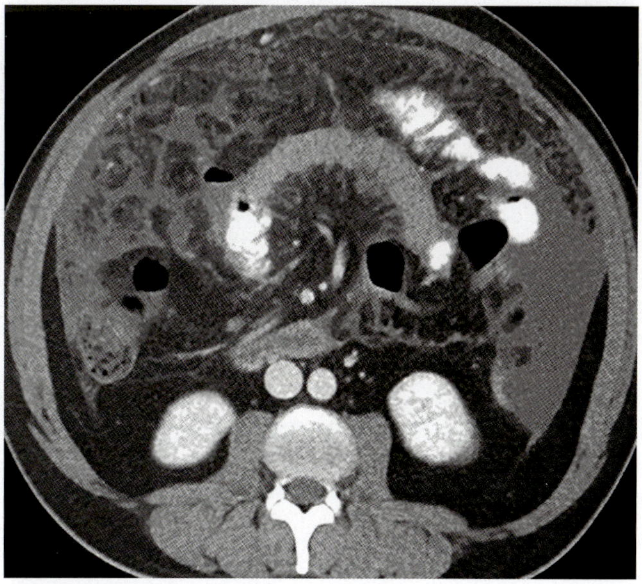

   A. Pseudomyxoma peritonei
   B. Omental infarction
   C. Tuberculous peritonitis
   D. Sclerosing mesenteritis

4. In this patient with a history of pelvic surgery, what is the likely diagnosis of the cystic lesion that was seen separate from the ovary?

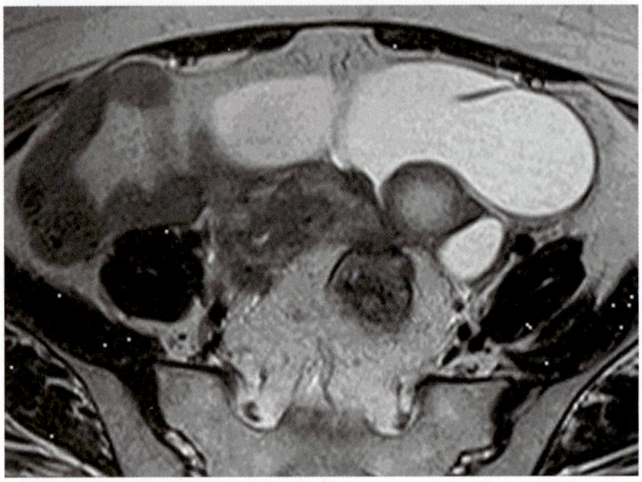

A. Peritoneal inclusion cyst
B. Mesenteric cyst
C. Mesenteric panniculitis
D. Desmoid

5. A 50-year-old male presents with abdominal distention. What is the most likely diagnosis?

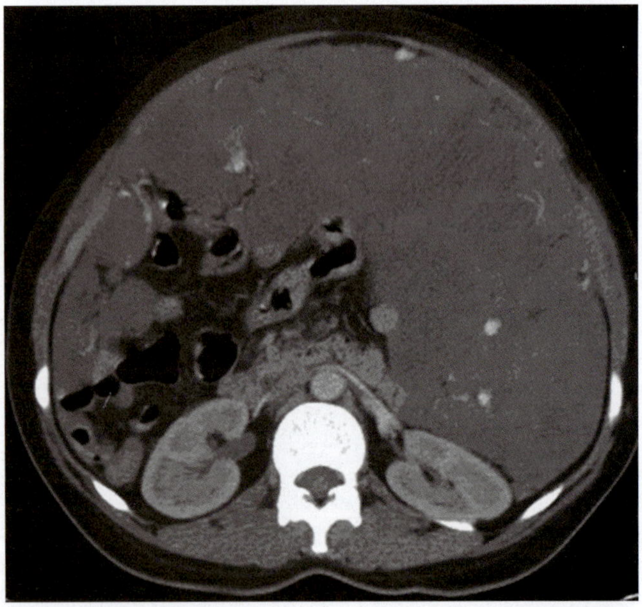

A. Mesenteric cyst
B. Peritoneal mesothelioma
C. Sclerosing mesenteritis
D. Omental infarction

## Answers to Self-Assessment Questions

**1. D.** Appendix. Pseudomyxoma peritonei can be caused by mucin-producing cells from ruptured appendiceal mucocele, mucinous ovarian cyst, or mucinous colorectal adenocarcinoma.

**2. B.** The CT (B) shows misty mesentery with fat sparing surrounding the mesenteric vessels (fat ring sign). C could represent calcified carcinoid or retractile mesenteritis. The lymphadenopathy in D could be secondary to lymphoma.

**3. C.** Tuberculous peritonitis. Omental infarction is a focal abnormality on CT and is most often in the right lower quadrant. Tuberculous peritonitis on the CT shows ascites and peritoneal nodularity, which would be indistinguishable from peritoneal metastases.

**4. A.** Peritoneal inclusion cyst. The CT depicts a fluid density cyst confirming to the contour of the peritoneum with no peripheral enhancement. The history of prior surgery is helpful in making the diagnosis in a premenopausal female.

**5. B.** Peritoneal mesothelioma. The CT demonstrates a large soft tissue density mass in the peritoneum, which is unlike the imaging findings expected with A, C, or D.

# Liver: Non-neoplastic Diseases

# 8A

*Sirote Wongwaisayawan, Rathachai Kaewlai, and Ajay K. Singh*

## LEARNING OBJECTIVE

**1.** Describe the imaging features of hepatic infections, vascular disorders, cirrhosis, and traumatic injuries.

## HEPATIC SEGMENTAL ANATOMY

The Couinaud-Bismuth system divides the liver into eight functional segments, each having a branch of hepatic artery, portal vein, and bile duct running in its center while hepatic vein branches in the periphery.[1] A vertical plane along the middle hepatic vein separates the right from the left hepatic lobe. The right lobe is further divided into the anterior and posterior segments by a vertical plane through the right hepatic vein, while a vertical plane through the left hepatic vein separates the medial and lateral segments of the left lobe (Fig. 8A.1). An imaginary line drawn transversely through the right and left portal veins further divides each of these four segments into the superior and inferior segments. These hepatic segments are numbered from I to VIII in a clockwise fashion within each lobe. Segment I, which represents caudate lobe, is located behind the ligamentum venosum.

Left lobe: Segments II to IV

- II: Lateral superior
- III: Lateral inferior
- IV: Medial

Right lobe: Segments V to VIII

- V: Anteroinferior
- VI: Posteroinferior
- VII: Posterosuperior
- VIII: Anterosuperior

## IMAGING TECHNIQUES AND NORMAL APPEARANCE

### US Anatomy

- The liver has homogeneous, moderate echogenicity (more echogenic than renal cortex but less echogenic than pancreas). Change in echogenicity can indicate disease process (Table 8A.1).
- There is echogenic wall around portal vein branches.
- There are no visible walls of hepatic veins.
- Hepatic artery is barely visible.
- Length is of less than 15.5 cm in the midclavicular line.

### Transplant Liver Doppler (Fig. 8A.2)

*Hepatic artery:*

- Continuous diastolic flow
- Acceleration time of less than 80 msec
- RI between 0.55 and 0.8

*IVC and hepatic veins:*

- Triphasic waveform but occasional biphasic or monophasic
- Main portal vein: helical flow (regular alternating or parallel red and blue bands on color Doppler, undulating flow above and below the baseline on spectral Doppler)

### CT Anatomy

- Homogeneous attenuation on both noncontrast and post-contrast portovenous-phase CT
- Attenuation 45 to 60 HU or 5 to 10 HU denser than the spleen on noncontrast CT
- Caudate to right lobe ratio: less than 0.6

### MR Anatomy

- T1WI: Signal intensity higher than the spleen but lower than the pancreas
- T2WI: Signal intensity lower than the spleen
- Chemical shift: Minimal difference of signal intensity on in-phase and opposed-phase images

## HEPATIC STEATOSIS

Hepatic steatosis or fatty liver is abnormal accumulation of lipids (particularly triglyceride) in hepatocytes. It is often associated with metabolic derangement (i.e., diabetes, obesity, hyperlipidemia, glycogen storage disease), hepatotoxins (alcohol, chemotherapy, amiodarone), or viral hepatitis. Although fat deposition is generally reversible if mild, steatosis associated with hepatocytic inflammation (i.e., steatohepatitis) can lead to cirrhosis.

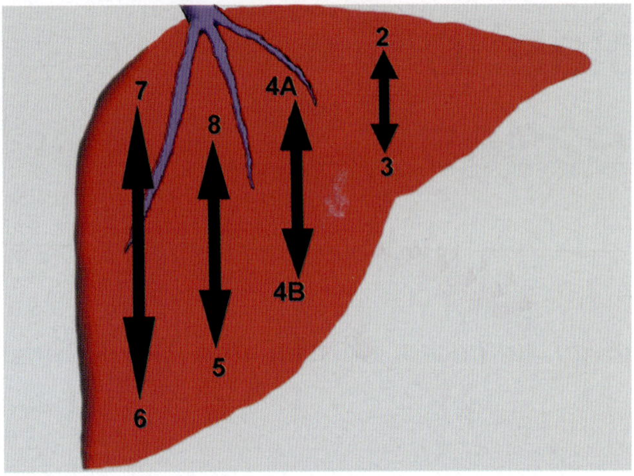


**FIG. 8A.1 • Normal liver anatomy (Couinaud-Bismuth system).** Schematic diagram depicts liver segments, separated by imaginary planes passing through the right, middle, and left hepatic veins.

On imaging, steatosis can involve an entire liver, segments, or a small area. There is no mass effect from steatosis and no displacement of intrahepatic vessels. Areas of steatosis are echogenic on US, hypoattenuating on noncontrast CT (absolute attenuation of less than 40 HU or at least 10 HU below that of the spleen), and hyperintense on T1WI. It loses the signal intensity on opposed-phase chemical shift MRI (Fig. 8A.4). *Diffuse steatosis* often results in hepatomegaly. If severe, intrahepatic vessels and diaphragm may not be visualized on US.[2] In a liver with diffuse steatosis, focal areas devoid of lipid accumulation (*focal fat sparing*) may be seen in the subcapsular region along the gall bladder fossa, adjacent to the falciform ligament and the posteromedial aspect of hepatic segment IV (Fig. 8A.5). Similar to *focal and segmental steatosis*, *focal fat* has sharp and geographical borders with the normal liver parenchyma. Common locations of focal fat and focal fat sparing are similar.

Table 8A.1 **DIFFERENTIAL DIAGNOSIS OF DIFFUSE LIVER DISEASE BY IMAGING PATTERN**

| Imaging Pattern | Differential Diagnosis |
|---|---|
| Mass with calcifications | Calcified metastasis (usually mucin-producing adenocarcinoma)<br>Adenoma<br>Hemangioma |
| Generalized hyperechoic liver (US) | Steatosis<br>Cirrhosis<br>Chronic hepatitis<br>Glycogen storage disease<br>Diffuse infiltrative malignancy |
| Periportal edema | Passive hepatic congestion<br>Viral hepatitis<br>Hepatic trauma<br>Post liver transplantation<br>Lymphatic obstruction |
| Generalized hypoattenuation (noncontrast CT) | Steatosis<br>Infiltrative malignancy<br>Budd-Chiari syndrome<br>Amyloidosis |
| Generalized hyperattenuation (noncontrast CT) | Hemosiderosis<br>Hemochromatosis<br>Glycogen storage disease<br>Amiodarone treatment (Fig. 8A.3) |
| Signal drop-off (chemical shift MRI) | Drop-off on opposed-phase images: steatosis<br>Drop-off on in-phase images: hemosiderosis, hemochromatosis |
| Generalized hypoechoic liver (US) | Acute hepatitis<br>Diffuse infiltrative malignancy |

## HEPATIC CIRRHOSIS AND CONFLUENT FIBROSIS

Cirrhosis, which represents end-stage chronic liver disease, is characterized by fibrotic destruction of the normal hepatic parenchyma with nodular regeneration. The most common etiology in the Western hemisphere and Japan is hepatitis C viral infection. In Asia and Africa, hepatitis B viral infection is the most frequent etiology.[3] Cirrhosis is known to increase the risk of hepatocellular carcinoma (HCC).

The imaging findings of cirrhosis are as follows:

- Earliest morphologic change is expansion of hilar periportal space, major interlobar fissure, and pericholecystic space.
- Late changes (Fig. 8A.6) are as follows:
  1. Hypertrophy of caudate and lateral segment of the left hepatic lobe. The normal ratio of the caudate lobe to the right lobe is less than 0.6. Caudate lobe hypertrophy can increase the ratio to greater than 0.65. The caudate lobe is measured from the left margin of the caudate lobe to a vertical plane passing through the right margin of the portal vein.
  2. Atrophy of the anterior segment of the right hepatic lobe and medial segment of the left hepatic lobe.
  3. Diffuse coarse heterogeneous hepatic parenchyma.
- There is demonstration of portal hypertension (recanalized umbilical vein, dilated portal vein, varices, splenomegaly, ascites, portal colopathy, etc.) (Fig. 8A.7).
- Surface nodularity represents multiple regenerative nodules (micronodular and macronodular cirrhosis). Micronodules are usually smaller than 3 mm and are commonly seen in alcoholic liver disease. Macronodular cirrhosis has nodules ranging from a few mm to 15 mm and is common in viral hepatitis (Fig. 8A.8).[4]
- Areas of fibrosis may show mild T2 hyperintensity on MRI. This is typically seen as fine, cobblestone appearance of the hepatic parenchyma (Fig. 8A.9).

In patients with long-standing cirrhosis, or less commonly early-staged compensated cirrhosis, focal fibrotic masses may develop in areas of hepatic parenchymal collapse and are called confluent hepatic fibrosis. The imaging features of confluent hepatic fibrosis (Fig. 8A.9) include the following:

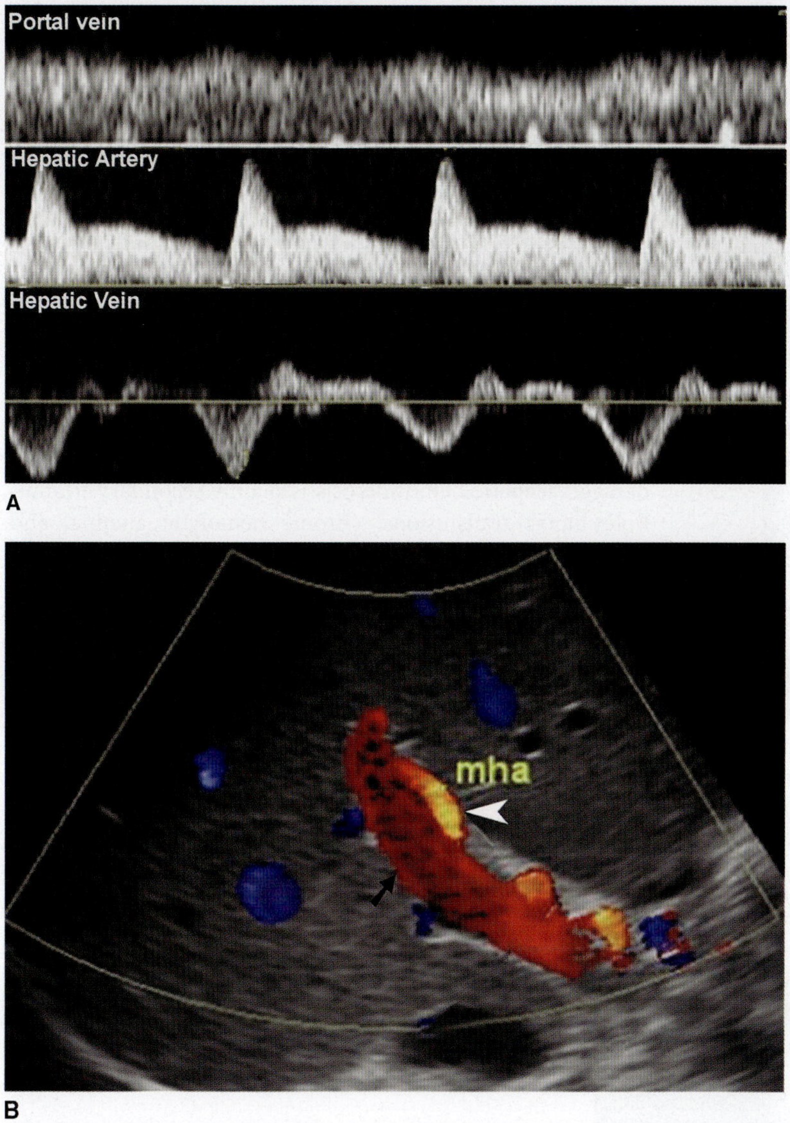


**FIG. 8A.2 • Normal Doppler ultrasound. A:** Spectral waveforms of the main portal vein (gently undulating waveform), hepatic artery (low resistance), and hepatic vein (triphasic waveform) are depicted. **B:** Color Doppler US demonstrates the main hepatic vein (*arrow*) at the porta hepatis, located posterior to the main hepatic artery (*arrowhead*).

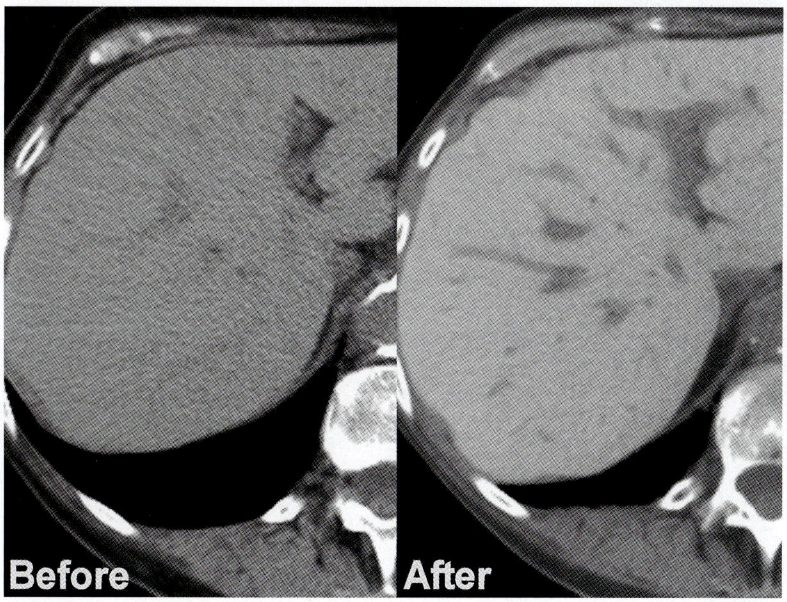


**FIG. 8A.3 • Amiodarone-induced increased liver density.** Noncontrast CT images before and 4 years after starting amiodarone treatment demonstrate more than 25 Hounsfield increase in the liver density, due to amiodarone and desethylamiodarone deposition in the liver parenchyma. Iodine constitutes 37% of the molecular weight of amiodarone.

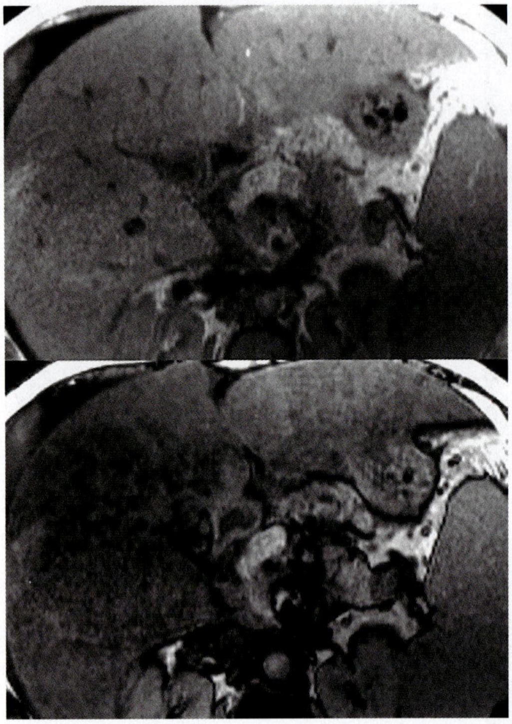

**FIG. 8A.4 • Fatty liver on MR.** In-phase and opposed-phase T1WI of the liver demonstrate heterogeneous loss of signal intensity most prominently in the right lobe of the liver. These are gradient echo sequences with same TR but different TE, which accentuates intracellular fat.

- Solitary or multiple wedge shape with a wide base toward the hepatic capsule, with capsular retraction and volume loss (vs. tumor).[3,5]
- Involvement of the segments IV and VIII is typical.
- Hypoattenuating on noncontrast CT, hypointense on T1WI, and hyperintense on T2WI.
- Enhancement on hepatic arterial and venous phases is either equal to or less than the surrounding hepatic parenchyma.
- Delayed enhancement is characteristic.

## HEPATIC PIGMENTARY DISORDERS

### Hemosiderosis

Hemosiderosis is a pathologic condition defined by tissue deposition of excess iron without the evidence of end organ damage. Hepatic hemosiderosis is mainly secondary to multiple blood transfusions, chronic hemolytic anemia, and chronic liver disease. The imaging findings resemble those of hemochromatosis.

### Hemochromatosis

Hemochromatosis is characterized by organ toxicity secondary to abnormal iron deposition in various organs, including the liver.

- *Primary hemochromatosis* is an autosomal recessive condition, characterized by abnormally increased intestinal

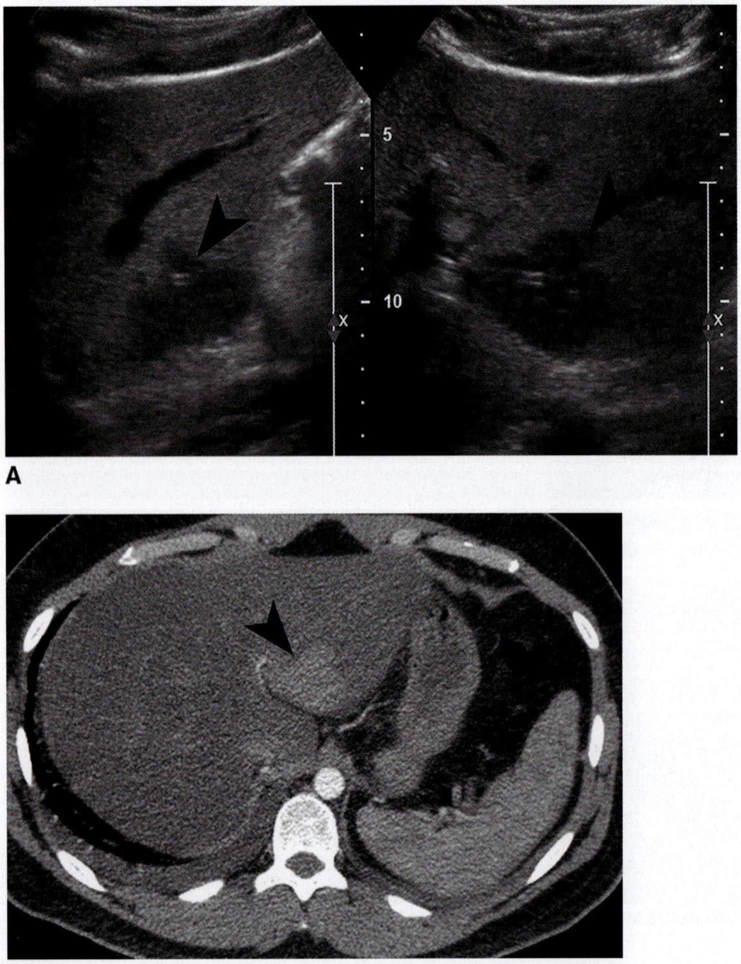


**FIG. 8A.5 • Fatty liver with focal fatty sparing. A:** US in a patient with fatty liver demonstrates diffusely increased liver echogenicity with a hypoechoic area of focal fatty sparing in the left lobe of the liver (*arrowheads*). **B:** CT of the abdomen demonstrates diffuse decrease in the liver density compared to the splenic parenchyma with a relatively higher density focal area located posteriorly in the left lobe (*arrowhead*), consistent with focal fatty sparing.

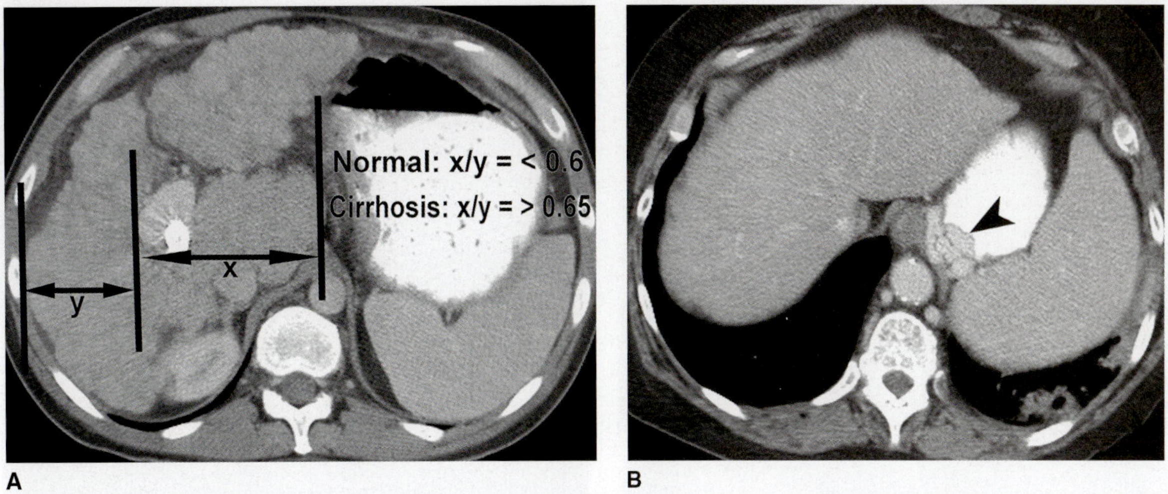


**FIG. 8A.6 • Cirrhosis and submucosal gastric varices. A:** Contrast-enhanced CT demonstrates enlargement of the caudate lobe of the liver. The ratio of the caudate lobe to the right lobe is normally less than 0.6. The caudate lobe is measured from the left margin of the caudate lobe to a vertical plane passing through the right margin of the main portal vein. The right lobe is measured from the right margin of the liver to the plane passing through the right margin of the main portal vein. **B:** Contrast-enhanced CT scan study demonstrates lobulated outline, left lobe hypertrophy, and submucosal gastric varices in the wall of posterior fundus (*arrowhead*).

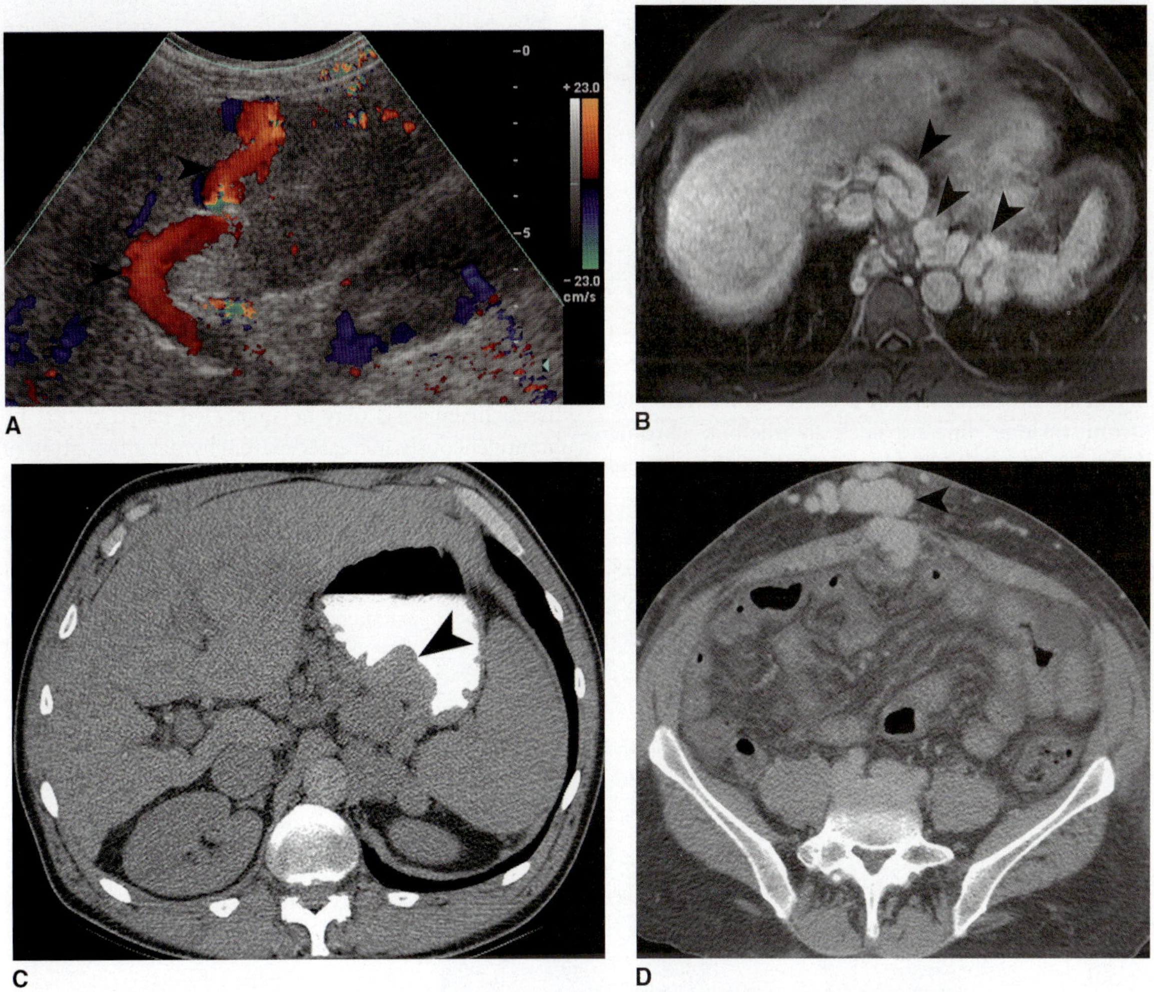


**FIG. 8A.7 • Cirrhosis with portal hypertension. A:** Color Doppler ultrasound demonstrates recanalized umbilical vein (*arrowheads*) in the ligamentum teres. **B:** Postcontrast T1WI demonstrates extensive upper retroperitoneal varices (*arrowheads*) in a patient with portal hypertension. **C:** Noncontrast CT of the abdomen demonstrates a lobulated submucosal mass in the posterior gastric wall (*arrowhead*), caused by multiple gastric varices. **D:** Contrast-enhanced CT in a patient with cirrhosis and portal hypertension demonstrates extensive dilated collateral vessels at the umbilicus (*arrowhead*).

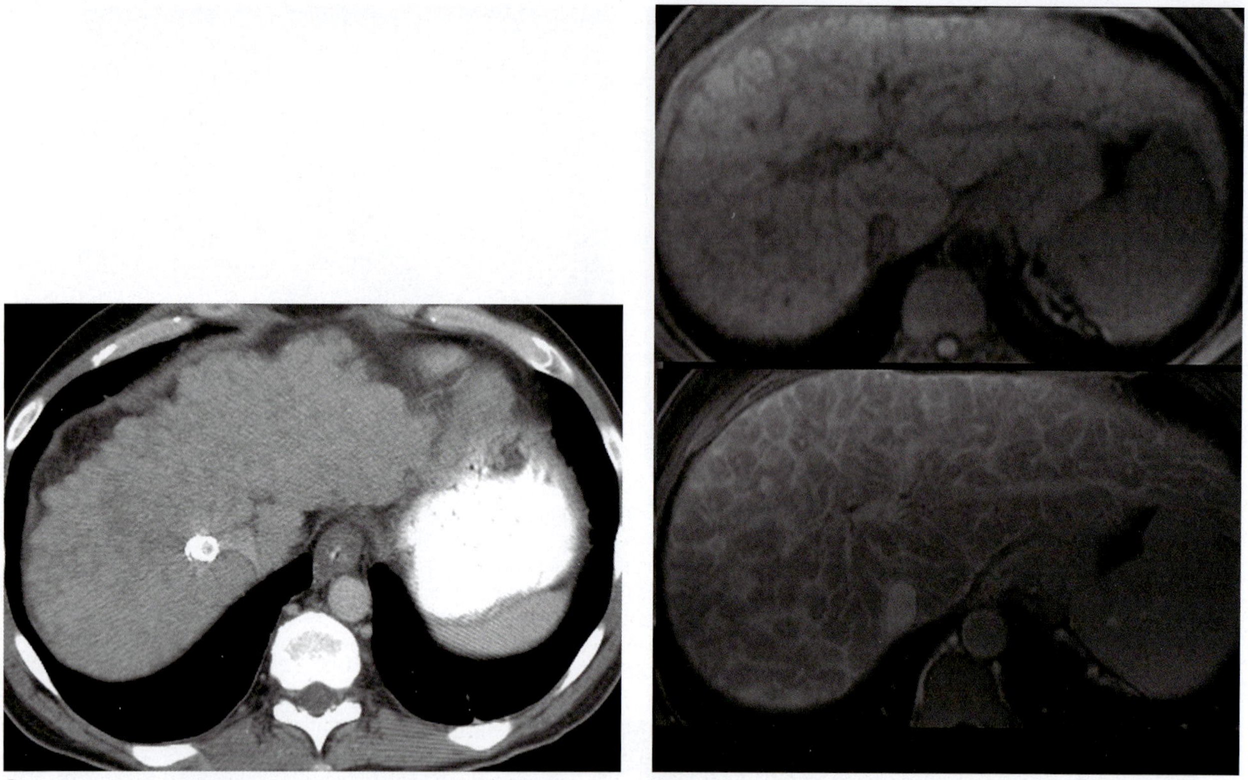


**FIG. 8A.8 • Cirrhosis (macronodular type). A:** Contrast-enhanced CT of the liver demonstrates extensive nodularity of the liver outline. A TIPS shunt is seen centrally in the liver. **B:** Noncontrast and postcontrast T1WI demonstrate nodular appearance of the liver and enhancement of the fibrous septa.

absorption of iron, resulting in excessive iron deposits in the liver, pancreas, heart, pituitary gland, thyroid, synovium, and skin. The spleen is typically not affected (Fig. 8A.10A).

- *Secondary hemochromatosis* is an acquired condition that results from various illnesses such as anemia, chronic liver disease, and multiple blood transfusions. Excess iron is taken up by the reticuloendothelial system, resulting in deposition in the liver, spleen, and bone marrow (Fig. 8A.10B).

CT is generally not used as an initial modality, although hemochromatosis may be suspected based on the finding of homogeneously increased parenchymal attenuation of greater

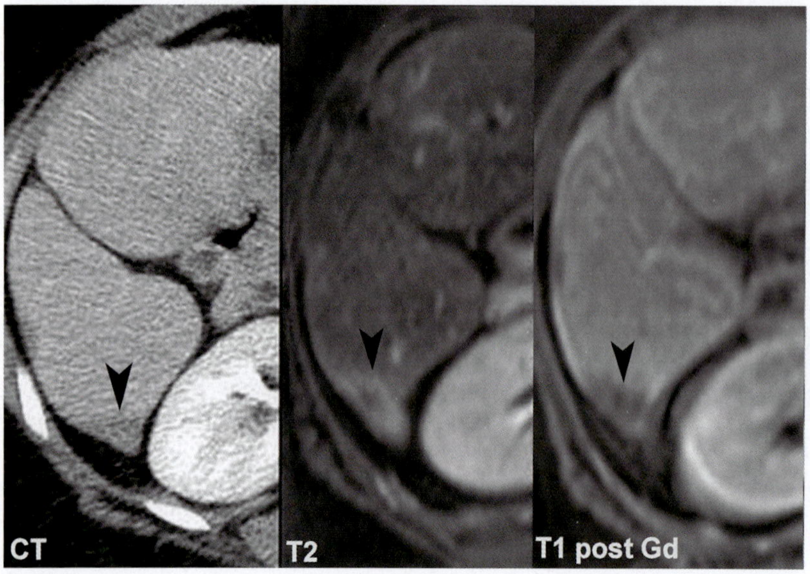


**FIG. 8A.9 • Confluent hepatic fibrosis.** Contrast-enhanced CT, T2WI, and postcontrast T1WI demonstrate capsular retraction (*arrowheads*) and volume loss at the site of confluent hepatic fibrosis.

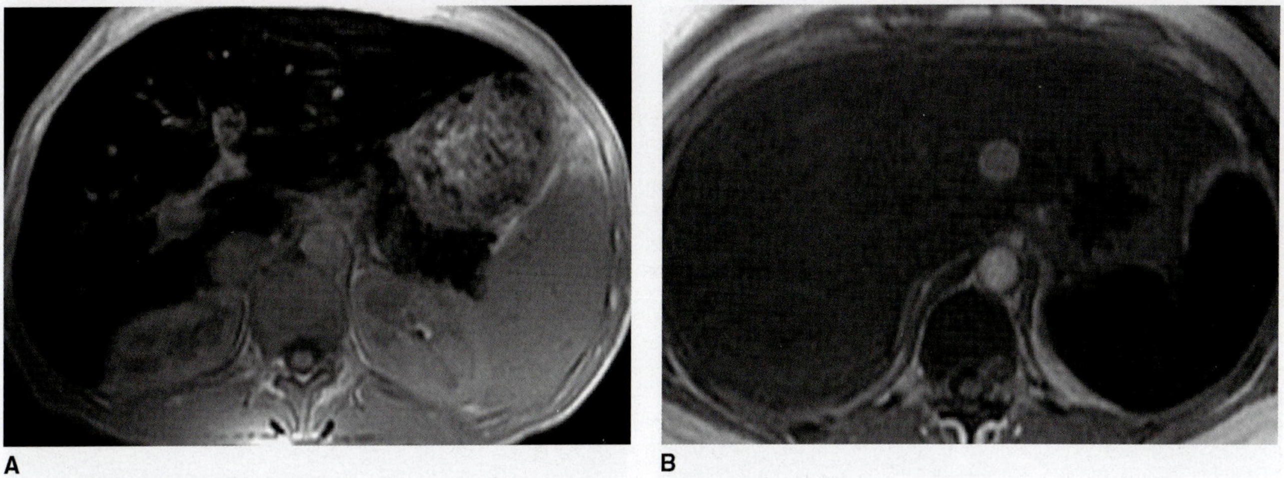

**FIG. 8A.10 • Hemochromatosis. A:** Primary hemochromatosis—In-phase T1WI demonstrates markedly hypointense liver, compared to splenic parenchyma in a patient with primary hemochromatosis. **B:** Secondary hemochromatosis—T1-weighted sequence demonstrates markedly decreased splenic parenchymal signal, compared to the liver parenchyma in a patient with secondary hemochromatosis.

than 70 HU on noncontrast CT. MRI is the best noninvasive method for detecting and quantifying iron deposits in the liver. Presence of iron causes a signal loss on all pulse sequences that is proportional to the amount of iron deposition. The iron deposits also cause signal drop-off on in-phase chemical shift images, which is the opposite of signal change seen with hepatic steatosis (Fig. 8A.11). Imaging also allows the diagnosis of cirrhosis and HCC.

Unlike iron, copper deposition has no ferromagnetic effect as it combines with proteins. Therefore, macronodular cirrhosis is the most common imaging manifestation of Wilson disease.[6,7]

## Glycogen Storage Disease

Glycogen storage disease is a heterogeneous group (12 subtypes) of metabolic disorders that results in abnormal accumulation of glycogen in the tissues. Majority of patients present with hepatomegaly, and the role of imaging is to evaluate for possible complication such as cirrhosis, HCCs, and hepatic adenomas.[8]

# VASCULAR DISEASES

## Transient Hepatic Intensity/Attenuation Difference

Transient hepatic intensity/attenuation difference (*THID/THAD*) is the result of regional heterogeneity in the proportion of arterial and portal venous flow to the liver. It is seen as a localized area of hepatic parenchyma that is hyperenhanced on arterial phase images and becomes isoattenuating or isointense to the adjacent liver parenchyma on portal venous and delayed images. THAD can be seen in patients with SVC obstruction, hepatic tumors, hemangiomas, FNH, liver abscess, and chronic cholecystitis.

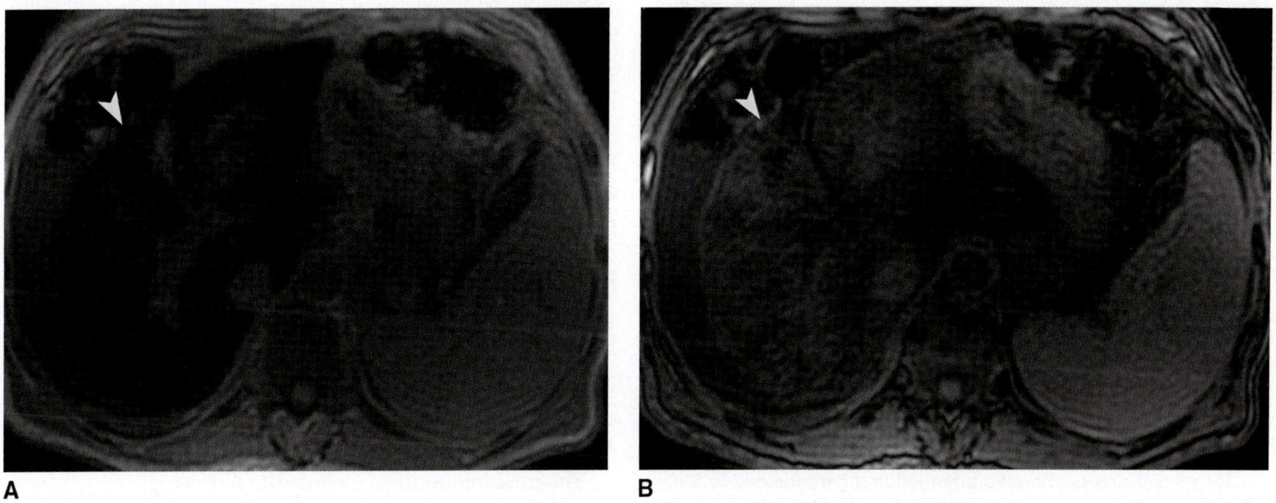

**FIG. 8A.11 • Primary hemochromatosis. A, B:** In-phase T1WI demonstrate loss of signal in the liver parenchyma (*arrowheads*), compared to opposed-phase T1WI.

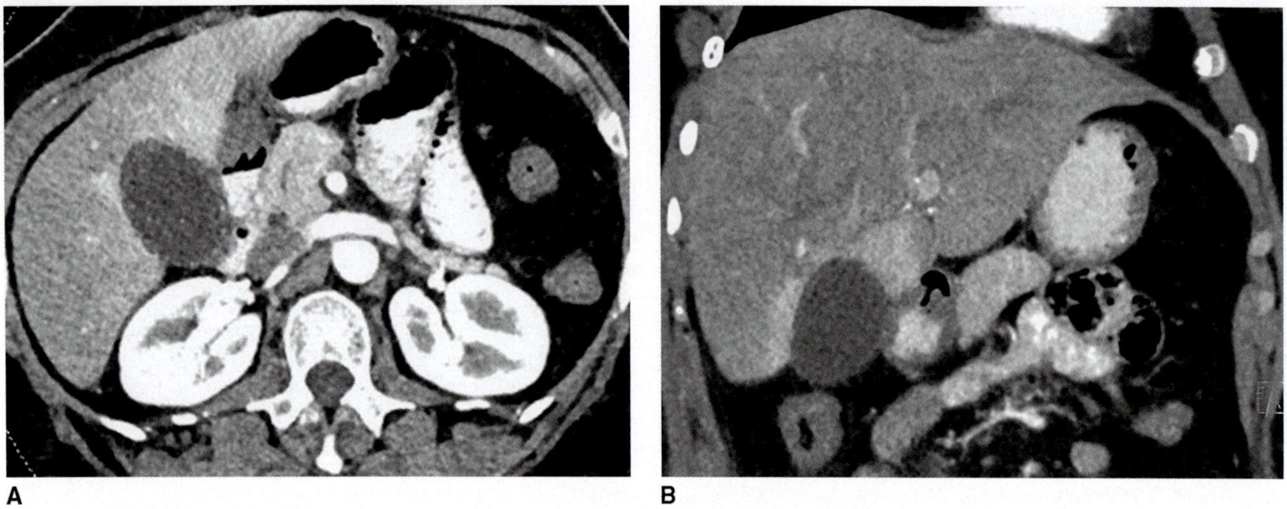

**FIG. 8A.12 • Transient hepatic attenuation difference due to chronic cholecystitis. A, B:** Axial and coronal contrast-enhanced CT in a patient with chronic calculus cholecystitis demonstrate increased density in the pericholecystic liver parenchyma.

The imaging findings are:

- There is hyperattenuation focus on arterial phase with no corresponding mass (Fig. 8A.12).
- The liver is normal on portal venous phase, noncontrast CT, and noncontrast MR sequences.
- It can be lobar, multisegmental, sectorial, polymorphous, or diffuse.[9]
- Arterial phase imaging in patients with *SVC obstruction* may show a focal area of hyperenhancement in the segment IV of the liver due to portosystemic shunt between the SVC and left main branch of the portal vein, via multiple enlarged subcutaneous collateral vessels (internal mammary vein, superficial epigastric vein, paraumbilical vein) (Fig. 8A.13).[10]

## Arterioportal Shunt

Arterioportal shunt is an intrahepatic communication between hepatic arterial branches and the portal system that results in redistribution of the arterial flow into a region of portal venous flow. It could be from neoplasm, trauma, biopsy, or radiofrequency ablation (RFA). Although most are asymptomatic, in rare cases, high-flow shunt may cause portal hypertension and hepatic failure.[11]

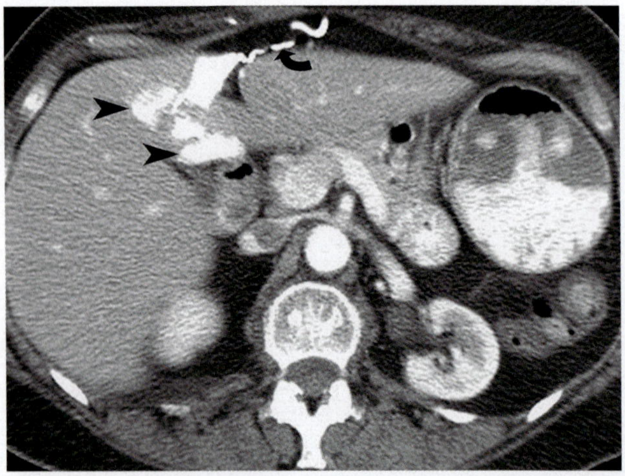

**FIG. 8A.13 • Transient hepatic attenuation difference due to SVC obstruction.** There is marked increased attenuation (*arrowheads*) in the segment IV of the liver, caused by collateral (*curved arrow*) circulation from the internal mammary vessels to the left branch of the portal vein.

Contrast-enhanced CT and MRI show a small, nonspherical focus of arterial enhancement in the periphery of the liver, which becomes indistinguishable from nearby normal hepatic parenchyma on portal venous phase. Early enhancement of the peripheral portal vein before central portal vein may be demonstrated (Fig. 8A.14). Most lesions do not show focal signal abnormality on other MRI sequences. Arterioportal shunts may accompany THID/THAD with the fistulous point of the shunt locating at the apex of the wedge-shaped hyperattenuation focus.[11,12]

## Hepatic Venoocclusive Disease or Sinusoidal Obstruction Syndrome

This is a potentially life-threatening complication of stem cell transplantation (usually in less than 30 days) or chemotherapy. Vascular endothelial injury leads to progressive obliteration of small hepatic venules, resulting in hepatic venous outflow obstruction.[13] Doppler US is the first modality used to screen patients at risk which may demonstrate decreased or reversed portal vein flow. Hepatomegaly, ascites, narrowing of hepatic veins, periportal edema, and gall bladder wall thickening may be seen on CT or MRI. Heterogeneous enhancement of the hepatic parenchyma can be observed on postcontrast images.[14–16]

## Passive Hepatic Congestion

Passive hepatic congestion is caused by stasis of blood within the liver resulting in hypoxia and necrosis of hepatocytes. It is secondary to cardiac problem (congestive heart failure and constrictive pericarditis) or compromised hepatic venous drainage.

The imaging findings include the following:

- On US, there is hepatomegaly, ascites, dilatation of IVC and hepatic veins, and cardiomegaly.

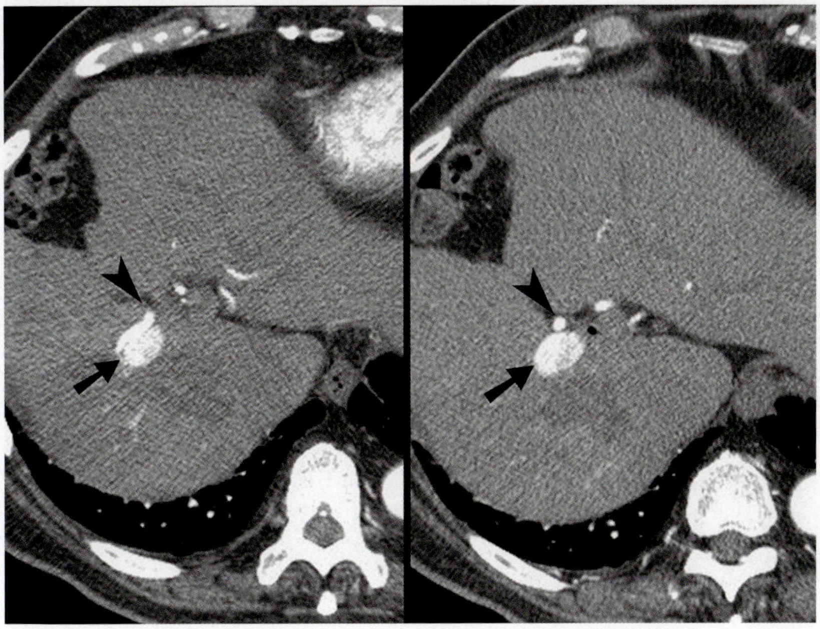

**FIG. 8A.14 • Arterioportal shunting after radiofrequency ablation.** Contrast-enhanced CT in arterial phase demonstrate intense enhancement of right portal vein with a right branch of the hepatic artery (*arrowheads*) communicating with the right branch of the portal vein (*straight arrows*) adjacent to the site of recent RFA.

- Decreased respiratory variation of the IVC, loss of triphasic waveform of hepatic veins with unidirectional continuous waveform, and increased pulsatility of the portal vein may be observed on Doppler US (Fig. 8A.15).
- On contrast-enhanced CT or MRI, there is reflux of contrast into the hepatic veins and IVC during the arterial phase, suggesting right-sided cardiac problem (Fig. 8A.16). The congested liver is enlarged and shows heterogeneous, mottled, mosaic pattern of contrast enhancement. Large patchy areas of delayed enhancement at the periphery of the liver may be seen. Decreased attenuation tends to be prominent along the perivascular zone with late enhancement of the affected parenchyma. Periportal edema may be present.[17]
- In late stage, morphologic change of cirrhosis occurs.

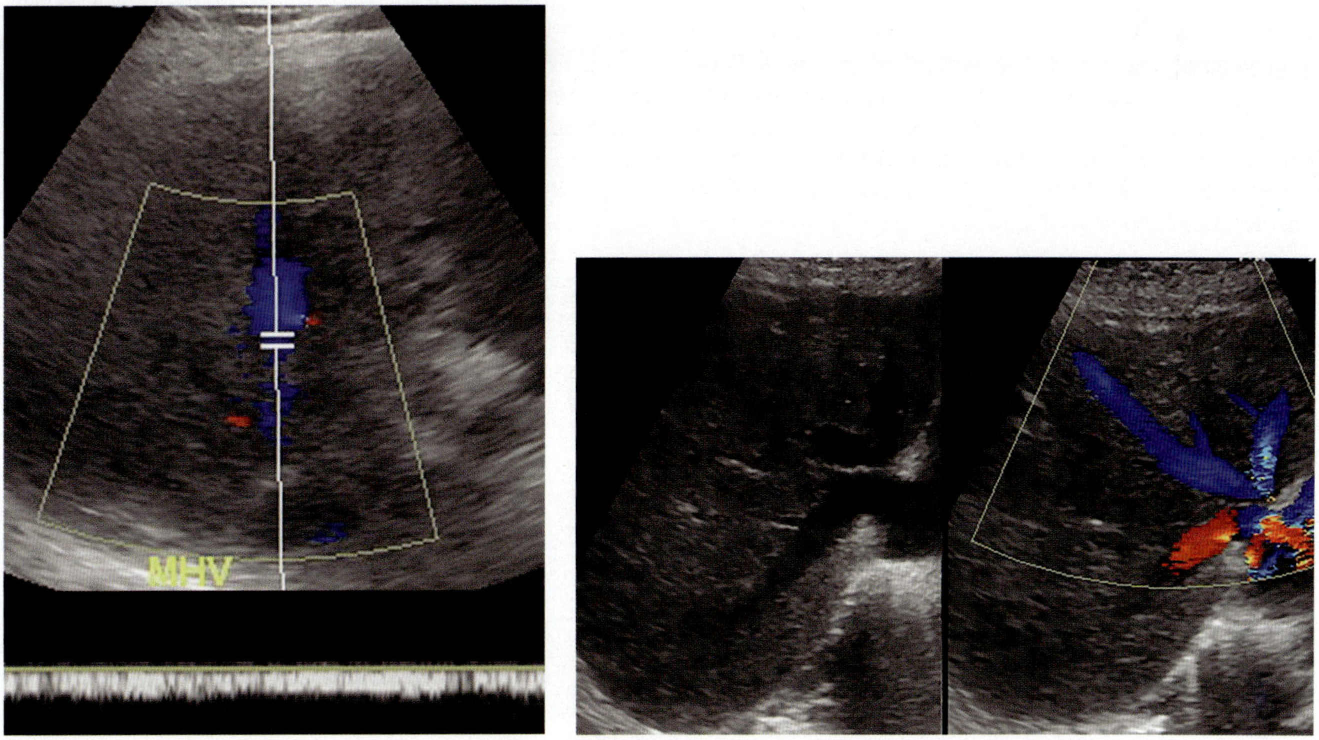


A B

**FIG. 8A.15 • Hepatic venous outflow obstruction from IVC stenosis. A:** Doppler US study of the middle hepatic vein demonstrates loss of triphasic waveform. **B:** Axial US study demonstrates dilatation of the right, middle, and left hepatic veins due to severe IVC narrowing.

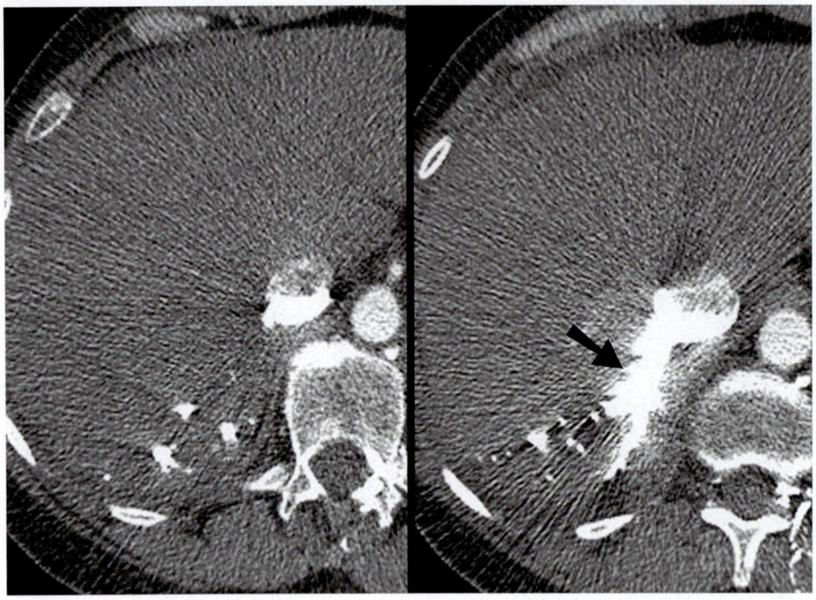

**FIG. 8A.16 • Hepatic venous congestion.** Contrast-enhanced CT in a patient with calcific constrictive pericarditis demonstrate reflux of contrast from the right atrium into the IVC and right hepatic vein (*arrow*).

## Portal Vein Occlusion

Portal vein occlusion is commonly caused by thrombosis, which may be due to cirrhosis, local infectious/inflammatory process, injury, and hypercoagulable state. Thrombus appears as a filling defect of varying echogenicity, attenuation, and intensity, within the portal vein (Fig. 8A.17). Peripheral rim of enhancement of the vessel wall can be seen on contrast-enhanced CT and MRI. Both modalities are more reliable than US for the evaluation of thrombus extension into the mesenteric vein.[16,18] *Cavernous transformation of the portal vein* occurs around the occluded portal vein. It is seen as a mass-like network of venous channels within the hepatoduodenal ligament and porta hepatis (Fig. 8A.18). *Recanalization of paraumbilical vein* bypassing blood from the left portal vein to the paraumbilical vein is seen as an enlarged, tortuous vascular structure between the left hepatic lobe and superficial epigastric veins that later drain into SVC or IVC.[19,20] Varices may be seen in other locations of portosystemic collateral circulation.

## Budd-Chiari Syndrome

Budd-Chiari syndrome (BCS) is a heterogeneous group of disorders characterized by hepatic venous outflow obstruction, regardless of the cause. In Western countries, BCS is frequently associated with hypercoagulable state, but in Asians, a membranous web-like obstruction of the hepatic vein and IVC is more common.[9] The condition can lead to portal hypertension, hepatic congestion, and, eventually, hepatocyte dysfunction. In acute BCS, there is hepatomegaly, abnormal hepatic parenchyma (heterogeneous echotexture on ultrasound, mottled appearance, decreased enhancement of the periphery of the liver but strongly enhanced caudate lobe on contrast-enhanced CT and MRI), and nonvisualization of hepatic veins or IVC. The thrombosed hepatic veins may be seen as cord-like filling defects (Fig. 8A.19) and may be associated with comma-shaped intrahepatic collaterals. In chronic BCS, there is atrophic change of the affected segment(s), enlarged caudate lobe, regenerative nodules, intra- or extrahepatic collaterals, or varices.[9,21]

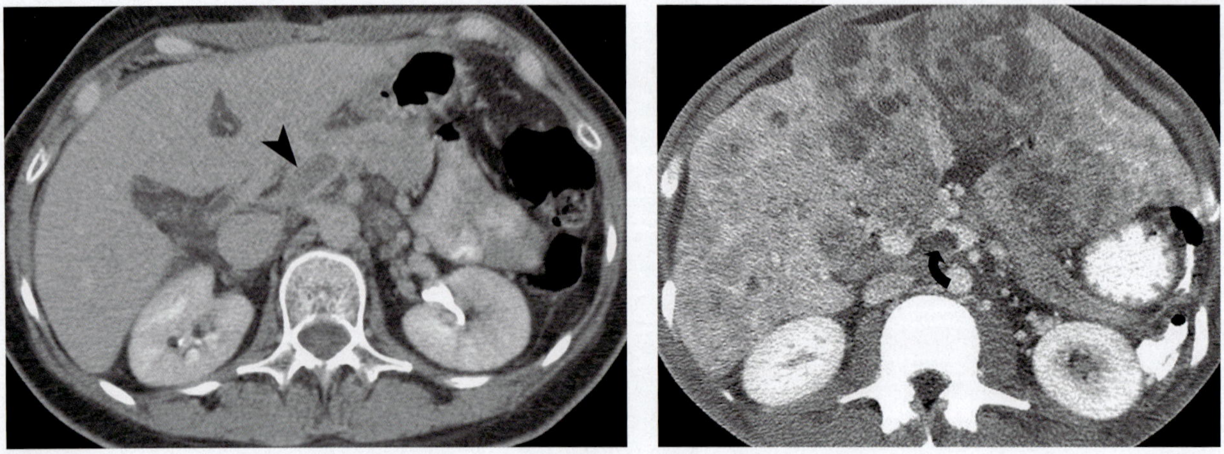

A B

**FIG. 8A.17 • Portal vein thrombosis. A:** Axial contrast-enhanced CT in portal venous phase demonstrates linear thrombus (*arrowhead*) in the main portal vein. **B:** Contrast-enhanced CT in a patient with infiltrating HCC demonstrates a tumor thrombus (*curved arrow*) in the portal vein.

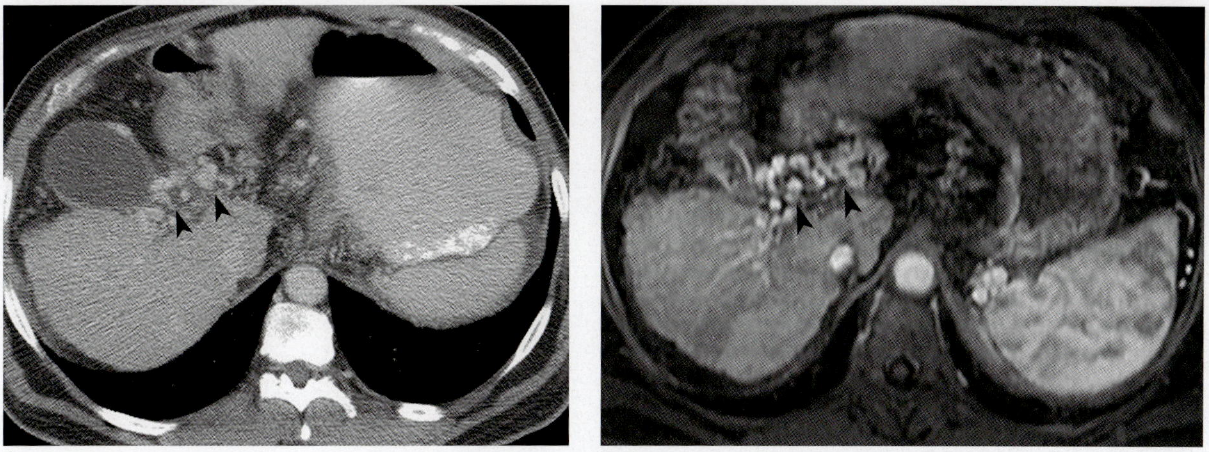

A B

**FIG. 8A.18 • Portal vein thrombosis with cavernous transformation. A, B:** Contrast-enhanced CT and postcontrast T1WI demonstrate chronic portal vein occlusion with extensive collateral circulation at the porta hepatis (*arrowheads*), consistent with cavernous transformation.

## Peliosis Hepatis

Peliosis hepatis is a rare benign disorder characterized by dilated blood-filled cystic cavities, representing sinusoids, within the liver. The exact pathogenesis is not well understood, but the condition is related to drugs, hepatotoxins, chronic wasting diseases, and AIDS. It rarely causes symptoms and is usually diagnosed incidentally. The most feared complication is hemorrhage and rupture into peritoneal cavity, which can be fatal.

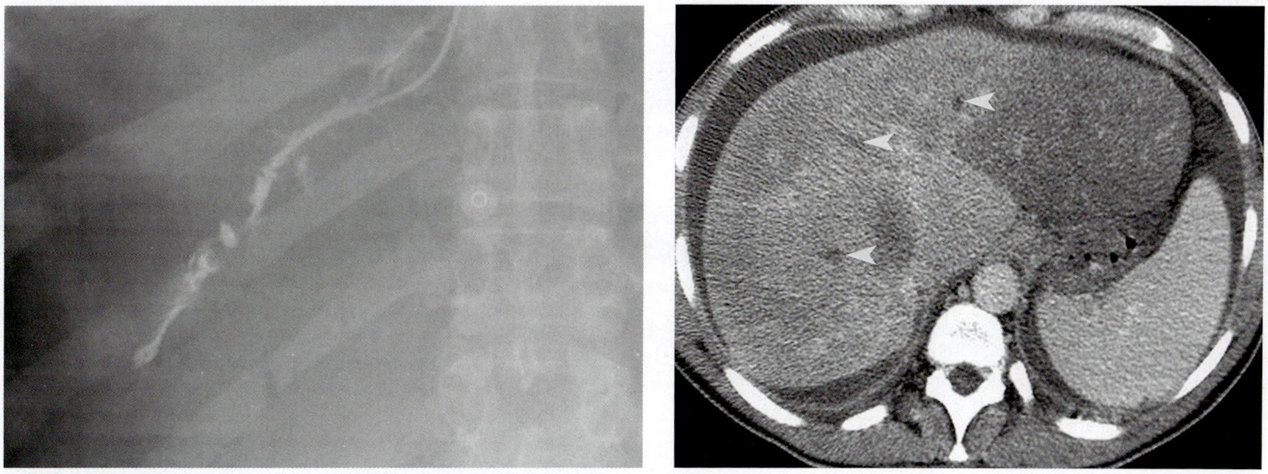

A B

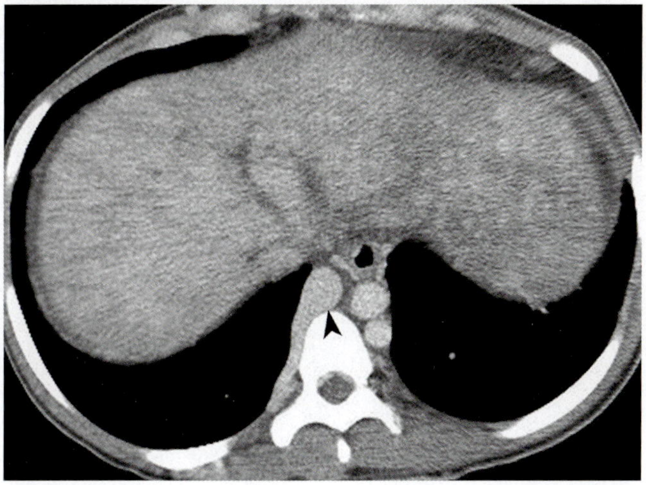

C

**FIG. 8A.19 • Budd-Chiari syndrome (BCS). A:** Hepatic venogram study demonstrates irregular thrombus in the lumen of the right hepatic vein. **B:** Contrast-enhanced CT reveals hepatomegaly, heterogeneous parenchymal enhancement, and thrombosed hepatic veins (*arrowheads*) in a patient with BCS. **C:** Contrast-enhanced CT demonstrates heterogeneous enhancement of the liver and chronically thrombosed hepatic veins. Prominent azygous vein (*arrowhead*) and hemiazygos vein are seen in the retroperitoneum.

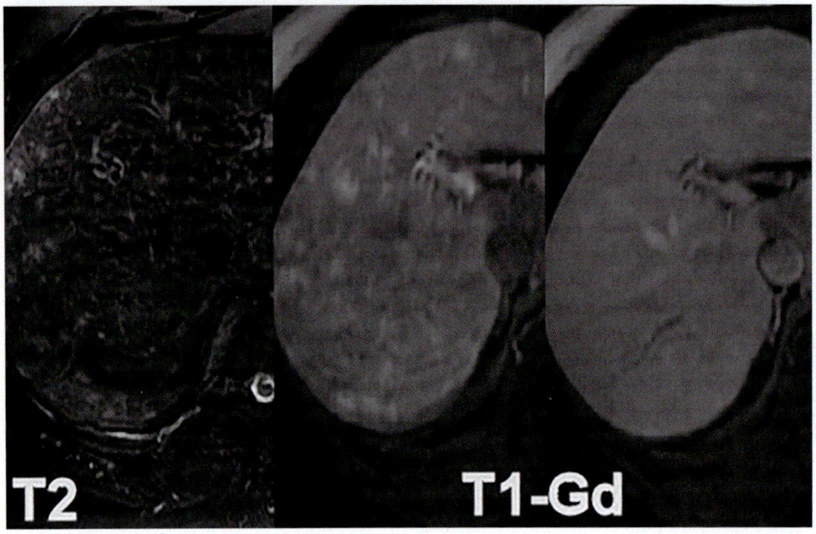


**FIG. 8A.20 • Peliosis hepatis.** T2WI and postgadolinium T1WI (arterial and portal venous phase) demonstrate multiple T2 hyperintense foci in the liver, which demonstrate arterial phase enhancement. On the portal venous phase, the focal lesions are isointense to the liver parenchyma.

Imaging appearance of peliosis depends on pathologic pattern, stages of hemorrhage within the lesions, and coexistent liver disease. The lesions can be solitary or multiple, with varying echogenicity, attenuation, intensity, and enhancement relative to the normal liver. Typical nonhemorrhagic lesions are hypoechoic on US, hypoattenuating on noncontrast CT, hypointense on T1, and hyperintense on T2WI (Fig. 8A.20). On contrast-enhanced images, typical peliotic lesions show early globular enhancement with multiple accumulations of contrast material in the center of the lesion (target sign). There is centrifugal pattern of enhancement during portal venous phase and late diffuse homogeneous hyperattenuation on delayed phase.[22]

## Hepatic Infarction

Hepatic infarction represents an area of coagulative necrosis of hepatocytes caused by diminished vascular supply of either hepatic artery or both arterial and portal venous system. Insults to the portal venous system alone generally do not cause hepatic infarction, because of dual blood supply and collateral pathways. Hepatic infarction may occur after liver transplantation, chemoembolization, ablation procedure, hepatobiliary surgery, or trauma.

On CT and MRI, hepatic infarction typically appears wedge-shaped and lacks mass effect. It is hypoattenuating on CT, hypointense on T1, and hyperintense on T2WI. On enhanced study, it manifests as a perfusion defect in geographical or segmental pattern in the periphery of the liver, abutting the hepatic capsule (Figs. 8A.21 and 8A.22).[5,23] Intralesional gas may be present in the minority of cases, which is not necessarily correlated to infection.

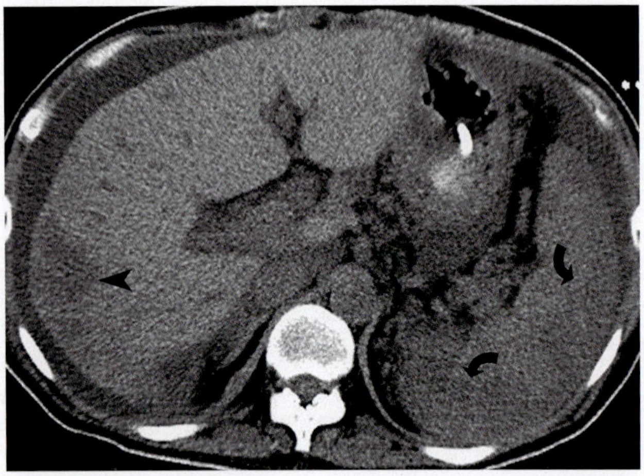

**FIG. 8A.21 • Liver infarct.** Noncontrast CT demonstrates wedge-shaped low density (*arrowhead*) seen peripherally in the right lobe, consistent with infarction. The patient also has multiple peripherally located infarcts (*curved arrows*) in the splenic parenchyma.

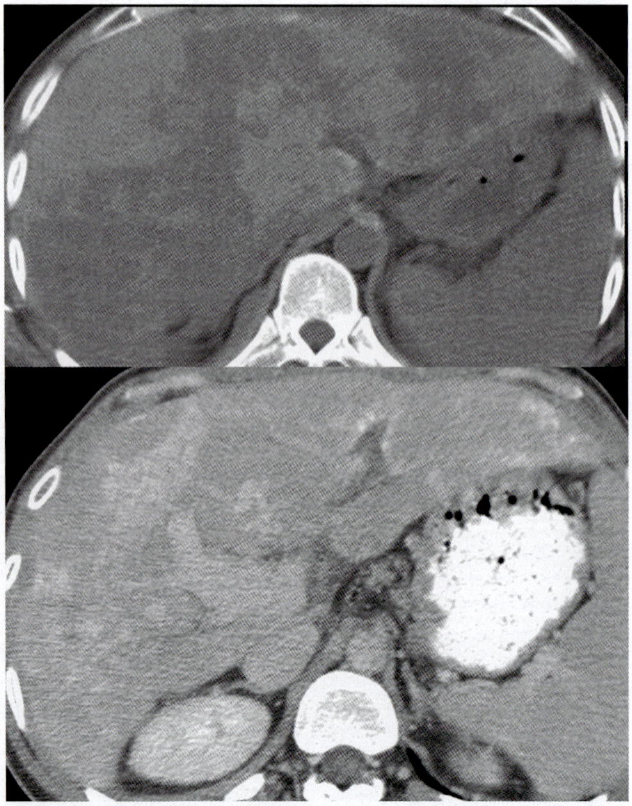

**FIG. 8A.22 • Liver infarcts in transplant liver.** Noncontrast and postcontrast CT of the liver demonstrate multiple heterogeneous areas of hyperdensity, consistent with liver infarcts in the transplant liver.

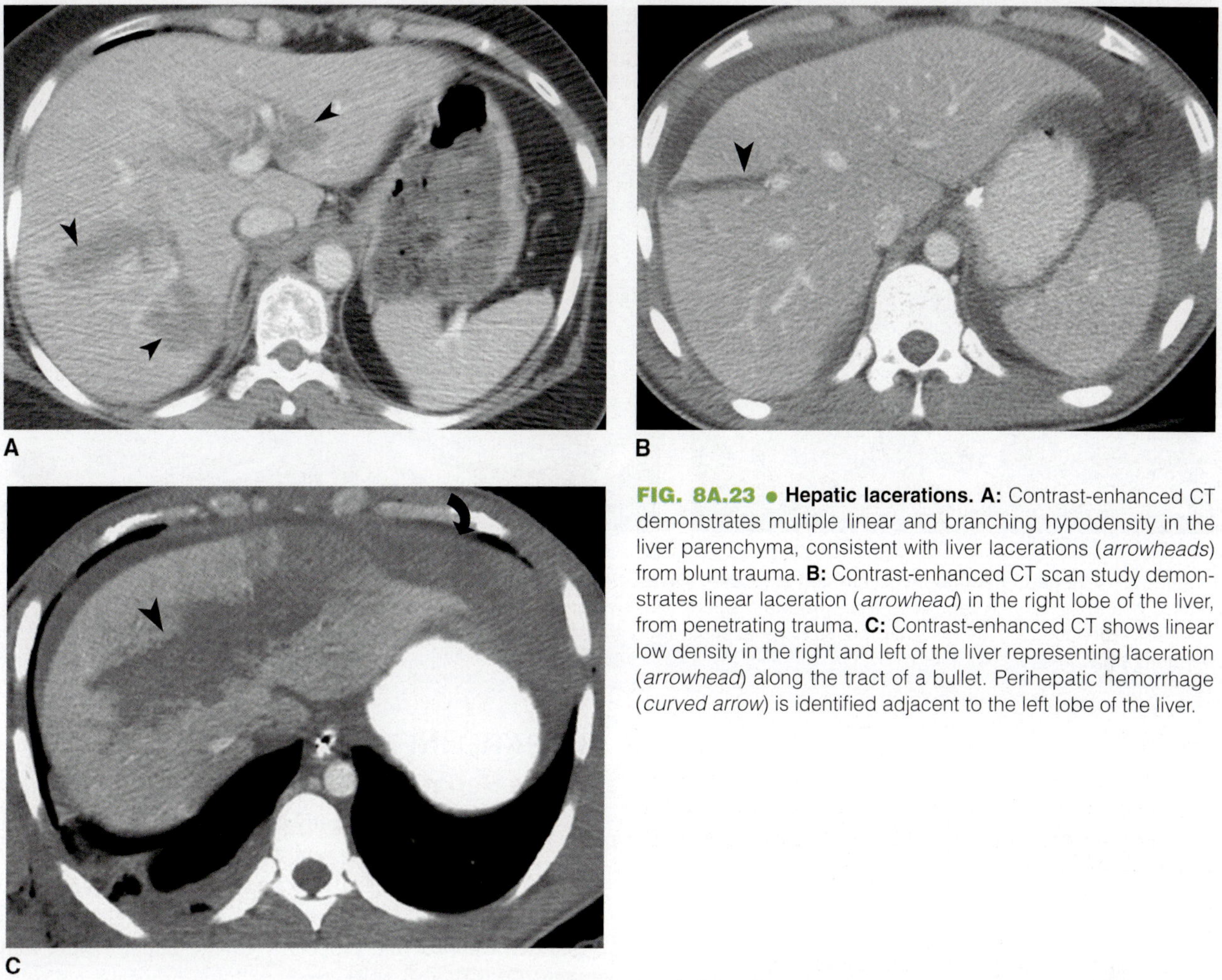

FIG. 8A.23 • **Hepatic lacerations. A:** Contrast-enhanced CT demonstrates multiple linear and branching hypodensity in the liver parenchyma, consistent with liver lacerations (*arrowheads*) from blunt trauma. **B:** Contrast-enhanced CT scan study demonstrates linear laceration (*arrowhead*) in the right lobe of the liver, from penetrating trauma. **C:** Contrast-enhanced CT shows linear low density in the right and left of the liver representing laceration (*arrowhead*) along the tract of a bullet. Perihepatic hemorrhage (*curved arrow*) is identified adjacent to the left lobe of the liver.

## TRAUMA

*Hepatic laceration* is the most common type of abdominal injury from penetrating trauma. CT is better than US, which can miss up to 25% of the liver lacerations.

The imaging findings of liver trauma include the following:

- Laceration is seen as irregular low-attenuation areas with linear or branching configuration on CT (Fig. 8A.23).
- Parenchymal hematoma is seen as a relatively low-attenuation focus with poorly defined margin on contrast CT.
- Subcapsular hematoma is seen as an elliptical hypoechoic or hypoattenuating collection between the hepatic capsule and liver parenchyma that indents or flattens the subjacent hepatic margin (Fig. 8A.24).
- Hepatic vascular injury can involve hepatic arterial and venous system. It is suspected when a laceration or hematoma extends into one or more major hepatic veins or IVC. Arterial phase imaging sometimes reveals active bleeding seen as a focal high-attenuation area in the laceration or hematoma and should prompt surgical or endovascular management (Fig. 8A.25).[24]

Traumatic liver injury is divided into six grades per American Association for the Surgery of Trauma:

- Grade I
  Hematoma: Subcapsular less than 10% surface area
  Laceration: Capsular tear less than 1 cm parenchymal depth
- Grade II
  Hematoma: Subcapsular 10% to 50% surface area; intraparenchymal less than 10 cm in diameter
  Laceration: Capsular tear 1 to 3 cm parenchymal depth, less than 10 cm in length

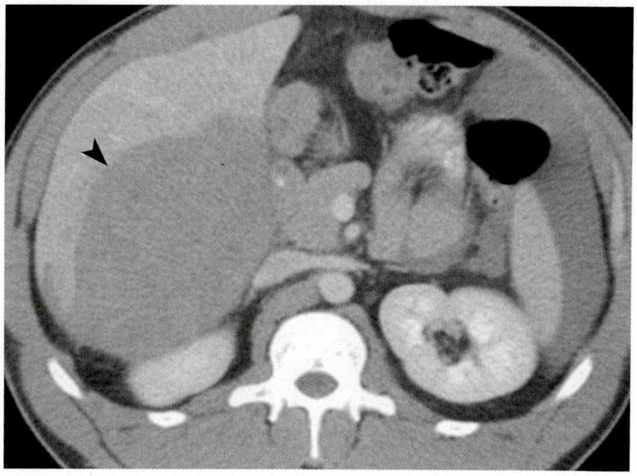

FIG. 8A.24 • **Subcapsular hematoma from blunt abdominal trauma.** Contrast-enhanced CT demonstrates a large biconvex subcapsular hematoma (*arrowhead*) posterior to the right lobe of the liver.

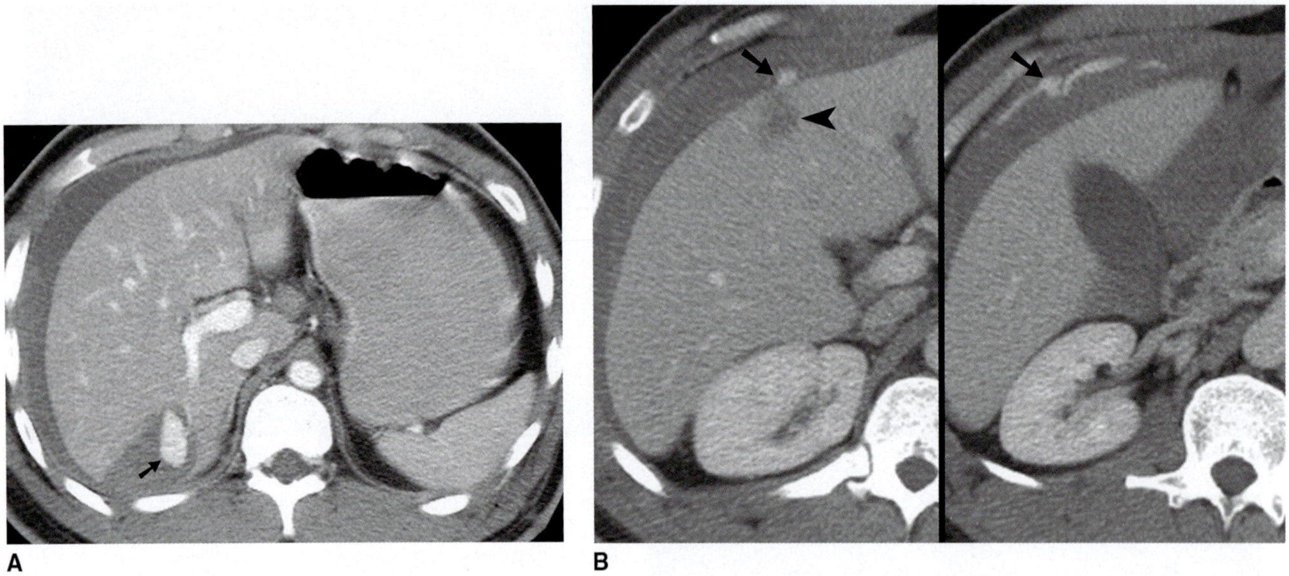

**FIG. 8A.25 • Hepatic pseudoaneurysm and arterial extravasation. A:** Contrast-enhanced CT demonstrates a pseudoaneurysm (*arrow*) within a wedge-shaped liver laceration caused by penetrating injury. **B:** Contrast-enhanced CT demonstrate active extravasation of contrast (*straight arrows*) arising from liver laceration (*arrowhead*).

- Grade III
  Hematoma: Subcapsular greater than 50% of surface area or ruptured subcapsular or parenchymal hematoma; intraparenchymal hematoma greater than 10 cm or expanding
  Laceration: Greater than 3 cm in depth
- Grade IV
  Laceration: Parenchymal disruption involving 25% to 75% of a hepatic lobe, or 1 to 3 Couinaud segments
- Grade V
  Laceration: Parenchymal disruption of greater than 75% of a hepatic lobe, greater than 3 Couinaud segments within a single lobe (Fig. 8A.26)
  Vascular: Juxtahepatic venous injuries (retrohepatic vena cava, central major hepatic veins)
- Grade VI
  Hepatic avulsion

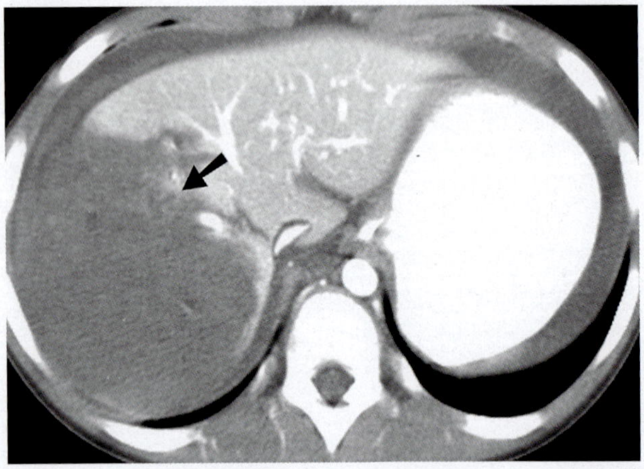

**FIG. 8A.26 • Grade V liver injury.** Contrast-enhanced CT demonstrates extensive laceration (*straight arrow*) and devascularization involving all segments of the right lobe of the liver.

## HEPATIC INFECTION

### Acute Hepatitis

Acute hepatitis is commonly caused by viral infection, which results in hepatomegaly and abnormal hepatic parenchyma. On US, decreased hepatic echogenicity causes accentuation of the venule wall (starry sky appearance) (Fig. 8A.27A). Gall bladder wall edema, especially of the hepatic side, may be seen. On CT and MRI, there is hepatomegaly, gall bladder wall thickening, and periportal edema (Fig. 8A.27B).[25]

### Hepatic Abscess

Hepatic abscess is a localized collection of necrotic inflammatory tissue in the liver with destruction of hepatic parenchyma caused by bacterial, parasitic, fungal, or mycobacterial organisms. ***Pyogenic abscess*** is bacterial seeding via hematogenous dissemination, ascending cholangitis, and direct extension from contiguous organ or direct trauma. *Escherichia coli* is the most common causative organism. Pyogenic abscesses can be classified as microabscess (less than 2 cm) or macroabscess (greater than or equal to 2 cm).[26]

US and CT can detect most abscesses with sensitivity greater than 90%. At US, small lesions are often hypoechoic while larger lesions can be hypo-, iso-, or hyperechoic (Fig. 8A.28). Gas within abscess cavity might be seen as linear or curvilinear hyperechoic lines with posterior reverberation artifacts. On CT and MRI, lesions are rounded, well circumscribed with surrounding edema. Faint rim enhancement is seen in hepatic venous and delayed phases.

*Cluster sign:* This represents smaller abscesses clustering around a dominant larger cavity (Fig. 8A.29A).

*Double target sign:* This refers to central low density pus surrounded with a rim of high-density wall, and another

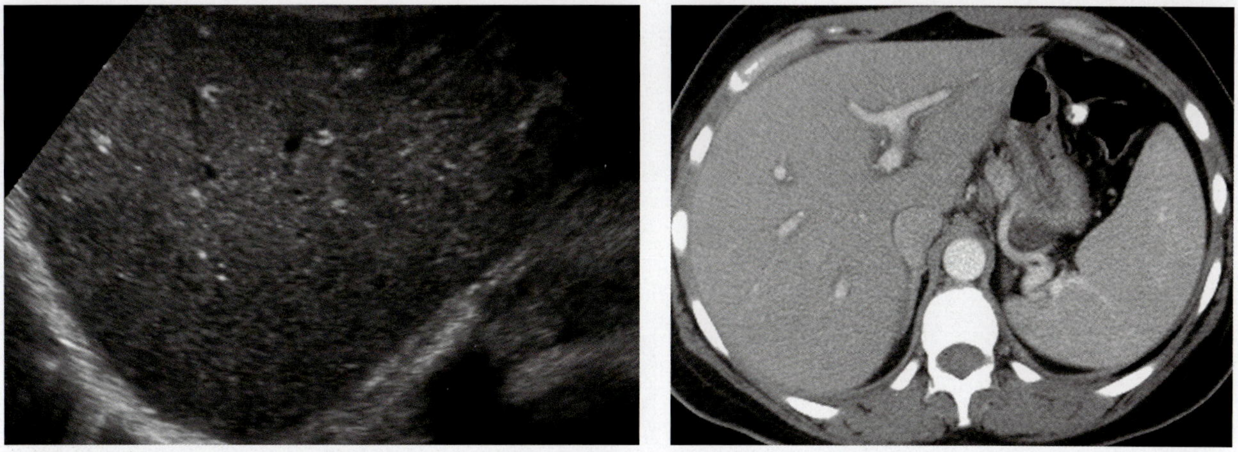

A B

**FIG. 8A.27 • Acute hepatitis. A:** US of the liver demonstrates echogenic portal triad in a background of edematous hepatic parenchyma, giving a starry sky appearance. **B:** Contrast-enhanced CT demonstrates periportal edema and gall bladder wall edema in a patient with acute hepatitis.

layer of low-density edema of the liver parenchyma (Fig. 8A.29B).

On MRI, pyogenic abscesses have variable T1 and T2 signal intensities depending on protein content. Diffusion-weighted imaging often shows restricted diffusion in the center of the lesions, in contrast to necrotic tumors.[25] *Klebsiella pneumoniae* is the most common organism resulting in air-containing abscess (Fig. 8A.30).

## Amebic Liver Abscess

Amebic abscess is the most common extraintestinal complication of amebiasis. The *Entamoeba* trophozoites enter the liver via the portal vein, forming an abscess.

The abscess is usually round or oval-shaped, large, and located near the liver capsule. Extrahepatic extension may involve the chest wall, pleural cavity, and pericardium. Amebic abscess appears hypoechoic with low-level internal echoes on US. On CT, it has complex fluid content that is hypoattenuating on CT and homogeneously T1 hypointense and T2 hyperintense on MRI (Fig. 8A.31). Peripheral rim of T2 hyperintensity may be seen. The wall is smooth and enhancing on portal venous and delayed phases of contrast-enhanced study.[25,26] It is difficult to differentiate amebic from pyogenic abscess based on imaging alone.

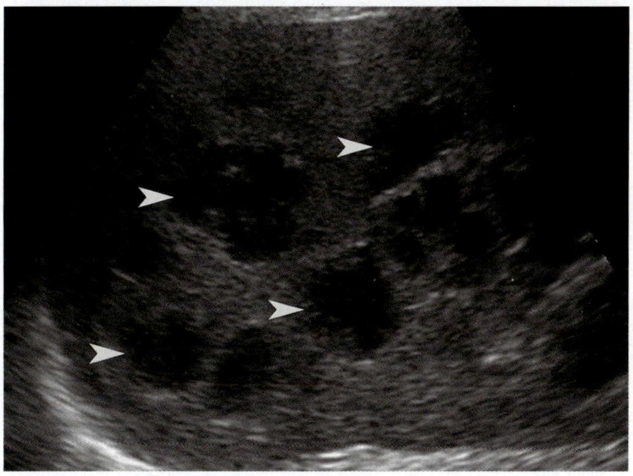

**FIG. 8A.28 • Pyogenic liver abscesses.** US study demonstrates a cluster of multiple small liver abscesses (*arrowheads*).

## Other Abscesses

*Fungal microabscesses* are disseminated disease usually caused by *Candida albicans* and occur in immunocompromised patients. The liver and spleen are the main sites of involvement. The most common but nonspecific US appearance is multiple small hypoechoic nodules. Other patterns include "wheel-within-a-wheel" appearance, bull's eye configuration, and echogenic focus with varying degree of posterior acoustic shadowing.[26] At CT, fungal microabscesses typically appear as multiple small, rounded, discrete lesions of low attenuation. Some of these lesions may have a central zone of high attenuation. At MRI, untreated lesions are T1 hypointense, markedly T2 hyperintense, and less enhanced than normal parenchyma. After treatment, signal intensity of these nodules return close to that of hepatic parenchyma.

*Tuberculous microabscesses* occur mostly in patients with disseminated tuberculosis. Hepatomegaly is the most common manifestation and may be the only imaging abnormality. Innumerable nodules of up to 2 mm in size may be found. Lesions are hypoechoic on US, hypoattenuating on CT, and T1 hypointense and T2 hypo- to isointense on MRI. Associated lymphadenopathy is common and characteristically seen as large lymph nodes with central low attenuation.[26] CT may demonstrate diffuse calcifications in the healed stage of tuberculosis.

*Echinococcosis* is a parasitic disease caused by infection with the larval stage of *Echinococcus granulosus* (most common) and *Echinococcus multilocularis*. The disease is characterized by cysts of variable size, either solitary or multiple, in the liver, lungs, brain, and other organs. US, CT, and MRI are used to detect a cyst-like mass, often in a person with a history of exposure to sheepdogs in an endemic area. Serologic tests may be used to confirm the diagnosis.

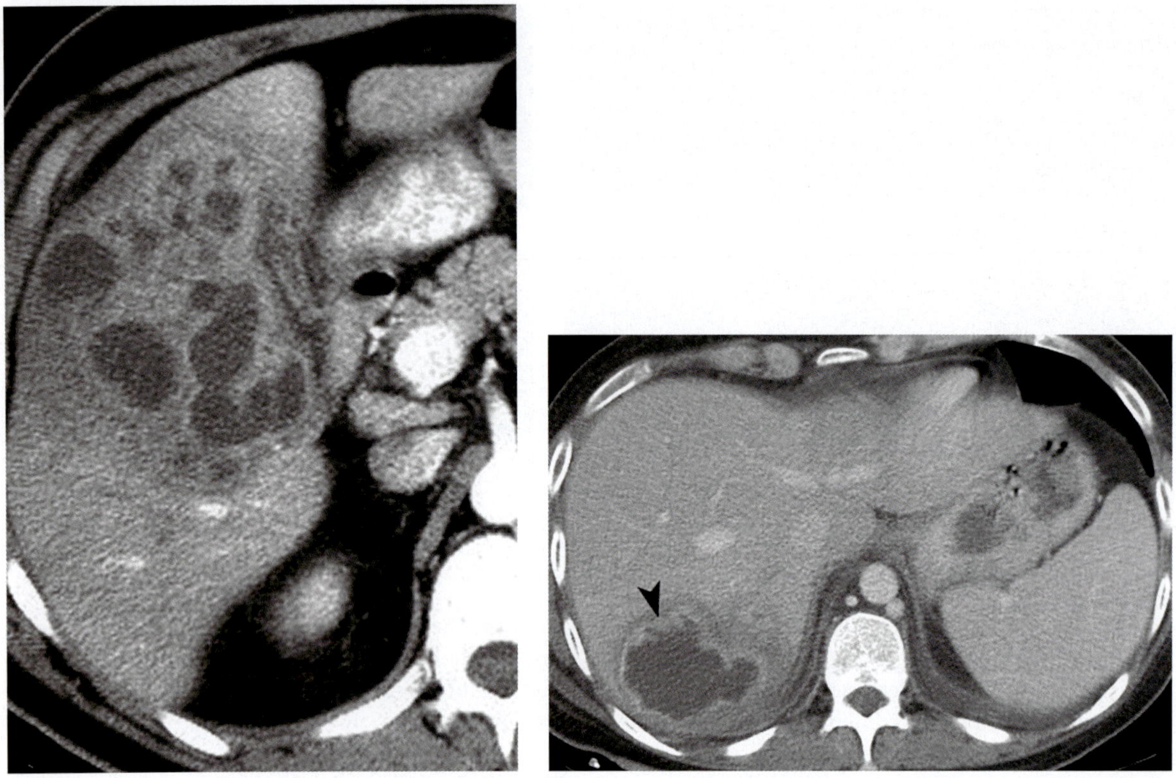

A B

**FIG. 8A.29 • Pyogenic liver abscesses. A:** Cluster sign—axial contrast-enhanced CT demonstrates multiple abscesses clustered in the right lobe of the liver, adjacent to larger abscesses. **B:** Double target sign—axial contrast-enhanced CT demonstrates irregular low-density liver abscess with a high-density wall and surrounding edema (*arrowhead*) in the liver.

The cyst caused by *E. granulosus* (*cystic echinococcosis*) is often solitary with an inner germinal layer and outer fibrous capsule forming the capsule. In chronic infection, curvilinear or nodular calcifications may develop in the capsule. Daughter cysts, found in approximately 75% of cases, bud off from the inner germinal layer and may remain attached or free floating in the cyst matrix. On imaging, cystic echinococcosis cysts are round or oval, with a smooth, thin, and well-defined wall (Fig. 8A.32). Daughter cysts appear honeycomb-like or wheel-like with internal wavy bands (water-lily sign). The cyst matrix is of variable echogenicity on US, hypoattenuation on CT, and T1 hypointense with markedly T2 hyperintense on MRI. Daughter cysts are hypointense on both T1- and T2-weighted images relative to the matrix. Due to the fibrous nature, the cyst wall appears T1 and T2 hypointense.[26]

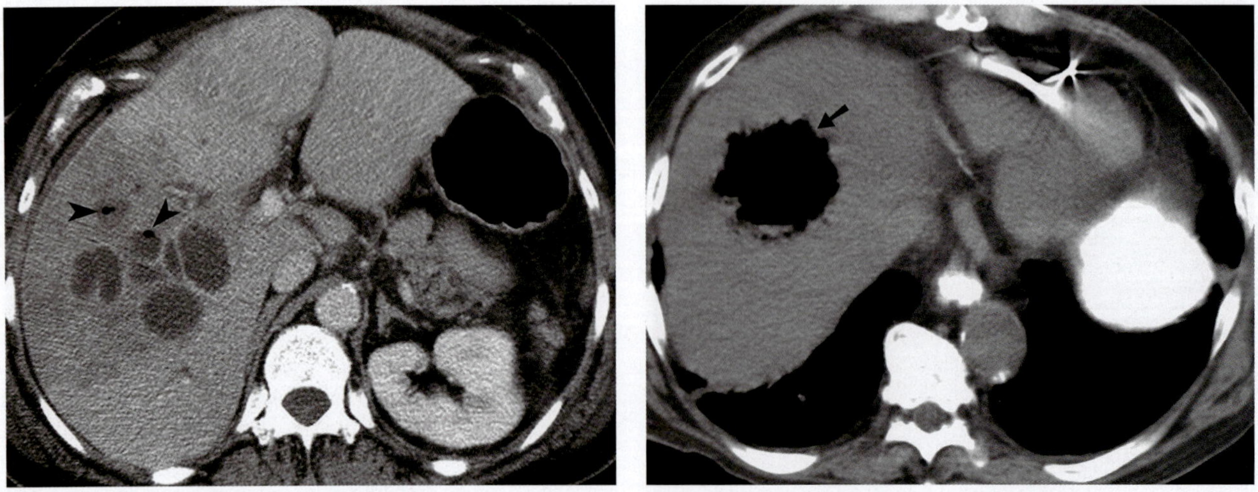

A B

**FIG. 8A.30 • Liver abscess containing air. A:** CT of the liver demonstrates multiple abscesses in the right lobe, some of which are containing foci of air (*arrowheads*). **B:** Noncontrast CT of the liver demonstrates a large air-containing abscess (*straight arrow*).

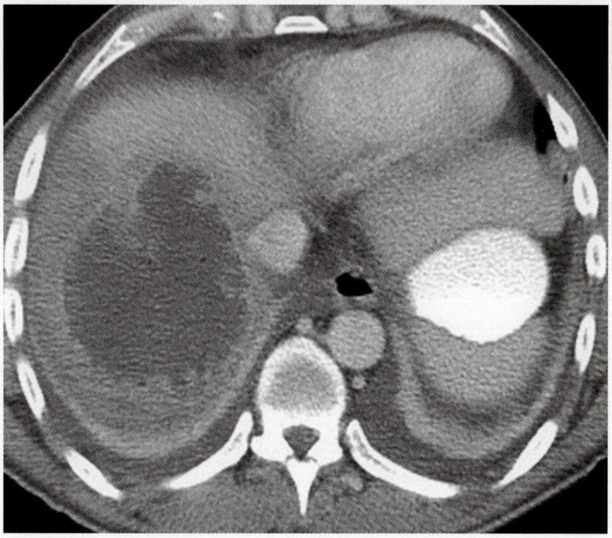

**FIG. 8A.31 • Amoebic liver abscess.** Contrast-enhanced CT demonstrates irregular large abscess in the right lobe of the liver with enhancing rim.

Cysts of *E. multilocularis* infection (*alveolar echinococcosis*) are numerous, irregular, small, and variable in size. They are multilocular, infiltrative, and aggressive appearing, mimicking malignancy.

## COMPLICATIONS OF LIVER TRANSPLANTATION

Early detection and prompt management of postoperative complications of liver transplantation are crucial for improving patient survival and preventing graft loss. Both gray-scale and Doppler US are the preferred method for postoperative screening. There are some recognized reversible postoperative findings, diagnosable on US, which eventually return to normal in the first postoperative week. These findings include starry sky appearance of the liver parenchyma due to periportal edema, transient foci of increased echogenicity of the liver parenchyma, pneumobilia, small perihepatic fluid collections or hematomas, pleural effusion, and temporarily increased velocity and resistive index (RI) of the hepatic artery, decreased RI of the hepatic artery with tardus parvus waveform, increased portal venous flow, and loss of triphasicity of the hepatic venous waveform.[27,28]

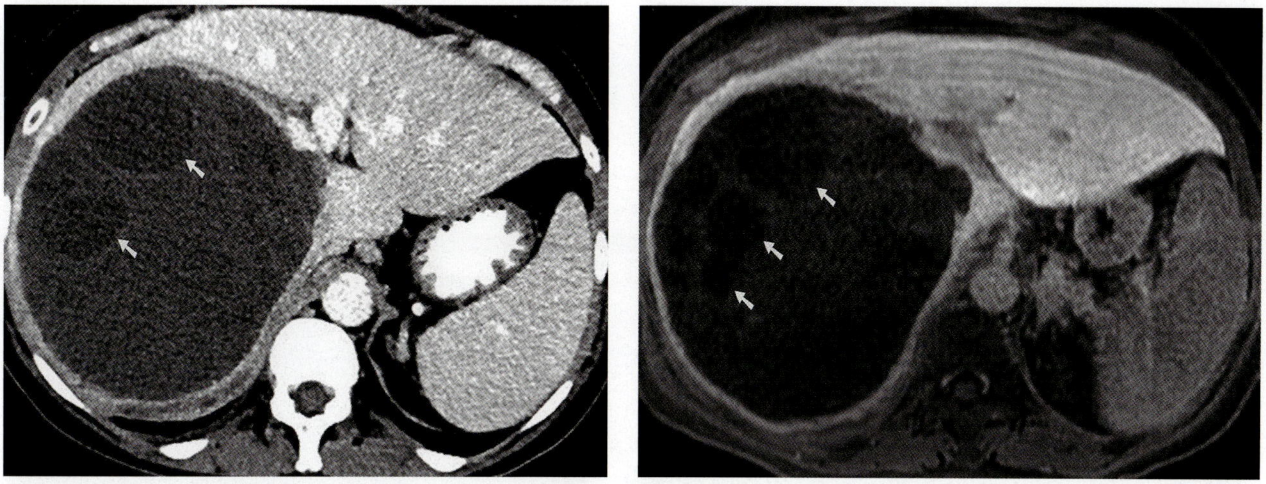

A

B

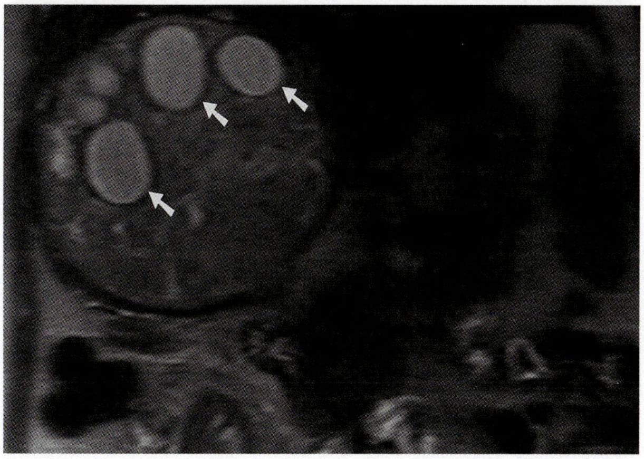

C

**FIG. 8A.32 • Hydatid cyst of liver. A–C:** Axial contrast-enhanced CT, axial contrast-enhanced T1WI, and coronal T2WI demonstrate a large hydatid cyst in the right lobe of the liver, containing multiple smaller daughter cysts (*straight arrows*).

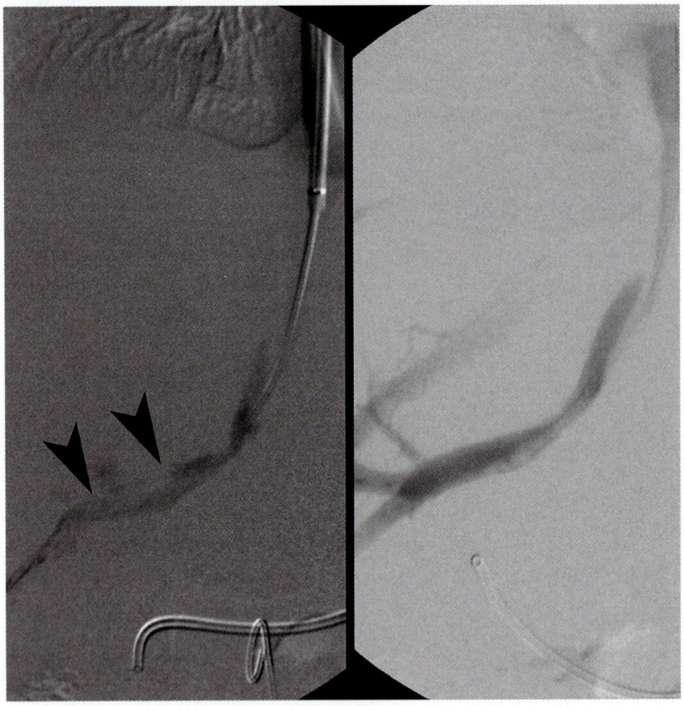

**FIG. 8A.33 • Hepatic vein thrombosis in transplant liver.** Right hepatic venogram study before and after thrombolysis demonstrates irregular thrombus (*arrowheads*) in the lumen of the vein, which markedly improved after thrombolysis with balloon angioplasty.

Complications after liver transplantation are classified into vascular, biliary, parenchymal, and other complications.

1. *Vascular complications:* Excluding graft rejection, vascular complication is the most common cause of graft failure. They range from stenosis, thrombosis, to pseudoaneurysm formation. *Hepatic artery thrombosis* is the most common vascular complication and can lead to hepatic infarction, biliary ischemia, and biloma formation (Figs. 8A.33 and 8A.34). Nonvisualization of hepatic artery on Doppler US prompts further evaluation for definite diagnosis. Nonopacification of the hepatic artery and findings of hepatic infarction can be seen on CT or MRI. *Hepatic artery stenosis* usually occurs at a median of 100 days after operation. Doppler US shows increased peak systolic velocity (PSV) at the stenotic point, low RI (less than 0.5), long acceleration time (greater than 80 msec), and tardus parvus waveform distal to the stenosis.

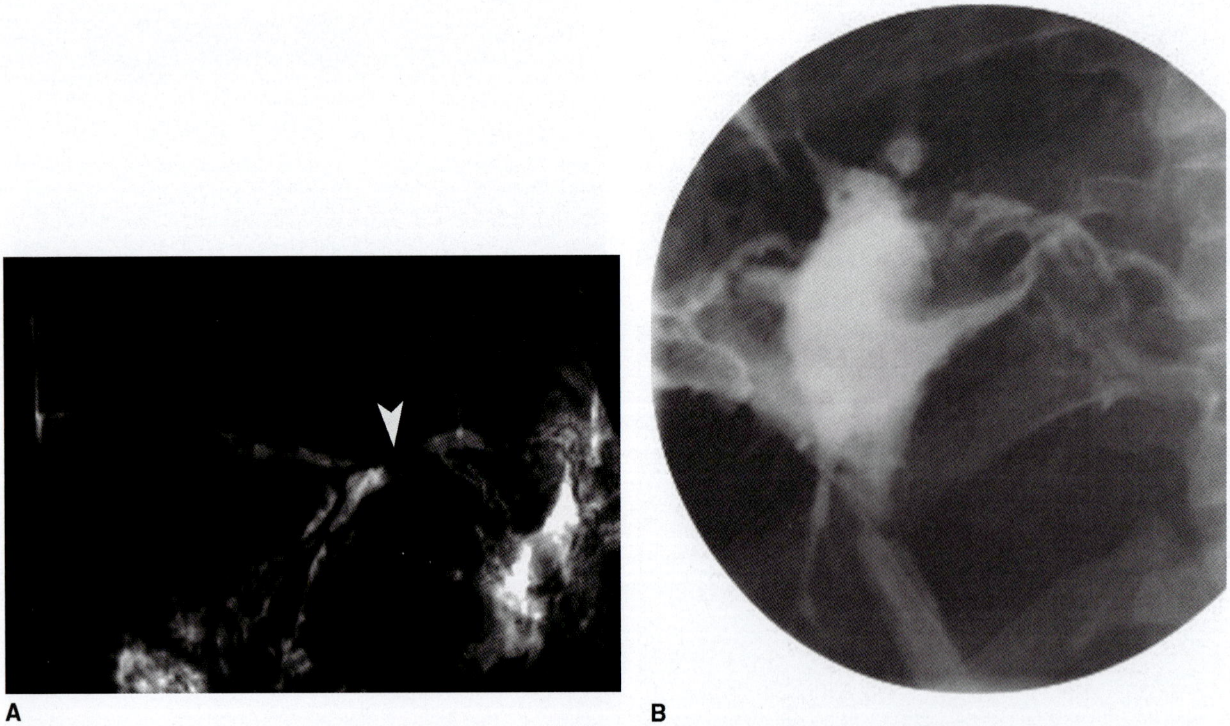

**FIG. 8A.34 • Biliary complications in transplant liver. A:** MRCP demonstrates chronic biliary stricture at the site of biliary anastomosis at the porta hepatis (*arrowhead*). **B:** ERCP demonstrates extensive irregularity and dilatation of the intrahepatic biliary tree, caused by biliary necrosis after hepatic artery occlusion.

CTA is most reliable in identification of the stenotic point. *Hepatic artery pseudoaneurysm* is most commonly extrahepatic at the arterial anastomosis. Intrahepatic pseudoaneurysms are mostly secondary to percutaneous biopsy, biliary procedure, or infection. The pseudoaneurysm may be seen on US as a cystic structure with disorganized arterial flow or bidirectional flow at the aneurysmal neck.

*Portal vein stenosis* usually occurs at the anastomosis. Visible focal narrowing of the portal venous anastomosis on gray-scale US can be seen. Since size discrepancy between the recipient and donor portal vein can produce this appearance, abnormal flow velocity on Doppler US is required for the diagnosis. There is increased PSV (greater than 125 cm/sec) or increased anastomosis to preanastomosis PSV ratio (greater than or equal to 3). *Portal vein thrombosis* usually occurs at the extrahepatic segment. Doppler US, CT, or MRI demonstrates portal vein with filling defects and lack of blood flow. *IVC stenosis/thrombosis* is an infrequent complication. They may result from an intrinsic anastomotic narrowing or extrinsic compression from graft swelling, hematoma, or fluid collection. Doppler US shows color aliasing and increased PSV of the IVC. Indirect findings that may be seen are distension of hepatic veins and dampening of waveform and loss of phasicity of the hepatic venous waveforms. *Hepatic vein stenosis/thrombosis* is also uncommon. Imaging may demonstrate reduced pulsatility or monophasic waveform of the hepatic vein. Intraluminal filling defect may be seen in hepatic vein and IVC thrombosis on US, CT, and MRI (Fig. 8A.33).

2. *Biliary complications* usually occur in early postoperative period (less than 3 months) (Fig. 8A.34). *Biliary obstruction*, seen as dilatation of the donor CBD, is often secondary to anastomotic stricture or stone formation. Dilatation and biliary stones are most reliably demonstrated on MRCP. Anastomotic stricture occurs at the extrahepatic segments of bile duct and is secondary to scar formation. Nonanastomotic stricture is secondary to biliary ischemia and can be multifocal and intrahepatic. *Bile leak* usually occurs at the biliary anastomosis. Localized leakage is called biloma and may be seen as a discrete, round hypoechoic or hypoattenuating fluid collection, often indistinguishable from other postoperative fluid collections. Radionuclide scintigraphy may be required for definitive diagnosis.
3. *Others: Perihepatic hematoma* may be detected within 2 weeks after an operation. It can be seen near the vascular anastomosis, in the perihepatic space or lesser sac. Most hematomas resolve within a few weeks. Acute-to-subacute hematomas appear echogenic at US, hyperattenuating at CT, and hypointense on T2-weighted MR images. *Abscess formation* can occur on the pre-existing hematoma as a result of superimposed infection or secondary to hepatic infarction. Imaging shows a complex fluid collection with or without an air–fluid level.

## References


1. Couinaud C. Liver anatomy: portal (and suprahepatic) or biliary segmentation. *Dig Surg.* 1999;16:459–467.
2. Hamer OW, Aguirre DA, Casola G, et al. Fatty liver: imaging patterns and pitfalls. *Radiographics.* 2006;26:1637–1653.
3. Willatt JM, Hussain HK, Adusumilli S, et al. MR imaging of hepatocellular carcinoma in the cirrhotic liver: challenges and controversies. *Radiology.* 2008;247:311–330.
4. Gupta AA, Kim DC, Krinsky GA, et al. CT and MRI of cirrhosis and its mimics. *AJR Am J Roentgenol.* 2004;186:1595–1601.
5. Ohtomo K, Baron RL, Dodd GD III, et al. Confluent hepatic fibrosis in advanced cirrhosis: appearance at CT. *Radiology.* 1993;188:31–35.
6. Boll DT, Merkle EM. Diffuse liver disease: strategies for hepatic CT and MR. *Radiographics.* 2009; 29:1501–1614.
7. Mergo PJ, Ros PR, Buetow PC, et al. Diffuse disease of the liver: radiologic-pathologic correlation. *Radiographics.* 1994;14(6): 1291–1307.
8. Colagrande S, Centi N, La Villa G, et al. Transient hepatic attenuation differences. *AJR Am J Roentgenol.* 2004;183:459–464.
9. Cura M, Haskal Z, Lopera J. Diagnostic and interventional radiology for Budd-Chiari syndrome. *Radiographics.* 2009;29:669–681.
10. Baba Y, Miyazono N, Inoue H, et al. Altered flow dynamics of intravascular contrast material to the liver in superior vena cava syndrome: CT findings. *Abdom Imaging.* 2000;25:146–150.
11. Choi BI, Lee KH, Han JK, et al. Hepatic arterioportal shunts: dynamic CT and MR features. *Korean J Radiol.* 2002;3:1–15.
12. Torabi M, Hosseinzadeh K, Federle MP. CT of nonneoplastic hepatic vascular and perfusion disorders. *Radiographics.* 2008;28:1967–1982.
13. Richardson PG, Ho VT, Cutler C, et al. Hepatic veno-occlusive disease after hematopoietic stem cell transplantation: novel insights to pathogenesis, current status of treatment, and future directions. *Biol Blood Marrow Transplant.* 2013;19:588–590.
14. Chung YE, Park MS, Park YN. Electronic clinical challenges and images in GI. Hepatic venoocclusive disease. *Gastroenterology.* 2008;135(1): e3–e4.
15. Erturk SM, Mortele KJ, Binkert CA, et al. CT features of hepatic venoocclusive disease and hepatic graft-versus-host disease in patients after hematopoietic stem cell transplantation. *AJR Am J Roentgenol.* 2006;186:1497–1501.
16. Ito K, Higuchi M, Kada T, et al. CT of acquired abnormalities of the portal venous system. *Radiographics.* 1997;17:897–917.
17. Gore RM, Mathieu DG, White EM, et al. Passive hepatic congestion: cross-sectional imaging features. *AJR Am J Roentgenol.* 1994;162: 71–75.
18. Ponziani FR, Zocco MA, Campanale C, et al. Portal vein thrombosis: insight into physiopathology, diagnosis, and treatment. *World J Gastroenterol.* 2010;16:143–155.
19. Kang HK, Jeong YY, Choi JH, et al. Three-dimensional multi-detector row CT portal venography in the evaluation of portosystemic collateral vessels in liver cirrhosis. *Radiographics.* 2002;22:1053–1061.
20. Moubarak E, Bouvier A, Boursier J, et al. Portosystemic collateral vessels in liver cirrhosis: a three-dimensional MDCT pictorial review. *Abdom Imaging.* 2012;37:746–766.
21. Brancatelli G, Vilgrain V, Federle MP, et al. Budd-Chiari syndrome: spectrum of imaging findings. *AJR Am J Roentgenol.* 2007;188(2):W168–W176.
22. Gouya H, Vignaux O, Legmann P, et al. Peliosis hepatis: triphasic helical CT and dynamic MRI findings. *Abdom Imaging.* 2001;26:507–509.
23. Smith GS, Birnbaum BA, Jacobs JE. Hepatic infarction secondary to arterial insufficiency in native livers: CT findings in 10 patients. *Radiology.* 1998;208:223–229.
24. Yoon W, Jeong YY, Kim JK, et al. CT in blunt liver trauma. *Radiographics.* 2005;25:87–104.
25. Kawamoto S, Soyer PA, Fishman EK, et al. Nonneoplastic liver disease: evaluation with CT and MR imaging. *Radiographics.* 1998;18:827–848.
26. Mortelé KJ, Segatto E, Ros PR. The infected liver: radiologic-pathologic correlation. *Radiographics.* 2004;24:937–955.
27. Sanyal R, Lall CG, Lamba R, et al. Orthotopic liver transplantation: reversible Doppler US findings in the immediate postoperative period. *Radiographics.* 2012;32:199–211.
28. Singh AK, Nachiappan AC, Verma HA, et al. Postoperative imaging in liver transplantation: what radiologists should know. *Radiographics.* 2010;30:339–351.

## SELF-ASSESSMENT QUESTIONS

1. Which of the following best represents the underlying cause of the CT imaging findings?

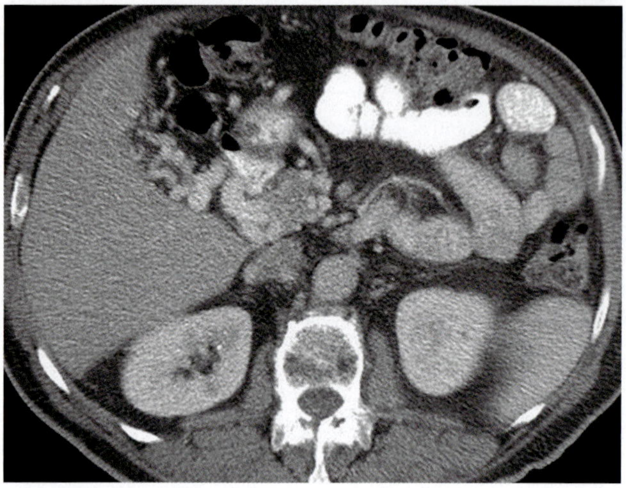

   A. Cirrhosis
   B. Portal vein thrombosis
   C. Hepatitis
   D. Cholangitis

2. Which of the followings best describes diffuse liver disease, as seen on the MR?

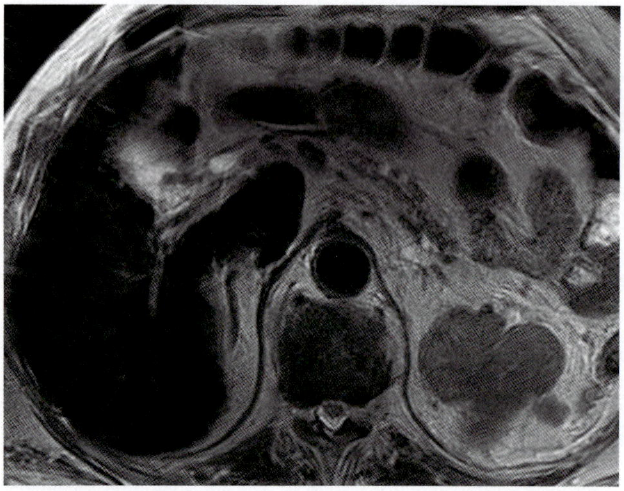

   A. Wilson disease
   B. Hemochromatosis
   C. Fatty liver
   D. Gaucher disease

3. Based on the CT, what is the most likely cause of the patient's symptoms?

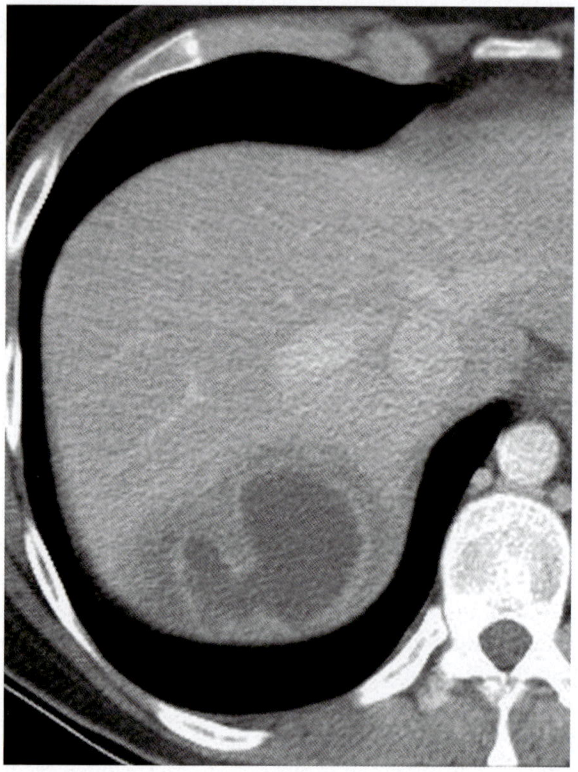

   A. Hydatid cyst
   B. Pyogenic abscess
   C. Hemangioma
   D. Infarction

### *Answers to Self-Assessment Questions*

**1. B.** Portal vein thrombosis. The contrast-enhanced CT demonstrates cavernous transformation of the portal vein, a finding which indicates portal vein thrombosis in the past.

**2. B.** Hemochromatosis. The T2WI depicts hypointensity of the liver parenchyma relative to muscles, due to iron deposition. There is sparing of the splenic parenchyma, a feature which suggests primary hemochromatosis.

**3. B.** Pyogenic abscess. The contrast-enhanced CT demonstrates double target sign, which refers to central low density surrounded with a rim of high-density wall, surrounded by low-density edema in the liver parenchyma.

# Liver: Neoplastic Diseases 8B

*Rathachai Kaewlai, Sirote Wongwaisayawan, and Ajay K. Singh*

## LEARNING OBJECTIVE

1. Describe the imaging features of neoplastic pathologies of the liver.

Secondary liver neoplasms are the most common hepatic neoplasm, far outnumbering primary hepatic neoplasm. Imaging plays an important part in diagnosing and characterizing focal hepatic lesions (Table 8B.1). The primary neoplasm arises from hepatocytes, biliary epithelium, or endothelium and is often associated with underlying chronic liver disease.

## PRIMARY HEPATIC MASSES

### Hepatocellular Adenoma

Hepatocellular adenoma (HCA) is a benign tumor of Kupffer cells that composes largely of hepatocytes with significant arteriovenous shunting, feeding arteries, and poor connective tissue support. It is frequently seen in young middle-aged women on long-term oral contraceptive pills.[1] Tumors are also seen in men who use anabolic steroids and in those with underlying glycogen storage disease, diabetes, obesity, and iron deposition disease. Greater than 80% of HCAs are solitary. When multiple and larger than 10 lesions, the condition is called adenomatosis.[2] Most tumors do not cause symptoms, although 10% may present with hemorrhage and rupture, especially for a large lesion. Surgical resection is the currently preferred treatment method for tumors larger than 5 cm because of an increased risk of hemorrhage, rupture, and malignant transformation. The estimated risks are 27.2%, 17.5%, and 4.2% of patients, respectively.[3]

On CT, HCA is seen as a circumscribed mass with smooth borders and homogeneous arterial enhancement that become isoattenuating on portal venous and delayed phases (Fig. 8B.1). Hemorrhage, fat, and calcifications are detected in the minority of cases on CT. Tumor rupture is diagnosed when hemorrhage is seen beyond the mass, into either the liver parenchyma or abdominal cavity (Fig. 8B.2).[1–3]

On MR, they are T1 hyperintense and T2 iso- to mildly hyperintense. HCA shows strong arterial enhancement and becomes hypointense on hepatobiliary phase (Fig. 8B.3). Hemorrhage, hemosiderin, and fat are easier to detect on MR in most tumors (Fig. 8B.4).

Although imaging appearance mimics that of HCC, the absence of underlying cirrhosis makes HCC less likely. Hypervascular metastasis would also be unlikely in young patients without history of known malignancy. Differentiation with focal nodular hyperplasia (FNH) can be made if HCAs show internal hemorrhage, fat or calcification, and hypointensity on hepatobiliary phase.

### Focal Nodular Hyperplasia

FNH is a benign, nonencapsulated nodule of hyperplastic hepatocytes with a central fibrous scar that occurs in response to pre-existing arterial malformation. The central fibrous scar usually contains abnormal vessels and proliferating bile ductules. FNH is seen predominantly in women between the ages of 30 and 50 and is rare in pediatric and elderly population. Most are found incidentally detected solitary tumors on imaging at the mean size of 4 to 5 cm. FNH has no known potential for malignant transformation and extremely low rate of rupture or hemorrhage. Its association with long-term oral contraceptive use is controversial.[4,5]

The imaging features of FNH are as follows:

- On US, there is a well-demarcated, homogeneous mass of slight hypoechogenicity or isoechogenicity and a central scar. Color Doppler imaging shows a classic, though nonspecific, spoke-wheel pattern of peripherally radiating aberrant vessels.
- On CT, there is homogeneous enhancement in arterial phase that becomes iso- to hypointense in portal venous phase. There is gradual enhancement of the central fibrous scar, which becomes hyperattenuating on delayed phase because contrast medium diffuses slowly into fibrotic tissues. Discontinuous peripheral vascular rim can be seen in 40% of FNH in delayed phase.

Table 8B.1 **DIFFERENTIAL DIAGNOSIS OF FOCAL LIVER LESIONS BASED ON IMAGING**

| Imaging Patterns | Differential Diagnoses |
|---|---|
| Focal hyperechoic lesion (US) | Focal fat<br>Benign neoplasm: hemangioma, adenoma, FNH<br>Abscess<br>Malignancy: metastasis, HCC |
| Focal hyperattenuating lesion (noncontrast CT) | Hematoma, laceration<br>Calcification<br>Lipiodol-stained tumors |
| Focal lesion with T1 hyperintensity (MRI) | Fat in the lesion<br>Blood degradation products in the lesion<br>Proteinaceous content in abscess<br>Melanoma metastasis<br>Lipiodol |
| Focal lesion with arterial enhancement (CT, MRI) | Transient hepatic attenuation difference<br>Arterioportal shunt<br>SVC obstruction (if in segment IV)<br>HCC<br>Hypervascular metastasis<br>Benign neoplasm (adenoma, FNH, and hemangioma) |
| Focal lesion with delayed enhancement (CT, MRI) | Hemangioma<br>Cholangiocarcinoma<br>Treated metastasis<br>Central scar of FNH<br>Capsule of HCC |
| Focal lesion with central scar | FNH<br>FLHCC<br>Cholangiocarcinoma<br>HCC<br>Large hemangioma |
| Focal lesion with calcification | Granuloma<br>Echinococcosis<br>Fibrolamellar HCC<br>Adenoma<br>Metastasis<br>Teratoma |
| Focal lesion with fat | Adenoma<br>HCC<br>Lipoma<br>AML<br>FNH<br>Focal fat |
| Focal lesion with iron | Siderotic nodule<br>Dysplastic nodule<br>HCC |

- On MR, FNH appears isointense on both T1WI and T2WI with a central scar, which is T1 hypointense and T2 hyperintense (Figs. 8B.5 and 8B.6). The tumor enhancement pattern is similar to that of CT.[4] In addition, FNH appears iso- to hyperintense on hepatobiliary phase when hepatocyte-specific contrast agent is used.

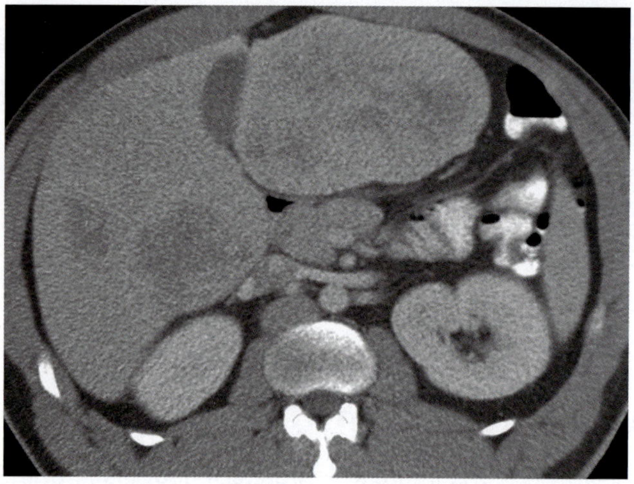

**FIG. 8B.1 • Hepatic adenoma.** Axial contrast-enhanced CT in portal venous phase demonstrates multiple heterogeneous, iso- to hypodense adenomas within the liver.

Two main differential diagnoses are HCA and fibrolamellar hepatocellular carcinoma (FLHCC). When the lesions have atypical features, such as presence of calcification, size greater than 10 cm, T2 hypointense scar, vascular invasion, and lymphadenopathy; further diagnostic tests are recommended.[4]

## Cirrhotic Nodules and Hepatocellular Carcinoma

Regenerative nodules, dysplastic nodules, and HCC represent a pathologic–radiologic continuum of cirrhotic-related nodules from benignity to malignancy. In general, the greater the degree of hepatic arterial supply to the nodules, the more likely they are malignant.

*Regenerative nodules (RN)* are hepatocellular nodules surrounded by fibrous septa present in all cirrhotic liver. They are categorized by size into micronodular (size 3 mm or less) and macronodular. Cirrhosis secondary to alcohol and biliary etiologies is usually micronodular while that associated with chronic active hepatitis B and C is macronodular. RNs are mainly supplied by portal veins with minimal contribution from hepatic artery. Small RNs are rarely visible on noncontrast CT and often indistinguishable from the background cirrhotic liver because of similar enhancement. Iron-containing RNs or siderotic nodules can be seen as a hyperattenuating nodule on noncontrast CT and T2 hypointense nodule on MRI.

*Dysplastic nodules (DN)* are hepatocellular nodules with dysplasia but lack of any pathologically malignant features. It is found in 15% to 25% of cirrhotic liver, showing variable attenuation/signal intensity on noncontrast CT and MRI. After contrast administration, low-grade DNs are generally unenhanced while high-grade ones may enhance in the arterial phase (Figs. 8B.7 and 8B.8). Similar to siderotic RNs, if the DNs contain iron, they will appear T2 hypointense.[6]

*HCC* represents the most malignant hepatocellular lesion on the spectrum of cirrhosis-related pathology. The annual incidence of HCC is 2% to 6.6% among cirrhotic patients and

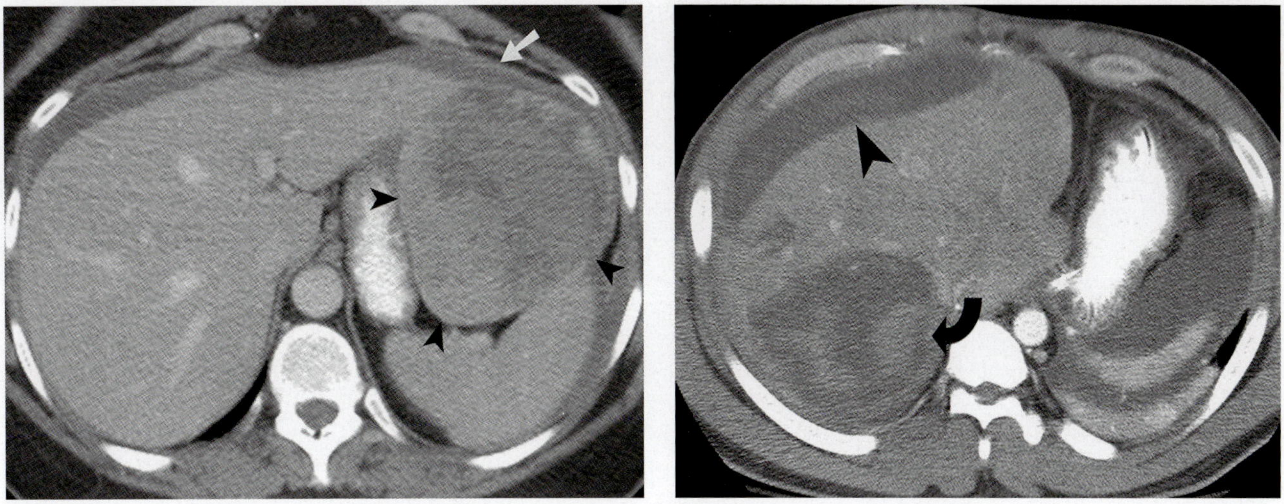

A B

**FIG. 8B.2 • Hepatic adenoma with hemorrhage. A:** Axial contrast-enhanced CT demonstrates a large hepatic adenoma (*arrowheads*) arising from the left lobe of the liver with intralesional blood clot. There is perihepatic high-density fluid (*arrow*) seen anterior to the adenoma. **B:** Axial contrast-enhanced CT demonstrates a large right hepatic adenoma with intralesional blood clots (*curved arrow*). There is perihepatic hemoperitoneum (*arrowhead*) identified anterior to the liver. There is also a smaller hepatic adenoma seen in the right lobe of the liver.

0.4% in patients without cirrhosis. They present as a focal mass (single large mass with or without small satellite nodules), multifocal nodules (multiple discrete nodules throughout the liver), or diffuse abnormality (multiple minute indistinct nodules throughout the liver).

The imaging features include the following:

- CT: Because of hepatic artery supply, the HCC is heterogeneous with strong arterial enhancement (Fig. 8B.9) with venous washout. Tumor of greater than 1 cm showing arterial hypervascularity and venous or delayed phase washout in patients with cirrhosis can be confidently diagnosed as HCC. For lesions less than 1 cm, imaging appearance may not be straightforward and a 3-month follow-up US is suggested to determine growth and changing character.[7] The outer rim of HCC may show delayed enhancement.
- MRI: HCCs are typically T1 hypointense and heterogeneously T2 hyperintense and show diffusion restriction and hypointensity on hepatobiliary phase (Figs. 8B.10 to 8B.12). Some HCCs are T1 hyperintense due to presence of fat, copper, glycogen, or zinc within the mass. Large HCCs are often T2 heterogeneous. Portal venous thrombosis, either bland or tumor, may be seen. Findings supportive of malignant thrombi include T2 hyperintensity, dilated portal vein, and enhancement (Fig. 8B.13).[6]

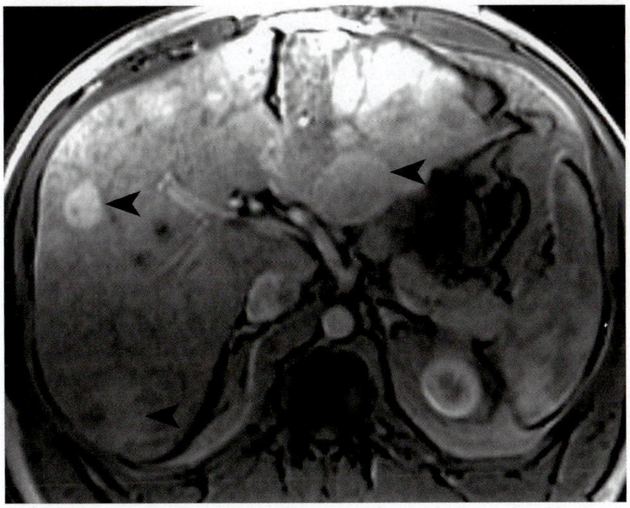

**FIG. 8B.3 • Hepatic adenoma.** Postgadolinium T1WI in arterial phase demonstrates multiple hyperenhancing adenomas (*arrowheads*) in the right and left lobe of the liver.

*Ruptured HCC* occurs when tumors grow expansively beyond the fibrous capsule, disrupting the feeding arteries. This occurs in 6% to 10% of all HCCs and results in intratumoral hemorrhage that extends beyond the capsule into adjacent perihepatic space and peritoneal cavity.[8,9] Rupture is often fatal because of uncontrolled bleeding due to coexistent coagulopathy. Maximum tumor diameter greater than 5 cm and high Child-Pugh grade are strongly associated with spontaneous rupture.[9] On imaging, ruptured HCCs are often very large, located in the periphery of the liver with a protruding contour, and are among many other lesions. US demonstrates hepatic masses with echoic perihepatic fluid collection. Signs of rupture on CT include discontinuity of the tumor surface, high-attenuation collection in the nearby perihepatic space, and hemoperitoneum (Fig. 8B.14). Enucleation sign describes a ruptured tumor that has central, nonenhancing portion separated from peripheral rim enhancement with a focal discontinuity of the tumor surface—mimicking an enucleated orbital globe.[8]

After treatment with *RFA*, HCC is usually followed with CT or MRI at 1 month. Complete lack of enhancement of the tumor ("tumor cavity") in all phases is expected due to coagulative necrosis. On MRI, three zones within the ablated

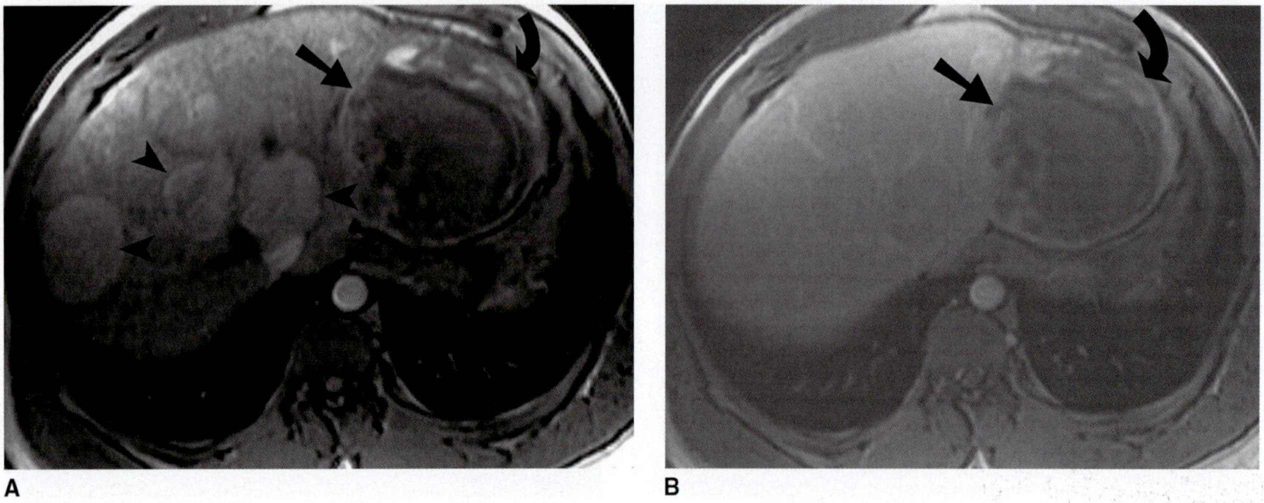


**FIG. 8B.4 • Hepatic adenoma with hemorrhage. A, B:** Postgadolinium T1WI in arterial and portal venous phase demonstrates multiple hyperenhancing adenomas (*arrowheads*), which become isointense to the liver on the later phase imaging. There is a large left hepatic lobe adenoma (*straight arrow*) with heterogeneous, T1 hyperintense perilesional hemorrhage (*curved arrow*).

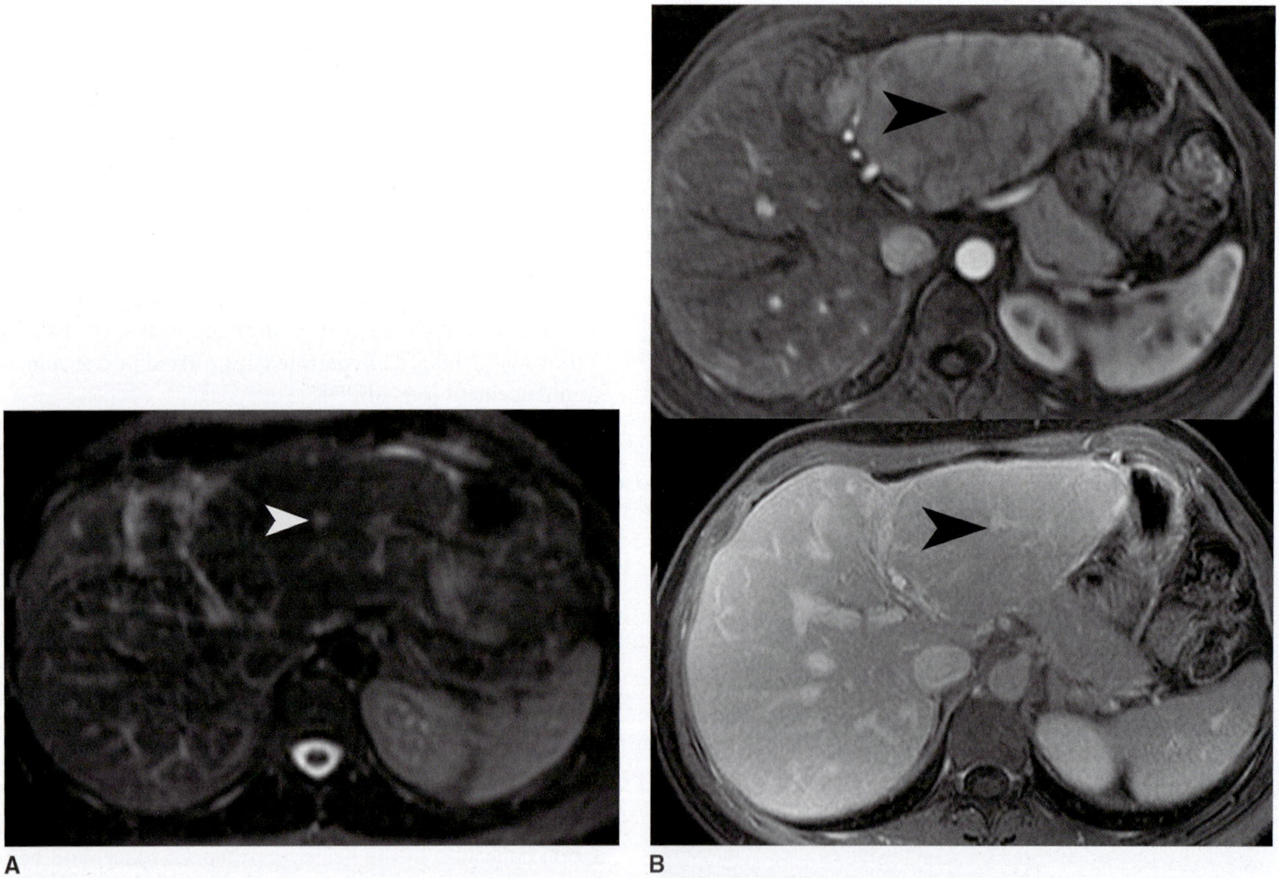


**FIG. 8B.5 • Focal nodular hyperplasia. A:** FSE T2WI shows large left lobe FNH, which is isointense to the liver, but demonstrates a T2 hyperintense central scar (*arrowhead*). **B:** Postgadolinium T1WI in arterial and portal venous phase demonstrates intense arterial phase enhancement of the FNH, which becomes isointense to the liver on the portal venous phase. The central scar (*arrowhead*) shows enhancement on the portal venous phase.

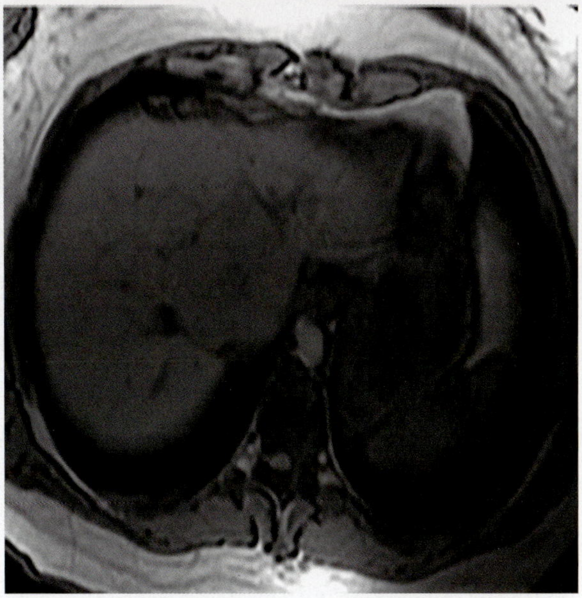

A

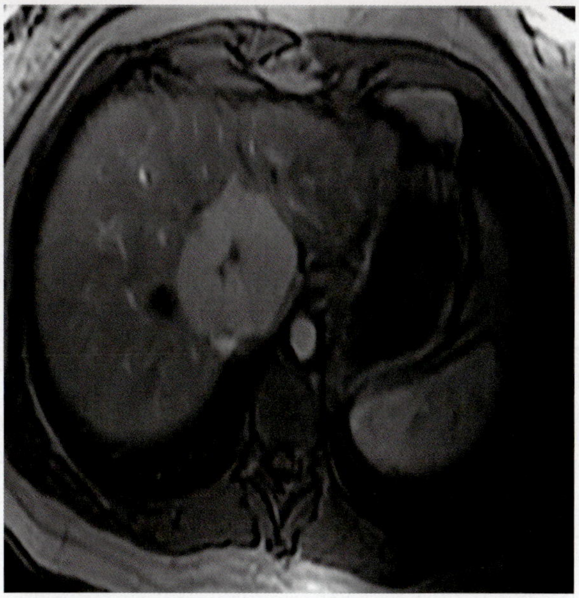

B

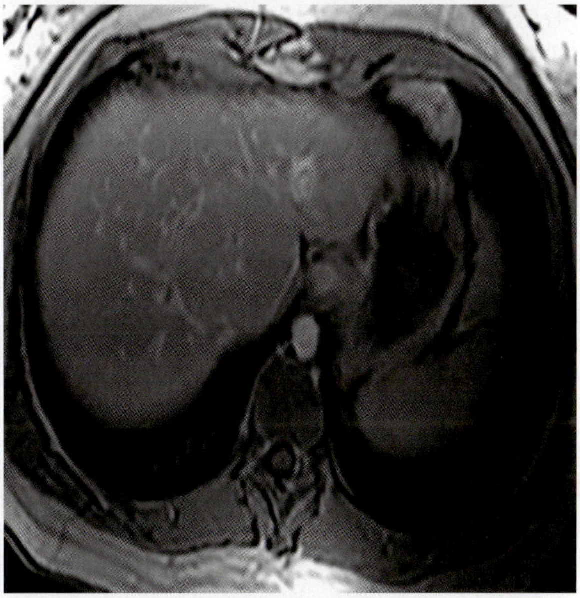

C

**FIG. 8B.6 • Focal nodular hyperplasia. A–C:** Noncontrast, postgadolinium MR in arterial (A) and portal venous (B) phase demonstrate an FNH, which is isointense on noncontrast and portal venous phase imaging. The FNH demonstrates intense enhancement on the arterial phase imaging with a central scar.

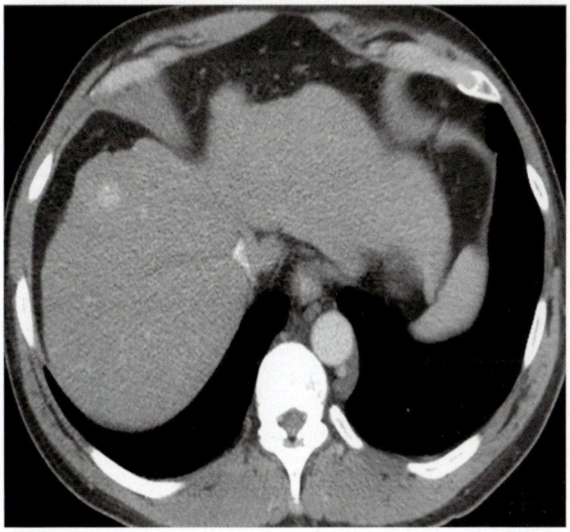

**FIG. 8B.7 • Dysplastic nodule with cirrhosis.** Axial contrast-enhanced CT in arterial phase demonstrates a 1-cm diameter enhancing focus in the right lobe in a patient with macronodular cirrhosis.

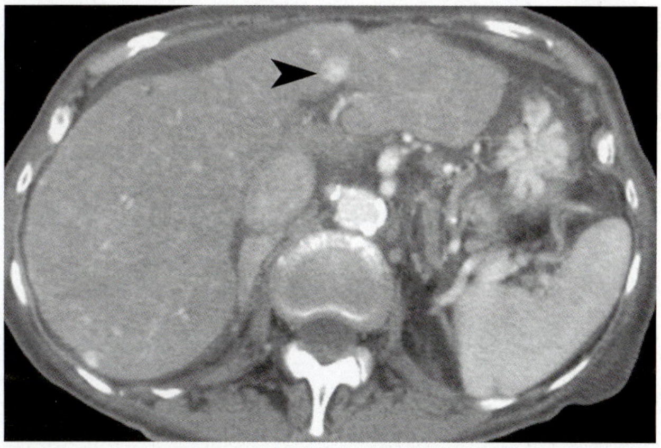

**FIG. 8B.8 • Dysplastic nodule with cirrhosis.** Axial contrast-enhanced CT in arterial phase demonstrates a hypervascular nodule (*arrowhead*) in the left lobe of the liver. A smaller hypervascular subcapsular nodule is seen in the segment VI of the liver.

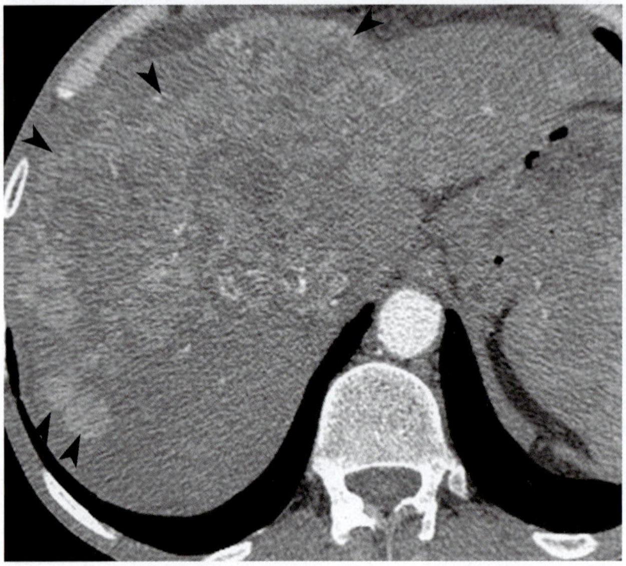

**FIG. 8B.9 • Multifocal hepatocellular carcinoma.** Contrast-enhanced CT an arterial phase demonstrates multiple discrete and confluent nodules (*arrowheads*) in the liver.

cavity are seen on T1W images, consisting of central hypointensity, middle hyperintensity, and outer hypointense band. The central and middle zones represent changes of coagulative necrosis while the outer band is secondary to sinusoidal congestion (acute phase) or fibrosis (subacute phase). This outer band may show mild, smooth, regular enhancement especially on delayed phase and should not be mistaken for recurrence. Signs of treatment failure include persistent enhancement of the tumor cavity, nodular/irregular arterial hypervascularity at the periphery of the cavity with venous washout, and enlarging tumor cavity.[6]

For HCC treated by *transarterial chemoembolization (TACE)*, response is suggested as development of necrosis within the tumor and reduced tumor volume on CT or MRI. Lipiodol at the site of tumor uptake appears intensely hyperattenuating on CT and hypointense on opposed-phase MR images (Fig. 8B.15). Residual or recurrent tumors appear as arterial enhancing focus that are best demonstrated on MRI because lipiodol may mask such enhancement on CT. Interestingly, the presence or absence of viable

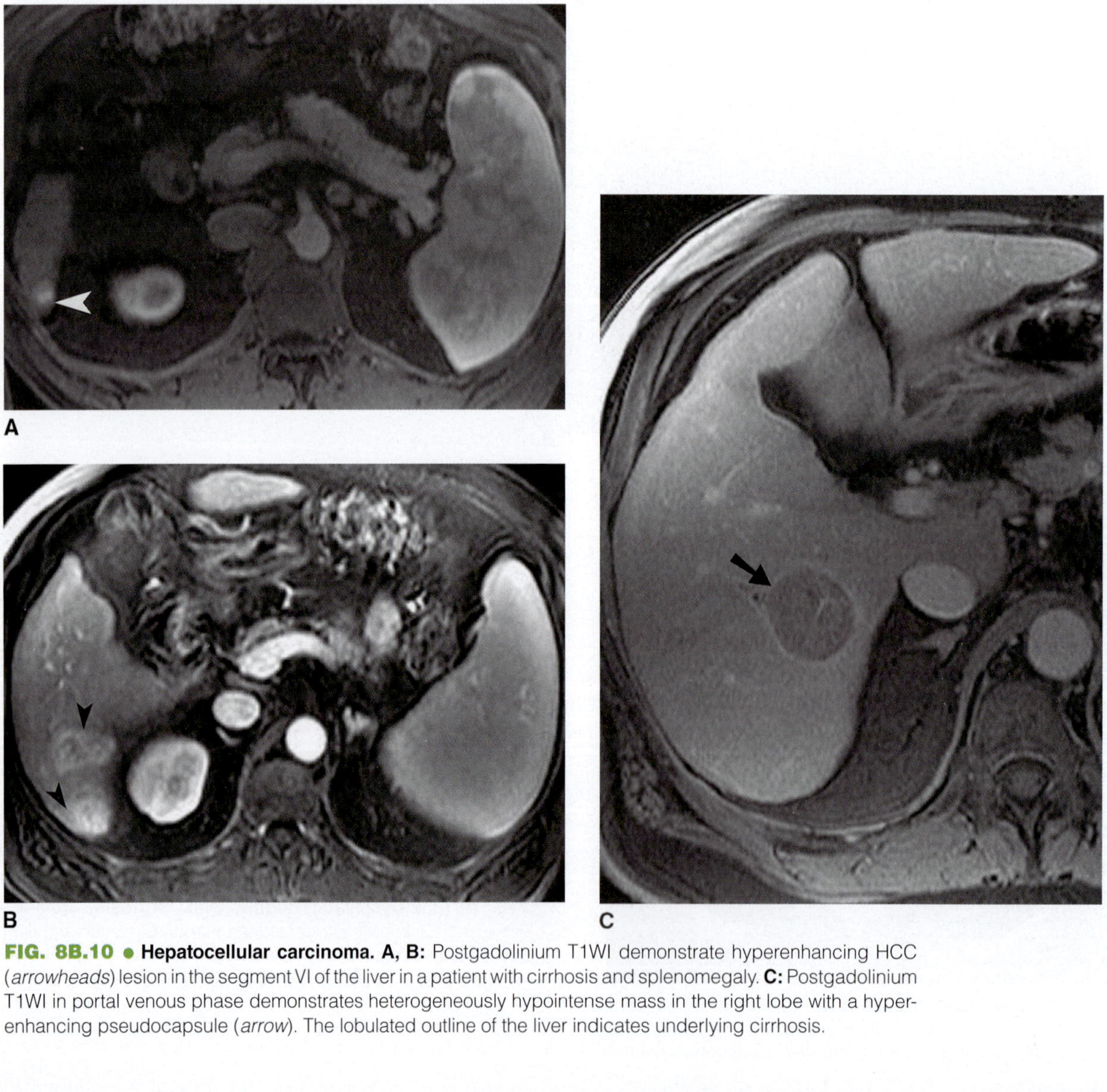

**FIG. 8B.10 • Hepatocellular carcinoma. A, B:** Postgadolinium T1WI demonstrate hyperenhancing HCC (*arrowheads*) lesion in the segment VI of the liver in a patient with cirrhosis and splenomegaly. **C:** Postgadolinium T1WI in portal venous phase demonstrates heterogeneously hypointense mass in the right lobe with a hyperenhancing pseudocapsule (*arrow*). The lobulated outline of the liver indicates underlying cirrhosis.

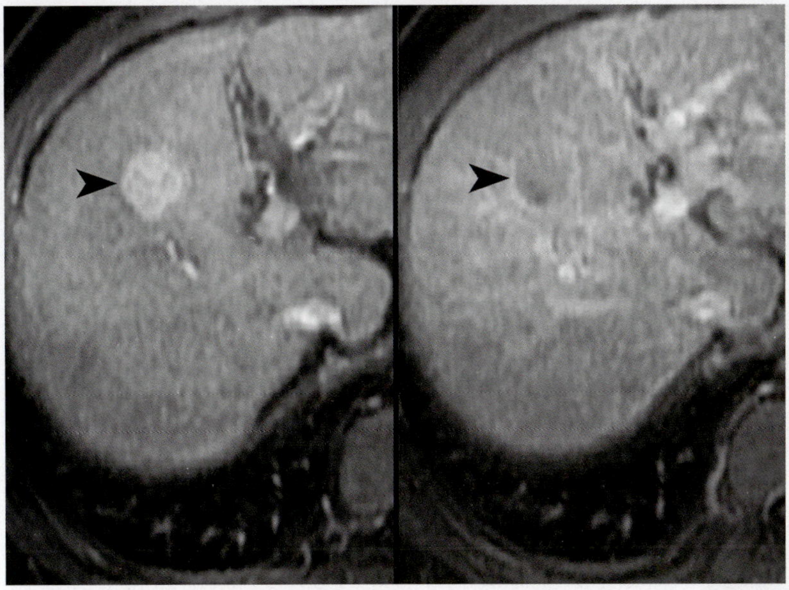

**FIG. 8B.11 • Hepatocellular carcinoma.** Postgadolinium T1WI in arterial and portal venous phase demonstrate an arterially hyperenhancing right lobe HCC (*arrowhead*), which is hypointense on the late phase imaging. There is a hyperenhancing pseudocapsule around the lesion on the late phase imaging.

tumor on MRI does not correlate with lipiodol uptake on CT.[6]

*Liver imaging reporting and data system* (LI-RADS) is a system for standardizing performance and interpretation of liver CT and MRI in patients at increased risk of HCC. Developed by the American College of Radiology (ACR) and launched in March 2011, LI-RADS consists of imaging terminology, illustrative atlas, diagnostic algorithm, and guidance for appropriate imaging technique, which is available in the ACR Web site. Liver nodules found on CT or MRI of an individual

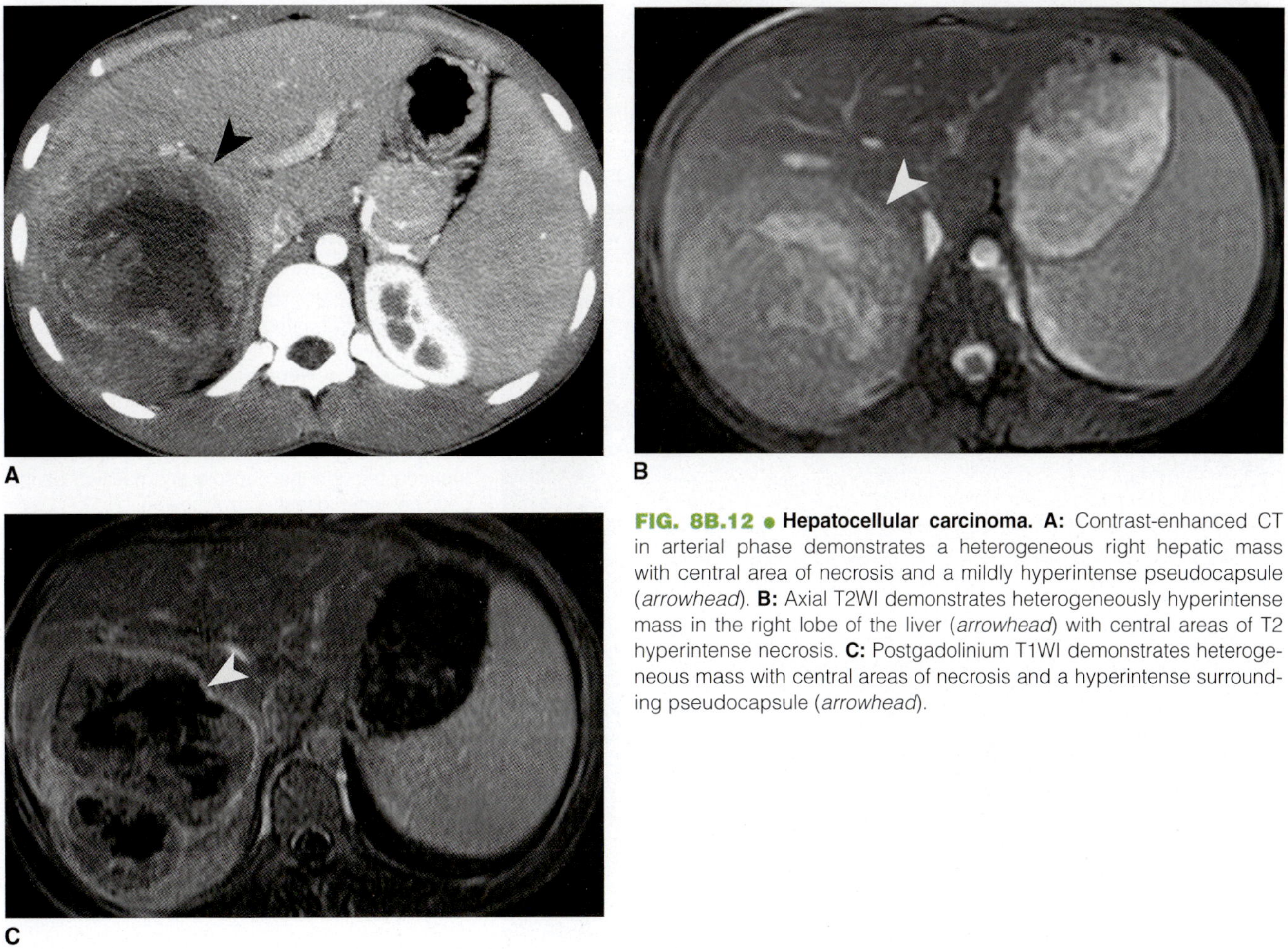

**FIG. 8B.12 • Hepatocellular carcinoma. A:** Contrast-enhanced CT in arterial phase demonstrates a heterogeneous right hepatic mass with central area of necrosis and a mildly hyperintense pseudocapsule (*arrowhead*). **B:** Axial T2WI demonstrates heterogeneously hyperintense mass in the right lobe of the liver (*arrowhead*) with central areas of T2 hyperintense necrosis. **C:** Postgadolinium T1WI demonstrates heterogeneous mass with central areas of necrosis and a hyperintense surrounding pseudocapsule (*arrowhead*).

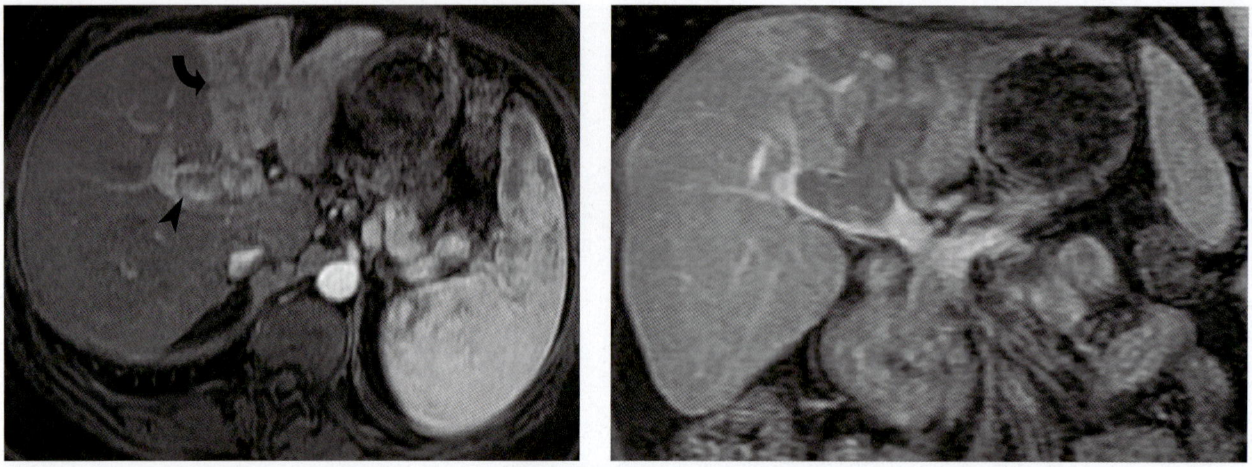

A B

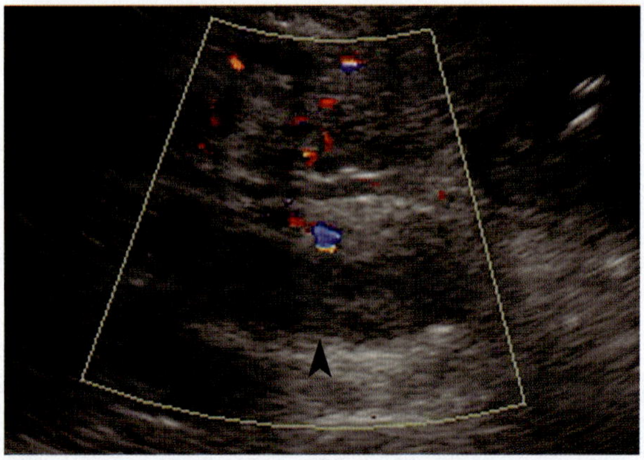

C

**FIG. 8B.13 • Hepatocellular carcinoma with portal venous invasion. A, B:** Postgadolinium T1WI in axial and coronal planes demonstrate infiltrating left hepatic mass (*curved arrow*) with direct extension of the tumor thrombus (*arrowhead*) into the portal vein. **C:** Color Doppler US study in a patient with HCC demonstrates occluding bland thrombus (*arrowhead*) occupying the main portal vein lumen.

at risk for HCC are categorized into five categories of LR-1 to LR-5 in order of increasing probability of HCC of a newly found nodule/mass. LR-M is assigned for probably malignant lesions that are not specific for HCC while LR-treated represents HCC that has been treated. Imaging categorization is based on the diameter and presence of four major imaging features, which include arterial phase hyperenhancement, washout appearance following hyperenhancement, capsule appearance, and threshold growth compared with previous imaging.[10]

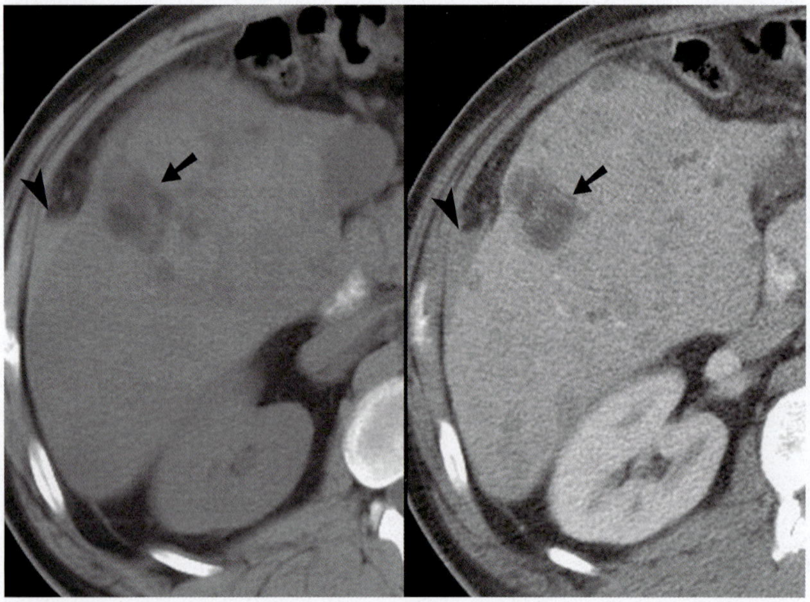

**FIG. 8B.14 • Hepatocellular carcinoma with rupture.** Noncontrast and postcontrast axial CT demonstrate multiple heterogeneously hypodense HCCs, the largest one (*straight arrow*) of which has ruptured through the capsule and causing perihepatic hemoperitoneum (*arrowheads*).

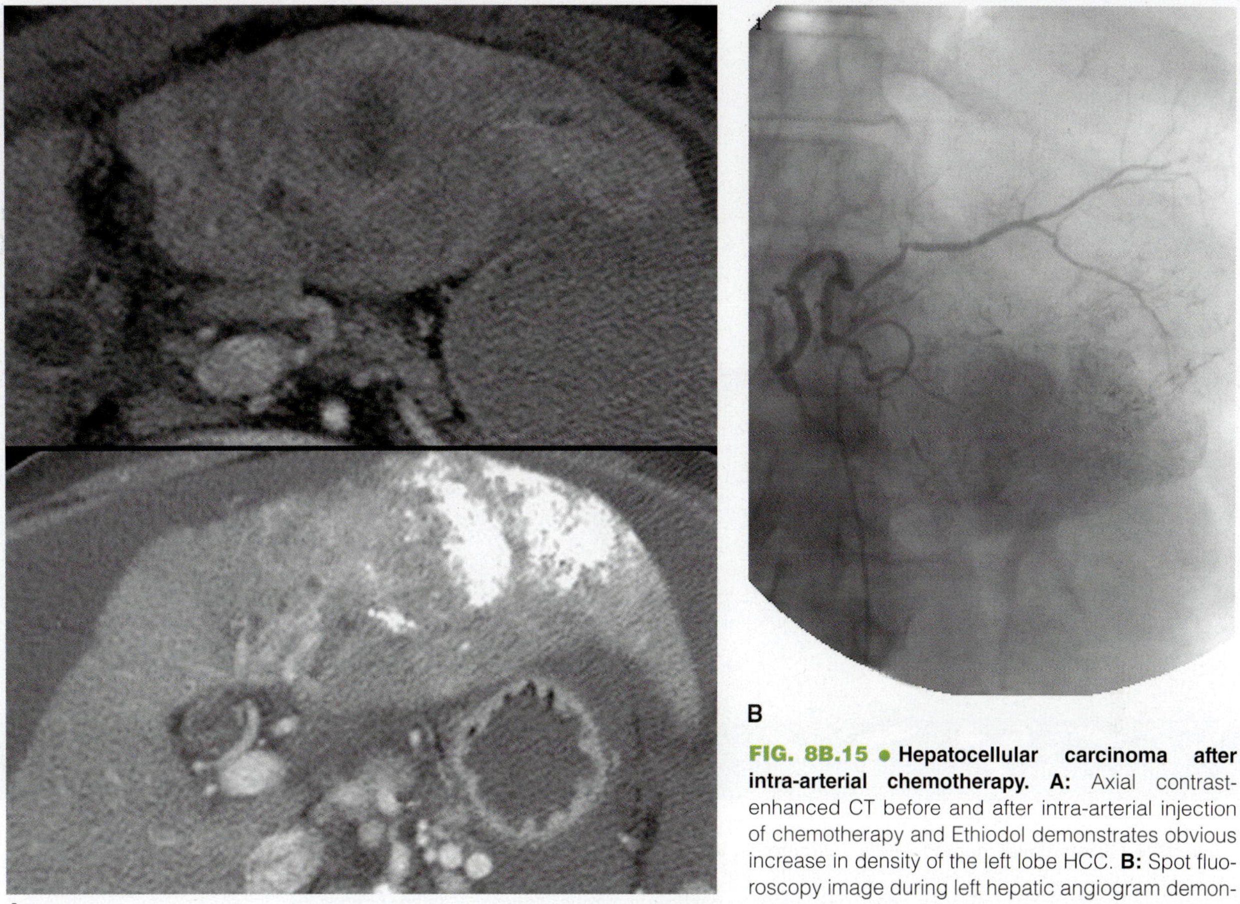

A B

**FIG. 8B.15 • Hepatocellular carcinoma after intra-arterial chemotherapy. A:** Axial contrast-enhanced CT before and after intra-arterial injection of chemotherapy and Ethiodol demonstrates obvious increase in density of the left lobe HCC. **B:** Spot fluoroscopy image during left hepatic angiogram demonstrates tumor neovascularity and blush in the HCC.

## Fibrolamellar Hepatocellular Carcinoma

FLHCC is a rare form of HCC, accounting for less than 1% of HCC, with distinctively different clinicopathologic features. Most (95%) occur in patients without any underlying hepatitis or cirrhosis. Young patients, generally below 40 years old, are mostly affected without gender predilection. Lesions are usually solitary and large with an average size at diagnosis of 13 cm. Central scar is present in 65% to 75% of cases. Nodal disease is found in 50% to 65% of cases, predominantly at the hepatic hilum and hepatoduodenal ligament. Serum alpha-fetoprotein is generally not elevated.[11]

The CT and MR imaging features of FLHCC include the following:

- There is a large, heterogeneous mass with well-demarcated borders and lobulated contour (Fig. 8B.16A).
- Calcification is seen in 40% to 68% of cases.
- There is heterogeneous enhancement on arterial phase and washout on portal venous and delayed phases.
- Central scar is hypoattenuating with or without enhancement.
- On MRI, the mass is T1 hypointense and T2 hyperintense and demonstrates diffusion restriction. On hepatobiliary phase, FLHCC is hypointense relative to liver parenchyma (Fig. 8B.16B). The scar is classically T1 and T2 hypointense.[11]

## Intrahepatic Cholangiocarcinoma

Intrahepatic cholangiocarcinoma is adenocarcinoma of the bile ducts that is confined to the liver without involvement of the hepatic duct bifurcation and extrahepatic ducts. They account for 6% of all cholangiocarcinomas and can be further divided into three subtypes with distinct patterns of spread, imaging features, and outcome.[12]

1. *Mass-forming cholangiocarcinoma* is the most common subtype, often presenting as a large, infiltrative mass in the periphery of the liver with irregular and lobulated margins (Fig. 8B.17A). Its central part contains fibrous stroma. The mass is hypoattenuating on CT and T1 hypointense and T2 hyperintense on MRI with maximal enhancement in the delayed phase due to delayed enhancement of the fibrotic tissues. Peripheral enhancement and focal dilatation of large intrahepatic duct (IHD) surrounding the mass may be seen.
2. *Periductal cholangiocarcinoma* represents tumors that longitudinally grow along the dilated or narrowed bile ducts without mass formation (Fig. 8B.17B). On imaging, there is thickening and enhancement of the periductal tissues with bile duct dilatation of the segment or lobe involved.
3. *Intraductal cholangiocarcinoma* is papillary or polypoid tumors that spread along the mucosal surface of the bile duct with or without confinement to the bile duct wall.

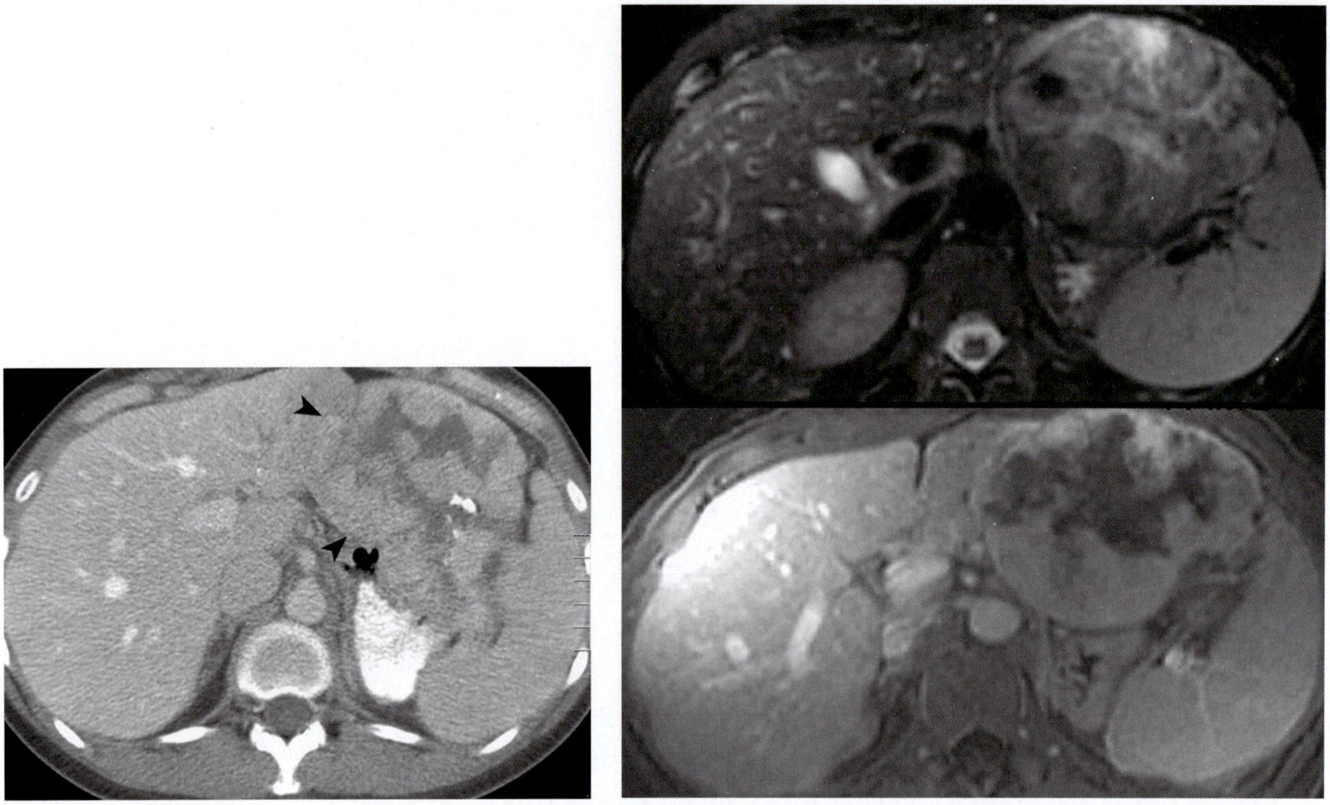

A B

**FIG. 8B.16 • Fibrolamellar hepatocellular carcinoma. A:** Contrast-enhanced axial CT demonstrates large heterogeneous mass lesion (*arrowheads*) with central areas of necrosis and calcifications in the left lobe of the liver. **B:** FSE T2WI and postgadolinium T1WI demonstrate heterogeneous large left hepatic mass lesion with central areas of necrosis and lobulated peripheral enhancement.

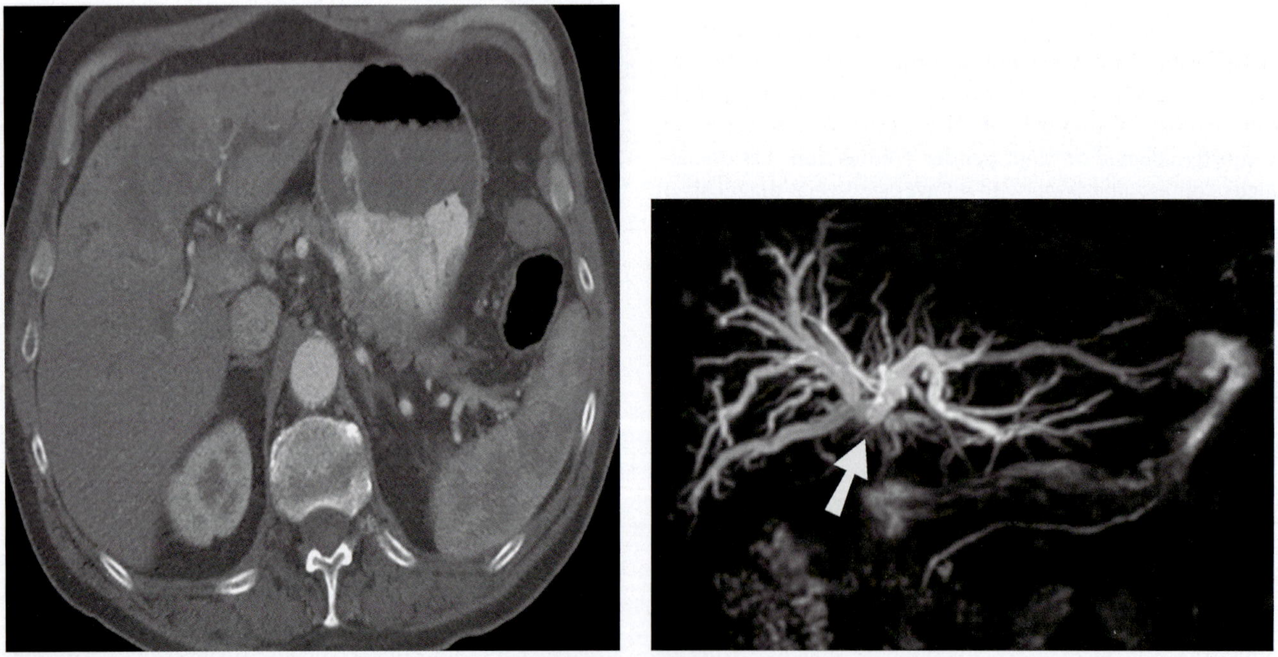

A B

**FIG. 8B.17 • Intrahepatic cholangiocarcinoma. A:** Axial contrast-enhanced CT scan study demonstrates a heterogeneously hypodense mass in the segment IV of the liver with associated intrahepatic biliary ductal dilatation in the left lobe of the liver. **B:** MRCP demonstrates intrahepatic biliary ductal dilatation due to the presence of an obstructing mass at the porta hepatis (*arrow*).

Tumors produce mucin and obstruct the bile duct, resulting in ductal dilatation both distal and proximal to the tumor. Mucin in dilated ducts may appear hyperattenuating on CT while the polypoid tumors show slight hypoattenuation. Delayed enhancement of the tumors is not seen because of lack of fibrous stroma.[13]

## Biliary Cystic Tumors

Biliary cystic tumors are cysts arising from biliary epithelium that account for less than 5% of all solitary hepatic cystic lesions.[14,15] They include biliary cystadenoma and cystadenocarcinoma. They are generally solitary, slow-growing lesions of varying size with multilocular cystic components and fluid content. Cyst walls can have dense fibrosis and even calcification. If direct communication with biliary tree exists, it is called biliary intraductal papillary mucinous neoplasm. The mean age at presentation of biliary cystadenoma is 45 to 50 years, while this is a decade later for cystadenocarcinoma. Malignant transformation of biliary cystadenoma is seen in as high as 20% of cases; therefore, surgical resection is generally recommended.[14]

On imaging, both biliary cystadenoma and cystadenocarcinoma demonstrate cystic appearance with internal contents (debris, hemorrhage), septation, papillary projections, mural/septal nodules, and enhancement of the septa, nodules, and walls (Fig. 8B.18). Fine punctate calcification of the cyst wall may be seen. Biliary cystadenocarcinoma generally has thicker, more irregular walls, more nodularity, and enhancement of the septa.

US is more sensitive than CT to detect septa in cystic lesions, while CT more accurately depicts lesion size, extent, and pattern of enhancement. The presence of upstream bile duct dilatation, lesion location in the left hepatic lobe, fewer than three coexistent cysts, and transient hepatic attenuation difference are suggestive of biliary cystic neoplasm.[16]

## Angiosarcoma

Angiosarcoma is a malignant tumor arising from mesenchymal tissue and constitutes only 2% of primary malignant tumors. It is most commonly seen in the 60 to 70 years age group and has been associated with thorotrast, vinyl chloride, and arsenic exposure. They have variable imaging appearance, often resembling hemangioma or metastases.

# SECONDARY HEPATIC MASSES

## Metastasis

High volume of blood flow, favorable microscopic anatomy, and rich biochemical environment of the liver make it the most common site of distant metastasis from extrahepatic primary malignancy.[17] Imaging is done to stage the disease after primary tumor is identified and characterize the lesion.[18]

Most metastases are *hypovascular* relative to the surrounding liver parenchyma. They are hypoattenuating on noncontrast CT and portal venous phase of contrast-enhanced CT. On MRI, most tumors are slightly T1 hypointense and slightly T2 hyperintense, showing diffusion restriction and

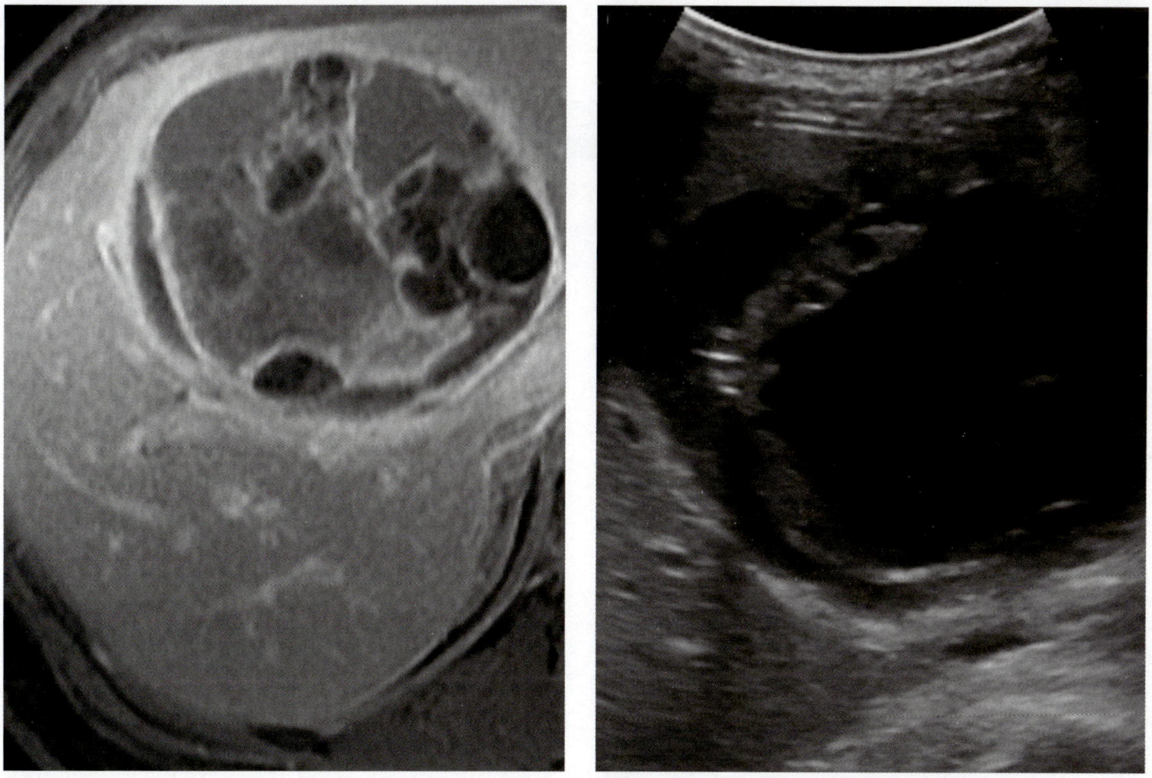

A B

**FIG. 8B.18 • Biliary cystadenoma. A:** Postgadolinium T1WI demonstrates large right hepatic complex cystic mass with enhancing internal septations and irregular capsule thickness. **B:** US study demonstrates a complex cystic mass in the liver with hyperechoic, irregularly thick capsule.

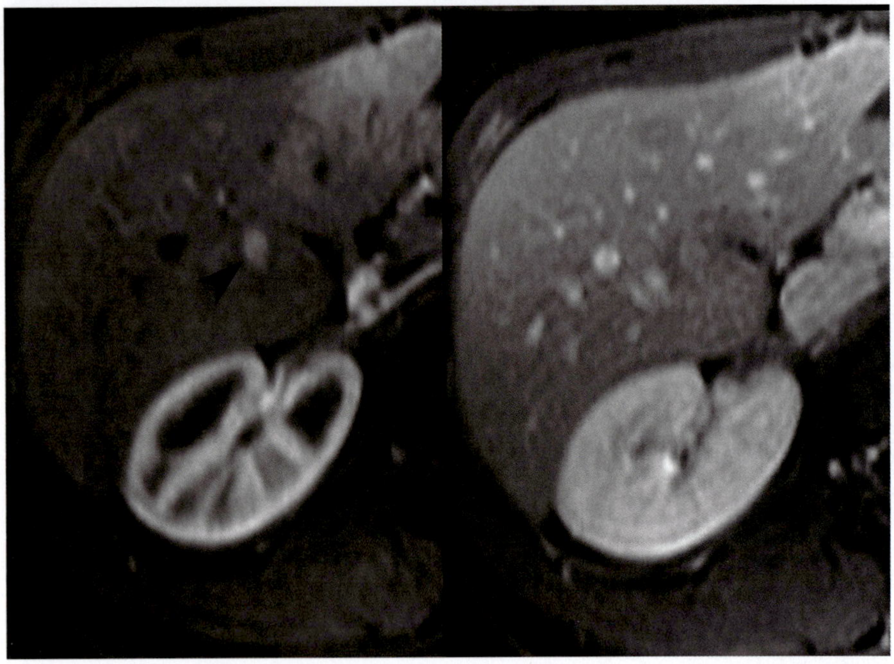

**FIG. 8B.19 • Hemangioma.** Postgadolinium T1WI in arterial and portal venous phase demonstrate small arterially enhancing right hepatic hemangioma (*arrowhead*), which becomes isointense to the liver on portal venous phase.

hypointense on hepatobiliary phase. Some metastases with central desmoplastic areas may demonstrate delayed enhancement in the equilibrium to delayed phases.[18,19]

*Hypervascular metastasis* demonstrates partial or total enhancement of tumors during the arterial phase imaging. Examples of primary malignancy with hypervascularity are breast, renal, thyroid, pancreatic, and neuroendocrine cell carcinoma, pheochromocytoma, melanoma, and carcinoid (Fig. 8B.19). Many of these lesions are obscured on routine CT with only portal venous phase imaging; therefore, an addition of arterial phase is recommended.

*Cystic metastases* show large areas of necrosis in the masses due to rapid growth and insufficient arterial supply. Cystic metastasis can be from either cystic or solid primary tumors. Examples include colonic adenocarcinoma; melanoma; carcinoid; breast, renal, and gastrointestinal tumors; and ovarian cancers. Imaging features indicative of malignant process generally exist (such as ill-defined margins, irregular walls, amputated nearby vessels, irregular and peripheral rim enhancement), making it distinguishable from other benign cysts (Fig. 8B.20).[15,19]

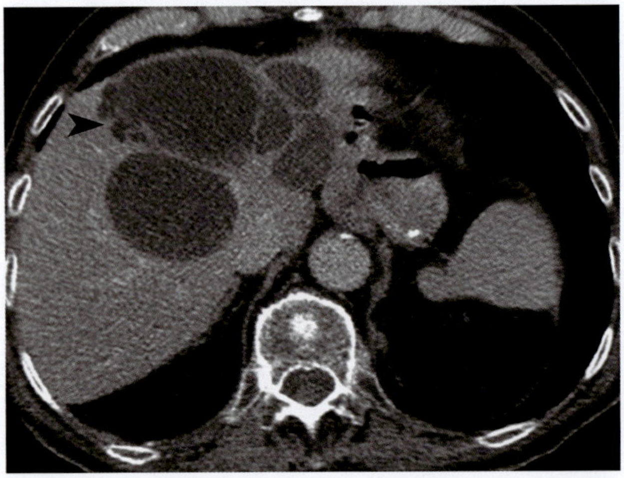

**FIG. 8B.20 • Cystic metastasis to the liver.** Axial contrast-enhanced CT demonstrates complex multicystic lesion (*arrowhead*) in the left lobe of the liver due to metastasis from gastric carcinoma.

*Calcified metastasis* is commonly from primary breast cancer, osteosarcoma, papillary thyroid carcinoma, and mucinous adenocarcinoma of the colon. Soft tissue component and peripheral edema are often present with calcification, allowing differentiation of calcified metastasis from benign hepatic calcification. *Metastases with fluid–fluid levels* are suggestive of primary neuroendocrine tumor. They are often multiple and disseminate throughout the liver. On MRI, they are strongly T2 hyperintense.[20]

### Hepatic Involvement in Lymphoproliferative Disorders

At initial imaging staging of lymphoma, leukemia, and multiple myeloma, hepatic involvement is seen in about 2% to 12% of cases with the highest prevalence in Hodgkin lymphoma. The most common pattern of hepatic involvement, regardless of disease, is multiple masses that are hypoechoic on ultrasound and hypoattenuating on CT. Later in the course of diseases, according to autopsy studies, hepatic involvement is very common with prevalence between 55% and 80% of cases.[21]

## NEOPLASM-LIKE CONDITIONS

### Simple Hepatic Cyst

Simple hepatic cysts are fluid-containing lesions with smooth, sharply defined, thin walls and lack of complex internal features. They are seen in up to 2.5% of general population, mostly between 5th to 7th decades of life. Cysts are often multiple without malignant potential. Simple cysts appear well circumscribed and completely anechoic and have posterior acoustic enhancement on ultrasound. At CT, they have water attenuation (−10 to 10 Hounsfield units). Homogeneous T1 hypointensity and T2 hyperintensity with increased signal intensity on heavily T2W images and lack of enhancement are characteristic of a simple cyst. Minimal thin septa, up to 2, may be seen.[16,22]

## Biliary Hamartoma

Biliary hamartoma or von Meyenburg complexes are multiple subcentimeter cysts due to failure of involution of small intrahepatic interlobular bile ducts that results in innumerable dilated bile ducts, which do not communicate with biliary system (vs. Caroli disease). On imaging, they present as multiple tiny subcentimeter lesions of uniform size. Characterization is better with MRI than CT or US, where lesions are strongly hyperintense on T2WI and heavily T2WI and usually demonstrate no enhancement (Fig. 8B.21).[15,23]

## Polycystic Liver Disease

Polycystic liver disease is a group of genetic disorders characterized by presence of multiple cysts in the liver only (autosomal dominant polycystic liver disease; ADPLD) or in combination with cysts in the kidneys (autosomal dominant polycystic kidney disease; ADPKD). Both have similar natural history with continuous growth expected at the annual rate of 0.9% to 3.2%. Advanced age, female gender, estrogen exposure, renal dysfunction, and higher cyst volume are associated with growth of these cysts. The distinction between ADPLD and ADPKD is made by number of renal cysts, age at presentation, and family history (Fig. 8B.22).[24]

## Caroli Disease

Caroli disease and syndrome are autosomal recessive disease spectrum linked by a common developmental pathogenesis of derangement in embryonic remodeling of intrahepatic bile ducts. It results in varying degrees of segmental, nonobstructive biliary ductal dilatation that are in direct communication with the rest of biliary system. Accumulation and stasis of bile in the dilated ducts increase the risk of stone formation, infection, and malignancy. If only IHDs are affected, the condition is termed Caroli disease. Caroli syndrome is another extreme of the spectrum with involvement of large IHDs and small intralobular bile ducts. The latter may result in congenital hepatic fibrosis and portal hypertension.[25]

On imaging, Caroli disease typically appears as multiple cystic liver lesions in a segmental distribution. Central to these cysts, there often is a small soft tissue structure that if seen on a transverse section appears dot-like. This central

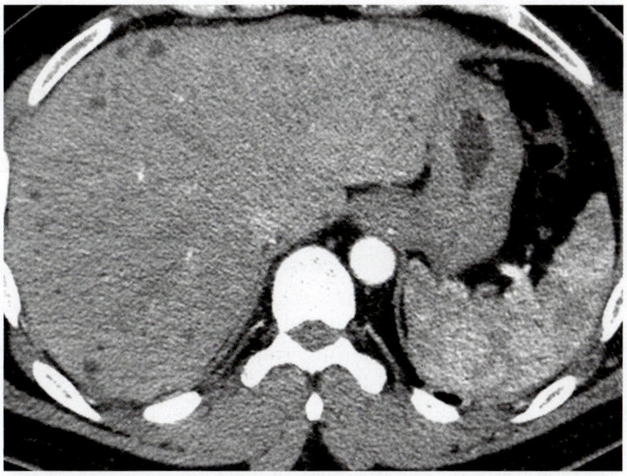

A

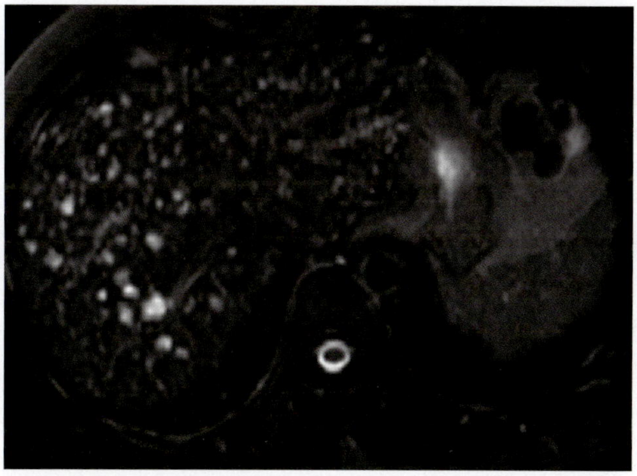

B

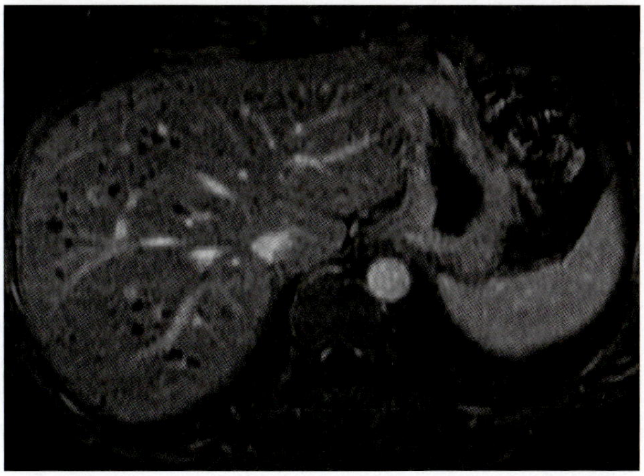

C

**FIG. 8B.21 • Biliary hamartoma. A:** Axial contrast-enhanced CT demonstrates multiple subcentimeter hypodense cysts scattered in both lobes of the liver. **B, C:** FSE T2WI and postgadolinium T1WI demonstrate multiple subcentimeter cysts scattered in the liver.

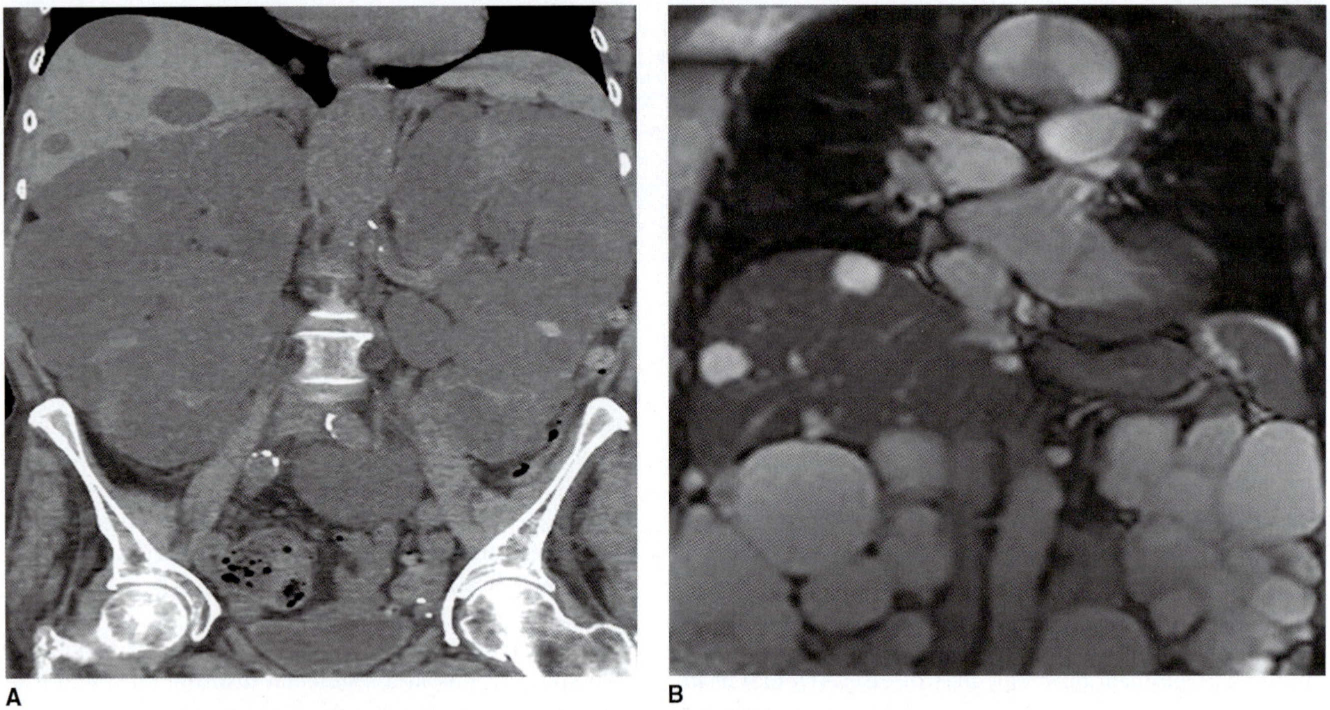


**FIG. 8B.22 • Autosomal dominant polycystic disease with liver involvement. A, B:** Coronal CT reformation and T2WI demonstrate multiple cysts in the liver, in a patient with autosomal dominant polycystic kidney disease. The coronal MR image also demonstrates aortic dissection flap in the aortic arch.

dot sign is present in most cases and represents a string of fibrovascular bundles consisting of portal vein radicle and hepatic artery branch surrounded by dilated IHDs. The central dot enhances vividly when intravenous contrast medium is used.[15,26] On coronal sections, demonstration of connection of these dilated ducts with the rest of biliary tree is diagnostic of Caroli disease. Most dilated IHDs in these disorders are saccular, in contrast to those seen in recurrent pyogenic cholangitis and primary sclerosing cholangitis (Fig. 8B.23). Because extrahepatic bile duct dilatation is present in 21% to 53% of cases, obstructive lesion may need to be excluded.[25]

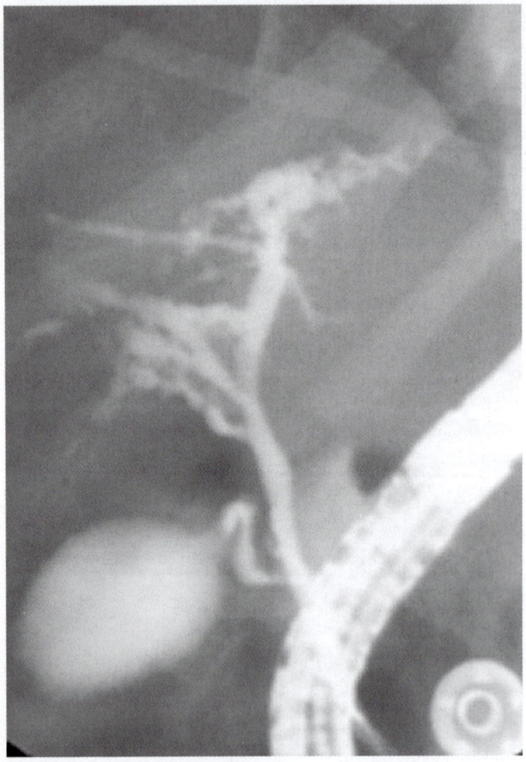

**FIG. 8B.23 • Caroli disease.** ERCP study demonstrates multifocal cystic dilatation of intrahepatic biliary ducts.

## Hemangioma

Hemangioma is a benign, neoplasm-like condition characterized by a group of numerous, dilated vascular channels that are lined by epithelial cells and separated by fibrous septae in an atypical or irregular arrangement. Most hemangiomas are diagnosed in adults between the ages of 30 and 50 years with 2:1 to 5:1 female predominance.

Typical hemangiomas are homogeneously hyperechoic on ultrasound and hypoattenuating on noncontrast CT and show peripheral interrupted nodular enhancement with progressive centripetal filling on delayed images (Fig. 8B.24). If larger than 5 cm, it is called giant hemangioma (Fig. 8B.25). On MRI, they are strongly hyperintense on T2W and heavily T2W images (Figs. 8B.26 and 8B.27). Because of the lack of hepatocytes, hemangiomas appear hypointense on hepatobiliary phase MRI. However, other typical imaging features are often helpful for diagnosis. Hemangiomas larger than 3 cm usually demonstrate incomplete filling of contrast on delayed phase because of central scarring. On the other hand, small hemangiomas are often filled with contrast rapidly on arterial phase imaging and are associated with arterioportal shunting in the adjacent hepatic parenchyma.[5] Approximately half of the hemangiomas do not show typical imaging features and cannot be reliably distinguished from malignant neoplasm of the liver (Fig. 8B.28).

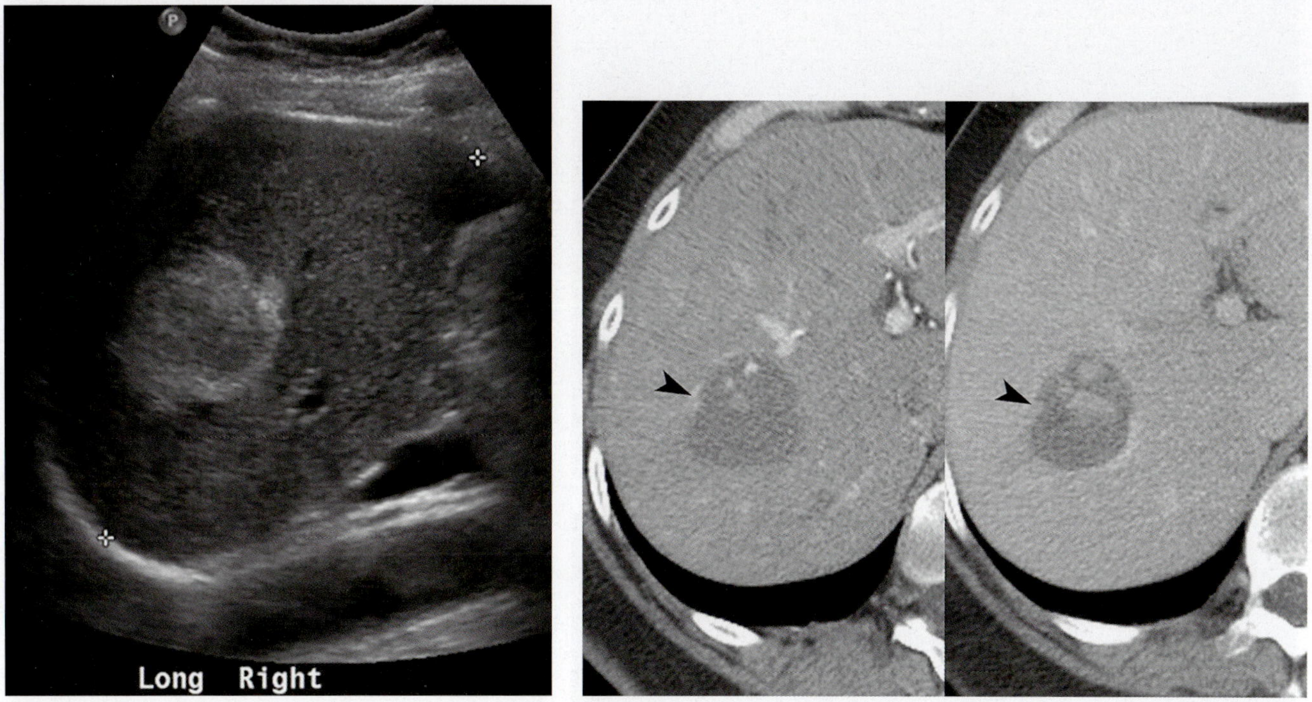


A B

**FIG. 8B.24 • Hemangioma. A:** US study demonstrates a 5-cm diameter hyperechoic mass in the right lobe of the liver. **B:** Axial contrast-enhanced CT in arterial and portal venous phase demonstrate right hepatic mass (*arrowheads*) with arterial phase peripheral nodular enhancement, which progressively blooms on portal venous phase.

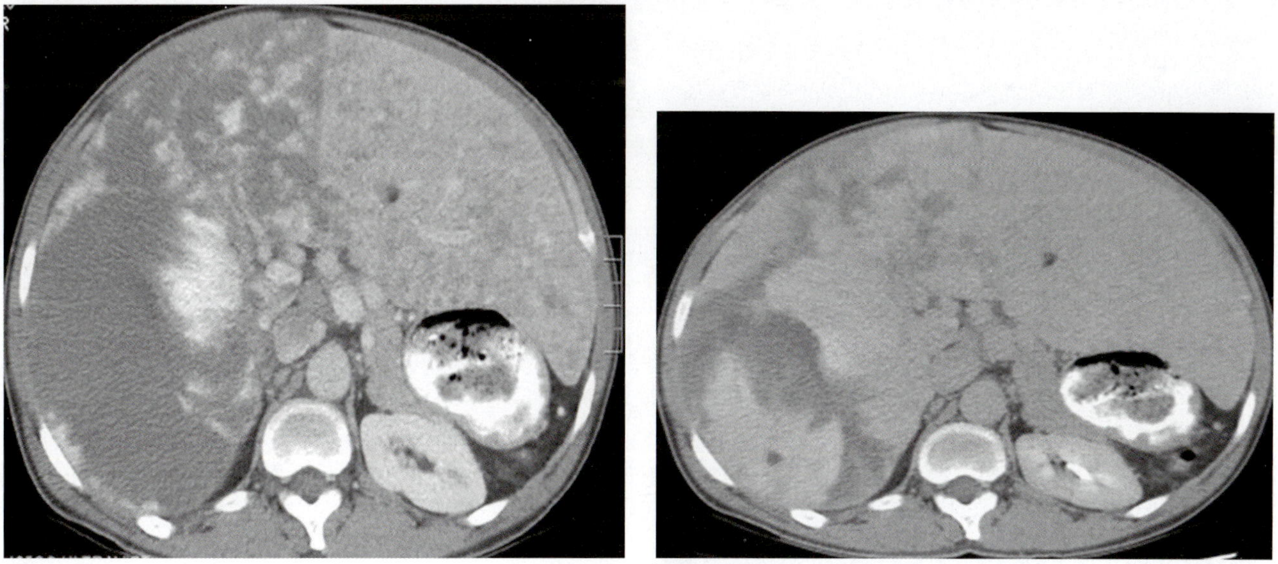

A B

**FIG. 8B.25 • Giant hemangioma. A, B:** Arterial phase and delayed phase contrast-enhanced axial CT demonstrate peripheral, discontinuous nodular enhancement of the giant hemangioma, which shows progressive filling on delayed phase CT. There are persistent areas of nonenhancement in the center of the hemangioma, indicating central necrosis.

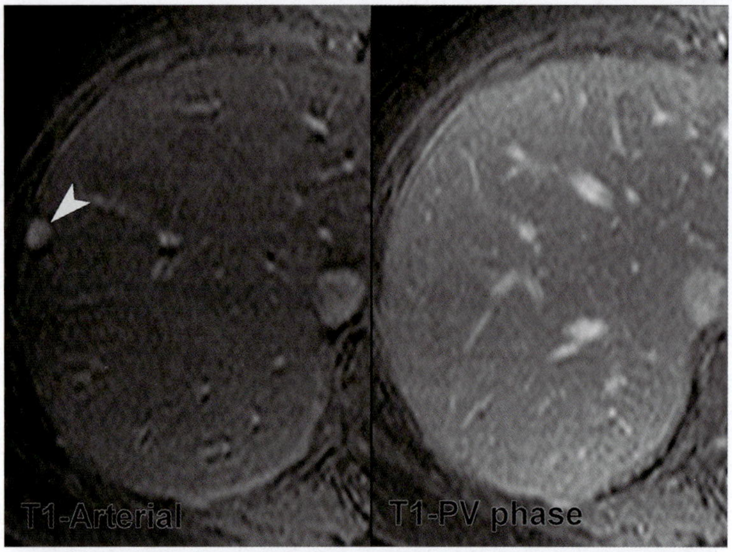


**FIG. 8B.26 • Hemangioma.** Axial contrast-enhanced T1WI in arterial and portal venous phase demonstrate arterially enhancing hemangioma (*arrowhead*), which is isointense to the liver on portal venous phase. The hemangioma was intensely hyperintense on T2-weighted sequence, thereby allowing separation from other liver pathologies, such as FNH and HCC.

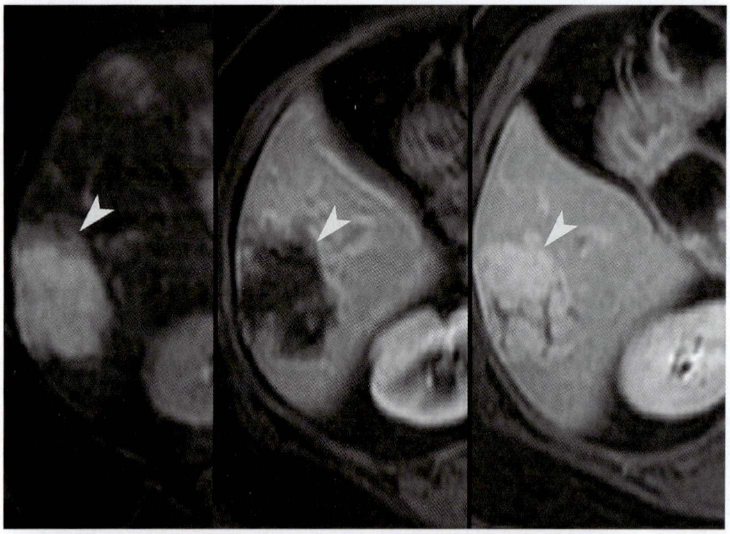

**FIG. 8B.27 • Hemangioma.** FSE T2WI and post-gadolinium T1WI (arterial and portal venous phase) demonstrate intensely T2 hyperintense hemangioma (*arrowhead*) in the right lobe, which demonstrates peripheral nodular enhancement on the arterial phase imaging. On venous phase imaging, there is progressive fill-in of the hemangioma with contrast.

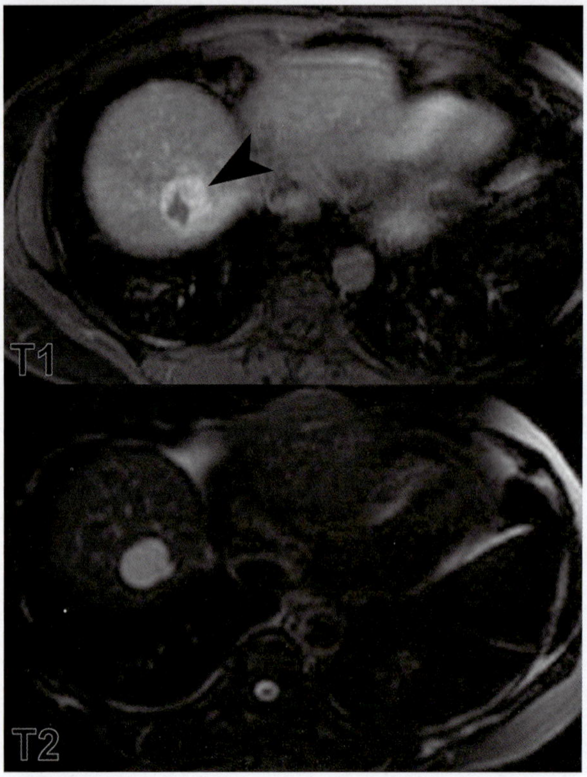


**FIG. 8B.28 • Hepatic metastasis misinterpreted as hemangioma.** Axial contrast-enhanced MR demonstrate right hepatic mass with peripheral enhancement of irregular thickness (*arrowhead*). This enhancement pattern is inconsistent with the appearance of a classical hemangioma. FSE T2WI demonstrates intense hyperintensity in the mass lesion in which the lesion was misinterpreted as a hemangioma.

## References


1. Denecke T, Steffen IG, Agarwal S, et al. Appearance of hepatocellular adenomas on gadoxetic acid-enhanced MRI. *Eur Radiol.* 2012;22: 1769–1775.
2. Raman SP, Hruban RH, Fishman EK. Hepatic adenomatosis: spectrum of imaging findings. *Abdom Imaging.* 2013;38:474–481.
3. van Aalten SM, de Man RA, IJzermans JN, et al. Systematic review of haemorrhage and rupture of hepatocellular adenomas. *Br J Surg.* 2012;99:911–916.
4. Nahm CB, Ng K, Lockie P, et al. Focal nodular hyperplasia—a review of myths and truths. *J Gastrointest Surg.* 2011;15:2275–2283.
5. Cogley JR, Miller FH. MR imaging of benign focal liver lesions. *Radiol Clin North Am.* 2014;52;657–682.
6. Willatt JM, Hussain HK, Adusumilli S, et al. MR imaging of hepatocellular carcinoma in the cirrhotic liver: challenges and controversies. *Radiology.* 2008;247:311–330.
7. Bruix J, Sherman M. Management of hepatocellular carcinoma: an update. *Hepatology.* 2011;53:1020–1022.
8. Choi BG, Park SH, Byun JY, et al. The findings of ruptured hepatocellular carcinoma on helical CT. *Br J Radiol.* 2001;74:142–146.
9. Aoki T, Kokudo N, Matsuyama Y; Liver Cancer Study Group of Japan. Prognostic impact of spontaneous tumor rupture in patients with hepatocellular carcinoma: an analysis of 1160 cases from a nationwide survey. *Ann Surg.* 2014;259:532–542.
10. Mitchell DG, Bruix J, Sherman M, Sirlin CB. LI-RADS (Liver Imaging Reporting and Data System): summary, discussion, and consensus of LI-RADS Management Working Group and future directions. *Hepatology.* 2015;61(3):1056–1065.
11. Ganeshan D, Szklaruk J, Kundra V, et al. Imaging features of fibrolamellar hepatocellular carcinoma. *AJR Am J Roentgenol.* 2014;202:544–552.
12. Nakeeb A, Pitt HA, Sohn TA, et al. Cholangiocarcinoma. A spectrum of intrahepatic, perihilar, and distal tumors. *Ann Surg.* 1996;224:463–473.
13. Lee JW, Han JK, Kim TK, et al. CT features of intraductal intrahepatic cholangiocarcinoma. *AJR Am J Roentgenol.* 2000;175:721–725.
14. Soares KC, Arnaoutakis DJ, Kamel I, et al. Cystic neoplasms of the liver: biliary cystadenoma and cystadenocarcinoma. *J Am Coll Surg.* 2014;218:119–128.
15. Del Poggio P, Buonocore M. Cystic tumors of the liver: a practical approach. *World J Gastroenterol.* 2008;14:3616–3620.
16. Kim JY, Kim SH, Eun HW, et al. Differentiation between biliary cystic neoplasms and simple cysts of the liver: accuracy of CT. *AJR Am J Roentgenol* 2010;195:1142–1148.
17. Robinson PJ. Imaging liver metastasis: current limitations and future prospects. *Br J Radiol.* 2000;73:234–241.
18. Danet IM, Semelka RC, Leonardou P, et al. Spectrum of MRI appearances of untreated metastases of the liver. *AJR Am J Roentgenol.* 2003;181:809–817.
19. Kanematsu M, Kondo H, Goshima S, et al. Imaging liver metastases: review and update. *Eur J Radiol.* 2006;58:217–228.
20. Sommer WH, Zech CJ, Bamberg F, et al. Fluid-fluid level in hepatic metastases: a characteristic sign of metastases of neuroendocrine origin. *Eur J Radiol.* 2012;81:2127–2132.
21. Bach AG, Behrmann C, Holzhausen HJ, et al. Prevalence and imaging of hepatic involvement in malignant lymphoproliferative disease. *Clin Imaging.* 2012;36:539–546.
22. Vachha B, Sun MR, Siewert B, et al. Cystic lesions of the liver. *AJR Am J Roentgenol.* 2011;196:W355–W366.
23. Yam BL, Siegelman ES. MR imaging of the biliary system. *Radiol Clin North Am.* 2014;52:725–755.
24. Abu-Wasel B, Walsh C, Keough V, et al. Pathophysiology, epidemiology, classification and treatment options for polycystic liver diseases. *World J Gastroenterol.* 2013;19:5775–5786.
25. Levy AD, Rohrmann CA Jr, Murakata LA, et al. Caroli's disease: radiologic spectrum with pathologic correlation. *AJR Am J Roentgenol.* 2002;179:1053–1057.
26. Lefere M, Thijs M, De Hertogh G, et al. Caroli disease: review of eight cases with emphasis on magnetic resonance imaging features. *Eur J Gastroenterol Hepatol.* 2011;23:578–585.

## SELF-ASSESSMENT QUESTIONS

1. A 35-year-old woman with cirrhosis has a contrast-enhanced MR. Which of the following is the most likely diagnosis?

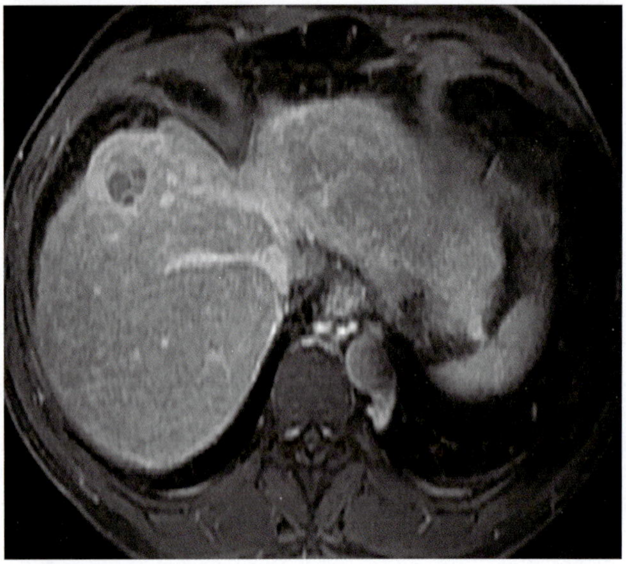

A. Focal fat
B. Hemangioma
C. Hepatocellular adenoma
D. Hepatocellular carcinoma

2. The MR of a 55-year-old man without any prior medical illness shows a focal mass. What is the most likely diagnosis?

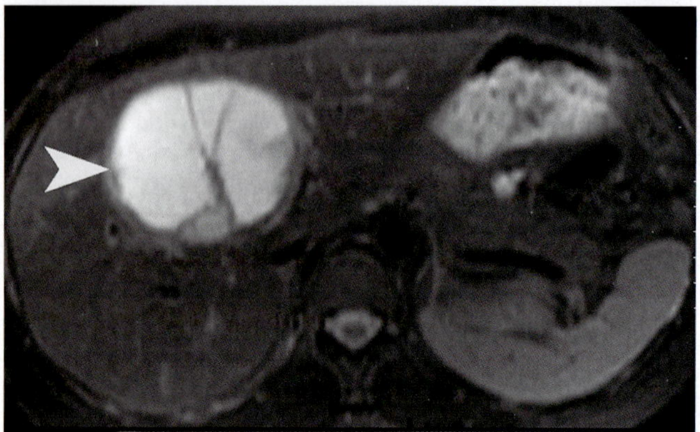

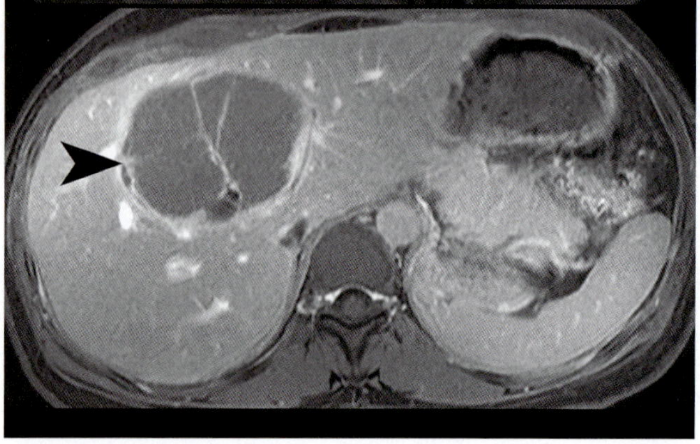

A. Carcinoid metastases
B. HCC
C. Biliary cystadenoma
D. Cholangiocarcinoma

### Answers to Self-Assessment Questions

**1. D.** The contrast-enhanced MR in portal venous phase depicts continuous enhancement of the peripheral pseudocapsule and relative hypointensity of the hepatocellular carcinoma.

**2. C.** The T2WI and contrast-enhanced T1WI show a complex cystic lesion with multiple enhancing septations, which would be atypical for A, B, and D.

# Gall Bladder and Bile Ducts 9

*Rathachai Kaewlai, Sirote Wongwaisayawan, and Ajay K. Singh*

## LEARNING OBJECTIVE

**1.** Describe the imaging features of gall bladder and biliary pathologies.

Networks of bile canaliculi form segmental and lobar intrahepatic ducts (IHDs) that drain the right and left lobes of the liver. The right and left IHDs join at the hepatic hilum to become a common hepatic duct (CHD), beginning the extrahepatic portion of bile duct. Below the confluence of right and left IHDs, the cystic duct (CD) of the gall bladder joins the CHD to become a common bile duct (CBD). The diameter of the IHD is generally 2 mm or less than one-and-a-half of the accompanying portal vein branch. The CHD and CBD are less than 7 mm in adults, and at the age of 70 and above, the cutoff for the normal CBD becomes 8 mm. After cholecystectomy, the normal CBD can be up to 10 mm.[1]

The gall bladder lies beneath the hepatic interlobar fissure and can measure up to 5 × 10 cm. The wall is less than 3 mm thick. It consists of the neck, body, and fundus. The neck is the narrowest part that is usually the site of obstruction secondary to stone disease. Occasionally, there is a fold at the junction between the body and fundus, which is called phrygian cap.[1] Normally, the CD joins the CHD just below the IHD confluence and into the right side of the CHD. Low or medial insertion of the CD into the CHD (insertions into distal third or the left of the CHD, respectively) occurs in 9% to 17% of population.[2]

## GALL BLADDER PATHOLOGIES

### Cholelithiasis and Biliary Sludge

Cholelithiasis or gallstones are precipitates of cholesterol, pigments, and calcium salts within the gall bladder. Risk factors include female gender, obesity, increased age, and diabetes (Table 9.1).

The gold standard noninvasive method for gallstone diagnosis is US, which has an accuracy of greater than 95%.[3] Echogenic focus with clean posterior acoustic shadow and gravitational dependence are the three main US features of gallstones. When stones occupy the entire gall bladder, a wall–echo–shadow (WES) sign (Fig. 9.1) can be appreciated. The WES sign consists of a rind of anechoic bile in between the more superficial hyperechoic anterior gall bladder wall and the deeper hyperechoic anterior surface of the gallstone.

On CT, stones may be hypo-, iso-, or hyperattenuating depending on the amount of calcium, cholesterol, and gas. While CT generally shows gallstones in only 75% of cases, MRI performs better because of marked contrast between gallstones and surrounding bile on T2WI.[4] Gallstones appear as signal void because of restricted water motion and cholesterol molecules in the lattice.

Biliary sludge represents thickened, viscous bile commonly seen in patients with critical illness, rapid weight loss, pregnancy, or total parenteral nutrition. It often appears, disappears, and reappears within months or years and may be related to gallstone formation. Sludge moves slower with gravity change than normal bile and does not show posterior acoustic shadowing on US.

### Acute Cholecystitis and Complications

Acute inflammation of the gall bladder occurs in the setting of obstructing gallstones in 90% to 95% of cases.[1,5] US is the initial imaging modality of choice. The imaging findings of acute cholecystitis include (Fig. 9.2):

1. Obstructive gallstone in the gall bladder neck or CD
2. Gall bladder wall thickening (greater than 3 mm) and striation
3. Sonographic Murphy sign
4. Gall bladder distension (greater than 4 cm transverse diameter)
5. Pericholecystic fluid

CT and MRI can show pericholecystic inflammatory changes better than ultrasound, including fat stranding and enhancement of liver parenchyma adjacent to the gall bladder (Figs. 9.3 and 9.4).

Table 9.1 **DIFFERENTIAL DIAGNOSIS OF GALL BLADDER DISEASE BY IMAGING PATTERN**

| Imaging Pattern | Differential Diagnoses |
|---|---|
| Gall bladder wall thickening: diffuse | Pseudothickening secondary to postprandial physiology<br>Primary gall bladder disease:<br>Cholecystitis<br>Infiltrative neoplasm<br>Diffuse adenomyomatosis<br>Secondary:<br>Cirrhosis<br>Hypoalbuminemia<br>Heart failure |
| Gall bladder wall thickening: focal | Benign:<br>Polyp<br>Focal adenomyomatosis<br>Xanthogranulomatous cholecystitis<br>Malignant:<br>Gall bladder carcinoma<br>Neoplasm (primary or metastasis) |
| Gall bladder wall hyperechogenicity | Porcelain gall bladder<br>Emphysematous cholecystitis<br>Wall–echo–shadow (WES) complex<br>Adenomyomatosis/ cholesterolosis |

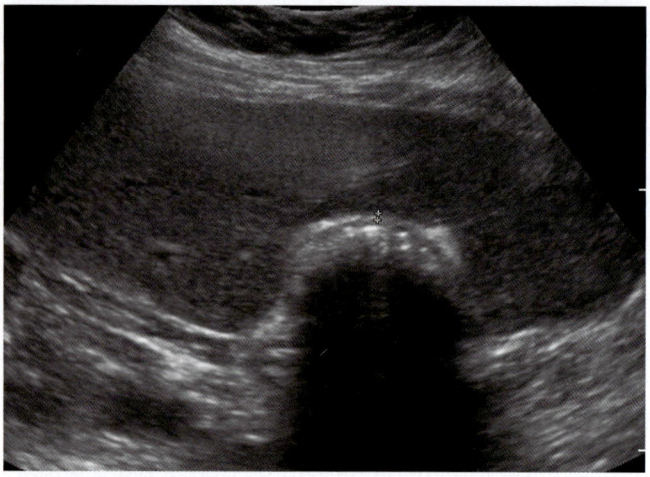

**FIG. 9.1 • Wall–echo–shadow sign of cholelithiasis.** US study demonstrates hyperechoic gall bladder wall and anterior margin of the gallstones, separated by a hypoechoic rim of bile.

### *Complications*

Complications include gangrene, hemorrhage, emphysematous change, empyema, and perforation. Increased gall bladder distention leads to mural ischemia, hemorrhage, and necrosis found in *gangrenous cholecystitis*. On ultrasound, the gall bladder wall is striated (alternating hypo- and hyperechogenicity) and has irregular inner surface with floating intraluminal membranes and irregular projections into the lumen (Fig. 9.5A, B). Sonographic Murphy sign is present in only 33% of cases.[4] Asymmetric wall thickness, focal wall defect, edema, and lack of wall enhancement are more specific but less sensitive signs seen on CT and MRI (Fig. 9.5C).[5,6] Rim sign on cholescintigraphy refers to a rim of increased radiotracer activity in the liver, adjacent to the gall bladder fossa. This sign has been shown to have a high positive predictive value for diagnosis of acute cholecystitis and is often associated with gangrenous cholecystitis (Fig. 9.5D).

*Emphysematous cholecystitis* is diagnosed when gas is present in the gall bladder lumen, wall, or pericholecystic tissues in the absence of fistula between the gall bladder and gastrointestinal tract. Ischemic change of the gall bladder wall with superimposed clostridia or *Escherichia coli* infection is the likely cause. Up to one-third of patients have no underlying gallstones. US shows ring-down or reverberation artifacts with dirty posterior shadow from gas in the lumen, wall, or pericholecystic

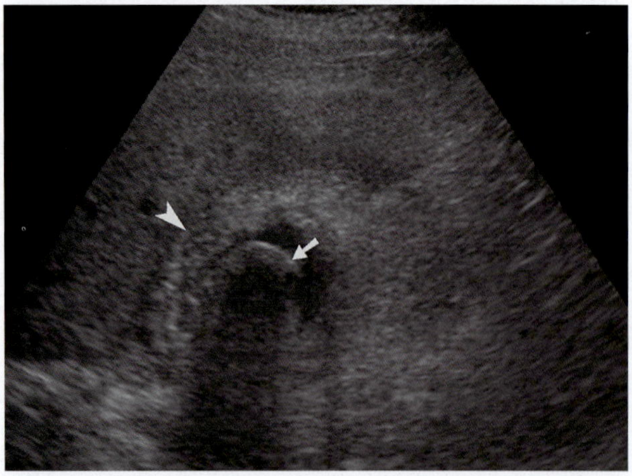

A

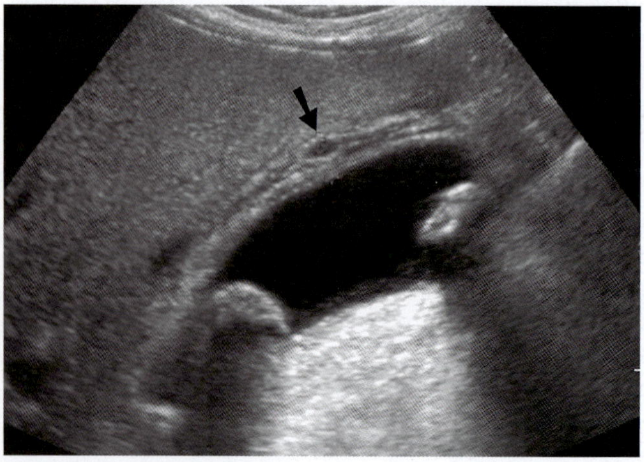

B

**FIG. 9.2 • Acute cholecystitis on US. A:** US demonstrates gall bladder wall thickening (*arrowhead*) in a patient with acute cholecystitis. A solitary large gallstone (*arrow*) is visualized in the gall bladder lumen. **B:** US demonstrates gall bladder wall thickening with stratification (*arrow*). Two gallstones are identified in the gall bladder lumen.

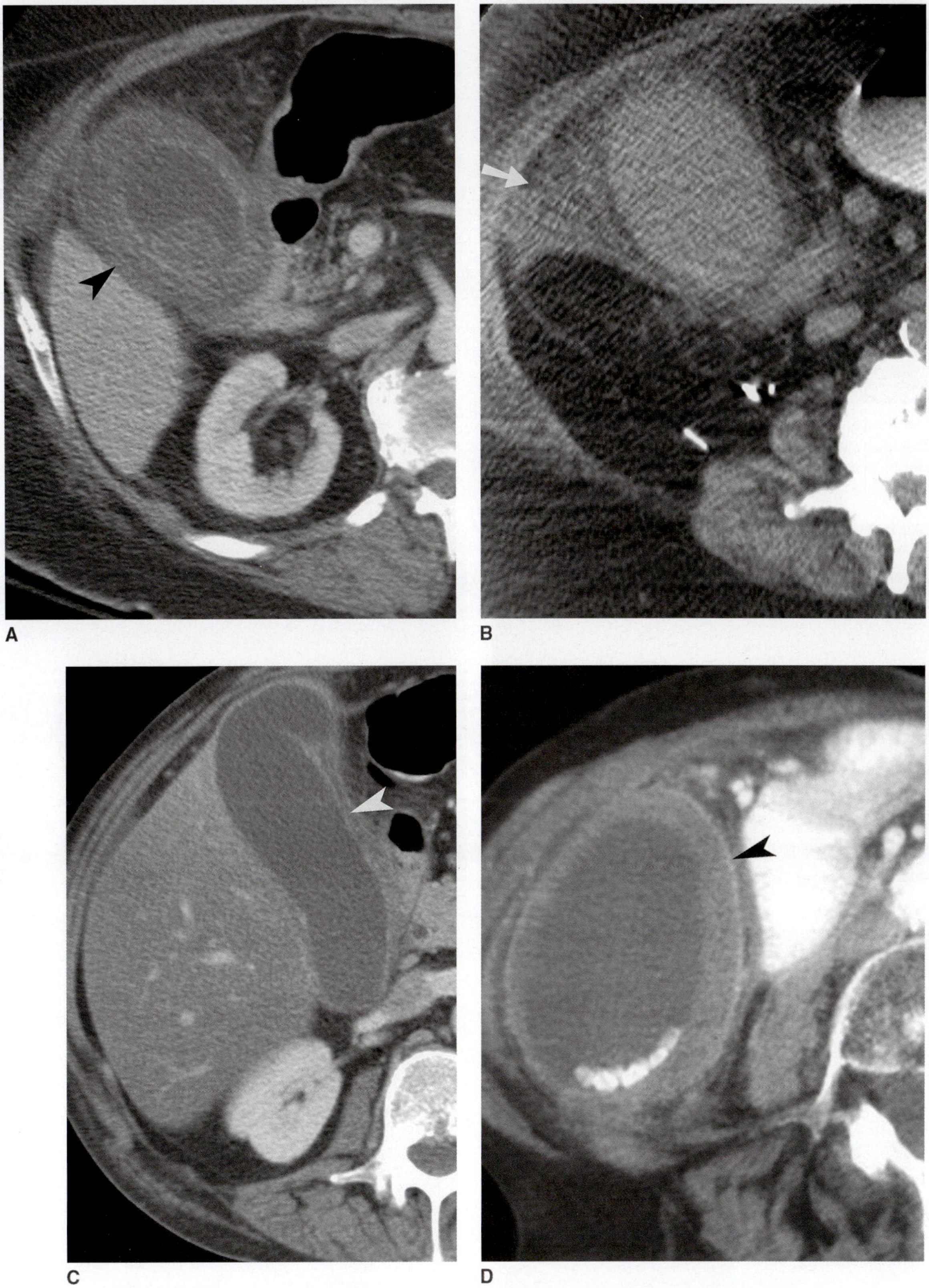

**FIG. 9.3 • Acute cholecystitis on CT. A–D:** Contrast-enhanced CT in three different patients demonstrating gall bladder wall thickening (*arrowheads*) from acute cholecystitis. There is serosal enhancement **(D)**, and pericholecystic inflammation (*arrow*) **(A–C)** and transient hepatic attenuation difference **(C)** are also identified.

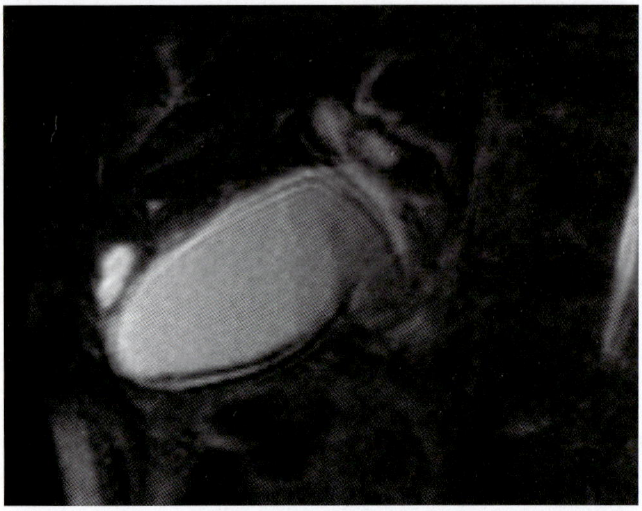

**FIG. 9.4 • Acute cholecystitis on MR.** MRCP study demonstrates intensely hyperintense wall of the gall bladder in a patient with obstructing gall bladder neck calculus. This patient also has dilatation of the biliary ducts due to the gall bladder neck stone.

tissues (Fig. 9.6A). The findings can be mistaken for calculi or porcelain gall bladder. CT has higher sensitivity and should be performed if the diagnosis is entertained (Fig. 9.6B, C).[4]

In patients presenting with biliary colic and hematemesis, one should suspect *hemorrhagic cholecystitis.* Mucosal ulceration, hemorrhage, and necrosis result in echogenic and hyperattenuating bile, with a fluid–fluid level (Fig. 9.7A).

*Gall bladder empyema or pus-filled gall bladder* can be difficult to diagnose on imaging because appearance of pus is indistinguishable from sludge (echogenic, hyperattenuating, T2 hypointense). Marked distention of the gall bladder with other imaging signs of acute cholecystitis and rapid progression of symptoms should lead to the diagnosis, which can be confirmed at percutaneous needle aspiration or cholecystostomy (Fig. 9.7B). Perhaps, the most dreadful complication of acute cholecystitis is *gall bladder perforation,* which can occur in the setting of gangrenous, hemorrhagic, emphysematous, acalculous cholecystitis, or empyema. Perforation releases infected bile salts and other materials into pericholecystic

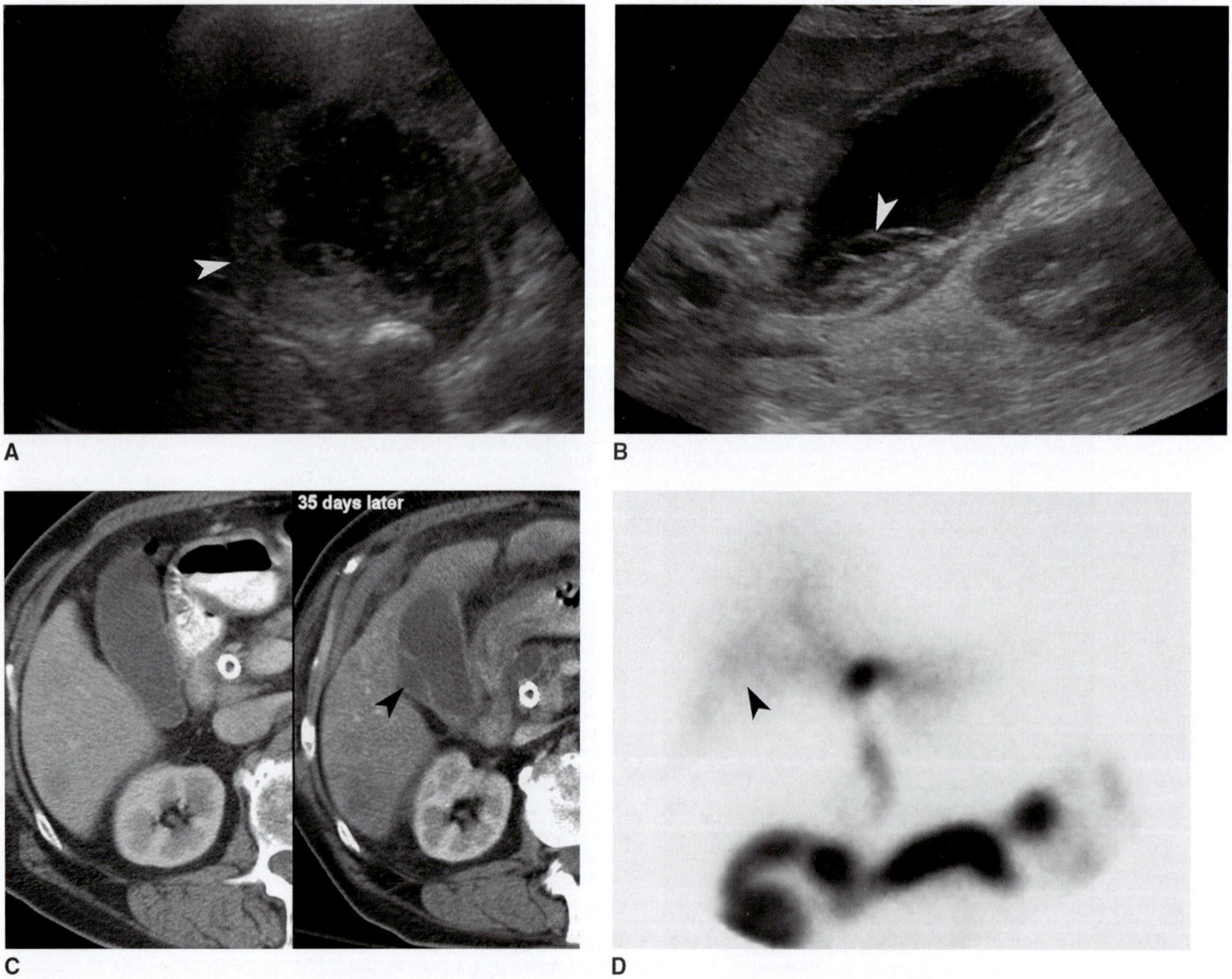


**FIG. 9.5 • Gangrenous cholecystitis. A:** US demonstrates gall bladder wall thickening and luminal irregularity caused by sloughing of the gall bladder wall (*arrowhead*). **B:** A patient with gangrenous cholecystitis demonstrates gall bladder wall thickening and dependent intraluminal membranes caused by sloughed off wall (*arrowhead*). **C:** Contrast-enhanced CT of a patient with gangrenous cholecystitis demonstrates fluid dissecting into the wall of the gall bladder (*arrowhead*). **D:** Cholescintigraphy study demonstrates curvilinear focus of increased radiotracer activity (*arrowhead*) in the pericholecystic liver. There is nonvisualization of the gall bladder caused by CD obstruction.

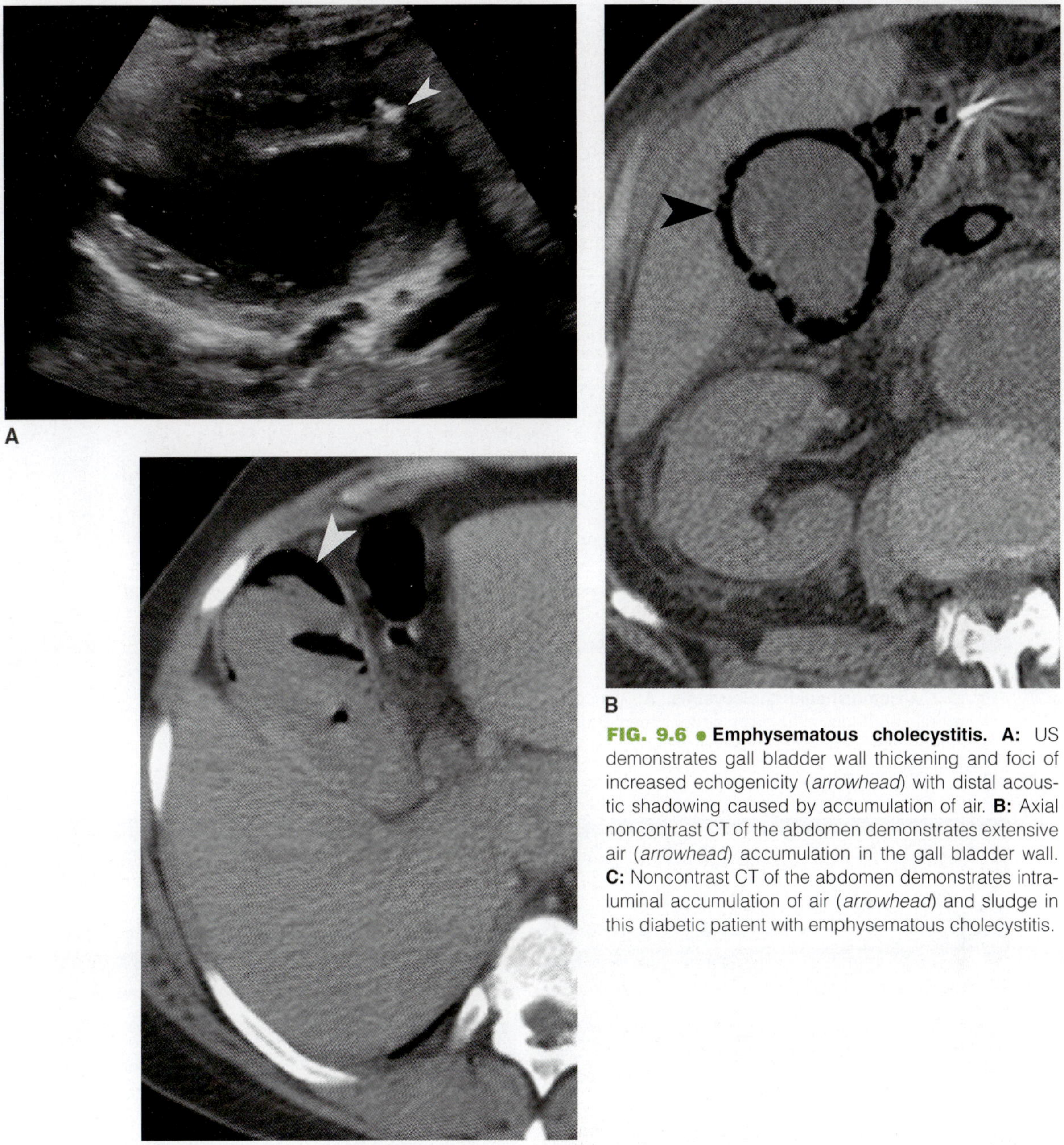

**FIG. 9.6 • Emphysematous cholecystitis. A:** US demonstrates gall bladder wall thickening and foci of increased echogenicity (*arrowhead*) with distal acoustic shadowing caused by accumulation of air. **B:** Axial noncontrast CT of the abdomen demonstrates extensive air (*arrowhead*) accumulation in the gall bladder wall. **C:** Noncontrast CT of the abdomen demonstrates intraluminal accumulation of air (*arrowhead*) and sludge in this diabetic patient with emphysematous cholecystitis.

tissues. Chronic, localized perforation can also manifest as cholecystoenteric fistula. Most perforations occur at the gall bladder fundus, and the majority results in pericholecystic abscess (Fig. 9.8). On imaging, a loss of normal ovoid shape of the gall bladder along with pericholecystic fluid or fluid collection should suggest this complication. Focal defects, seen in 70% of cases, are better shown on CT than ultrasound. Extraluminal location of gallstone is a specific but insensitive sign.[4,5]

In the absence of gallstones, gradual increase in bile viscosity can lead to functional obstruction of the CD and later inflammatory and ischemic change of the gall bladder, resulting in *acalculous cholecystitis*.[7] This condition should be considered in hospitalized patients with sepsis after surgery, burn, or significant trauma. Imaging features mirror those of calculous cholecystitis, but there is lack of gallstone.

## Chronic Cholecystitis

Chronic cholecystitis is characterized by low-grade inflammation and fibrosis of the gall bladder wall, which disrupts normal motility. The most common imaging findings are cholelithiasis, wall thickening, and contracted gall bladder in the absence of pericholecystic inflammation. Transient hepatic attenuation difference, referring to linear or wedge-shaped area of hyperattenuation on contrast-enhanced CT, adjacent to the gall bladder, is most often associated with chronic cholecystitis (Fig. 9.9). Acute cholecystitis, gall bladder carcinoma, cholecystoenteric fistula, and gallstone ileus (Figs. 9.10 and 9.11) may further complicate chronic cholecystitis.

*Xanthogranulomatous cholecystitis* is an uncommon form of chronic cholecystitis that is secondary to bile extravasation into the gall bladder wall and superimposed infection.[6,7]

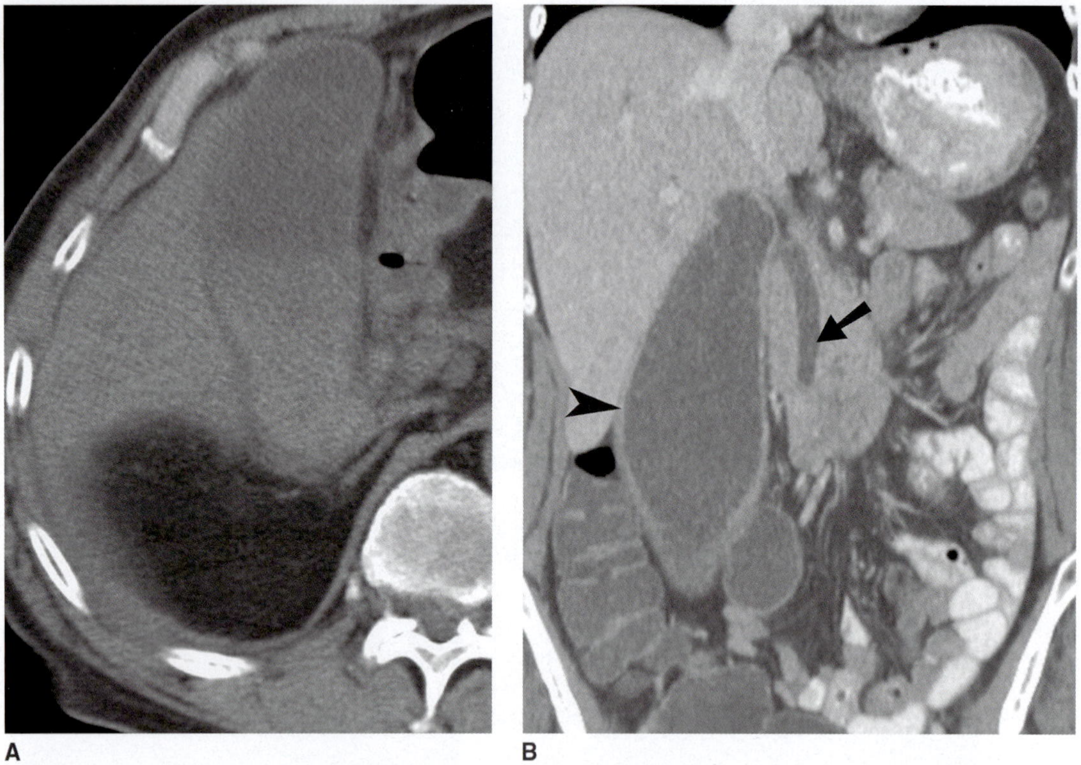

**FIG. 9.7 • Hemorrhagic cholecystitis. A:** Noncontrast CT of the abdomen demonstrates dependent hemorrhagic products in the gall bladder lumen. **B:** Gall bladder empyema seen on coronal CT reformation, indicated by grossly distended gall bladder (*arrowhead*) with wall thickening. The CBD is dilated (*arrow*) due to choledocholithiasis.

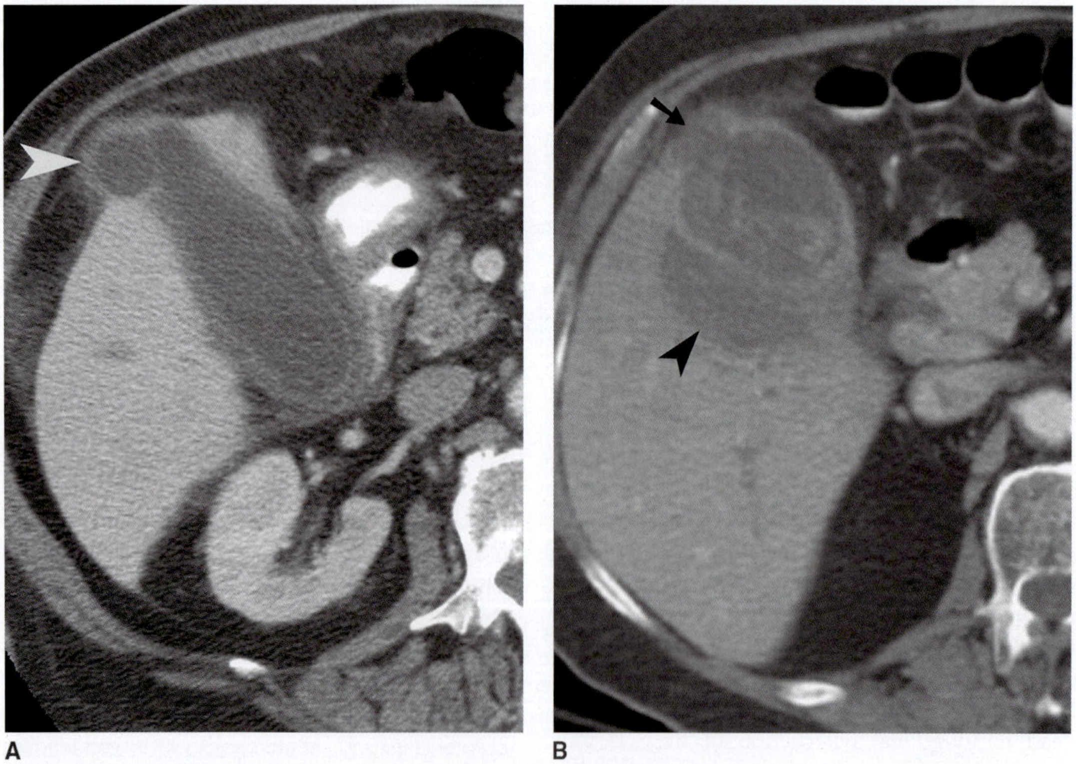

**FIG. 9.8 • Gall bladder perforation. A:** Contrast-enhanced CT demonstrates gall bladder wall inflammation, pericholecystic fluid, as well as a focal localized perforation (*arrowhead*) from the gall bladder fundus. **B:** Contrast-enhanced CT demonstrates findings of acute cholecystitis and a focal breech in the gall bladder wall seen at the fundus resulting in a small intrahepatic collection (*arrow*). There is a larger pericholecystic liver abscess (*arrowhead*) seen in the segment 5 of the liver.

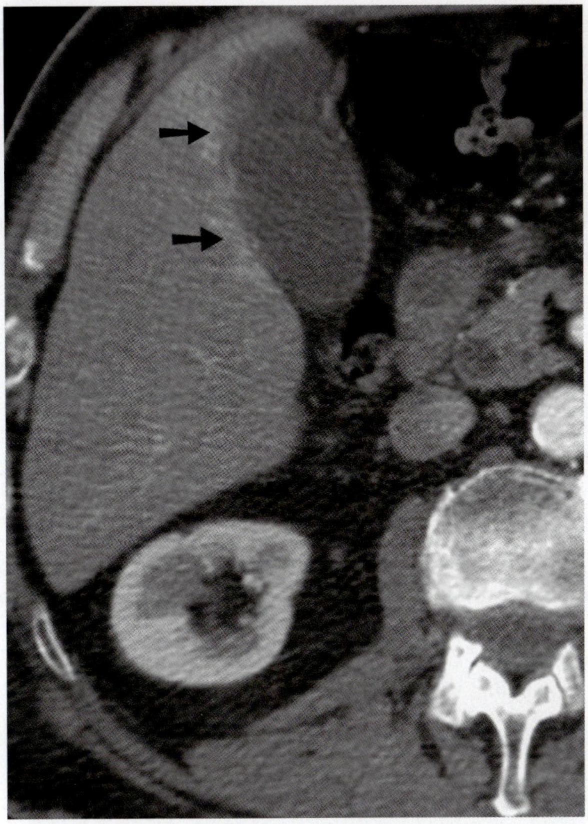

**FIG. 9.9 • Chronic cholecystitis.** Contrast-enhanced CT of the abdomen demonstrates linear band of increased attenuation (transient hepatic attenuation difference) (*arrows*) in the pericholecystic hepatic bed.

It is commonly seen in elderly individuals, and preoperative diagnosis is often difficult. Imaging findings mimic carcinoma of the gall bladder with infiltrative mass, irregular/asymmetric gall bladder wall thickening, and cholelithiasis.[5]

*Porcelain gall bladder* represents calcification in the gall bladder wall associated with cholelithiasis and chronic cholecystitis. It is found in 0.06% to 0.8% of cholecystectomy specimen.[3] Calcified gall bladder wall, which can involve the entire or part of the wall, is best visualized on CT. Ultrasound may show a hyperechoic, linear/curvilinear structure with posterior acoustic shadowing (Fig. 9.10). Although recent studies dispute the association between porcelain gall bladder and developing carcinoma, prophylactic cholecystectomy is still suggested.[5]

## Gallstone Ileus

The gallstones may pass into the bowel lumen in patients with recurrent cholecystitis, sometimes resulting in mechanical obstruction. The fistulous communication is most often to the duodenum and most often occurs in elderly females with history of gallstones. Although majority of the stones pass through bowel without causing bowel obstruction, in one-fourth of the cases, the gallstone can cause bowel obstruction (Fig. 9.12). Rarely, bowel obstruction may occur in the distal stomach or proximal duodenum (Bouveret syndrome).

The common sites of bowel obstruction from obstructing gallstone are:

1. Terminal ileum (60%)
2. Proximal ileum (30%)

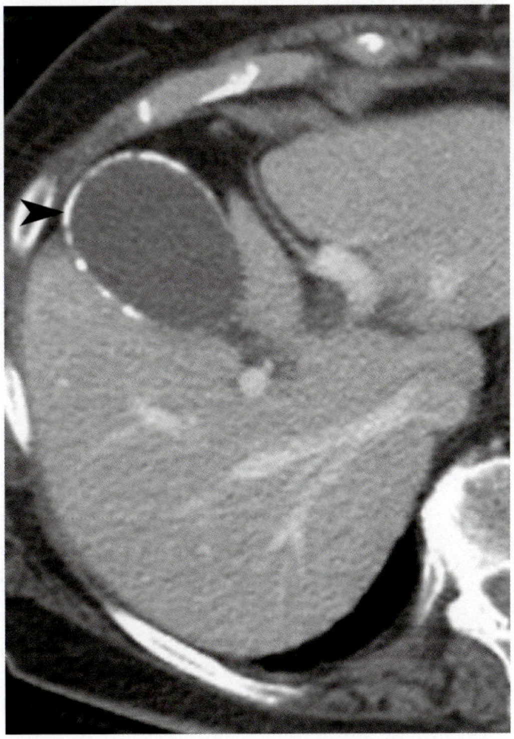

A

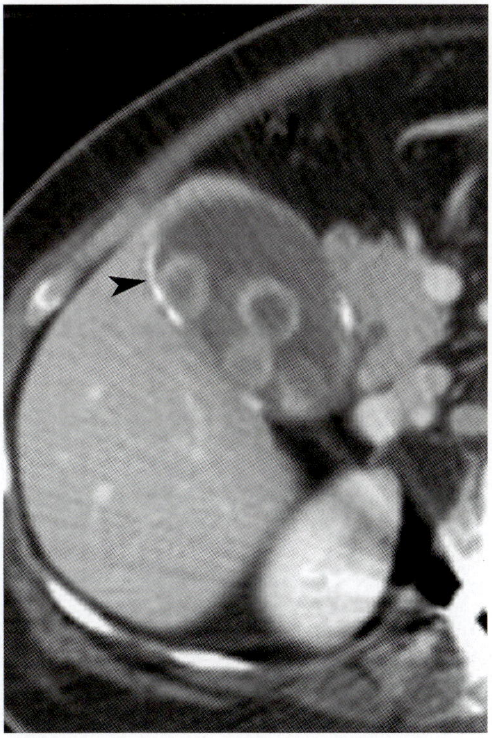

B

**FIG. 9.10 • Porcelain gall bladder. A, B:** Axial contrast-enhanced CT demonstrates calcification (*arrowheads*) in the wall of the gall bladder.

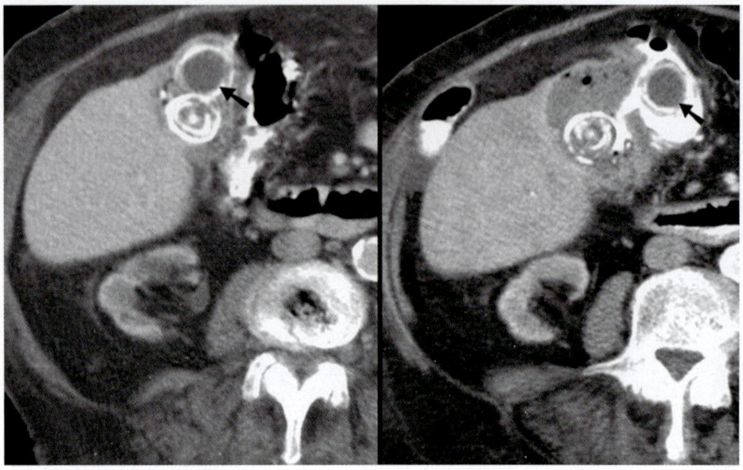

**FIG. 9.11 • Cholecystocolonic fistula.** Contrast-enhanced CT studies performed a week apart demonstrate a gallstone (*arrow*) seen in the gall bladder lumen on the first CT and in the colonic lumen on the second CT.

3. Distal jejunum (5%)
4. Colon or rectum (3%)
5. Duodenum (2%)

The radiographic findings include pneumobilia and dilated small bowel loops. The CT findings include Rigler's triad of distended small bowel loops, pneumobilia, and obstructing gallstone. The larger the gallstone, the more proximal is the bowel obstruction.

## Postcholecystectomy Bile Leak

Postoperative bile leak is most often seen after laparoscopic cholecystectomy and is due to anatomic variation of the bile ducts, which may directly communicate with the gall bladder bed (ducts of Luschka) or injury to the larger biliary or CD remnant (Fig. 9.13). US and CT can help localize the biloma, which may become secondarily infected and require drainage.

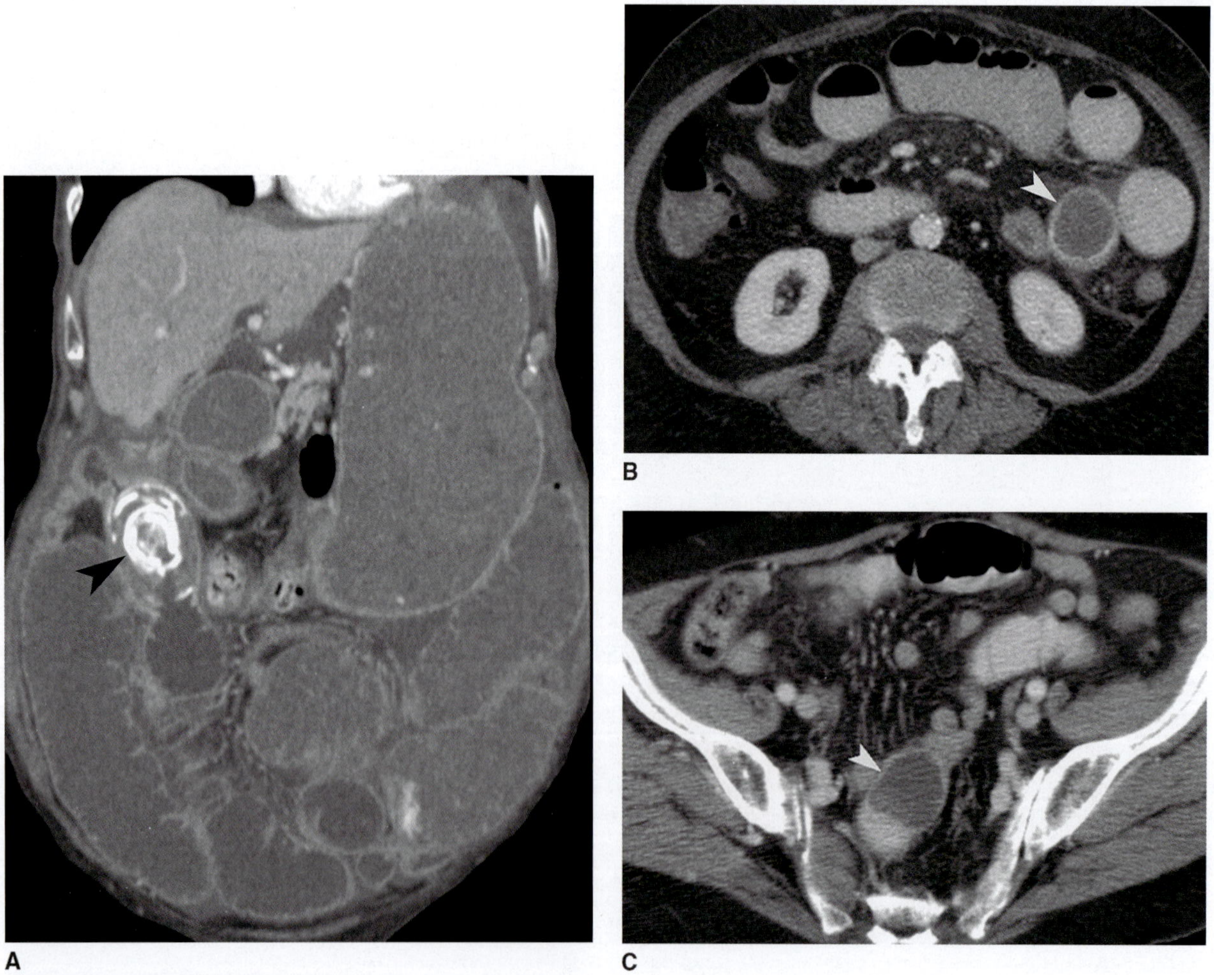

**FIG. 9.12 • Gallstone ileus. A–C:** CT in three different patients demonstrates dilated small bowel lumen, caused by a gallstone (*arrowheads*) located in the small bowel.

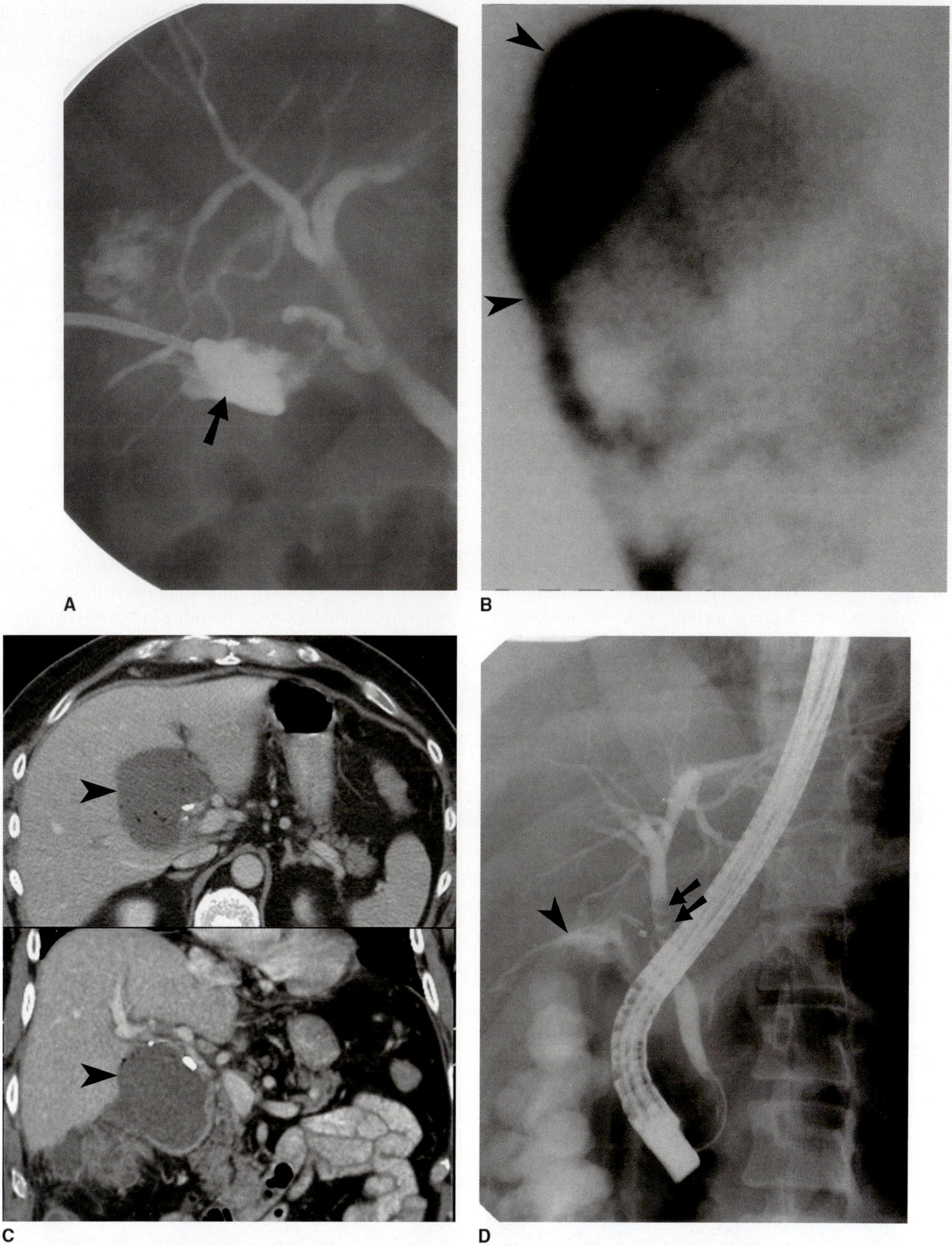

**FIG. 9.13 • Postcholecystectomy bile leak. A:** Fluoroscopy spot image after injection through a pigtail drainage catheter placed in the gall bladder fossa demonstrates communication of the biloma (*arrow*) in the gall bladder fossa with IHDs through the ducts of Luschka. **B:** Cholescintigraphy study demonstrates extensive leakage (*arrowheads*) of radiotracer into the perihepatic and right subdiaphragmatic space. **C:** Contrast-enhanced CT demonstrates fluid accumulation along with tiny foci of air in the gall bladder fossa (*arrowheads*), also extending into the Morison pouch. **D:** ERCP demonstrates filling defects in the CBD lumen (*arrows*) and frank leakage of contrast from the CD stump into the gall bladder fossa (*arrowhead*).

Cholescintigraphy study can detect leakage of bile from the biliary ducts into the gall bladder fossa and perihepatic region. Endoscopic retrograde cholangiopancreatography (ERCP) allows diagnoses as well as therapeutic intervention in patients with suspected bile leak. It can pinpoint the exact site of the bile leak more accurately than cholescintigraphy and cross-sectional imaging.

## Dropped Gallstone

Dropped gallstones and resulting abscesses are most often seen in the Morrison pouch. More than half of the cases of dropped gallstones seen on CT are associated with abscess formation (Fig. 9.14). Unlike dropped gallstones, retained surgical clips rarely cause abscess formation. Dropped gallstone is a possible cause of Morrison pouch abscess in patients with history of cholecystectomy.

## Gall bladder Adenomyomatosis

Adenomyomatosis is an acquired, hyperplastic noninflammatory condition of the gall bladder. It is characterized by hyperplasia of the gall bladder wall resulting in deepened Rokitansky-Aschoff sinuses that may be filled with cholesterol crystals (Fig. 9.15A). Wall thickening with immobile echogenic foci casting posterior ring-down artifacts are shown on ultrasound (Fig. 9.15B). T2WI may show a characteristic string-of-pearls appearance. CT findings include cystic wall thickening and enhancing inner surface of the gall bladder (Fig. 9.15C, D). Segmental adenomyomatosis usually occurs at the body, which results in annular narrowing and segmentation of the gall bladder lumen, in which gallstones might be trapped in the fundus. The localized form most often occurs in the gall bladder fundus.[7]

## Gall bladder Polyp

Gall bladder polyps are usually incidentally seen on US, immobile, nonshadowing projections from the gall bladder wall. Most polyps are nonneoplastic, though some have malignant potential. Size is the most useful determinant of malignant potential of polyps. Generally, polyps of less than 5 mm are considered unlikely to be malignant, while those greater than 10 mm are suspicious for malignancy (Figs. 9.16 and 9.17). Those in between should be followed up at 3 to 6 months interval. Malignant potential is higher if polyps are larger than 16 mm, found in elderly individual, and there is coexisting gall bladder wall thickening and invasion of the adjacent liver surface on imaging.[8]

## Gall bladder Carcinoma

Adenocarcinoma represents 98% of all gall bladder malignancy.[1] It is commonly found in elderly women with cholelithiasis, which is an established risk factor seen in 80% of all carcinomas.

On imaging, it most frequently manifests as an infiltrating mass replacing the entire gall bladder. The necrotic mass is ill-defined, heterogeneously enhancing, often invading hepatic parenchyma and bile ducts, resulting in bile duct obstruction. The second, less common, presentation is a polypoid mass within the gall bladder, which is homogeneous and confined

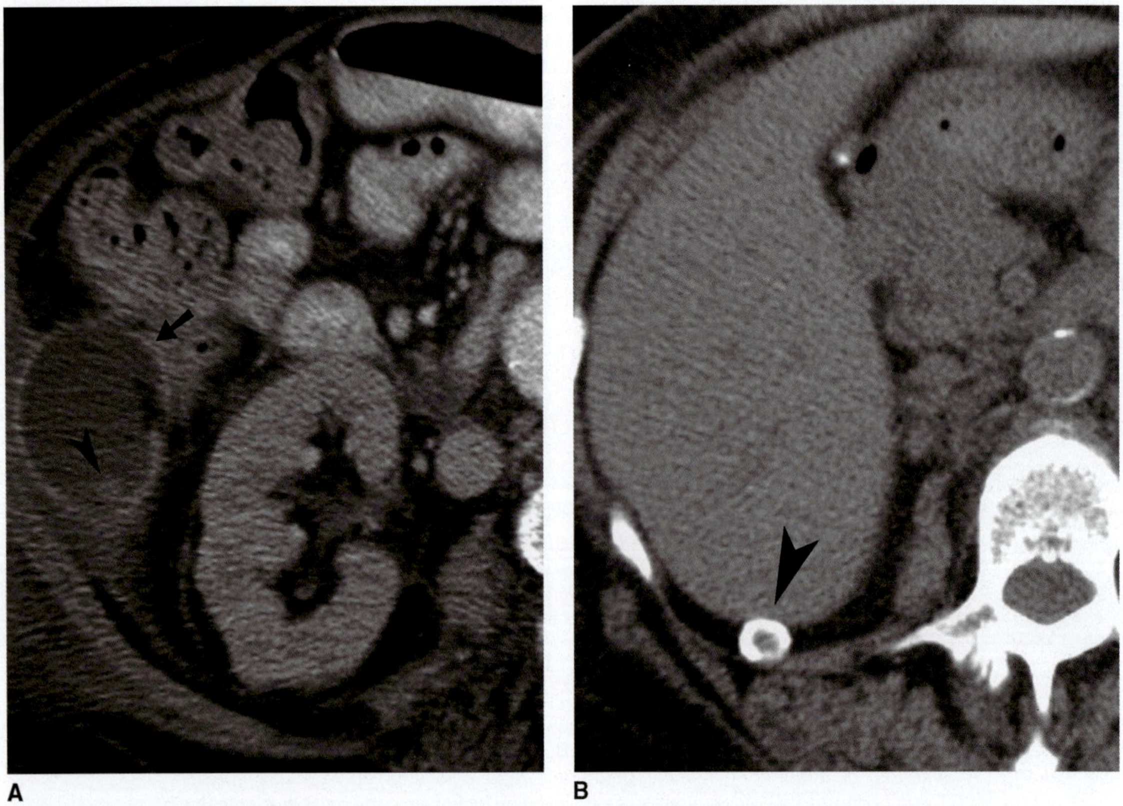


**FIG. 9.14 • Dropped gallstones.** Axial CT images **(A, B)** demonstrate dropped gallstone (*arrowheads*). There is a right paracolic gutter abscess (*arrow*) associated with a dropped gallstone in the first patient.

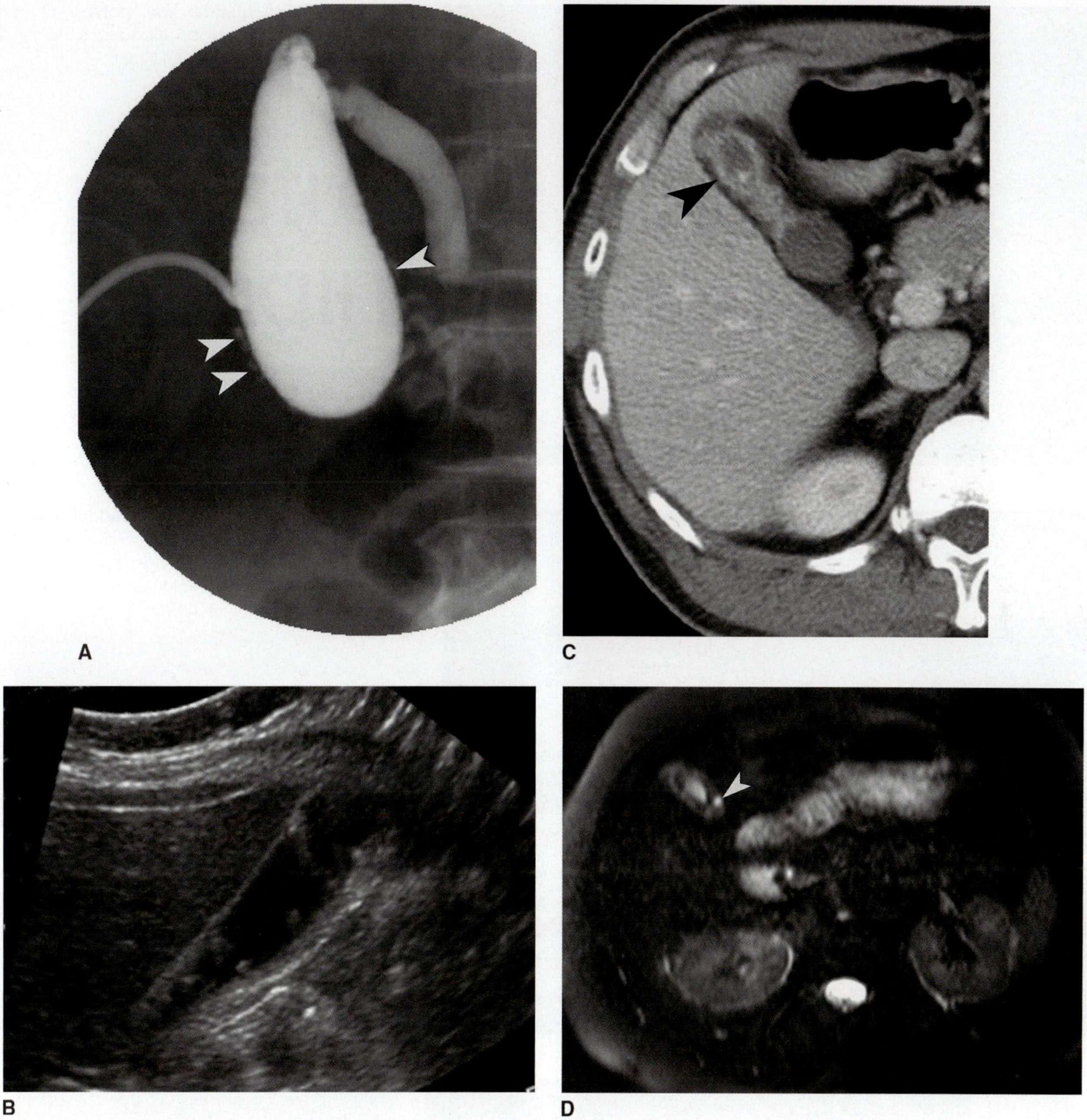

**FIG. 9.15 • Adenomyomatosis of the gall bladder. A:** Cholecystostomy tube injection demonstrates multiple small flask-shaped outpouchings of contrast from the gall bladder lumen, consistent with prominent Rokitansky-Aschoff sinuses (*arrowheads*). **B:** US demonstrates ring-down artifacts caused cholesterol crystals located in the Rokitansky-Aschoff sinuses. **C:** Axial contrast-enhanced CT shows contracted gall bladder with segmental irregular wall thickening (*arrowhead*) and a tiny intraluminal stone. **D:** SSFSE T2WI demonstrates foci of T2 hyperintensities (*arrowhead*) in the wall of the gall bladder.

to the gall bladder wall. The least common imaging pattern is asymmetric mural thickening, irregularity, and enhancement. Gall bladder carcinoma is generally hypo- to isoechoic on ultrasound, hypo- to isoattenuating on CT, or mildly T2 hyperintense on MRI. Radiologic staging is best done with CT, where lymphadenopathy, local spread to the liver, porta hepatis, and adjacent structures are assessed (Figs. 9.18 to 9.21).

Metastasis to gall bladder is rare and is most often reported in patients with malignant melanoma and renal cell carcinoma (Fig. 9.22).

## Gall bladder Trauma

Traumatic gall bladder injuries are most commonly secondary to motor vehicle collision but can also be seen in the setting of penetrating trauma. The injury ranges from laceration, contusion, perforation, to avulsion. Gall bladder perforation is the most common injury pattern. Total avulsion represents the extreme of gall bladder injuries in which the CD and the cystic artery are torn from the liver bed. Many gall bladder injuries are life threatening because of associated injuries to the abdominal viscera/vessels (liver, colon, duo-

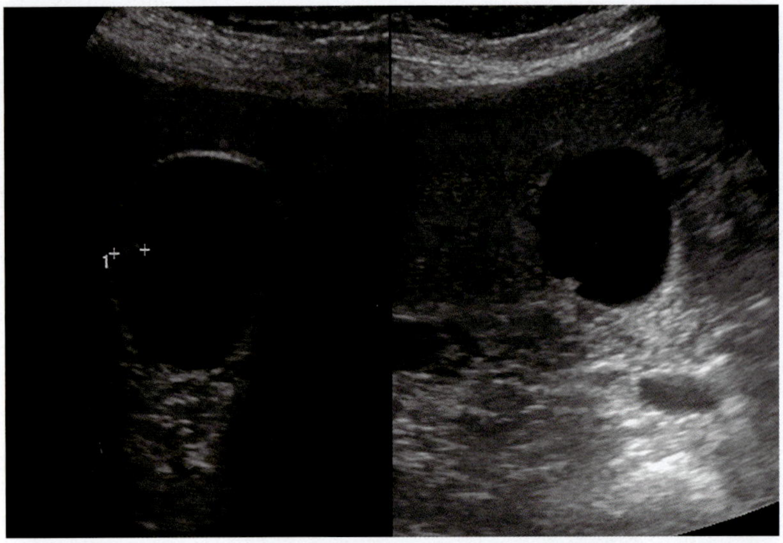

**FIG. 9.16 • Gall bladder wall polyp.** US demonstrates nondependent polyps arising from the gall bladder wall and protruding into the lumen.

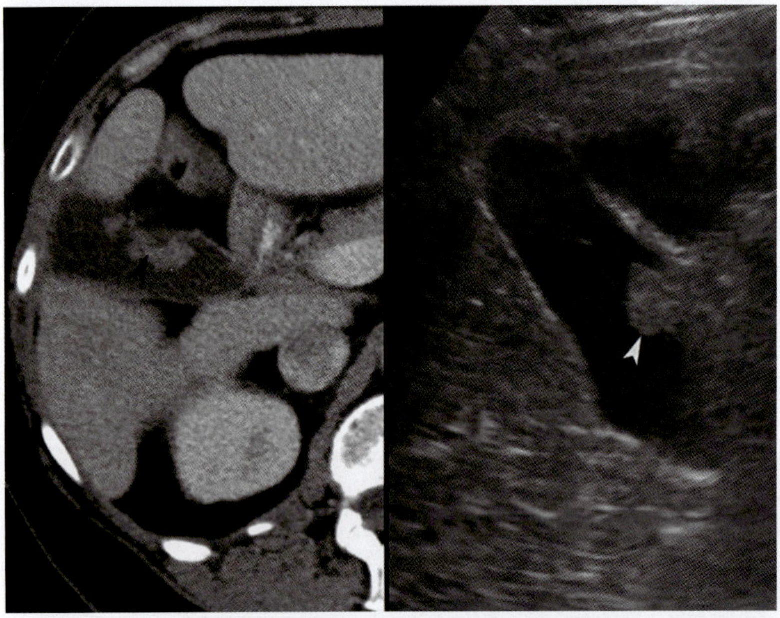

**FIG. 9.17 • Adenomatous gall bladder polyp.** Axial CT and the corresponding US demonstrate irregular polypoidal lesion (*arrowheads*) projecting into the lumen of the gall bladder, which on surgery was found to represent adenomatous polyp.

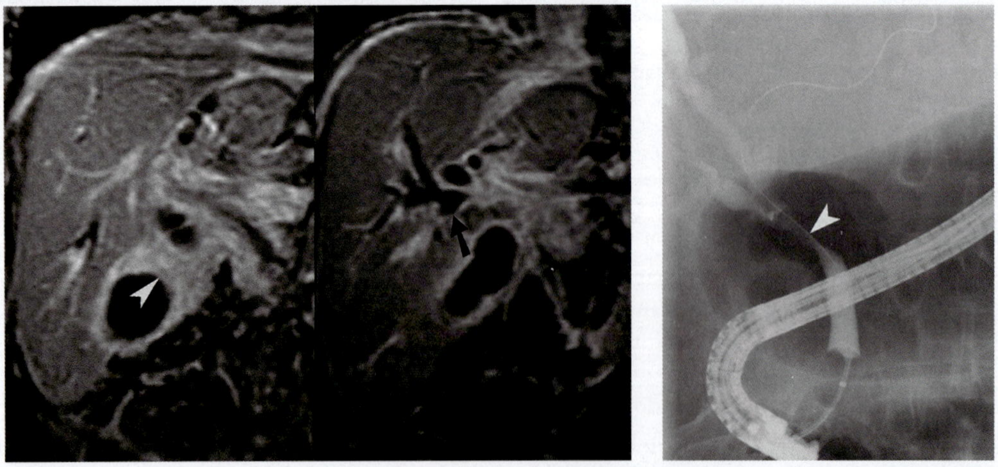

A B

**FIG. 9.18 • Gall bladder adenocarcinoma. A:** Postgadolinium T1WI demonstrates thickening of the gall bladder wall (*arrowhead*) from infiltrating mass extending to the porta hepatis, resulting in biliary ductal dilatation (*arrow*). **B:** ERCP demonstrates smooth narrowing of the proximal CBD from extrinsic impression (*arrowhead*) from gall bladder adenocarcinoma.

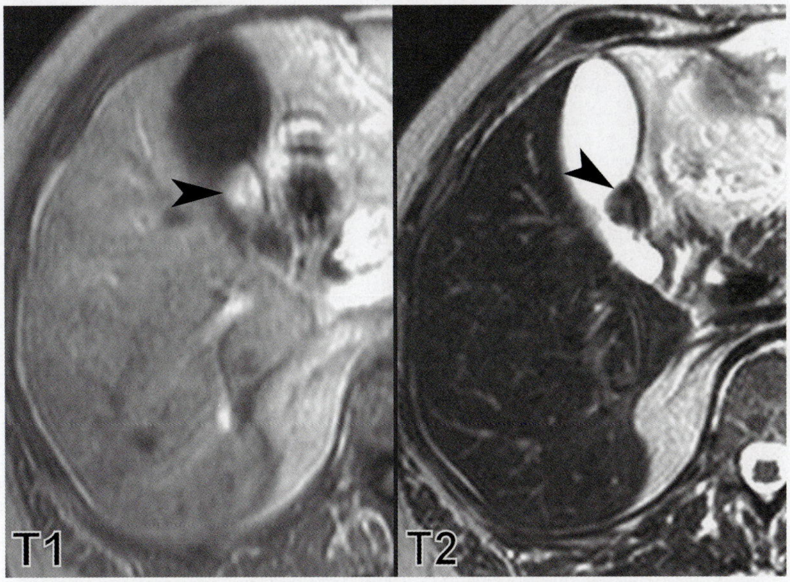


**FIG. 9.19 • Gall bladder adenocarcinoma.** T1WI and T2WI demonstrate a 1.5-cm-diameter polypoidal focal mass lesion (*arrowhead*) without pericholecystic or intrahepatic extension.

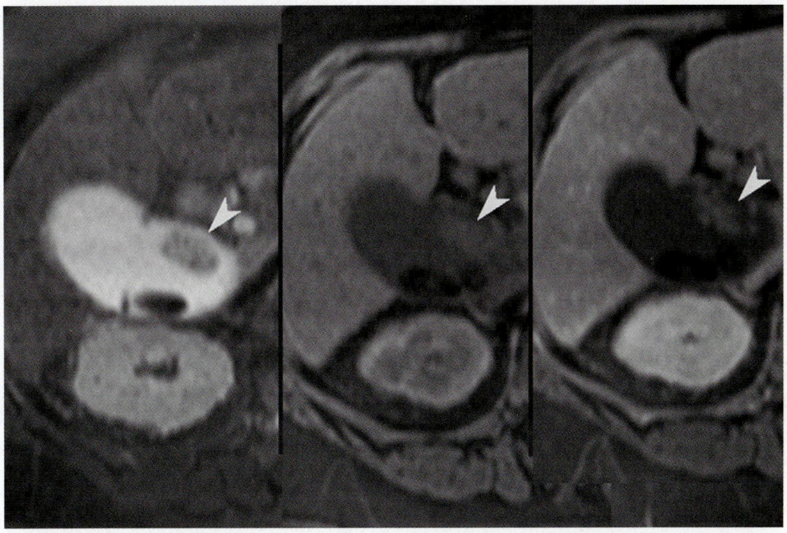

**FIG. 9.20 • Gall bladder adenocarcinoma.** Post-gadolinium T1WI demonstrates a 2-cm-diameter polypoidal mass (*arrowheads*) projecting into the gall bladder lumen.

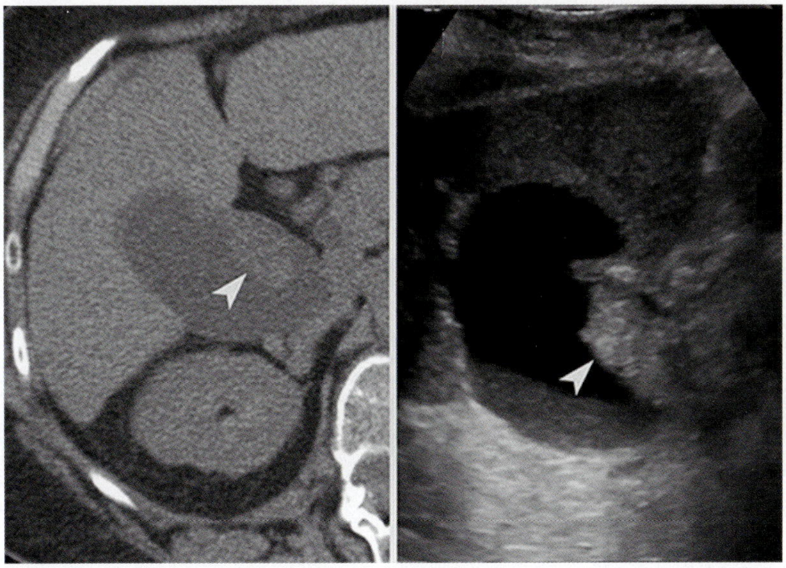

**FIG. 9.21 • Gall bladder adenocarcinoma.** Noncontrast axial CT and US demonstrate irregular lobulated mass (*arrowheads*) projecting into the lumen of the gall bladder.

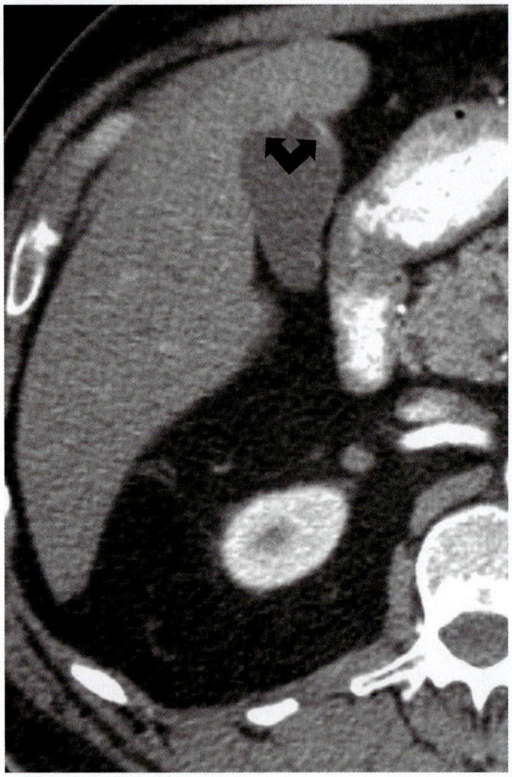

**FIG. 9.22 • Melanoma metastasis to gall bladder.** Axial contrast-enhanced CT demonstrates two foci of focal gall bladder wall thickening in the fundus (*bifid arrow*) caused by melanoma metastatic deposits.

denum, kidney, pancreas) and outside the abdomen (cardiothoracic, brain, and multiorgan failure).[9] Ultrasound, as a part of focused examination, can demonstrate free fluid. Contrast-enhanced CT is performed in hemodynamically stable patients and can help detect high-attenuating blood in the gall bladder lumen, collapsed gall bladder, gall bladder wall thickening, pericholecystic fluid, and active contrast extravasation (Fig. 9.23).[10]

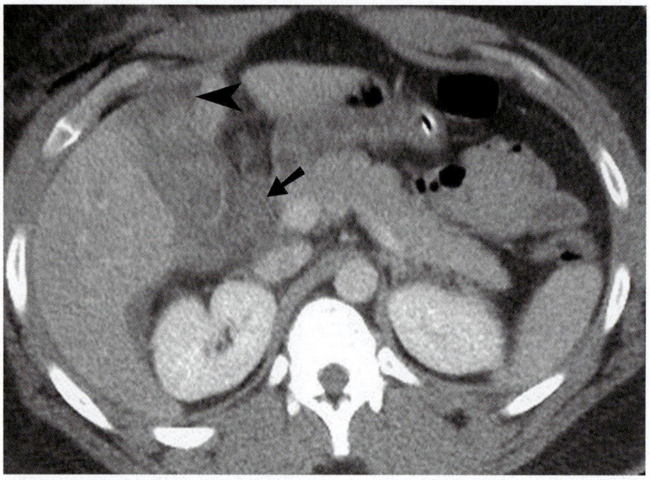

**FIG. 9.23 • The gall bladder traumatic injury.** Axial contrast-enhanced CT demonstrates liver laceration (*arrowhead*) and gall bladder rupture caused by bullet injury. There is high-density fluid (*arrow*) present posterior to the gall bladder.

## BILE DUCT PATHOLOGIES

### Choledocholithiasis

Stones in bile ducts may develop within the ducts (primary choledocholithiasis) or in the gall bladder (secondary choledocholithiasis). It is found in 7% to 20% of patients undergoing cholecystectomy and 2% to 4% after cholecystectomy.[3] Most stones are small; therefore, they can pass spontaneously into the duodenum. Stones larger than 5 mm are more difficult to pass and often located near the ampulla of Vater, resulting in biliary obstruction and potential development of cholangitis and pancreatitis.

Imaging detection of choledocholithiasis is greater if stones are larger, located more proximally within the CBD, and biliary ductal dilatation is present. On US, stones appear echogenic with or without posterior acoustic shadowing, distal to dilated, fluid-filled duct. Overall, US (18% to 45%) has lower sensitivity than CT (75% to 80%) for choledocholithiasis (Fig. 9.24). Magnetic Resonance

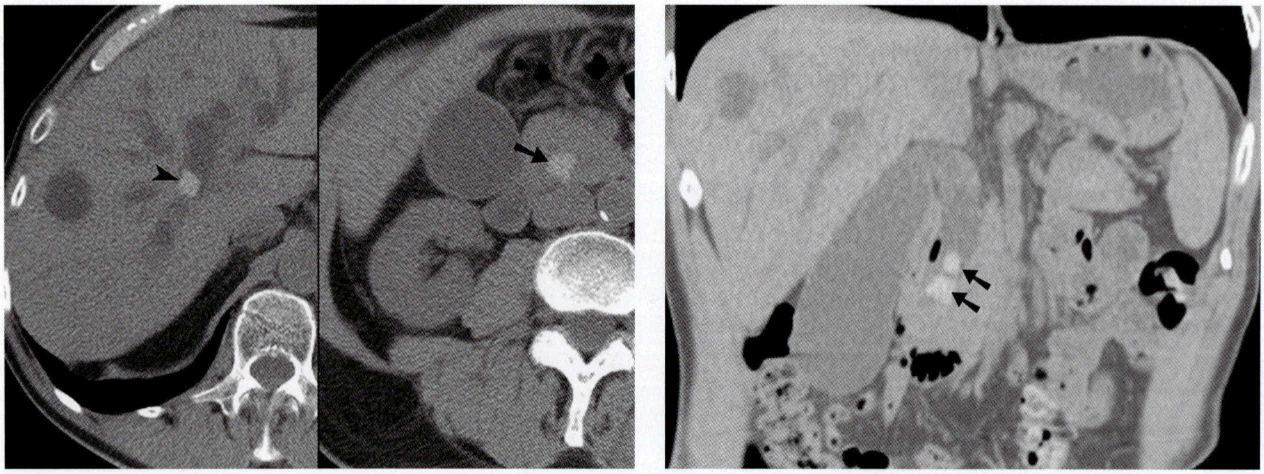

A B

**FIG. 9.24 • Choledocholithiasis on CT.** Axial **(A)** and coronal **(B)** noncontrast CT demonstrates multiple faceted stones located in the right intrahepatic hepatic duct (*arrowhead*) and distal CBD (*arrows*).

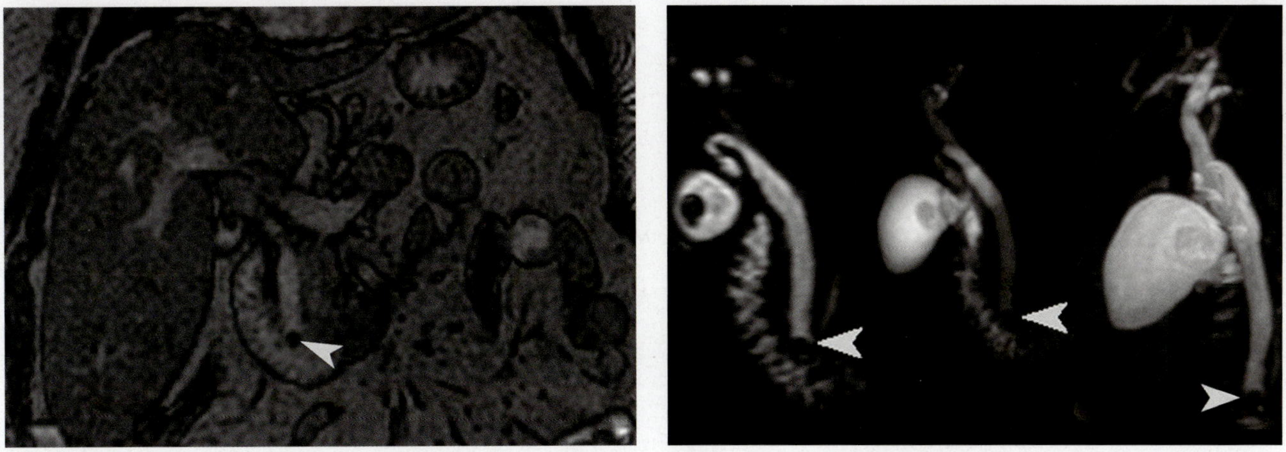

A B

**FIG. 9.25 • Choledocholithiasis on MRCP. A:** Scout image for MR study demonstrates a focal 9-mm-diameter calculus (*arrowhead*) located at the lower end of the CBD. **B:** MRCP study demonstrates calculus (*arrowheads*) at the lower end of the CBD (*arrowheads*).

Cholangiopancreatography (MRCP) is the most sensitive noninvasive method with ability to detect stones as small as 2 mm and with high sensitivity (81% to 100%) and specificity (85% to 99%) (Fig. 9.25).[3] MRCP is increasingly utilized because it provides greater level of diagnostic confidence and helps identify patients who require therapeutic intervention.

## Acute Cholangitis

Ascending cholangitis secondary to gram-negative enteric bacteria is a common complication of biliary obstruction, which is, associated with choledocholithiasis in greater than 80% cases. It is a medical emergency that requires imaging to document the presence of biliary tract obstruction, etiology of obstruction, and complications such as hepatic abscess. US is generally employed as the first imaging method with CT and MRI/MRCP as a problem-solving tool. Findings of cholangitis, in addition to biliary dilatation and its etiology, include ductal wall thickening, enhancement, transient hepatic attenuation differences, and hepatic abscess (Fig. 9.26).

*HIV cholangiopathy* is a type of cholangitis seen in advanced HIV-positive patients. Opportunistic infection of the bile ducts is usually secondary to cryptosporidium or cytomegalovirus. On imaging, there is irregular biliary ductal dilatation, wall thickening, and alternating areas of strictures and dilatations.

*Recurrent pyogenic cholangitis* is characterized by intrahepatic pigmented stones and recurrent cholangitis believed to be associated with chronic parasitic infestation of bile ducts. IHD stones cause obstruction and recurrent attacks of cholangitis, abscesses, biliary ductal strictures, hepatic atrophy, and cirrhosis. This condition is commonly seen in East Asian descents, and there is an increased risk of cholangiocarcinoma. On imaging, there is biliary ductal dilatation that is usually diffuse and disproportionately involves the first- and second-order ducts. IHD stones, periductal parenchymal changes (hyperechogenicity, abnormal enhancement), and pneumobilia can also be seen.[1,11]

## Primary Sclerosing Cholangitis

Primary sclerosing cholangitis is chronic cholestatic inflammatory liver disease of unknown etiology characterized by destruction and fibrosis of the bile ducts (intrahepatic, extrahepatic, or both). It is common in men with onset of disease in the fourth decade of life, often in patients with inflammatory bowel disease.[12] The patients are at risk of cholangiocarcinoma with a lifetime prevalence of 10% to 30%.[13]

On cholangiography and MRCP, the findings include irregular circumferential bile duct wall thickening and alternating segments of bile duct strictures as well as dilatations (Figs. 9.27 and 9.28). Evidence of cirrhosis with portal hypertension may be seen later in the course of the disease.

## Mirizzi Syndrome

Chronically impacted gallstones can directly compress the adjacent CHD/CBD, resulting in biliary obstruction. In some cases, choledochoenteric fistula may develop. This is a rare complication of long-standing cholelithiasis that should be suspected in patients presenting with symptoms of cholelithiasis and obstructive jaundice. Imaging shows dilatation of the IHDs and collapsed CBD with stone impacted in the CD (Fig. 9.29).

## Cholangiocarcinoma

Cholangiocarcinoma is the primary malignant tumor of the bile duct that usually occurs in elderly patients. Tumors are most often in the extrahepatic ducts, and most are moderate-to-well differentiated adenocarcinoma. Extrahepatic tumors are mostly located at the hepatic hilum, so-called Klatskin tumor (60%), or more distally in the CBD (25%). Intrahepatic tumors are less common (15%). *Klatskin tumors* originate

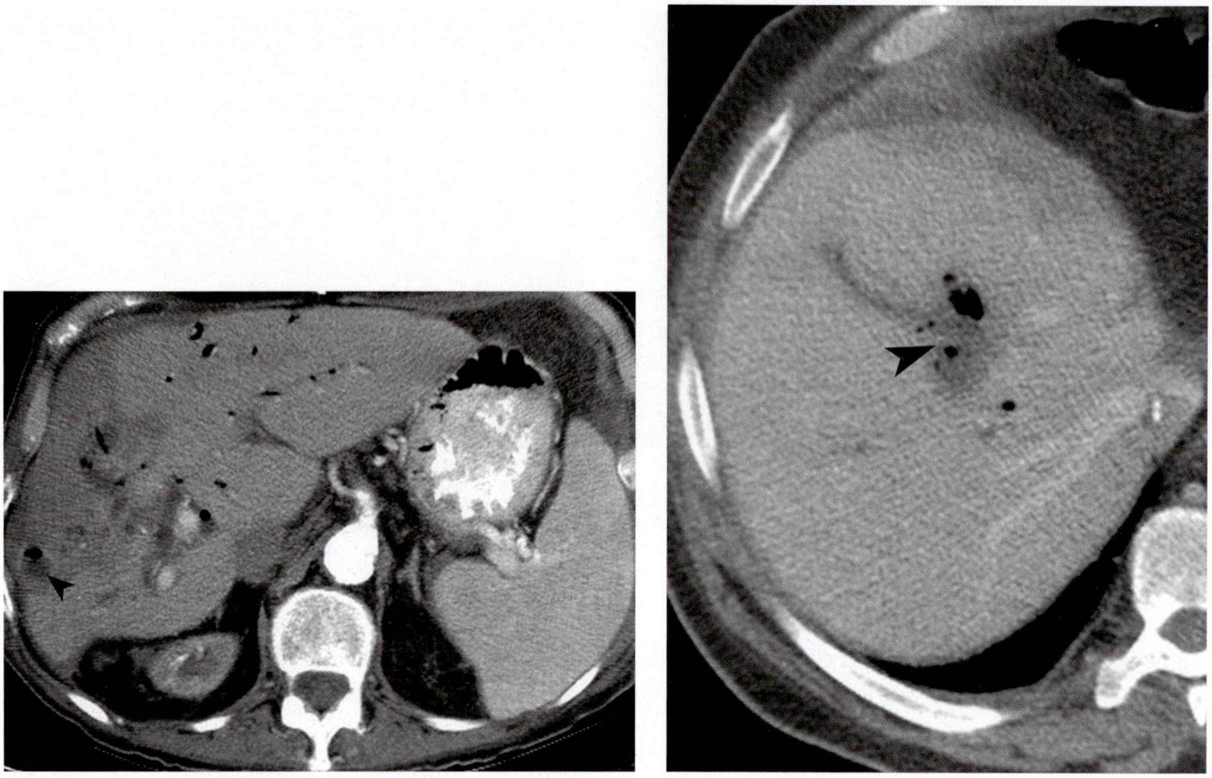

A B

**FIG. 9.26 • Cholangitis and biliary necrosis.** Axial contrast-enhanced CT scan study in two patients **(A, B)** with history of liver transplant demonstrates irregularity of the biliary ducts and abscess (*arrowheads*) caused by biliary necrosis and superimposed infection.

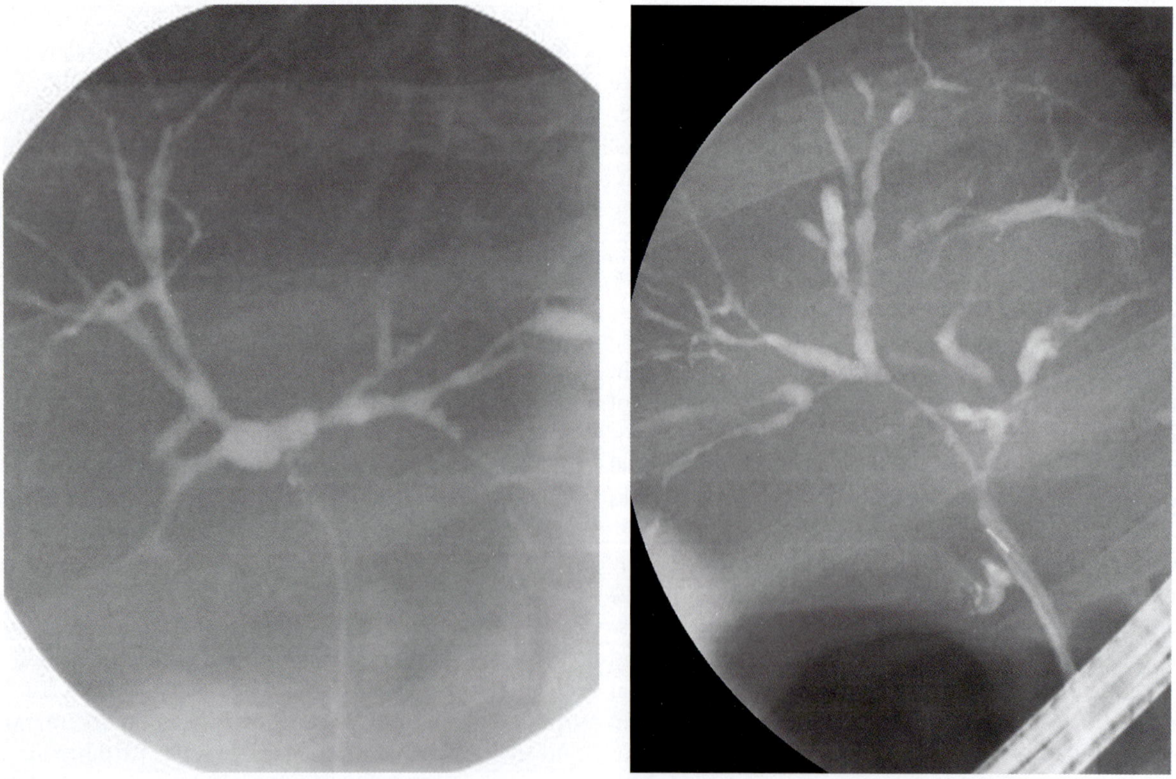

A B

**FIG. 9.27 • Sclerosing cholangitis on ERCP.** ERCP study in two patients **(A, B)** with sclerosing cholangitis demonstrates alternating areas of narrowing and dilatation of the intrahepatic biliary ducts.

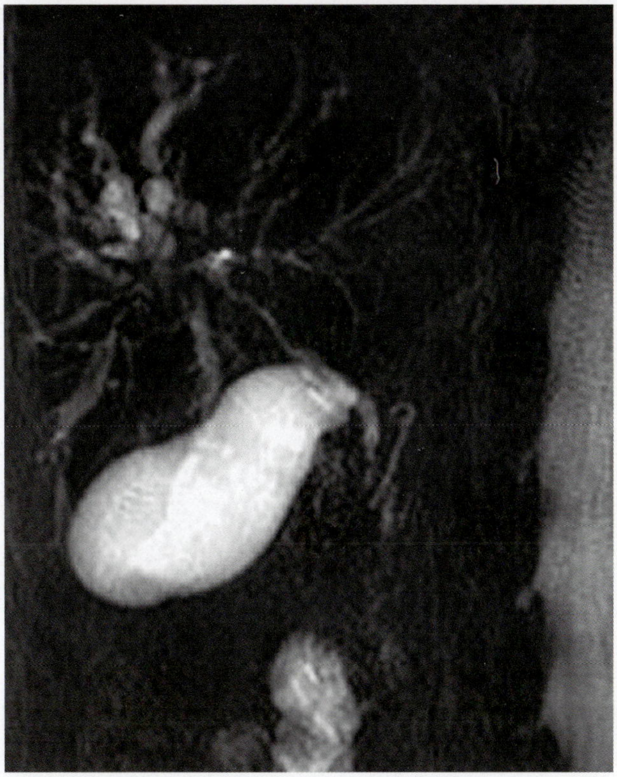

**FIG. 9.28 • Sclerosing cholangitis on MR.** MRCP study demonstrates multiple intrahepatic strictures in the IHDs, most prominently present near the porta hepatis.

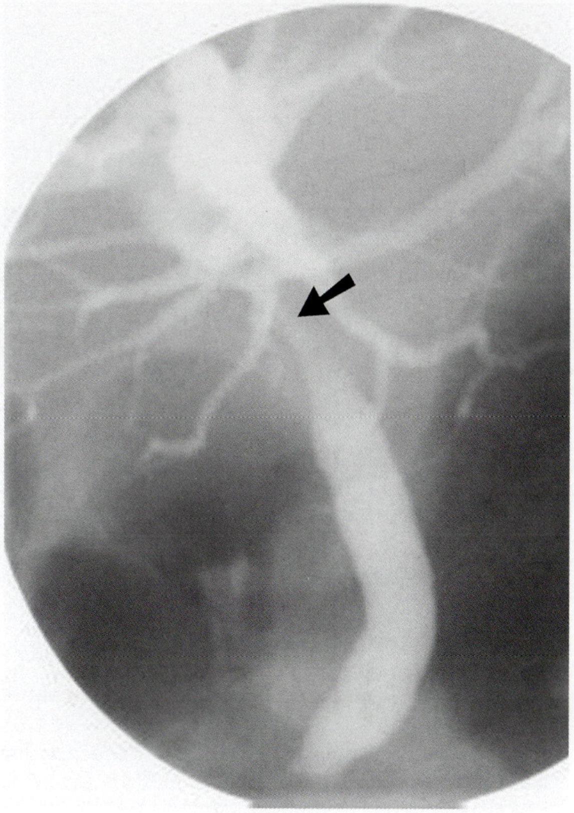

**FIG. 9.29 • Mirizzi syndrome.** ERCP study demonstrates smooth extrinsic impression (*arrow*) on the proximal CBD caused by obstructing stone located in the neck of the gall bladder.

from the right/left IHD or CHD. They mostly present as an infiltrative mass causing diffuse dilatation of IHD and atrophy–hypertrophy complex secondary to tumor invasion of the ipsilateral portal vein.[14] The tumor mass itself can be difficult to visualize on ultrasound and even on CT scan. MRI usually depicts the mass having ill-defined border, mild/moderate T1 hypointensity, T2 iso- to hyperintensity, and variable enhancement. Tumors with significant fibrosis demonstrate delayed enhancement.

*Distal CBD carcinomas* are also mostly infiltrative, growing intramurally, and appears as an irregular, asymmetric, long segmental stricture of the CBD with delayed-enhancing nodular mass at the site of stricture. *Periampullary tumors* occur within 2 cm of the major duodenal papilla. Beside distal CBD cholangiocarcinoma, the term includes tumors of the ampulla, pancreas, and duodenum. The exact organ of origin can be difficult to determine on imaging or even at pathology (Figs. 9.30 and 9.31).

## Choledochal Cyst

Choledochal cyst is a cystic dilatation of the biliary tree, more commonly found in the patients from East Asia. Most choledochal cysts are diagnosed during childhood, but up to 20% are found in adults.[1,2] This condition is believed to be congenital but may be predisposed by reflux of pancreatic juice into the CBD via a common channel of the pancreatic duct and distal CBD (aberrant pancreaticobiliary junction).

Todani classification describes five morphologic types of choledochal cyst, which mirrors findings at CT and MRI.

- Type 1 cyst is segmental dilatation of the CBD, either diffuse or focal.
- Type 2 cyst is true diverticulum of the CBD.
- Type 3 cyst or choledochocele refers to dilatation localized to the intraduodenal segment of the CBD.
- Type 4 cysts show multiple dilatations (fusiform or saccular) of the extrahepatic bile duct with or without intrahepatic ductal dilatation.
- Type 5 cysts are purely intrahepatic dilatations of bile ducts.

## Bile Duct Trauma

*Injuries to the bile ducts* are less common than those of the gall bladder. Injuries may present as biloma, biliary ascites, fistula, or stricture. *Biloma* is a loculated collection of bile most commonly in subhepatic space, caused by bile extravasation that may present hours or days after the initial injury. *Biliary ascites* represent freely mobile bile within the peritoneal cavity resulting from disruption of the major bile duct. *Fistulas* can develop from the bile duct to thoracic (pleura, bronchus) and vascular structures (hepatic artery/vein, portal vein) and result in fluid collections or hematobilia, respectively.[15]

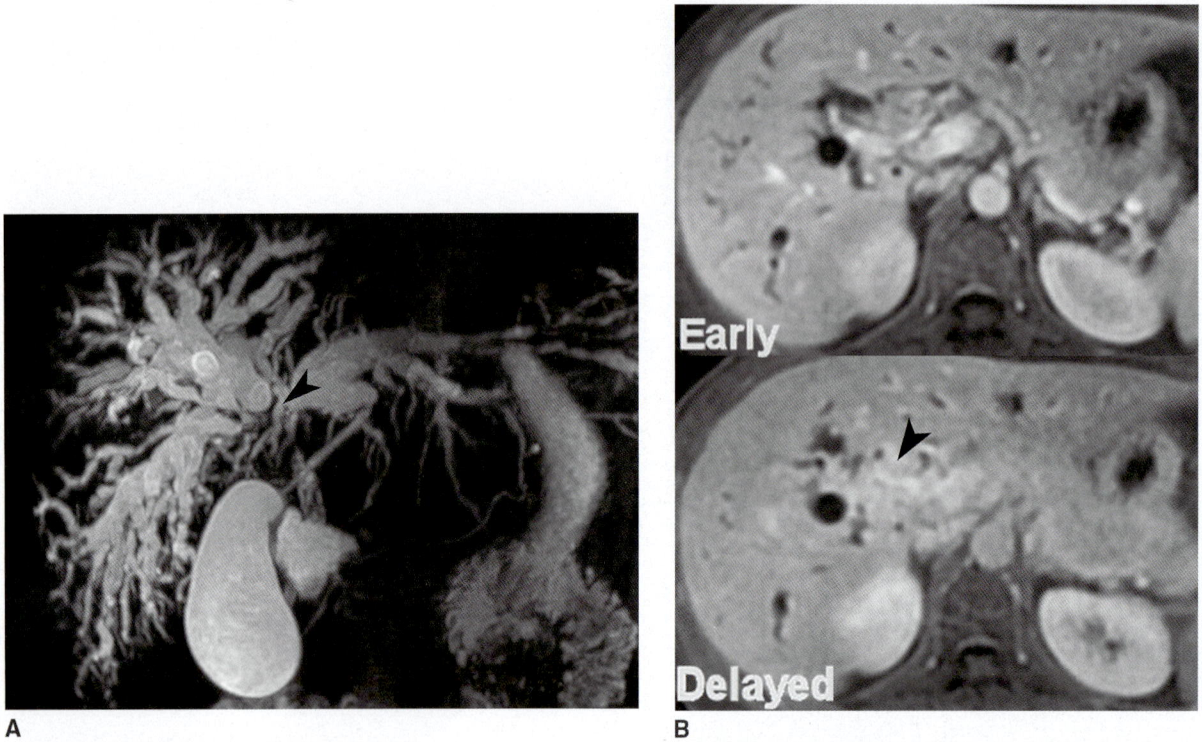


**FIG. 9.30 • Cholangiocarcinoma. A:** MRCP demonstrates marked intrahepatic biliary ductal dilatation with obstruction at the confluence of CHDs (*arrowhead*) caused by cholangiocarcinoma (Klatskin tumor). **B:** Early and delayed postgadolinium T1WI demonstrates biliary ductal dilatation from infiltrating tumor, which demonstrates delayed enhancement (*arrowhead*).

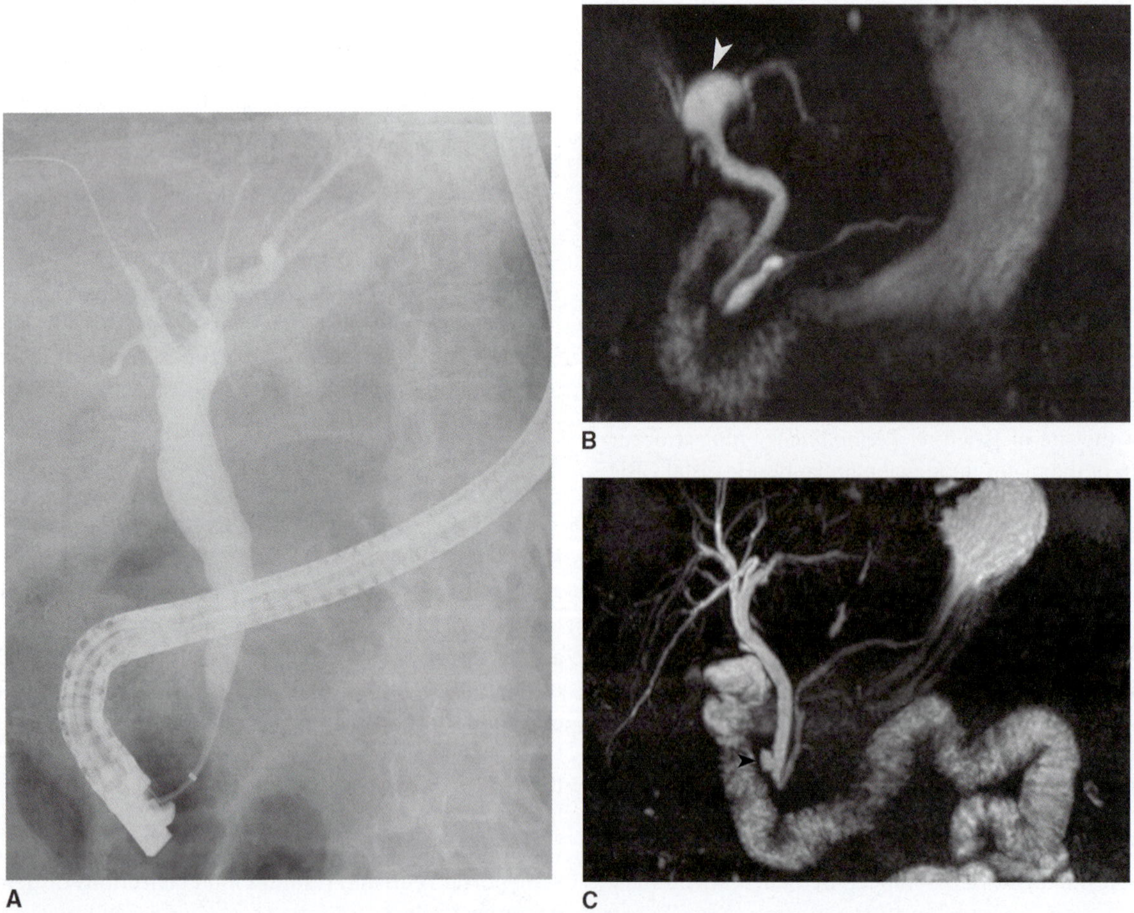

**FIG. 9.31 • Choledochal cyst.** ERCP **(A)** and MRCP **(B, C)** demonstrate type 1 (A), 2 (B), and 3 (C) cysts (*arrowheads*).

## References


1. Boyd B, Lee ER. Ultrasound of the gallbladder and biliary tree: back to basics. *Ultrasound Clin.* 2014;9:567–586.
2. Yam BL, Siegelman ES. MR imaging of the biliary system. *Radiol Clin North Am.* 2014;52:725–755.
3. Gore RM, Thakrar KH, Newmark GM, et al. Gallbladder imaging. *Gastroenterol Clin North Am.* 2010;39:265–287.
4. Bennett GL, Balthazar EJ. Ultrasound and CT evaluation of emergent gallbladder pathology. *Radiol Clin North Am.* 2003;41: 1203–1216.
5. O'Connor OJ, Maher MM. Imaging of cholecystitis. *AJR Am J Roentgenol.* 2011;196:W367–W374.
6. Smith EA, Dillman JR, Elsayes KM, et al. Cross-sectional imaging of acute and chronic gallbladder inflammatory disease. *AJR Am J Roentgenol.* 2009;192:188–196.
7. Runner GJ, Corwin MT, Siewert B, et al. Gallbladder wall thickening. *AJR Am J Roentgenol.* 2014;202:W1–W12.
8. Konstantinidis IT, Bajpai S, Kambadakone AR, et al. Gallbladder lesions identified on ultrasound. Lessons from the last 10 years. *J Gastrointest Surg.* 2012;16:549–553.
9. Ball CG, Dixon E, Kirkpatrick AW, et al. A decade of experience with injuries to the gallbladder. *J Trauma Manag Outcomes.* 2010;4:3.
10. Wittenberg A, Minotti AJ. CT diagnosis of traumatic gallbladder injury. *AJR Am J Roentgenol.* 2005;185:1573–1574.
11. Heffernan EJ, Geoghegan T, Munk PL, et al. Recurrent pyogenic cholangitis: from imaging to intervention. *AJR Am J Roentgenol.* 2009;192:W28–W35.
12. Karlsen TH, Schrumpf E, Boberg KM. Primary sclerosing cholangitis. *Best Pract Res Clin Gastroenterol.* 2010;24:655–666.
13. Mendes FD, Lindor KD. Primary sclerosing cholangitis. *Clin Liver Dis.* 2004;8:195–211.
14. Matos C, Serrao E, Bali MA. Magnetic resonance imaging of biliary tumors. *Magn Reson Imaging Clin N Am.* 2010;18:477–496.
15. Williamson JM. Traumatic injuries to the biliary tree. *Br J Hosp Med (Lond).* 2013;74:138–143.


## SELF-ASSESSMENT QUESTIONS

1. What is the cause of fever and abdominal pain on the CT of a patient with recent history of cholecystectomy?

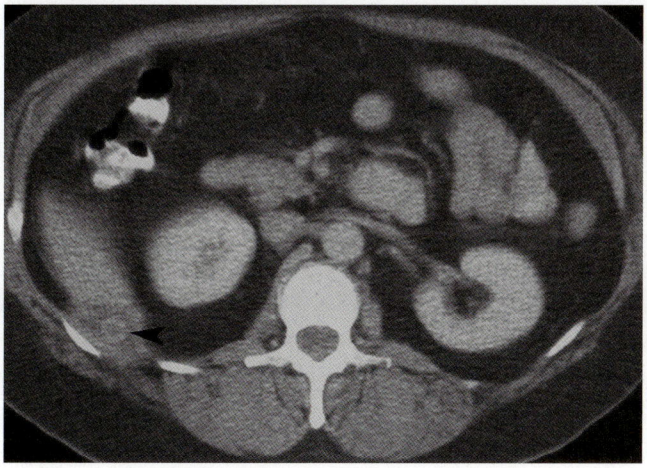

A. Dropped gallstone
B. Dropped clip
C. Dropped stone with abscess
D. Peritoneal carcinomatosis

2. Which of the following findings of acute cholecystitis is better demonstrated on CT than US?

A. Gallstone
B. Gall bladder wall thickening
C. Murphy sign
D. Pericholecystic fat inflammation

3. A 70-year-old diabetic woman presents to the emergency department with sepsis and right upper quadrant pain. Based on the CT, which of the following is the most likely diagnosis?

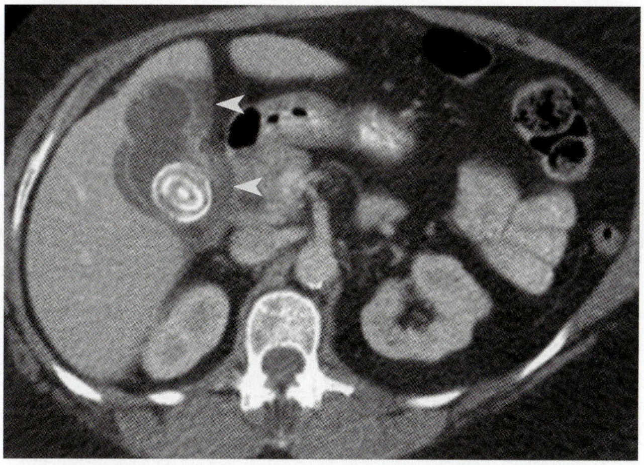

A. Emphysematous cholecystitis
B. Acute cholecystitis
C. Hydropic gall bladder
D. Gall bladder perforation

4. Which of the following is the most likely diagnosis on the MR study?

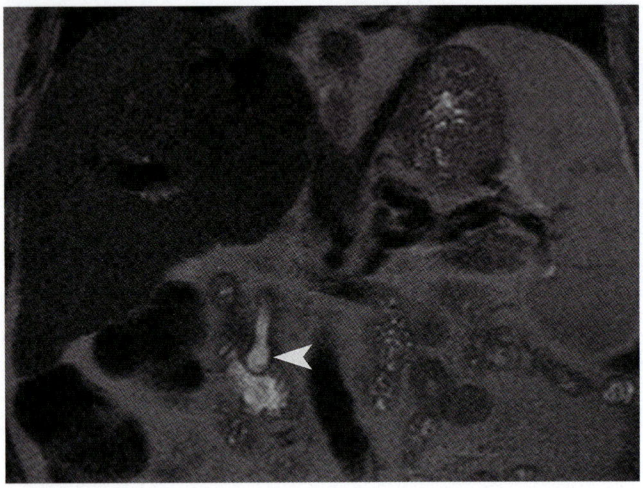

   A. IPMN
   B. Periampullary cancer
   C. Serous cystadenoma
   D. Choledochocele

5. What is the cause (arrowhead) of nausea and vomiting seen on the CT of an elderly patient?

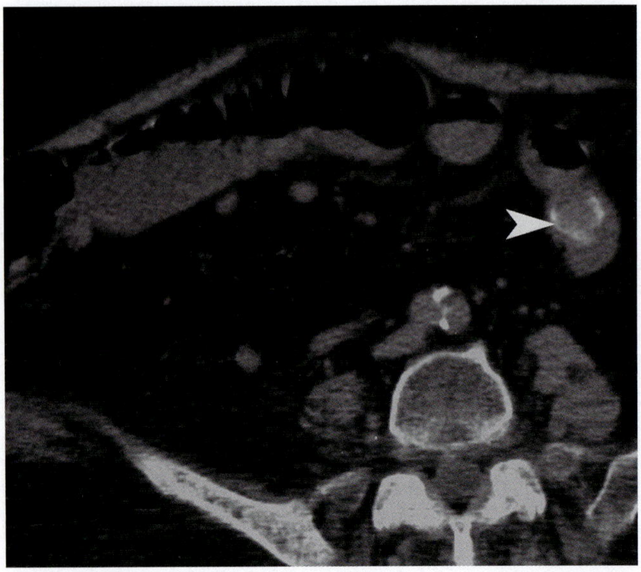

   A. Adhesions
   B. Gallstone
   C. Carcinoid
   D. Foreign body

## *Answers to Self-Assessment Questions*

**1. C.** Dropped stone with abscess. The contrast-enhanced CT demonstrates a dropped gallstone in the Morrison pouch with surrounding abscess.

**2. D.** Pericholecystic fat inflammation. CT is better than US in depicting inflammation in the pericholecystic fat, compared to US study.

**3. B.** Acute cholecystitis. The contrast-enhanced CT shows gallstone, wall thickening, pericholecystic inflammation, and discontinuous mucosal enhancement, suggesting the diagnosis of acute cholecystitis.

**4. D.** Choledochocele. The coronal SSFSE series demonstrates bulbous dilatation at the intramural portion of the CBD, consistent with choledochocele.

**5. B.** Gallstone. The noncontrast CT shows dilated small bowel and an obstructing, rim-calcified gallstone located in a jejunal loop.

# Pancreas: Non-neoplastic Diseases

# 10A

*Akshya Gupta, Alexander Kessler, and Shweta Bhatt*

## LEARNING OBJECTIVES

1. Review the normal anatomy and physiology of the pancreas.
2. Discuss the imaging appearance of congenital and inflammatory disorders of the pancreas.
3. Review the imaging appearance of uncommon nonneoplastic pancreatic conditions including posttraumatic injury.

The pancreas is located in the anterior pararenal space in the retroperitoneum; it is typically evaluated with computed tomography (CT) (Fig. 10A.1A) and magnetic resonance imaging (MRI) (Fig. 10A.1B), with MRCP and ERCP offering methods of evaluating the pancreatic duct. A normal pancreas measures approximately 12 to 15 cm in length, while a normal pancreatic duct measures up to 3 to 4 mm at the pancreatic head.

Anatomically, the pancreas is divided into the head, neck, body, and tail. The head lies in close approximation to the 2nd and 3rd portion of the duodenum and extends posterior to the SMV as the uncinate process. The neck is the thinnest portion of the pancreas and lies anterior to the superior mesenteric vessels. The body of the pancreas is the main component of the gland and lies to the left of the superior mesenteric vessels, while the tail is typically in close approximation to the splenic hilum. The head is typically supplied from branches of the gastroduodenal artery and the superior mesenteric artery, while the body and tail are supplied by the splenic artery.

The pancreas functionally is an accessory digestive gland with both exocrine and endocrine roles. Pancreatic acinar cells secrete digestive enzymes, which are secreted into the duodenum via the pancreatic duct. The pancreatic islet cells secrete insulin, glucagons, and various polypeptides into the systemic circulation via the portal venous system.

## PANCREAS DIVISUM

Pancreas divisum represents the most common congenital anatomic variant of the pancreas.[1] During gestation, the ventral pancreas must rotate posteriorly in relation to the duodenum and fuse with the dorsal pancreas. In pancreas divisum, the ventral and dorsal pancreatic buds fail to fuse normally, resulting in the absence of communication between the ventral and dorsal pancreatic ducts. The head and uncinate process of the pancreas are drained by the duct of Wirsung via the major papilla, while the body and tail of the pancreas are drained by the duct of Santorini via the minor papilla (Fig. 10A.2). There is increased risk of pancreatitis given the lack of proper drainage of the pancreatic body and tail; however, most patients are asymptomatic.

On CT, the pancreatic head can be enlarged with an irregular contour, and the separate ductal systems can be seen on MRCP and ERCP (Figs. 10A.3 and 10A.4).[2] The ventral duct is seen as a shorter structure, entering the major papilla, without any communication with the longer dorsal duct.

## ANNULAR PANCREAS

The majority of cases present with persistent vomiting in infancy or a history of polyhydramnios in utero. The pancreatic head encircles and narrows the second portion of the duodenum, causing bowel obstruction. In adults, annular pancreas can cause peptic ulcer disease, pancreatitis, or obstruction.[3]

Radiographs can classically demonstrate the double-bubble sign with narrowing of the duodenum (Fig. 10A.5). UGI barium studies can identify focal narrowing in the second portion of the duodenum with a dilated proximal GI tract (Fig. 10A.6A). On ERCP and MRCP, a small duct draining the pancreatic head encircles the descending duodenum and joins the normal-appearing main pancreatic duct in the body and tail (Fig. 10A.6B). CT and MRI will demonstrate the normal-appearing pancreatic parenchyma, encircling the duodenum below the ampulla of Vater (Fig. 10A.7).

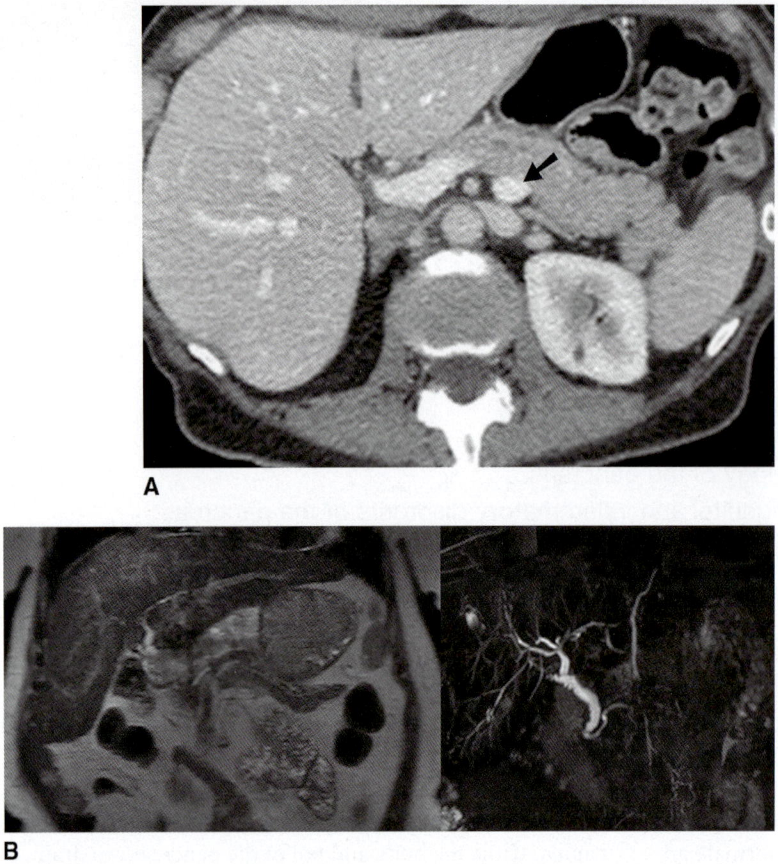

**FIG. 10A.1 • The normal pancreas on CT and MR. A:** Axial contrast-enhanced CT demonstrates the normal pancreas (*arrow*), anterior to the portal vein. **B:** Coronal T1WI demonstrates a normal pancreas, with corresponding MRCP image demonstrating a normal caliber of biliary ducts and pancreatic duct.

## PANCREATIC LIPOMATOSIS

Pancreatic lipomatosis is the most common pathologic condition of the adult pancreas.[4] It can be diffuse or complete (Fig. 10A.8) and can occasionally present as a focal lesion mimicking a pancreatic mass. The exact pathogenesis behind fatty replacement of the pancreas is not known; however, several predisposing factors have been linked to this benign condition, including obesity, diabetes mellitus, chronic pancreatitis, hereditary pancreatitis, chronic pancreatic duct obstruction, and cystic fibrosis.[5] The syndromes associated with pancreatic lipomatosis include Shwachman-Diamond syndrome, Cushing syndrome, cystic fibrosis, and Johanson-Blizzard syndrome.

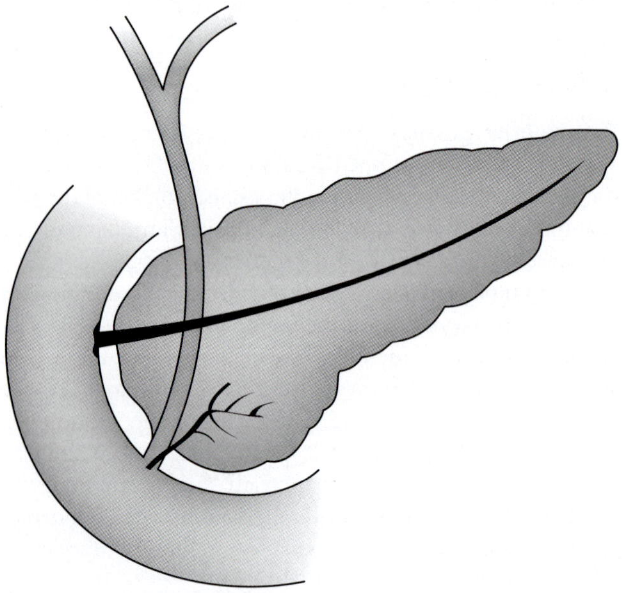

**FIG. 10A.2 • Pancreatic divisum.** Schematic diagram depicts drainage of the pancreatic body and tail through the duct of Santorini via the minor papilla. The pancreatic head is drained by the duct of Wirsung via the major papilla.

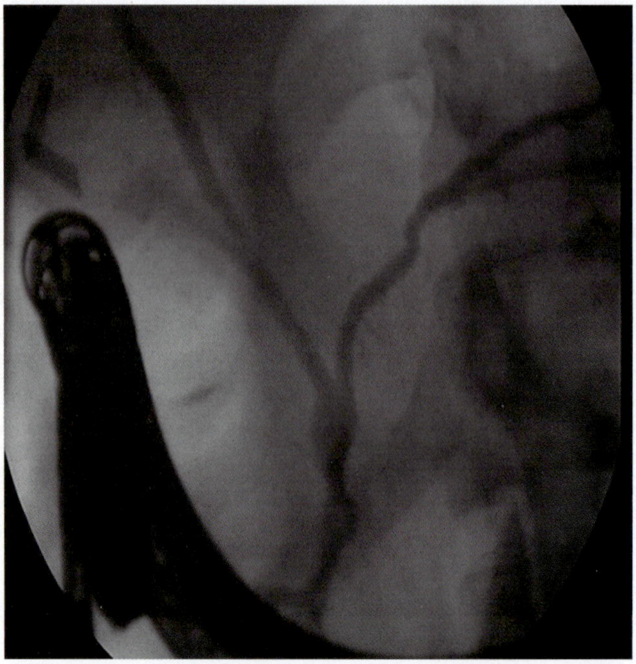

**FIG. 10A.3 • Pancreatic divisum.** ERCP demonstrates separate drainage of the main pancreatic duct and common bile duct.

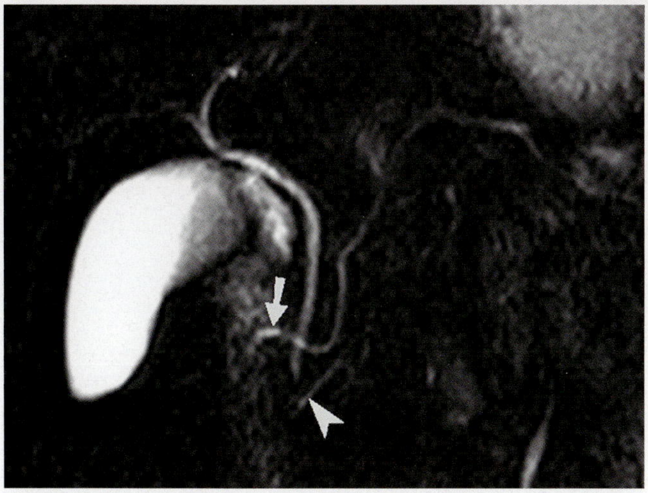

**FIG. 10A.4 • Pancreatic divisum.** MRCP image demonstrates the separate drainage of main pancreatic duct (dorsal duct) (*arrow*) and ventral duct (*arrowhead*) through the minor and major papilla, respectively.

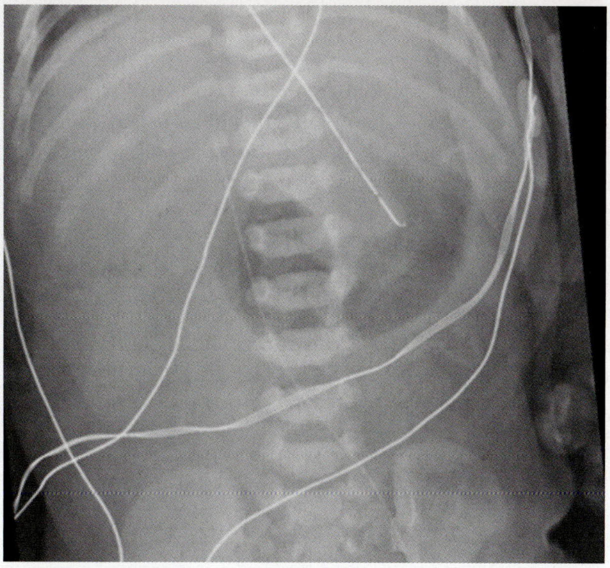

**FIG. 10A.5 • Annular pancreas.** Plain film demonstrates a double-bubble sign with gas in the dilated stomach and proximal duodenum, without evidence of bowel gas distally. The patient was found to have an annular pancreas and duodenal atresia.

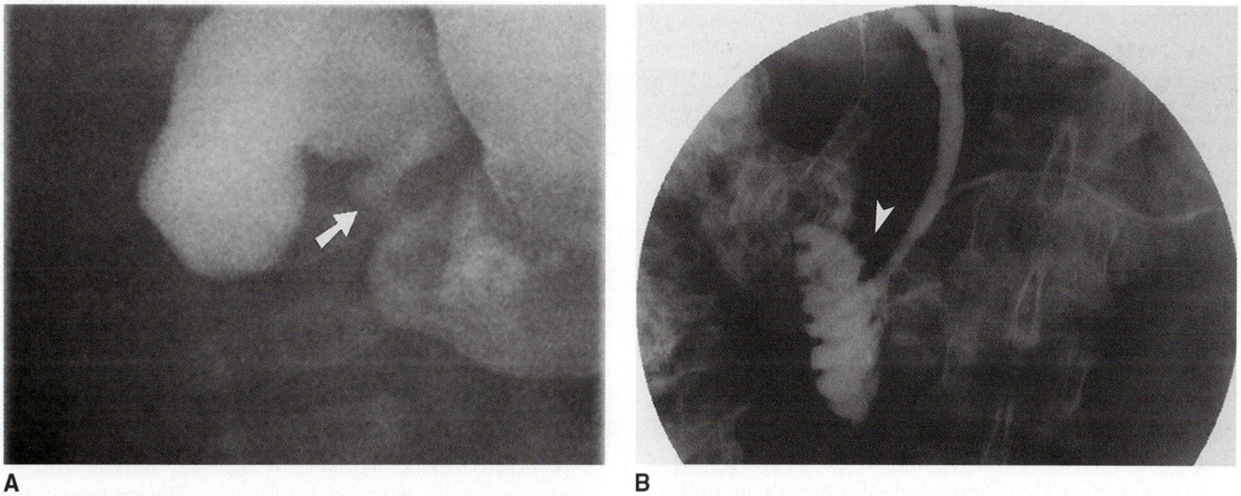

**FIG. 10A.6 • Annular pancreas. A:** Upper GI barium study demonstrates stricture (*arrow*) at the level of the second portion of the duodenum with proximal dilatation. **B:** ERCP demonstrates pancreatic duct encircling (*arrowhead*) the second portion of the duodenum.

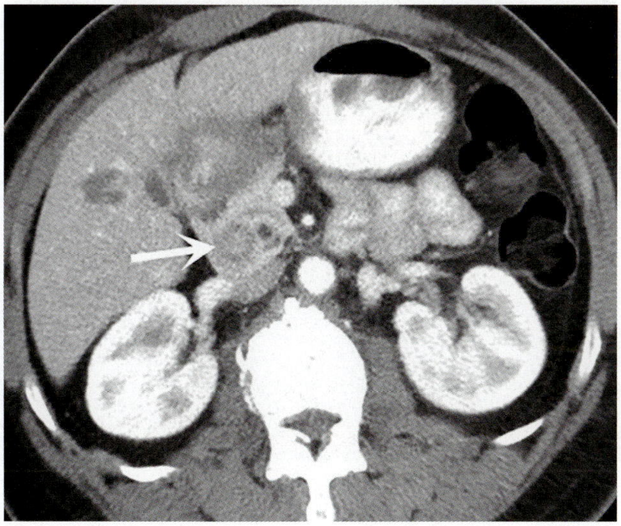

**FIG. 10A.7 • Annular pancreas.** Axial contrast-enhanced CT demonstrates the pancreas (*arrow*) encircling and narrowing the proximal duodenum.

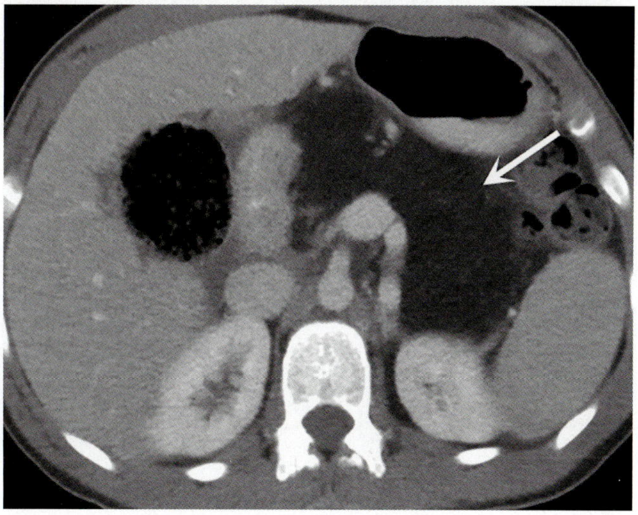

**FIG. 10A.8 • Diffuse pancreatic lipomatosis in cystic fibrosis.** Axial contrast-enhanced CT image demonstrates complete fatty replacement (*arrow*) of the pancreatic parenchyma.

Complete fatty replacement of the pancreatic bed can result in severe pancreatic enzyme insufficiency, which can lead to malabsorption, steatorrhea, or hypoproteinemia. Focal fatty replacement can be patchy or consist of multiple tiny fatty nodules throughout the pancreas. It may mimic a pancreatic neoplasm. Although CT can detect the fat in the majority of these lesions, chemical shift MRI has been found to be more specific and helpful in the diagnosis of milder degrees of fat attenuation.[6] On US, fatty infiltration will appear hyperechoic relative to the normal pancreas, while CT will show typical fat attenuation distributed within the pancreas. MR will demonstrate increased T1 signal with decreased signal on fat-suppressed images.

## PANCREATITIS

Imaging is helpful in determining the severity of the disease and presence of complications or in excluding other potential causes for abdominal pain. The presence of at least two of the following three conditions is required to fulfill the clinical criteria for the diagnosis of acute pancreatitis: acute upper abdominal or epigastric pain, serum amylase or lipase of at least three times the normal levels (ranges: lipase, 30 to 210 IU/L; amylase, 30 to 110 IU/L), or typical CT findings.[7] There are numerous causes, including alcohol abuse, gallstone impaction (Fig. 10A.10), metabolic disturbances, trauma, idiopathic, infection, and malignancy. The inflamed pancreatic tissue subsequently leaks pancreatic enzymes into the surrounding tissues causing further inflammation. Mortality can vary based on the severity and subtype, ranging from 3% edematous pancreatitis to 15% with necrotizing pancreatitis.

### Acute Pancreatitis

Routine utilization of CT for the diagnosis of acute pancreatitis is not warranted, and the diagnosis is primarily based on the typical clinical presentation along with laboratory

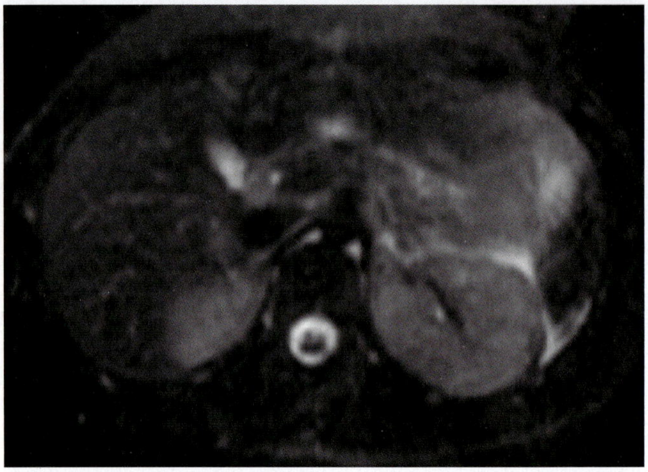

**FIG. 10A.9 • Acute pancreatitis.** T2WI with fat suppression demonstrates mild pancreatic edema and peripancreatic T2 hyperintensity due to inflammation.

parameters. CT is, however, indicated to exclude malignancy in patients older than 40 years of age presenting with pancreatitis for the first time without an identifiable cause. The optimal time for assessing acute complications of acute pancreatitis is approximately 72 hours after symptom onset.[8] Contrast-enhanced CT is the ideal method of assessment of pancreatitis. Unenhanced and contrast enhanced in the pancreatic phase (40 seconds after injection) is used for the assessment of necrosis and complications. US is the most appropriate test for evaluation of gallstones for initial presentation of acute pancreatitis in patients with typical clinical presentation and elevated amylase levels. MRI may be used as adjuncts, mainly for detection of gallstones or common bile duct stones, or for characterization of fluid collections (Figs. 10A.9 and 10A.10).

Typically, the pancreas will appear enlarged and edematous and will have surrounding inflammatory changes

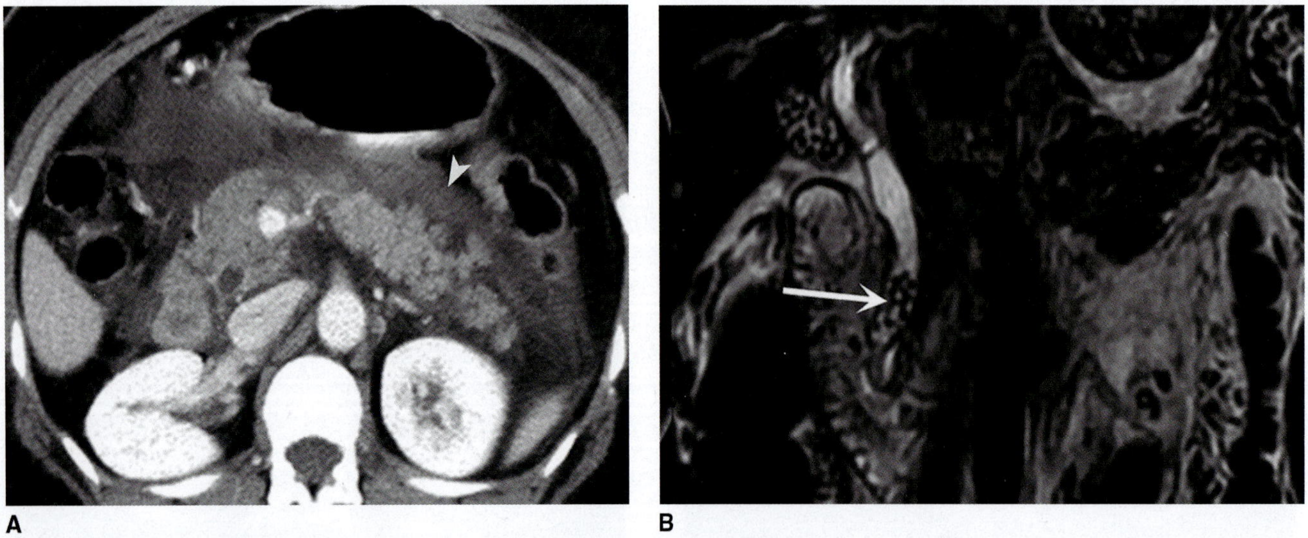

**FIG. 10A.10 • Acute gallstone pancreatitis. A:** Axial contrast-enhanced CT demonstrates peripancreatic edema and inflammation (*arrowhead*). **B:** Corresponding coronal MRCP image demonstrates numerous filling defects within the gall bladder and distal common bile duct (*arrow*), with dilatation of the common bile duct.

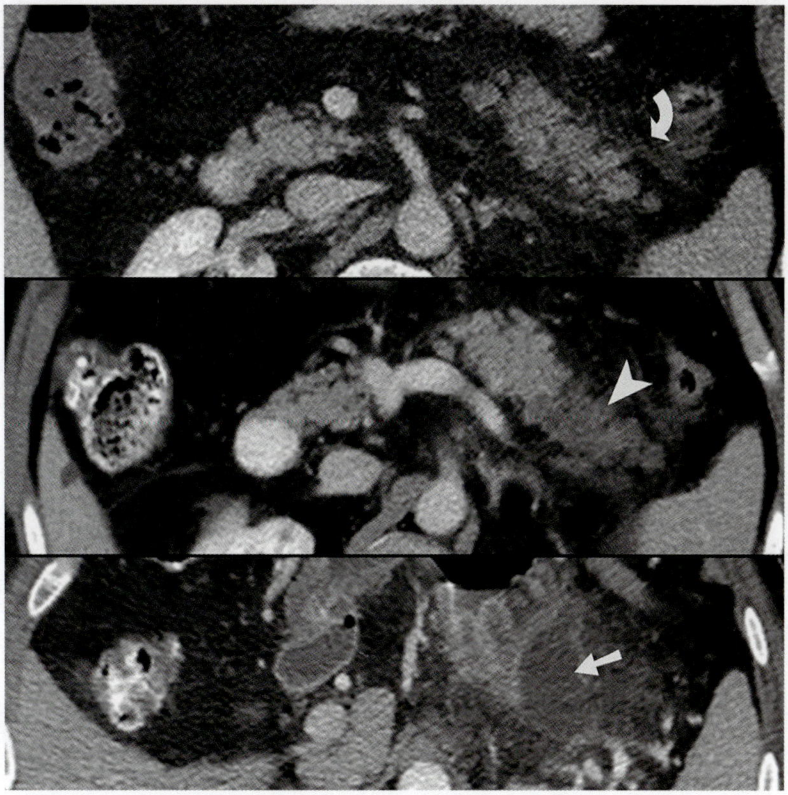

**FIG. 10A.11 • Acute pancreatitis.** Axial contrast-enhanced CT performed few weeks apart shows peripancreatic inflammation (*curved arrow*) on the first, pancreatic necrosis (*arrowhead*) on the second, and subsequent pseudocyst (*arrow*) formation on the third image.

blurring the mesenteric fat planes. Additional imaging findings are based on the presence or absence of local complications (Fig. 10A.11). CT is also used to stratify the severity of pancreatitis and is the only imaging modality, which correlates with clinical severity of the disease. Acute pancreatitis severity is divided into mild, moderate, and severe varieties based on the presence of organ failure or the presence of local or systemic complications.[9]

- Mild pancreatitis: no end organ dysfunction or local complications; good prognosis; no imaging required
- Moderate pancreatitis: end organ failure lasting less than 48 hours with or without complications
- Severe pancreatitis: end organ failure lasting for more than 48 hours with local complications

## Complications of Pancreatitis

Necrotizing pancreatitis: It occurs in approximately 20% of cases of acute pancreatitis. There are three subtypes of necrotizing pancreatitis: necrosis of pancreatic parenchyma with sparing of peripancreatic tissues (5%), necrosis of peripancreatic tissue with parenchymal sparing (20%), or involvement of both (75%). CT detects necrosis best after 72 hours of symptom onset. Necrosis of the pancreas can be focal (Fig. 10A.12) or segmental or involve the majority of the gland and can be sterile or infectious. Necrosis is identified as areas of nonenhancing, intermediate attenuation pancreatic tissue in a background of heterogeneously enhancing parenchyma. It appears hyperintense on T2-weighted MR imaging with no enhancement on postcontrast MRI (Fig. 10A.13). The percentage of necrotic parenchyma has a prognostic significance and must be estimated.

Peripancreatic necrosis involves the retroperitoneal fat and is more difficult to detect with imaging. Contrast-enhanced CT will depict areas of heterogeneous peripancreatic enhancement, which may contain liquefied or nonliquefied contents. Fluid collections occurring in or around the pancreas within the first 4 weeks of the onset of necrotizing pancreatitis are termed acute necrotic collections.[10] On CT, they appear as a heterogeneous collection containing hemorrhage, fat, or necrotic fat in the presence of acute necrotic pancreatitis (Fig. 10A.14). With time, a well-defined wall develops around these collections,

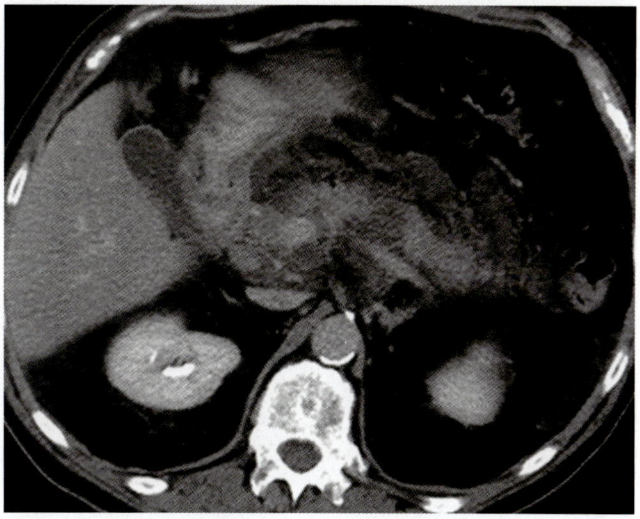

**FIG. 10A.12 • Focal pancreatic necrosis.** Axial contrast-enhanced CT demonstrates changes of acute pancreatitis with a focal nonenhancing area in the pancreatic body, consistent with focal necrosis.

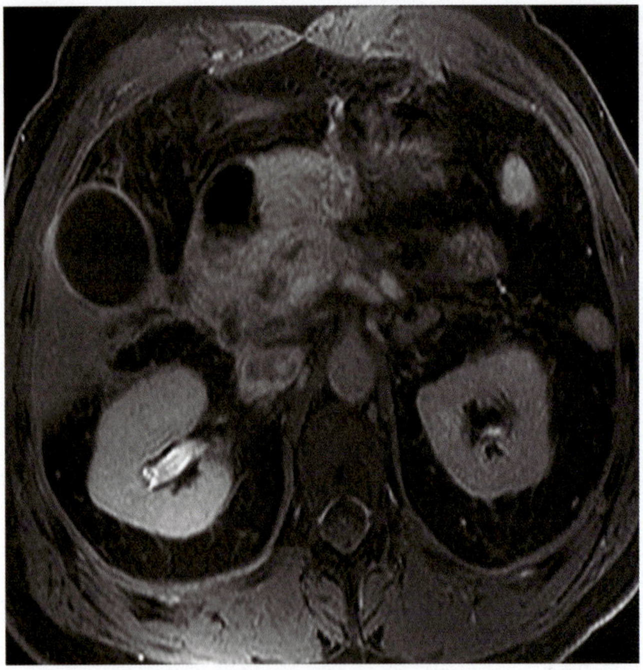

**FIG. 10A.13 • Necrotizing pancreatitis.** Axial contrast-enhanced T1WI shows foci of hypointensity in the pancreatic head from necrosis.

and after 4 weeks, the collection is referred to as walled-off necrosis (Fig. 10A.15). Infection may further complicate these collections, more likely in necrotizing pancreatitis than in acute interstitial pancreatitis associated fluid collections, and is suggested by the presence of gas within the collections along with suggestive clinical findings (Fig. 10A.16).

Hemorrhage: High attenuation on noncontrast CT scans involving either the pancreatic parenchyma or the surrounding fatty tissue is concerning for hemorrhage. MRI will demonstrate increased signal on fat-suppressed T1WI and typically decreased signal on T2WI.

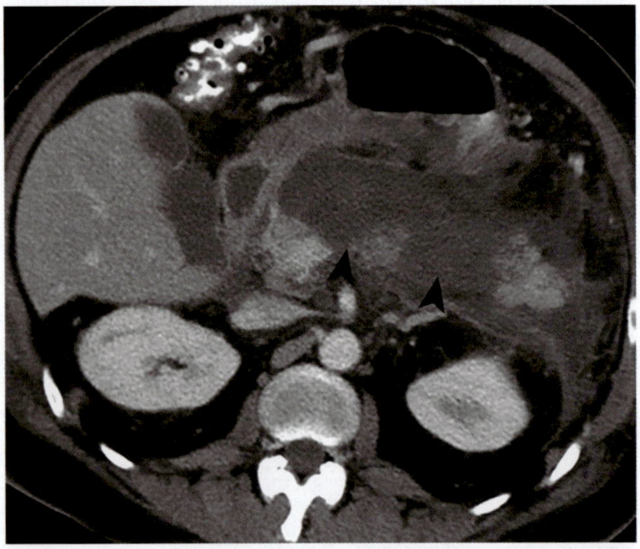

**FIG. 10A.14 • Acute necrotic collection.** Axial contrast-enhanced CT demonstrates a heterogeneous fluid collection encompassing the majority of the pancreatic and peripancreatic tissues, with surrounding fat stranding and inflammation. There are areas of nonenhancement in the pancreas from necrosis (*arrowheads*).

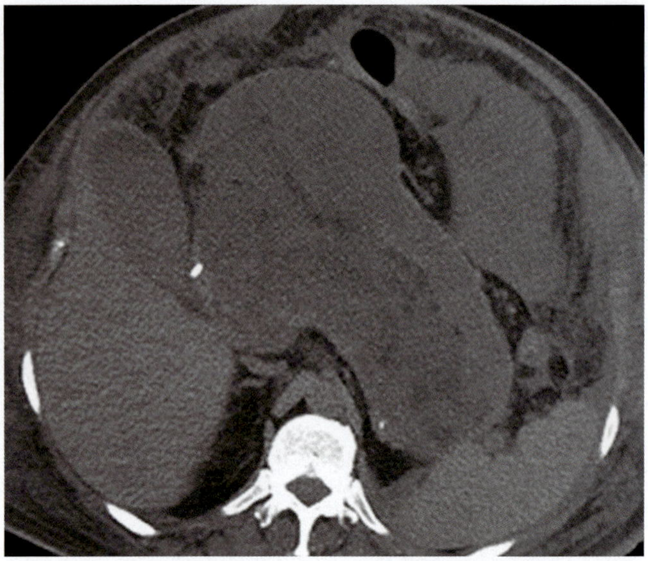

**FIG. 10A.15 • Walled-off pancreatic necrosis.** Axial noncontrast CT demonstrates the formation of a walled-off peripancreatic fluid collection in this patient with necrotizing pancreatitis. Imaging was obtained greater than 4 weeks after the initial presentation.

Pseudocyst (described below): A pseudocyst can typically form 4 weeks after an episode of acute pancreatitis.

Abscess: Infected collections around the pancreas are usually secondary to infection of liquefactive tissue necrosis, although infected pancreatic pseudocysts can have a similar appearance. They typically appear as a well-circumscribed fluid collection, with or without internal gas. Like abscesses in other locations, rim enhancement and surrounding inflammatory changes are helpful in making the diagnosis with contrast-enhanced CT. Terms such as "phlegmon," "pancreatic abscess," "organized necrosis," "sequestration," or "necroma" should no longer be used in relation to pancreatitis. MRI will typically demonstrate low T1 and high T2 signal, without internal enhancement. Diffusion-weighted imaging (DWI) will demonstrate restricted diffusion within the infected collection.

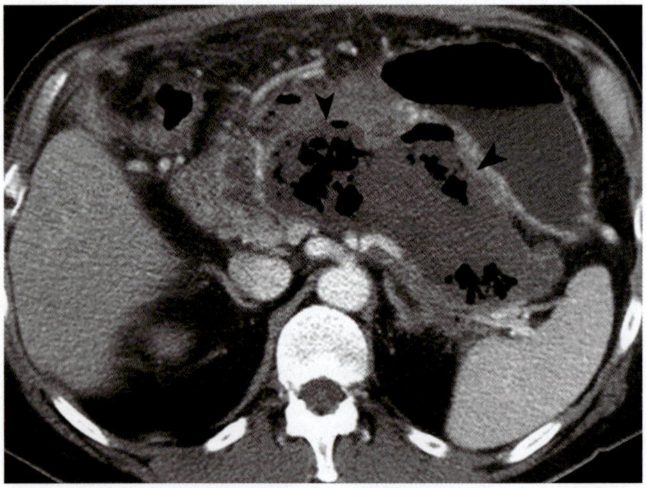

**FIG. 10A.16 • Infected fluid collection in necrotizing pancreatitis.** Contrast-enhanced CT demonstrates a large peripancreatic fluid collection (*arrowheads*) with internal foci of air and surrounding inflammatory changes.

Percutaneous drain insertion is required in the treatment of any infected collection.

Pseudoaneurysm: Pancreatic enzymes can erode vessel walls, resulting in the formation of a pseudoaneurysm. This typically will affect the splenic and gastroduodenal arteries and can occur in up to 10% of cases of acute pancreatitis. Color Doppler US can depict the to-and-fro spectral waveform at the neck of the pseudoaneurysm and a yin–yang pattern in the sac (Fig. 10A.17A). CT or MR angiography will demonstrate a well-circumscribed enhancing structure arising from the artery. This can appear hyperdense on nonenhanced scans if the pseudoaneurysm is thrombosed, or it can fill with contrast on postcontrast images (Figs. 10A.17B and 10A.18).

Venous thrombosis: Pancreatitis can result in thrombosis of the surrounding venous structures, including the portal, splenic, and superior mesenteric veins. This typically appears as a low attenuating filling defect on a contrast-enhanced CT (Fig. 10A.19). Enhancement of the thrombus on both CT and MR raises concern for tumor thrombus, as opposed to bland thrombus related to pancreatitis.

## Chronic Pancreatitis

Chronic pancreatitis is defined by irreversible damage to the pancreas from recurrent episodes of pancreatitis. The persistent inflammation causes a fibrotic response with subsequent atrophy and abnormal function. Although alcohol abuse is the most common etiology, gallstones and autoimmune pancreatitis also play a role. On imaging, CT and MR can demonstrate a beaded appearance of the pancreatic duct, with alternating areas of dilatation and constriction. This is in contrast to pancreatic carcinoma, where a smooth dilatation of the pancreatic duct is often seen. There is atrophy of the pancreatic

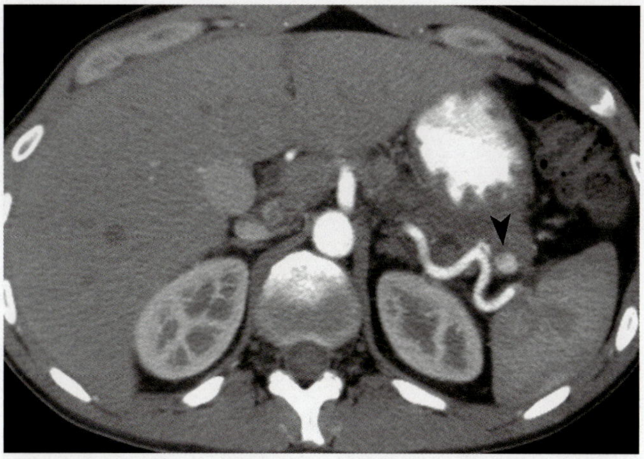

**FIG. 10A.18 • Splenic artery pseudoaneurysm.** Axial contrast-enhanced CT demonstrates a 1 cm pseudoaneurysm (*arrowhead*) supplied by a splenic artery branch.

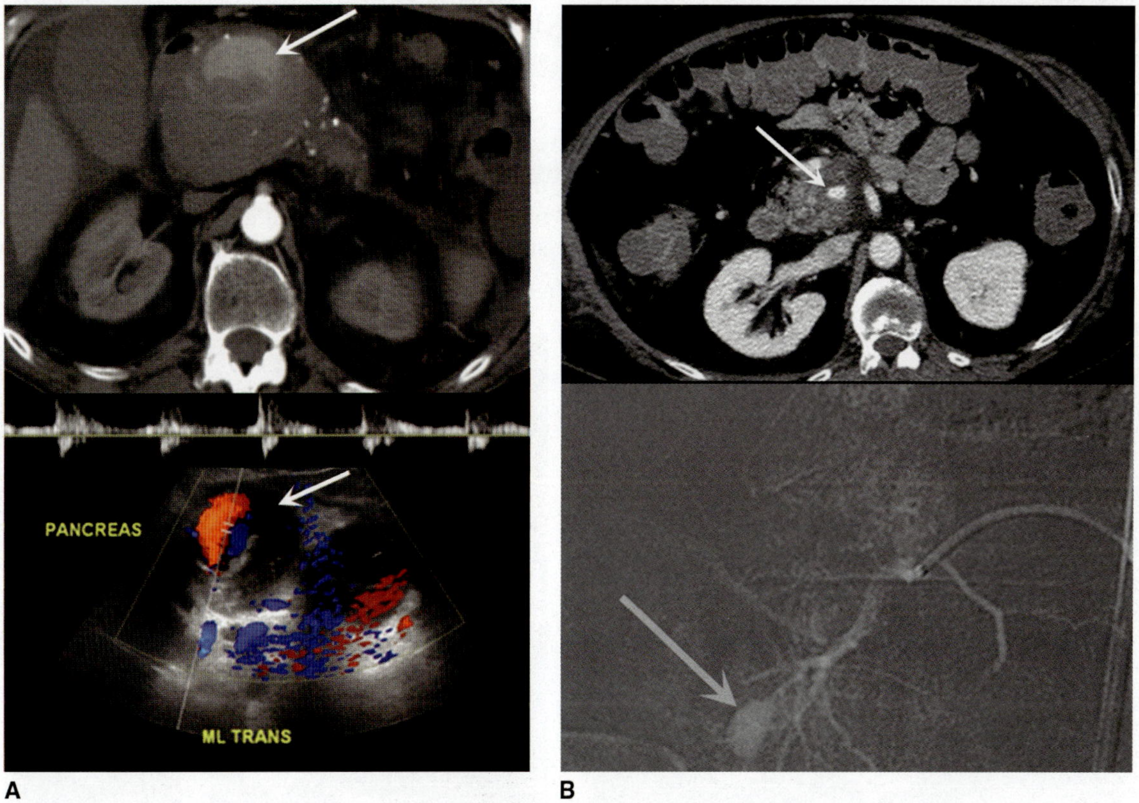


**FIG. 10A.17 • Gastroduodenal artery pseudoaneurysm. A:** Axial arterial phase CT demonstrates a large enhancing vessel in relation to pancreatic head, which is partially thrombosed (*arrow*). Corresponding color Doppler image demonstrates "yin–yang" color flow appearance within the aneurysmal sac (*arrow*). **B:** Contrast-enhanced CT demonstrates an abnormally enhancing focus within the pancreatic parenchyma (*arrow*), in this patient with history of recurrent pancreatitis. Contrast angiogram demonstrates pseudoaneurysm (*arrow*) supplied by gastroduodenal artery branch.

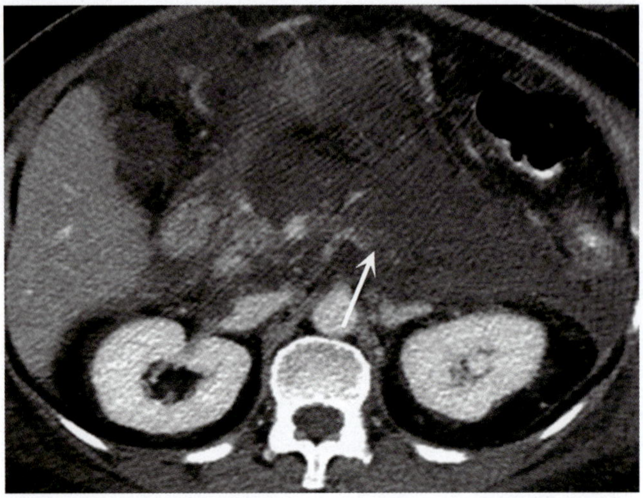

**FIG. 10A.19 • Splenic vein thrombosis.** Axial CT demonstrates a filling defect in the region of the splenic vein (*arrow*), located to necrotizing pancreatitis.

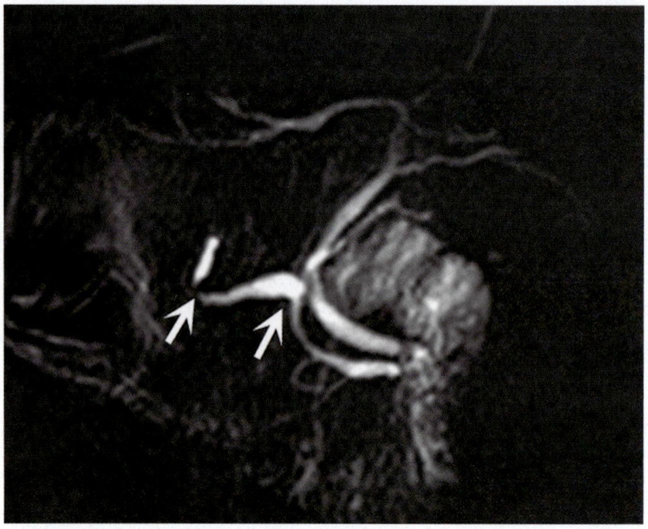

**FIG. 10A.21 • Chronic pancreatitis.** Coronal MRCP image demonstrates areas of focal narrowing (*arrows*) and dilatation of the pancreatic duct, secondary to a patient's history of chronic pancreatitis.

parenchyma, often with calcifications (Fig. 10A.20). There can also be focal fibrous enlargement that can mimic a mass lesion, typically in the pancreatic head. Biliary obstruction occurs in up to 3% to 23% of patients secondary to narrowing of the common bile duct within the pancreatic head.[11] MRCP can demonstrate dilatation of the pancreatic duct (Fig. 10A.21) with filling defects from intraductal stones. There is typically loss of the normal T1 hyperintense signal seen in the pancreatic parenchyma, with a variable enhancement pattern depending on the presence of long-term complications such as pseudocyst formation.

*Groove pancreatitis* is a subtype of chronic pancreatitis involving the pancreaticoduodenal groove. This is bordered by the pancreatic head medially, the second portion of the duodenum laterally, and the distal common bile duct posteriorly. Clinically, a purely groove pancreatitis can result in stenosis of the pancreatic duct and lead to a more diffuse pancreatitis. On CT, this will manifest as a hypodense mass within the groove, with inflammatory changes of the adjacent duodenum. There can be narrowing of both the pancreatic and common bile ducts. MRI will characteristically demonstrate a sheet-like mass within the groove that is hypointense on T1WI and of variable signal intensity on T2WI. Postcontrast images will demonstrate heterogeneous enhancement secondary to the associated fibrosis.

*Autoimmune pancreatitis* is an additional form of pancreatitis, possibly related to IgG4. These patients often have other autoimmune disorders such as Sjogren syndrome and ulcerative colitis. Imaging features include diffuse enlargement of the pancreas with a peripheral halo of hypoattenuation on CT (Fig. 10A.22) or hypointense signal on T2WI.

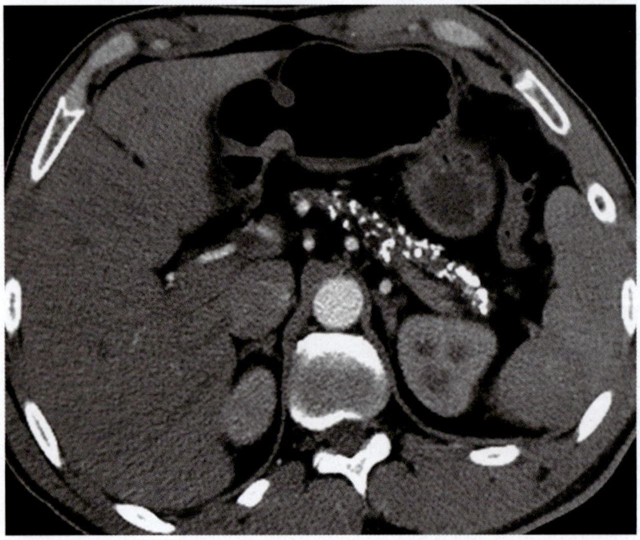

**FIG. 10A.20 • Chronic pancreatitis.** Axial CT image demonstrates atrophied pancreatic parenchyma, containing several coarse calcifications.

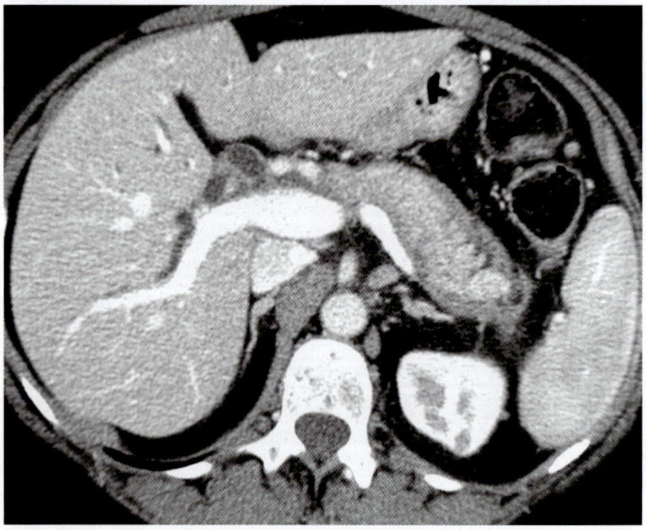

**FIG. 10A.22 • Autoimmune pancreatitis.** Axial contrast-enhanced CT demonstrates the enlarged pancreas with a hypoattenuating rim seen adjacent to the splenic vein.

There is typically no vascular involvement, calcification, or pseudocyst formation, and the pancreatic duct is diffusely narrowed. Enhancement on CT can be variable, and there is characteristically a lack of peripancreatic fatty stranding. MRCP can demonstrate multiple strictures of the biliary and pancreatic ducts, similar to findings seen in primary sclerosing cholangitis.[12] The patients typically respond well to steroid administration.

## PANCREATIC PSEUDOCYST

Collections associated with acute interstitial pancreatitis can be subclassified on the basis of the length of time between symptom onset and development of the collection, the presence of a wall surrounding the collection, or the presence of infection.

In the first 4 weeks after development of acute interstitial pancreatitis, nonencapsulated fluid can be seen surrounding the pancreas and is termed an acute peripancreatic fluid collection. On CT, the contents of this collection are uniformly hypoattenuating without solid components or internal enhancement. These collections usually resolve spontaneously without needing drainage.

About 4 weeks after the onset of acute pancreatitis, these fluid collections may develop a capsule around them and are termed pseudocysts (Fig. 10A.23). Fluid collections associated with acute interstitial pancreatitis should always develop in the peripancreatic tissues rather than the pancreatic parenchyma, in which case it should be considered a necrotizing process. These cysts can communicate with the pancreatic duct, and patients will have symptoms based on the size and associated mass effect.

On US, these cysts will typically appear well circumscribed with posterior enhancement. Complicated pseudocysts will have internal echoes and septations and can appear multilocular. On CT, these are typically hypodense lesions with water attenuation. The fibrous capsule may enhance, and internal foci of air raise the possibility of infection, although rare. Increased internal density also raises suspicion for internal hemorrhage. On MR, the pseudocyst is hypointense on T1WI with well-defined enhancing margin (Fig. 10A.24). On MRI, mostly fluid-containing cysts are hyperintense on T2WI, while those with internal debris and other contents have mixed signal intensity. Identifying internal mural nodules on MRI can be helpful in distinguishing between a benign pseudocyst and a malignant cystic lesion.

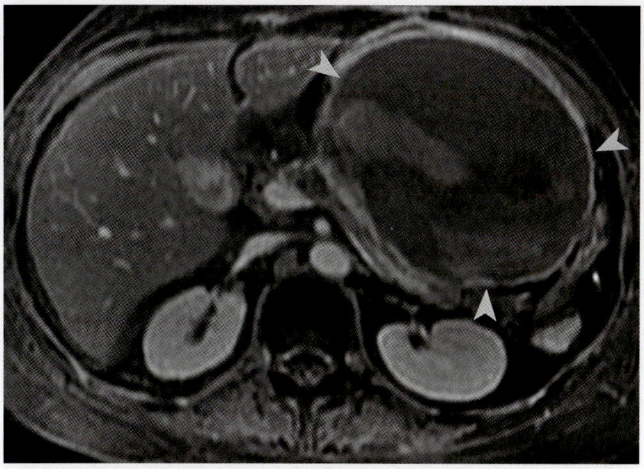

**FIG. 10A.24 • Pancreatic pseudocyst.** Postcontrast T1WI demonstrates a large pseudocyst (*arrowheads*) with enhancing rim. There is a dependent clot within the pseudocyst.

## TRAUMA

Pancreatic injuries secondary to blunt abdominal trauma are rare, with a relative incidence of 1% to 2%.[13] They are graded based on the presence of contusion, parenchymal injury, major ductal injury, or crush injury.

CT can demonstrate abnormal pancreatic contours with increased size, surrounding fatty infiltrative changes, variable

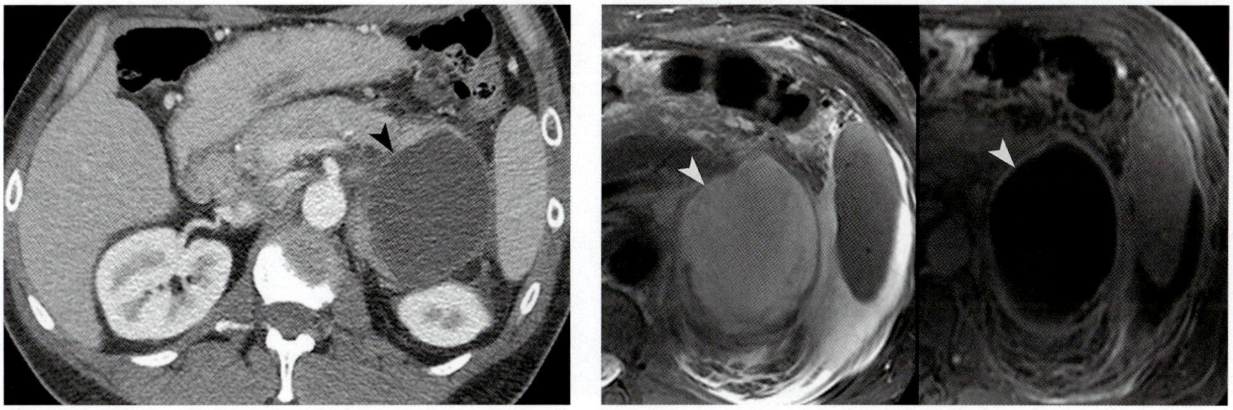

A B

**FIG. 10A.23 • Pancreatic pseudocyst. A:** Axial contrast-enhanced CT demonstrates a large hypoattenuating fluid collection (*arrowhead*) adjacent to the pancreatic tail, with enhancing capsule, in a patient with a history of pancreatitis 2 months prior. **B:** T2WI and postcontrast T1WI of the same patient demonstrate T2 hyperintense signal with enhancing rim (*arrowheads*), consistent with pseudocyst formation.

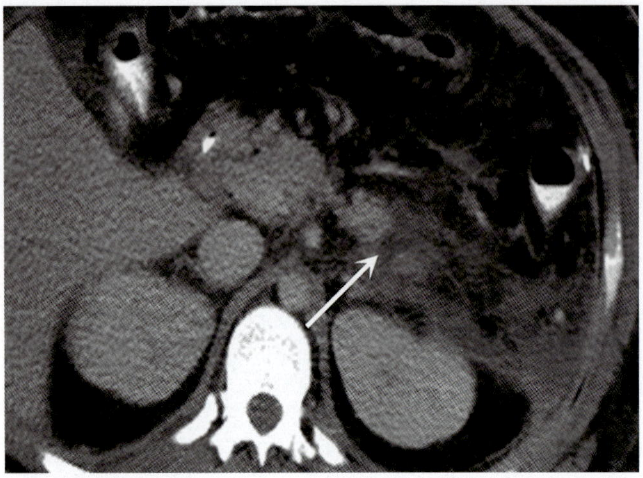

**FIG. 10A.25 • Pancreatic trauma.** Axial CT image in a patient with a history of motor vehicle accident demonstrates a laceration (*arrow*) through the pancreatic tail with fluid and surrounding inflammatory changes.

attenuation of the parenchyma, laceration, or fracture (Fig. 10A.25). MRCP can be helpful in evaluating ductal integrity, while MRI will demonstrate decreased T1 signal intensity and heterogeneous enhancement on postcontrast images. If initial injuries are not detected at admission, there is increased risk of further complications including abscess, fistula, and pseudocyst formation. Mortality rates can approach 30% with most deaths occurring within 48 hours of the traumatic event.

## PANCREATIC SARCOIDOSIS

Sarcoidosis is a granulomatous disease that can involve multiple different organ systems. Pancreatic sarcoidosis, although extremely rare, has been reported both with pancreatic parenchymal or peripancreatic lymph node involvement. The mass can mimic pancreatic adenocarcinoma and is more commonly seen in the pancreatic head. There can be associated obstruction of the common bile or pancreatic ducts, with patients presenting with abdominal pain and obstructive jaundice. The lesions will appear hypoechoic on US and hypoattenuating on CT. MRI demonstrates T1 hypointense signal and T2 hyperintense signal, without contrast enhancement.

## INTRAPANCREATIC ACCESSORY SPLEEN

Ectopic splenic tissue within the pancreatic parenchyma is rarely detected on imaging due to its small size. However, the pancreatic tail is a frequent location demonstrated on up to 10% to 30% of autopsies.[14] When visible, these lesions will appear as well-defined masses with imaging characteristics similar to splenic parenchyma. They will be isodense to the spleen on all phases of CT and subsequently will appear hyperdense to the pancreas (Fig. 10A.26). On MRI, intrapancreatic accessory spleens will appear hypointense on T1WI and hyperintense on T2WI, relative to the pancreas. Diagnosis can be confirmed with nuclear medicine sulfur colloid scans, demonstrating increased radiotracer uptake in the suspected accessory spleen.

## PANCREATIC HEMANGIOMA

Pancreatic hemangiomas are rarely seen. CT typically demonstrates well-circumscribed hypoattenuating lesions, which enhance after contrast administration.[15] Similar to cavernous hemangiomas, they will appear isointense on T1WI and hyperintense on T2WI.

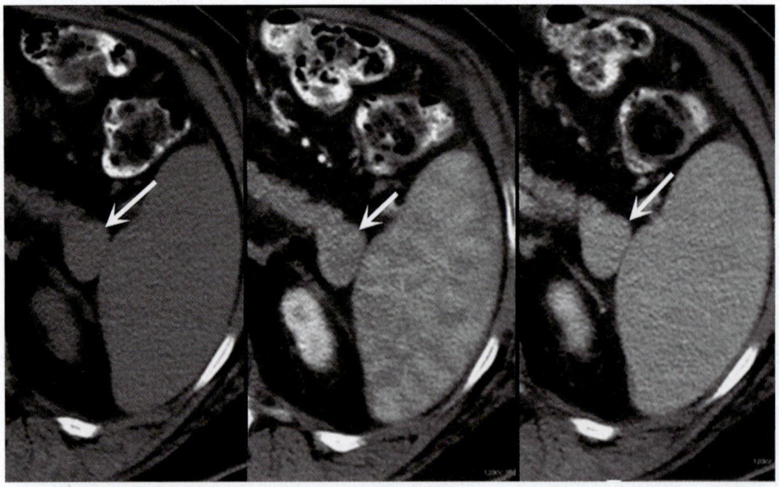

**FIG. 10A.26 • Accessory spleen mimicking pancreatic mass.** Noncontrast, arterial phase, and portal venous phase CT images demonstrate a focal lesion (*arrows*) within the pancreatic tail that is isodense to the spleen in all phases.

## References


1. Borghei P, Sokhandon F, Shirkhoda A, et al. Anomalies, anatomic variants, and sources of diagnostic pitfalls in pancreatic imaging. *Radiology.* 2013;266(1):28–36.
2. Soto JA, Lucey BC, Stuhlfaut JW. Pancreas divisum: depiction with multi-detector row CT. *Radiology.* 2005;235(2):503–508.
3. Mortelé KJ, Rocha TC, Streeter JL, et al. Multimodality imaging of pancreatic and biliary congenital anomalies. *Radiographics.* 2006;26(3):715–731.
4. Olsen TS. Lipomatosis of the pancreas in autopsy material and its relation to age and overweight. *Acta Pathol Microbiol Scand.* 1978;86: 367–373.
5. Soyer P, Spelle L, Pelage JP, et al. Cystic fibrosis in adolescents and adults: fatty replacement of the pancreas—CT evaluation and functional correlation. *Radiology.* 1999;210(3):611–615.
6. Kim HJ, Byun JH, Park SH, et al. Focal fatty replacement of the pancreas: usefulness of chemical shift MRI. *AJR Am J Roentgenol.* 2007;188(2):429–432.
7. Sarr MG. IAP guidelines in acute pancreatitis. *Dig Surg.* 2003;20: 1–3.
8. Thoeni RF. The revised Atlanta classification of acute pancreatitis: its importance for the radiologist and its effect on treatment. *Radiology.* 2012;262:751–764.
9. Dellinger EP, Forsmark CE, Layer P, et al. Determinant-based classification of acute pancreatitis severity: an international multidisciplinary consultation. *Ann Surg.* 2012;256:875–880.
10. Banks PA, Bollen TL, Dervenis C, et al. Classification of Acute Pancreatitis-2012: Revision of the Atlanta classification and definitions by international consensus. *Gut.* 2013;62:102–111.
11. Dumonceau, J-M, Carlos M-G. Endoscopic management of complications of chronic pancreatitis. *World J Gastroenterol.* 2013;19(42): 7308–7315.
12. Khandelwal A, Shanbhogue AK, Takahashi N, et al. Recent advances in the diagnosis and management of autoimmune pancreatitis. *AJR Am J Roentgenol.* 2014;202(5):1007–1021.
13. Gupta A, Stuhlfaut JW, Fleming KW, et al. Blunt trauma of the pancreas and biliary tract: a multimodality imaging approach to diagnosis. *Radiographics.* 2004;24(5):1381–1395.
14. Low G, Panu A, Millo N, et al. Multimodality imaging of neoplastic and nonneoplastic solid lesions of the pancreas. *Radiographics.* 2011;31(4):993–1015.
15. Mundinger GS, Gust S, Micchelli ST, et al. Adult pancreatic hemangioma: case report and literature review. *Gastroenterol Res Pract.* 2009;2009:839730.


## SELF-ASSESSMENT QUESTIONS

1. What is the pathology (arrowhead) depicted on the CT study of a patient with a recent history of pancreatitis?

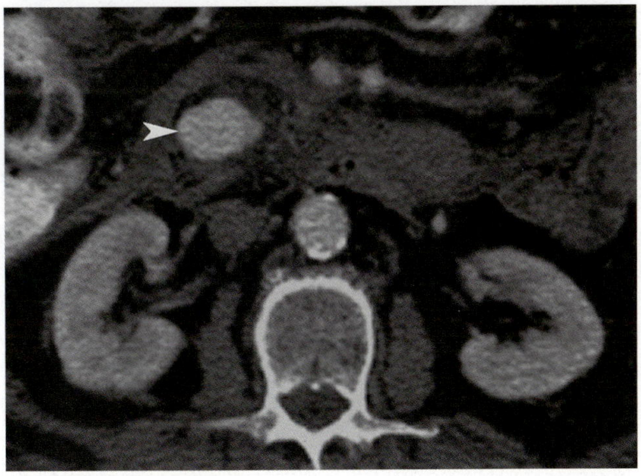

A. Islet cell tumor
B. Pseudoaneurysm
C. Accessory spleen
D. Metastases

2. What is the CT finding in a patient with abdominal pain after a motor vehicle accident?

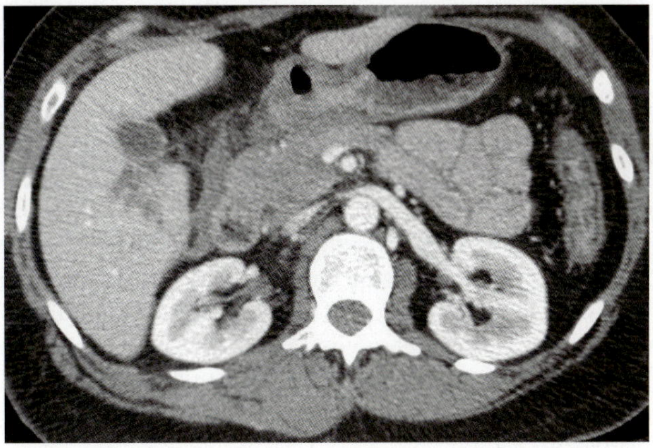

A. Liver laceration and pancreatic contusion
B. Acute pancreatitis
C. Portal vein thrombosis
D. Aortic rupture

### Answers to Self-Assessment Questions

**1. B.** Aneurysm. The contrast-enhanced CT depicts a gastroduodenal artery pseudoaneurysm (arrowhead), which is most often seen with pancreatitis or trauma.

**2. A.** Liver laceration and pancreatic contusion. The contrast-enhanced CT shows branching hepatic laceration located posterior to the gall bladder fossa. There is edema in the pancreatic head and peripancreatic fluid.

# Pancreas: Neoplastic Diseases

# 10B

*Caterina Missiroli and Ajay K. Singh*

## LEARNING OBJECTIVE

**1.** Describe the indications and important imaging features of neoplastic conditions of the pancreas.

Pancreatic tumors have a very poor prognosis, with a 4-month mean survival after diagnosis. An early and accurate diagnosis is important in the management of pancreatic lesions to exclude nonneoplastic diseases. Because an accurate evaluation of the lesions can be challenging, multimodality imaging approach is often necessary for diagnosis, including radiologic imaging modalities.[1,2]

CT is the imaging modality of choice for the detection and staging of the pancreatic neoplasm.[3] The aim of imaging is to detect the neoplastic mass as well as investigate vascular encasement and extrapancreatic extension. A pancreatic protocol CT is a dual-phase CT, consisting of pancreatic parenchymal phase (at 40 seconds, best to detect tumor in pancreatic parenchyma), followed by portal venous phase imaging at 60 to 70 seconds.[4] CT slice thickness of 2.5 mm is the most important parameter in evaluation of suspected pancreatic neoplastic lesions, allowing the detection of the tumor and the depiction of vascular invasion for determination of respectability of the tumor.[3] MR can be a problem-solving tool in patients who have suspected pancreatic cancer with nonconclusive US or CT investigation and in the follow-up for pancreatic tumor (primarily cystic).[5]

## ADENOCARCINOMA

Adenocarcinoma accounts about 90% of pancreatic neoplastic lesions, being the fourth cause of deaths in oncology patients. They are most commonly seen in 60- to 80-year-old males (M:F = 2:1).[2]

Location: Head of the pancreas is 60% to 70%, body is 10% to 20%, and tail is 5% to 10%. The prognosis of adenocarcinoma is poor (less than 20% of survivors at 1 year and less than 5% at 5 years).[2] The only treatment potentially curative that can increase the prognosis is surgery (20% survival within 5 years),[7] but unresectable disease is seen at presentation in 75% of patients and metastases (liver, lymph nodes, and peritoneum) are present in 85% of these patients.[2] CT has an accuracy of 85% to 95% for tumor detection, with a positive predictive value of 89% to 100% for unresectability and a negative predictive value of 45% to 79% for resectability.[2]

The CT findings include visualization of a hypovascular solid lesion ranging 1.5 to 10 cm in diameter (mean size 3 cm, with the body tumors larger than the head-located lesions) (Fig. 10B.1). Approximately 10% of tumors are isoattenuating and can be suspected by mass effects such as abnormal convex contour of the pancreas, ductal obstruction, vascular invasion, perivascular invasion, vascular thrombosis, and collateral vessels (Fig. 10B.2). On MR, adenocarcinoma has low signal intensity both on T1- and T2WI due to the scirrhous fibrotic nature and is hypovascular at postcontrast images. MR is superior than CT in detecting small tumors and liver metastases: the accuracy of MR imaging staging adenocarcinoma is 90% to 100%[2] (Fig. 10B.3).

Imaging features, which indicate unresectability (T4 disease) of pancreatic adenocarcinoma include (Fig. 10B.4) the following:

1. Celiac, superior mesenteric artery, common hepatic artery, or hepatic artery proper involvement. More than 180 degrees contact between the artery and tumor indicates arterial encasement.
2. Distant metastases.
3. Extrapancreatic invasion of adjacent organs. Pancreatic tail masses are mostly unresectable because of delay in diagnosis.
4. Tumors are more than 3 cm in size.

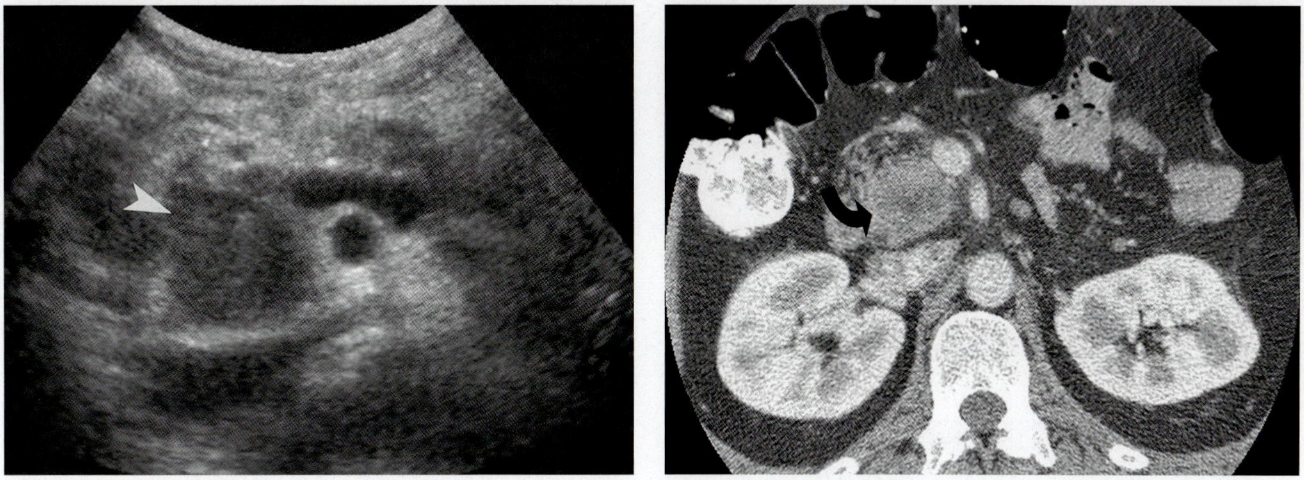

A B

**FIG. 10B.1 • Pancreatic adenocarcinoma. A:** US abdomen demonstrates a solid mass (*arrowhead*) in the pancreatic head without pancreatic ductal dilatation. **B:** Axial contrast-enhanced CT demonstrates a heterogeneous mass lesion (*curved arrow*) in the head and uncinate process of the pancreas with ill definition of the outer margin.

## CYSTIC PANCREATIC TUMORS

Cystic tumors seen in the pancreas include intraductal papillary mucinous neoplasm (IPMN), mucinous cystic neoplasm, serous cystadenoma, and solid lesions with cystic degeneration (e.g., neuroendocrine tumors, solid pseudopapillary neoplasms, and adenocarcinoma). CT and MR are not so accurate in histologic diagnosis (50%), but are useful in distinguishing aggressive from benign diseases (75% to 90%).[4]

### Intraductal Papillary Mucinous Neoplasm

IPMN arise from the mucinous epithelium of pancreatic ducts and growth intraductally, with mucin production, leading to ductal dilatation.[4] Most pancreatic cysts seen on imaging are presumed to be IPMN because these tumors are widely prevalent in patients with cystic pancreatic lesions (Fig. 10B.5). They are classified into:

1. Main-duct IPMN (higher malignancy risk)
2. Side-branch IPMN (most often in head and neck)

They occur more commonly in men (M:F = 3:2), with a mean age of 65 years (range 36 to 84 years).[4,8] The main imaging features are listed in Table 10B.1. Increased prevalence (about 30%) of synchronous or metachronous malignant neoplasms of other organs (e.g., stomach, colon, rectum, lung, breast, and liver) has been described in literature by some authors.[4] Treatment involve surgical resection of main-duct, mixed-type, and side-branch IPMN (measuring greater than 3 cm). Surgical resection of asymptomatic side-branch IPMN smaller than 3 cm is recommended only if mural nodules, positive cytologic findings, or rapid cyst growth are present. Small less than 1 cm side-branch IPMN without malignant degeneration features may be followed up by imaging (EUS, CT, or MR)[4] (Fig. 10B.5C).

### Mucinous Cystic Neoplasm

Mucinous cystic neoplasms are mucin production tumors with malignant potential, almost exclusively seen in middle-aged females (mean age of 47 years). They are more common

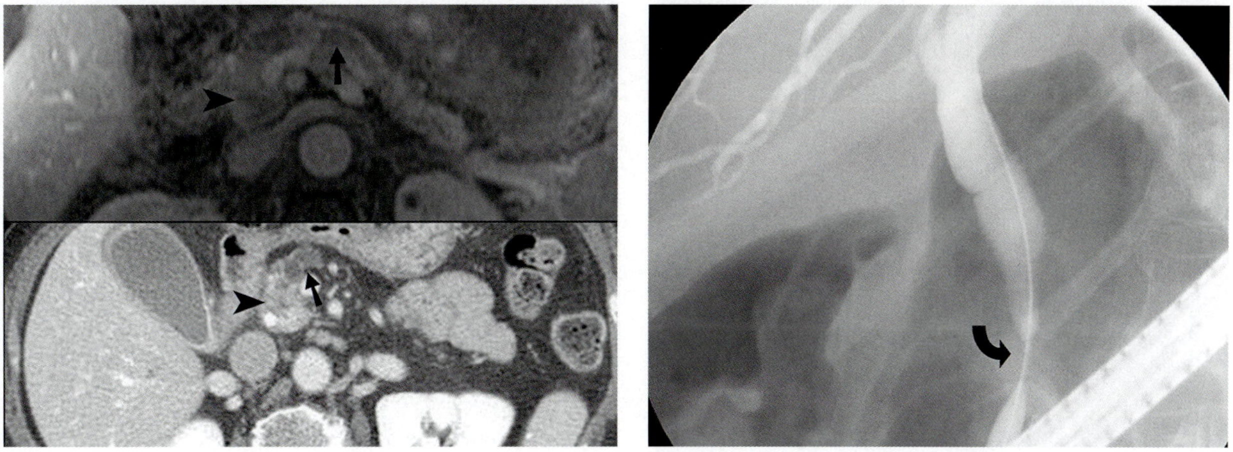

A B

**FIG. 10B.2 • Adenocarcinoma of the pancreas with biliary obstruction.** Axial contrast-enhanced T1WI and contrast-enhanced CT (**A**) demonstrate a heterogenous pancreatic head mass (*arrowhead*) with pancreatic ductal dilatation (*straight arrow*). Spot fluoroscopy image (**B**) demonstrates the narrowing (*curved arrow*) at the lower end of the common bile duct due the pancreatic head neoplasm.

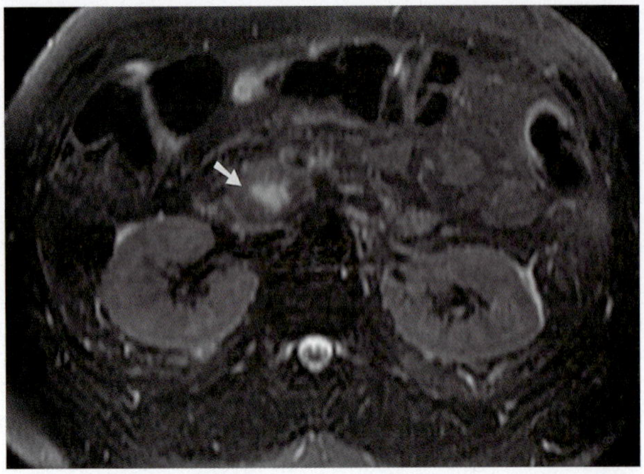

A

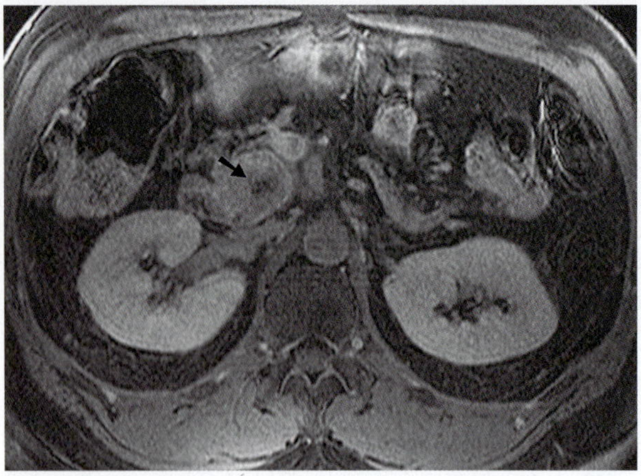

B

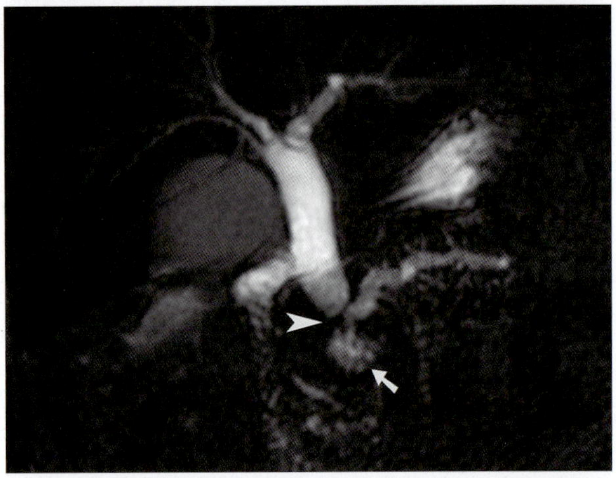

C

**FIG. 10B.3 • Adenocarcinoma of the pancreas on MRI.** **A, B:** T2WI and postgadolinium T1WI demonstrate a heterogeneous signal intensity mass lesion in the pancreatic head with central area of necrosis (*arrow*). **C:** MRCP study of the same patient demonstrates the dilated CBD and pancreatic duct with blunt tapered narrowing in the pancreatic head (*arrowhead*) due to the pancreatic head mass lesion. The necrosis within the pancreatic head mass lesion is visualized on the MRCP sequences as hyperintense lesion (*arrow*).

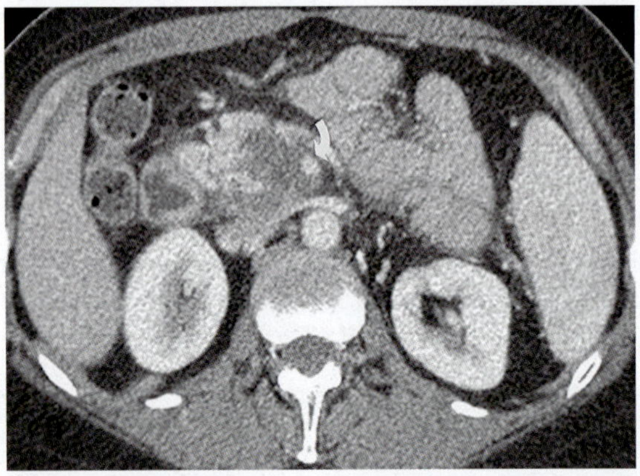

A

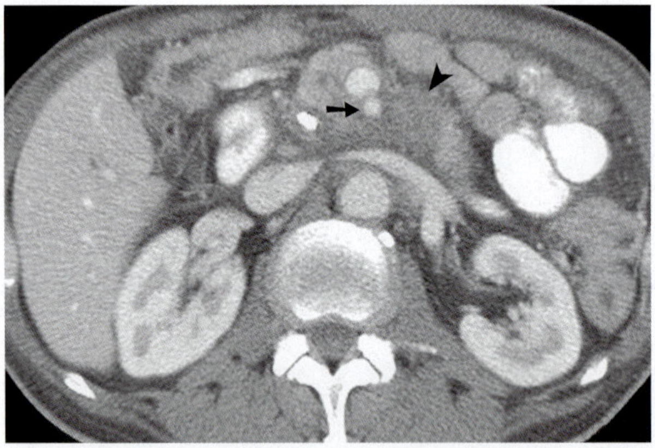

B

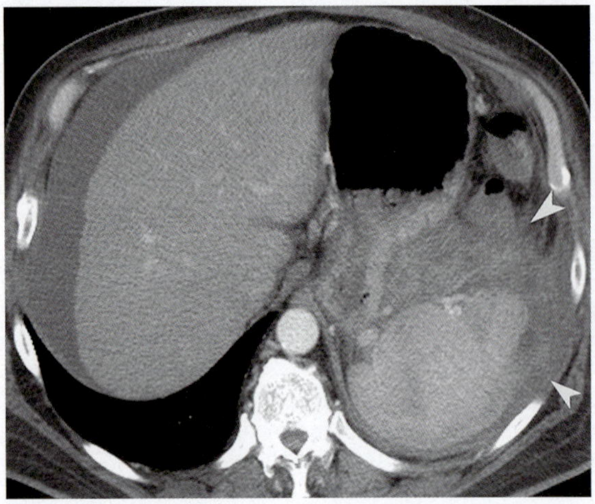

C

**FIG. 10B.4 • Unresectable pancreatic adenocarcinoma.** **A:** Axial contrast-enhanced CT demonstrates a heterogeneous pancreatic head mass lesion encasing the superior mesenteric artery (*curved arrow*). The superior mesenteric vein is not visualized as it was occluded by the mass. **B:** Axial contrast-enhanced CT scan study demonstrates a hypodense mass lesion in the pancreatic body (*arrowhead*), encasing the superior mesenteric artery (*straight arrow*). **C:** Axial contrast-enhanced CT in a patient with unresectable pancreatic tail adenocarcinoma demonstrates the tumor (*arrowheads*) invading the gastric wall as well as the spleen.

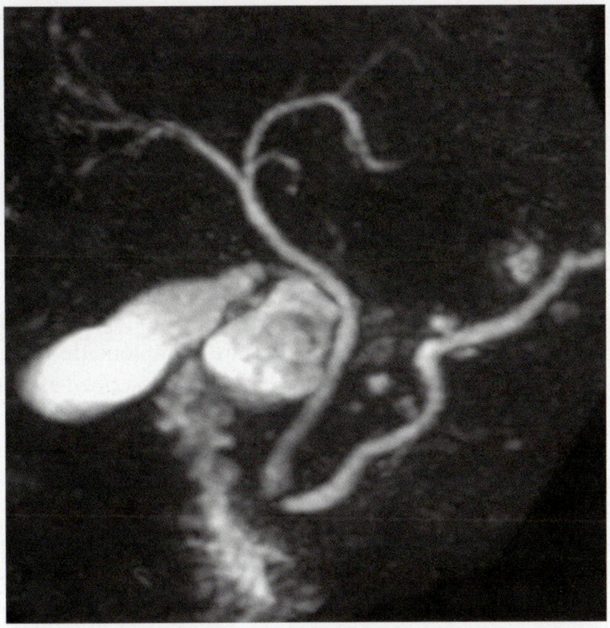

A

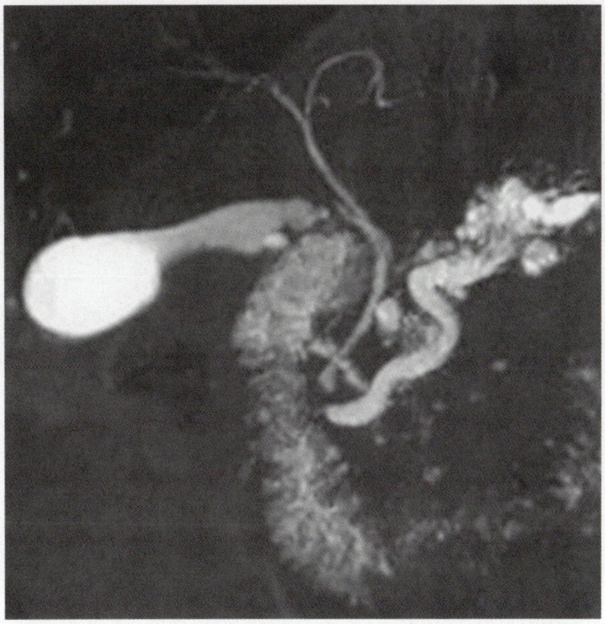

B

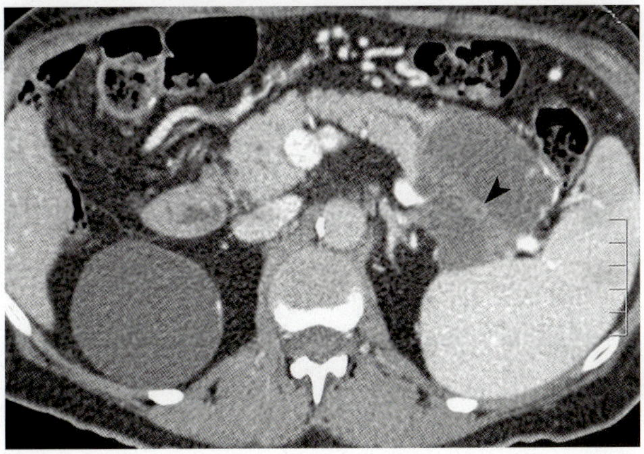

C

**FIG. 10B.5 • Intraductal papillary medullary neoplasm.** **A:** MRCP demonstrates multiple side-branch IPMN, some of which are seen to communicate with the pancreatic duct. **B:** MRCP study demonstrates multiple side-branch IPMN and dilated main pancreatic duct in a patient also has main-duct IPMN. **C:** Contrast-enhanced CT of a patient with IPMN in the pancreatic tail, containing a thickened septation (*arrowhead*), which represented malignant transformation of the IPMN.

Table 10B.1 **INTRADUCTAL PANCREATIC MUCINOUS NEOPLASM: IMAGING FEATURES**

| IPMNs | CT | MR |
|---|---|---|
| Type 1 (main-duct IPMN) | Main-duct dilatation (diffuse or segmental)<br>Hypodense | Papillary bulging with mucinous globule<br>Hypointense T1<br>Hyperintense T2 |
| Type 2 (side-branch IPMN) | *Microcystic* (multiple septations)<br>*Macrocystic* (uni-/multiloculated lesion with few septa)<br>Hypodense and heterogeneous even after contrast | Small rounded lobulated mass not involving the main pancreatic duct<br>Hypointense after contrast agent |

than serous cystadenoma. They are composed of atypical epithelial cells and ovarian-type stroma. They are most frequently located within the tail or the body (Fig. 10B.6).

On CT and MR, their imaging features are (Fig. 10B.7):

1. Unilocular or septated cystic lesion
2. Smooth outline
3. Enhancing wall and septations
4. No communication with the main pancreatic duct
5. Peripheral calcifications (15% of cases) and soft tissue–enhancing nodules sometimes detected
6. No central scar

These are premalignant lesions and contain foci of carcinoma in 17% of patients. Large size (greater than 6 cm), peripheral eggshell calcifications, irregular nodular wall, and involvement of the main duct are findings of malignant degeneration.[4] The treatment of mucinous cystic neoplasms is

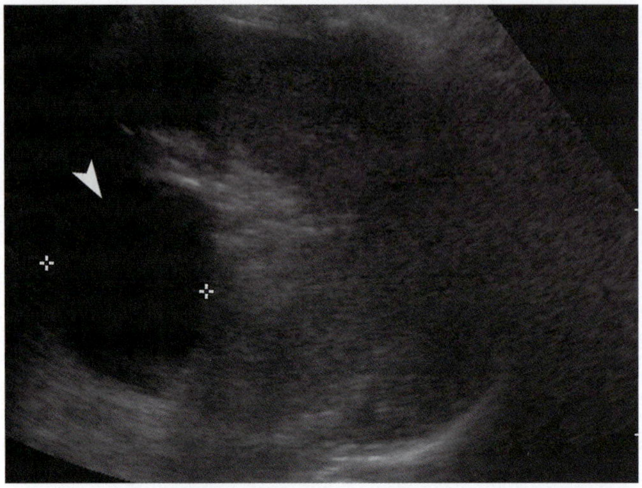

**FIG. 10B.6 • Intraductal medullary neoplasm.** Ultrasound demonstrates a cystic lesion in the pancreatic tail (*arrowhead*) without any nodularity in the wall or internal septations.

always surgical resection; no recurrence is known when resection is complete, so that follow-up is not necessary.

### Serous Cystadenoma

Serous cystadenomas of the pancreas are benign lesions accounting for 20% of all pancreatic cystic lesions. The tumor has a female prevalence (75%) and older age of occurrence (mean, 61.5 years) than mucinous cystadenoma.[4] It is seen in 75% of patients with von Hippel-Lindau syndrome. The most frequent location of serous cystoadenoma is in the head.

On imaging, the typical serous cystadenoma is most often microcystic and is seen as follows:

1. Cluster of several subcentimeter cysts (usually 1 to 5 mm in the center and larger at the periphery) (Fig. 10B.8A). MR demonstrates tiny hyperintense cysts on T2WI with septations and central scar, which enhance on delayed postcontrast images (Fig. 10B.8B, C).
2. Seventy percent of lesions have external lobulation and central fibrous scar. Less than 10% of cystadenomas have oligocystic or macrocystic pattern, consisting of one or more of the cystic lesions larger than 2 cm in diameter.[2,9,10]
3. Calcification of the central stellate scar is seen in 30% of cases.
4. There is no communication with the main pancreatic duct.

Malignant transformation is rare, so nonoperative management has been recommended to asymptomatic patients. Approximately 0.8% of tumors have been described as clearly malignant (with distant metastases).[4]

## NEUROENDOCRINE TUMORS

These arise from ductal pluripotent stem cell and account for 1% to 5% of all pancreatic neoplastic lesions. They can be differentiated into functioning (65% to 85%) or nonfunctioning tumors (Table 10B.2). Insulinoma is the most common functioning neuroendocrine tumor and is benign in 90% of cases. They usually arise in the fourth to sixth decades of life (mean range of age 51 to 57 years), and only the 1% to 2% are associated with familial syndromes like MEN type 1, von Hippel-Lindau syndrome, NF type 1, and tuberous sclerosis.[2,11]

On contrast-enhanced CT and MR, the lesions are hyperenhancing compared to pancreatic parenchyma (Fig. 10B.9). They are usually homogeneous when small and heterogeneous when larger, because of necrosis, calcification, fibrosis, and cystic areas.[2,11] On US, they are hypoechoic with smooth margins and hypervascular after contrast agent administration. On MR, they are hypointense, circumscribed masses on T1WI and hyperintense compared to the normal pancreas on T2WI. Hepatic metastases and lymphadenopathy may occur with malignant neuroendocrine tumors.

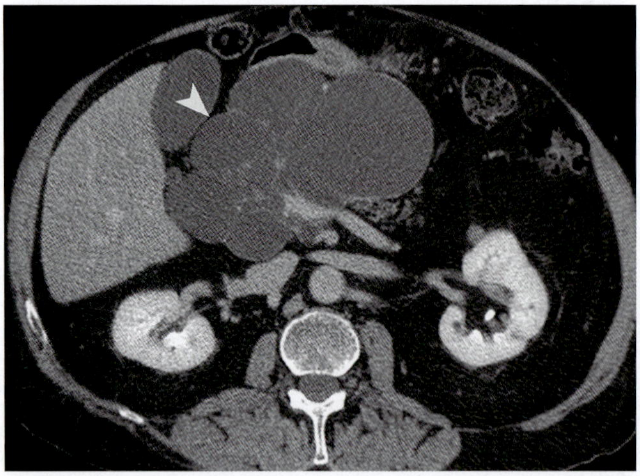

A

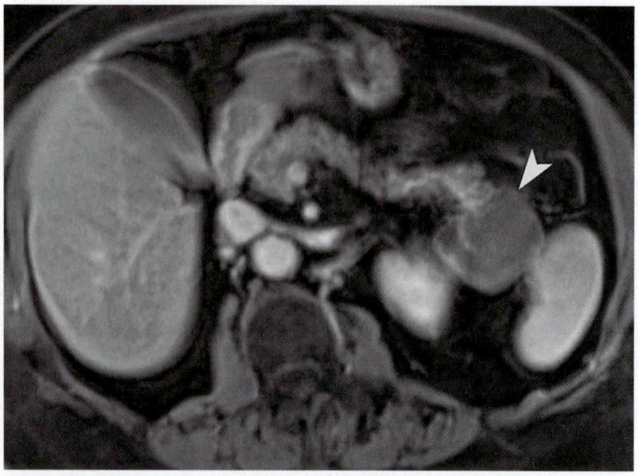

B

**FIG. 10B.7 • Mucinous cystadenoma of the pancreas. A:** Contrast-enhanced CT demonstrates a large multilobulated cystic mass lesion (*arrowhead*) in the pancreatic head. The individual cysts within the cystic mass lesion are more than 2 cm in diameter. **B:** Postgadolinium T1WI demonstrates a septated cystic lesion (*arrowhead*) in the pancreatic tail.

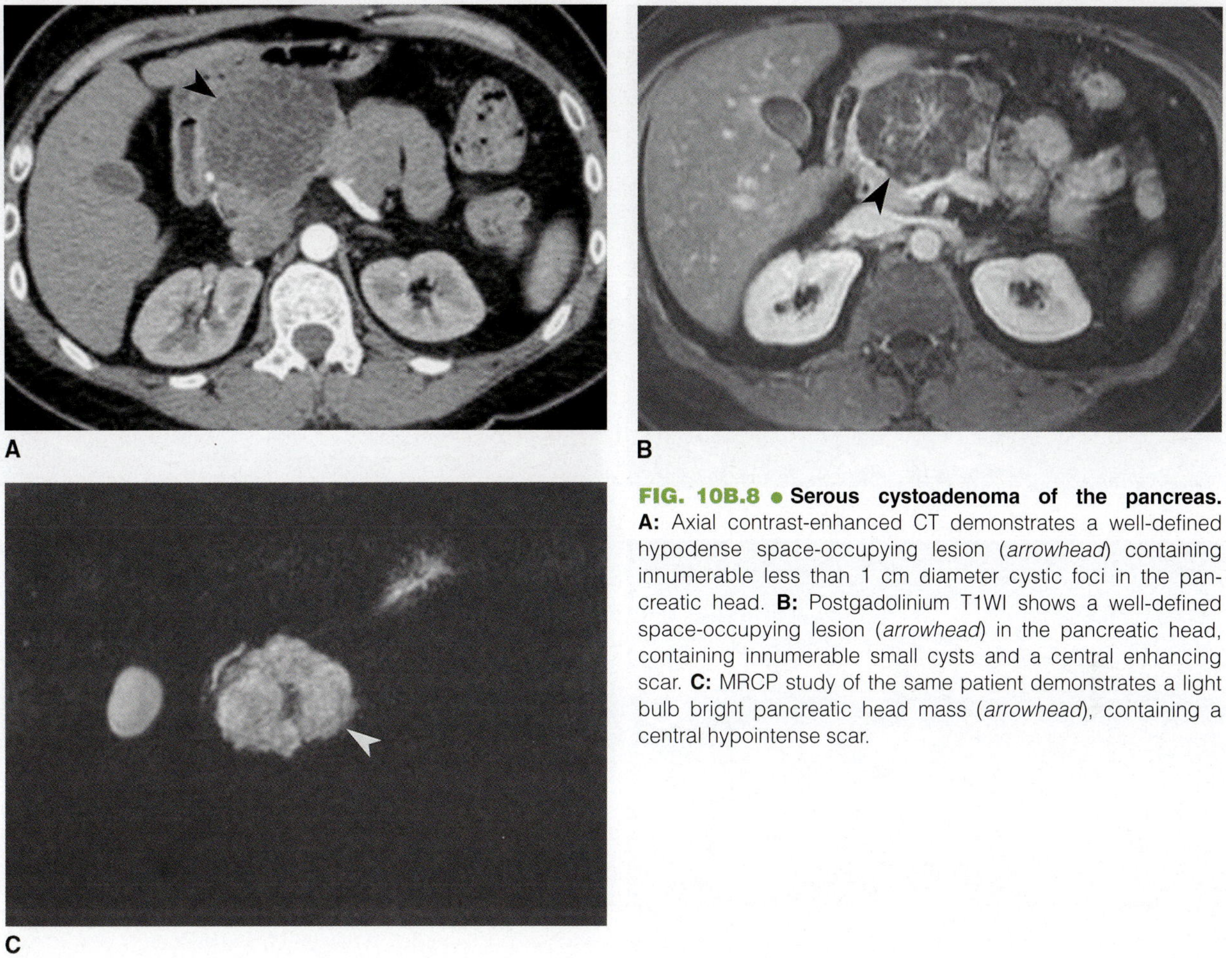

**FIG. 10B.8 • Serous cystoadenoma of the pancreas.** **A:** Axial contrast-enhanced CT demonstrates a well-defined hypodense space-occupying lesion (*arrowhead*) containing innumerable less than 1 cm diameter cystic foci in the pancreatic head. **B:** Postgadolinium T1WI shows a well-defined space-occupying lesion (*arrowhead*) in the pancreatic head, containing innumerable small cysts and a central enhancing scar. **C:** MRCP study of the same patient demonstrates a light bulb bright pancreatic head mass (*arrowhead*), containing a central hypointense scar.

## PSEUDOPAPILLARY TUMOR

Although this tumor has been called in the past by many different names (e.g., solid cystic papillary epithelial tumor, papillary cystic tumor, solid and cystic tumor), in 1996, the World Health Organization renamed it solid pseudopapillary tumor. These lesions are rare and account for 1% to 2% of all pancreatic tumors and are most common in young adult (mean age 25 years) non-Caucasian (African and Asian) females.[2,12–14] The tumor is usually benign, but malignant degeneration is seen in 15% of cases, so the best treatment is complete resection. Metastases are uncommon (7% to 9% of cases) and usually involve the liver (frequently solitary and resectable), omentum, peritoneum, lymph node, and vascular/neural sheath.

Table 10B.2 **SALIENT FEATURES OF PANCREATIC NEUROENDOCRINE TUMORS**

| Tumor Type | Malignancy | Location | Symptoms |
|---|---|---|---|
| Insulinoma (50%)<br>(90% <2 cm) | 10% | Pancreas (90%) | Hypoglycemia |
| Gastrinoma (20%)<br>(mean 4 cm) | 60% | Pancreas (25%–60%)<br>Gastrinoma triangle (90%) | Zollinger-Ellison syndrome |
| Glucagonoma (1%)<br>(usually 2–6 cm) | 70% | Pancreas (>90%)<br>(body or tail) | Necrolytic migratory erythema, diabetes, diarrhea |
| Vipoma (3%)<br>(mean 5 cm) | 75% | Pancreatic tail (90%)<br>Extrapancreatic (10%–20%) (retroperitoneal sympathetic chain and adrenal gland) | Werner-Morrison syndrome |
| Somatostatinoma (<1%)<br>(usually >5 cm) | 50% | Pancreas (50%)<br>Duodenum (50%) | Gallstones, diarrhea, diabetes |
| Nonfunctioning tumors (30%)<br>(range 3–24 cm; 30% >10 cm) | 90% | Pancreatic head | Abdominal pain, jaundice<br>GI bleeding |

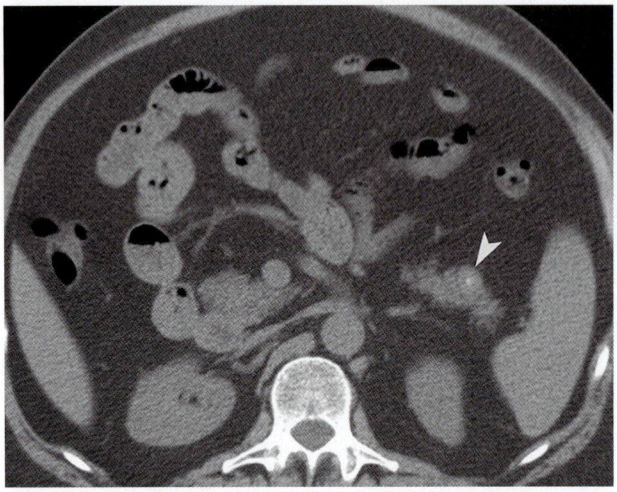

A

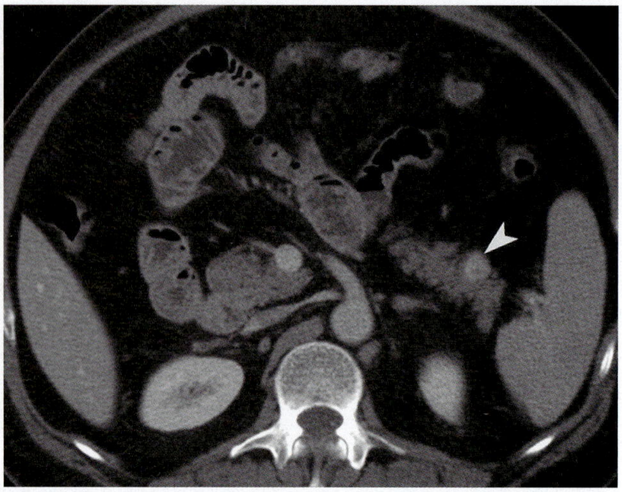

B

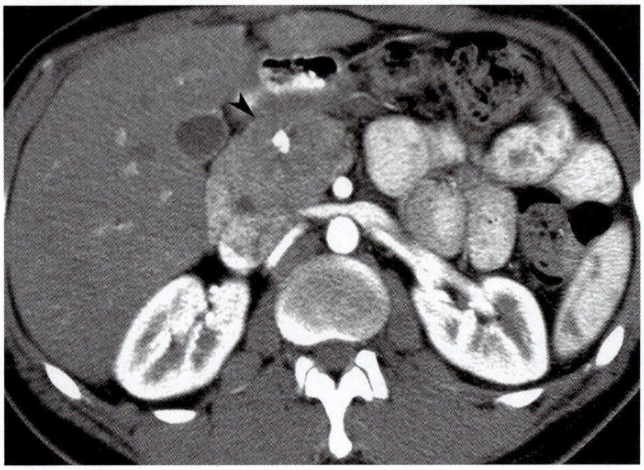

C

**FIG. 10B.9 • Neuroendocrine tumor of the pancreas. A, B:** Noncontrast and postcontrast CT demonstrate a well-defined 1.5-cm diameter lesion (*arrowhead*) in the tail with central calcification. This lesion demonstrates intense enhancement on the postcontrast CT study. **C:** Axial contrast-enhanced CT scan study demonstrates a pancreatic head mass lesion (*arrowhead*) with central calcification.

The imaging features of pseudopapillary tumors are as follows:

1. Typically, it is large low attenuation lesion (mean, 9 cm), slow-growing, and well-encapsulated mass with variable solid and cystic regions.
2. Most commonly in the pancreatic tail that generates symptoms in 15% of cases (Fig. 10B.10).

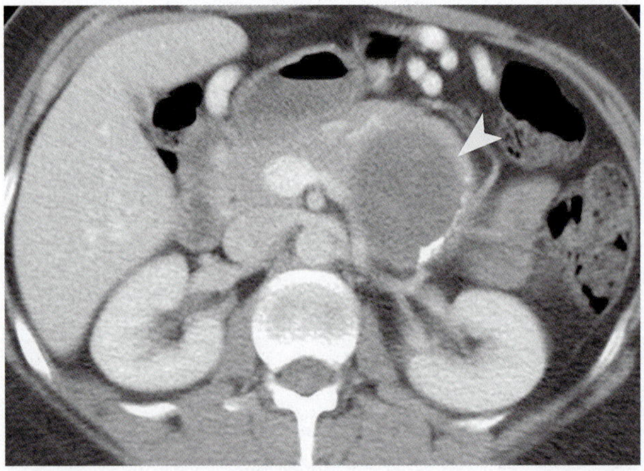

**FIG. 10B.10 • Solid and cystic papillary tumor of the pancreas.** Contrast-enhanced CT of the abdomen demonstrates a well-defined cyst (*arrowhead*) with peripheral calcification in the pancreatic body in a young adult female patient.

3. The tumor displaces rather than invades the surrounding structures, so it rarely causes obstruction of the bile or pancreatic ducts.
4. Internal hemorrhagic areas, necrosis, and cystic degenerative alterations are frequent and usually centrally located, due to the fragile vascular network in the tumor.
5. Central and rim calcifications are seen in 29% of cases.
6. Subacute hemorrhage in the tumor is hyperintense on T1 and variable signal intensity on T2WI. Sometimes (30% of cases), peripheral calcification may be detected.[2,13] They show peripheral heterogeneous enhancement (arterial phase) with progressive filling-in effect.[2,13]

## PANCREATOBLASTOMA

Pancreatoblastoma is seen in pediatric patients (mean age 5 years) and accounts for 0.2% of all pancreatic tumors.[2,14] Histologically, it arises from incompletely differentiated acini of fetal pancreatic tissue, and it is classified into tumors originating either ventral anlage or dorsal anlage. The first have a good prognosis and are right sided, well encapsulated, and free from calcification; the second have a poor prognosis and are left sided, infiltrative, and with intratumoral islet cells and calcification. In most cases, the slow growth of the tumor is asymptomatic and results in a large mass (mean 10 cm) at diagnosis.

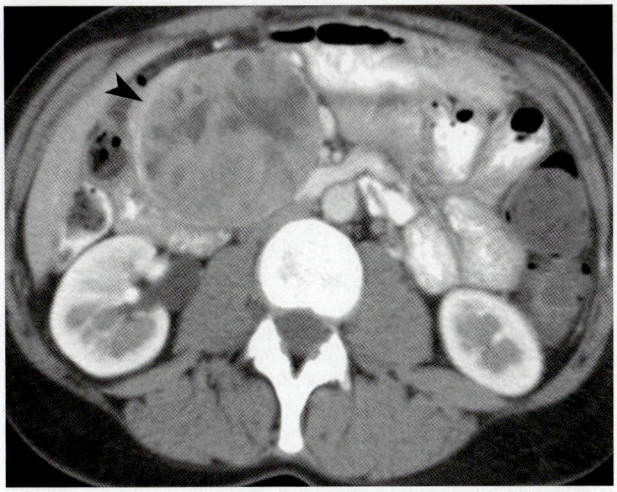

**FIG. 10B.11 • Pancreatoblastoma.** Axial contrast-enhanced CT scan study demonstrates a well-defined mass lesion (*arrowhead*) in the pancreatic head with multiple areas of low density.

In some cases, hormone-related syndromes like Cushing syndrome and syndrome of inappropriate antidiuretic hormone have been observed (paraneoplastic production of hormone). Rarely, an aggressive behavior, local or to distance spread, has been observed: metastases occur to the liver, lymph nodes, lung, bone, posterior mediastinum, peritoneum, and omentum.[2]

On cross-sectional imaging, they may appear circumscribed, lobulated, partially cystic, or calcified mass with septa that enhance after contrast agent injection (Fig. 10B.11). Vascular involvement (arterial encasement and venous invasion) has been described.[2] On US, it is seen a heterogeneous mass with cystic or hypoechoic areas and hyperechoic septa.[2,14] At MR, the tumor has low to intermediate signal intensity on T1WI and high signal intensity on T2WI, with a mild contrast enhancement after contrast injection.[2,14] Invasion of adjacent organs and distant metastases (most often to liver and lymph nodes) may occur in poorly marginated tumors. The best treatment is surgical (75% resectability), which may be difficult in the body or tail tumors.

## LYMPHOMA

Pancreatic lymphoma is most commonly a non-Hodgkin lymphoma, classified as either primary (rare) or secondary (most frequent). The secondary lymphoma is most frequent and originates from the direct extension of pathology from peripancreatic lymphadenopathy. The mean age at presentation is 55 years (range, 35 to 75 years) and patients are usually immunocompromised (e.g., HIV, transplant recipients).[2]

Two morphologic patterns of this pathology include the following:

1. Focal and well-circumscribed type (80% of cases), which occurs into the pancreatic head (mean size of 8 cm). It is homogeneously hypoattenuating on CT. It is low signal intensity on T1WI and intermediate signal intensity on T2WI, with faint enhancement on postcontrast images (Fig. 10B.12).
2. The second form is infiltrative, poor defined, and mimicking the appearance of acute pancreatitis (glandular enlargement). On MR, it is hypointense on T1WI and T2WI, with homogeneous contrast enhancement.[2]

Differentiation from adenocarcinoma is possible by identifying a bulky localized tumor without significant biliary dilatation, enlarged lymph nodes below the level of the renal vein, and a growth that does not respect anatomic boundaries (infiltrating into retroperitoneal or upper abdominal organs and gastrointestinal tract).

Chemotherapy is the first-line treatment and usually leads to a long-term regression or remission of the disease.[2]

## METASTASES

Metastases to the pancreas account for 2% to 5% of all pancreatic neoplasms and are most frequently from renal cell carcinoma and lung cancer. The prognosis is better than pancreatic adenocarcinoma, and surgery is an option when there is a long disease-free interval between resection of primary

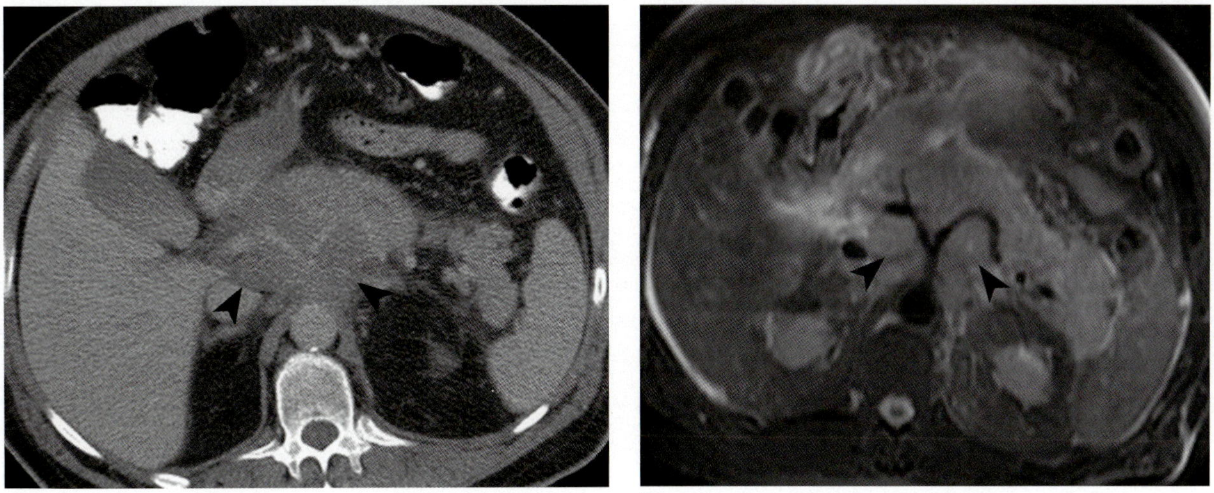

A B

**FIG. 10B.12 • Pancreatic lymphoma (large cell type).** Axial contrast-enhanced CT **(A)** and axial T2WI **(B)** demonstrate an infiltrating mass lesion (*arrowheads*) infiltrating into the pancreatic head and around celiac artery bifurcation.

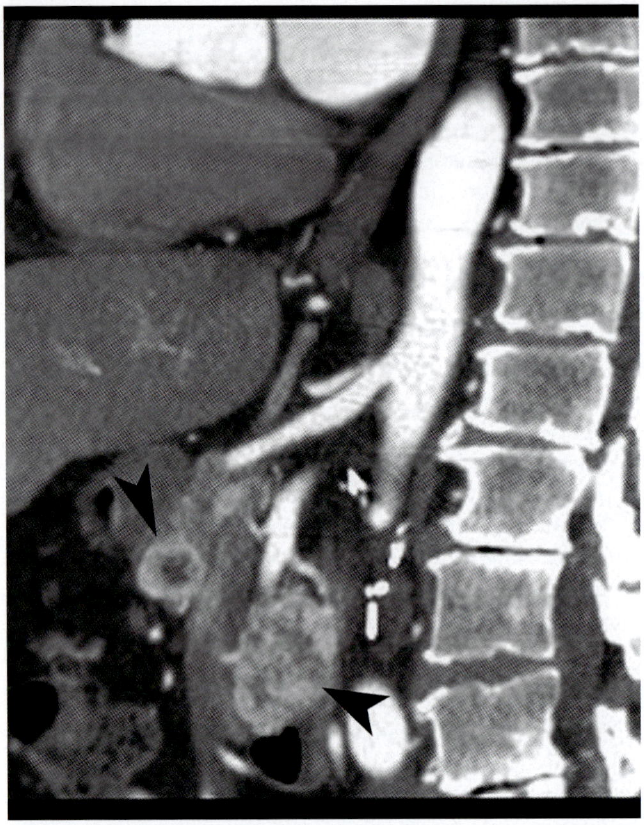

**FIG. 10B.13 • Metastases to the pancreas.** Sagittal contrast-enhanced CT reformation demonstrates two mass lesions (*arrowheads*) in the pancreas in this patient with a history of renal cell carcinoma and nephrectomy.

carcinoma and the development of pancreatic metastases or when the metastases are confined to the pancreas. Three morphologic patterns of involvement may be recognized: solitary (50% to 70% of cases), multifocal (5% to 10%) (Fig. 10B.13), and diffuse (15% to 44%) metastases.[2] On imaging, there is often a well-defined mass, hypo- or hyperechoic at US, hypo- or isoattenuating on CT, hypointense on T1WI, and hyperintense on T2WI. The main differential diagnosis of metastases to pancreas is neuroendocrine tumor and pancreatic adenocarcinoma.

## References


1. Karlson B-M, Ekbom A, Lindgren PG, et al. Abdominal US for diagnosis of pancreatic tumors: prospective cohort analysis. *Radiology.* 1999;213:107–111.
2. Low G, Panu A, Millo N, et al. Multimodality imaging of neoplastic and nonneoplastic solid lesions of the pancreas. *Radiographics.* 2011;31(4):993–1015.
3. Fletcher JG, Wiersema MJ, Farrell MA, et al. Pancreatic malignancy: value of arterial, pancreatic and hepatic phase imaging with multidetector row CT. *Radiology.* 2003;229:81–90.
4. Kucera JN, Kucera S, Perrin SD, et al. Cystic lesions of the pancreas: radiologic-endosonographic correlation. *Radiographics.* 2012;32: E283–E301.
5. Sandrasegaran K, Lin C, Akisik FM, et al. State-of-the-art pancreatic MRI. *AJR Am J Roentgenol.* 2010;195:42–53.
6. Fukukura Y, Takumi K, Kamimura K, et al. Pancreatic adenocarcinoma: variability of diffusion-weighted MR imaging findings. *Radiology.* 2012;263(3):732–740.
7. McNulty NJ, Francis IR, Platt JF, et al. Multi-detector row helical CT of the pancreas: effect of contrast-enhanced multiphasic imaging on enhancement of the pancreas, peripancreatic vasculature and pancreatic adenocarcinoma. *Radiology.* 2001;220:97–102.
8. Ishigami K, Yoshimitsu K, Irie H, et al. Imaging of intraductal tubular tumors of the pancreas. *AJR Am J Roentgenol.* 2008;191:1836–1840.
9. Kim HJ, Lee DH, Ko YT, et al. CT of serous cystadenoma of the pancreas and mimicking masses. *AJR Am J Roentgenol.* 2008;190:406–412.
10. Kim SY, Lee JM, Kim SH, et al. Macrocystic neoplasms of the pancreas: CT differentiation of serous oligocystic adenoma from mucinous cystadenoma and intraductal papillary mucinous tumor. *AJR Am J Roentgenol.* 2006;187:1192–1198.
11. Lewis RB, Lattin GE Jr, Paal E, et al. Pancreatic endocrine tumors: radiologic-clinicopathologic correlation. *Radiographics.* 2010;30: 1445–1464.
12. Coleman KM, Doherty MC, Bigler SA. Solid-pseudopapillary tumor of the pancreas. *Radiographics.* 2003;23:1644–1648.
13. Choi J-Y, Kim M-J, Kim JH, et al. Solid pseudopapillary tumor of the pancreas: typical and atypical manifestations. *AJR Am J Roentgenol.* 2006;187:W178–W186.
14. Chung EM, Travis MD, Conran RM. From the archives of the AFIP: pancreatic tumors in children: radiologic-pathologic correlation. *Radiographics.* 2006;26:1211–1238.

## SELF-ASSESSMENT QUESTIONS

1. What is the most likely pathologic diagnosis of the focal pathology seen on CT?

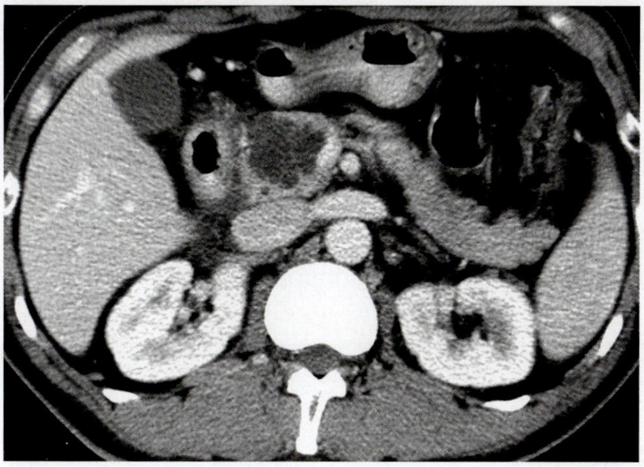

A. Serous cystadenoma
B. Mucinous cystoadenoma
C. Solid and cystic papillary tumor
D. Adenocarcinoma

2. What is the most likely pathologic diagnosis of the focal pancreatic lesion seen on CT?

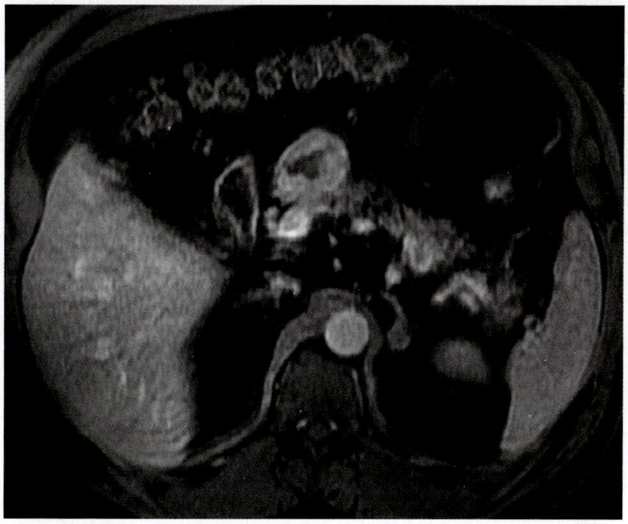

A. Macrocystic tumor
B. Neuroendocrine tumor
C. IPMN
D. Adenocarcinoma

3. In the pancreatic neoplasm depicted on the CT scan study, involvement of what structure makes it unresectable?

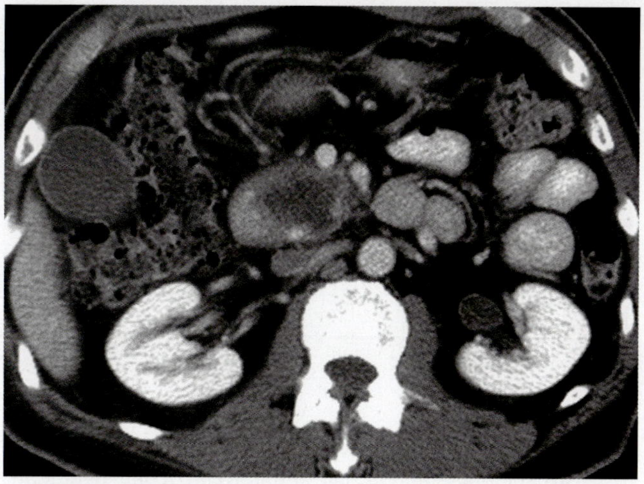

A. Superior mesenteric artery
B. Pancreatic duct
C. Superior mesenteric artery
D. Gastroduodenal artery

### Answers to Self-Assessment Questions

**1. A.** Serous cystadenoma. The CT demonstrates a serous cystadenoma, infected by the presence of a microcystic tumor. The tumor has lobulated outline and several subcentimeter cysts.

**2. B.** Neuroendocrine tumor. The contrast-enhanced MR shows a hyperenhancing mass compared to pancreatic parenchyma with central area of necrosis. The hyperenhancement distinguishes neuroendocrine tumor from adenocarcinoma.

**3. C.** Superior mesenteric artery. CT evidence of the involvement of celiac, superior mesenteric artery, common hepatic artery, or hepatic artery properly indicates unresectability.

# Spleen 11

*J. Paul Nielsen and Ajay K. Singh*

## LEARNING OBJECTIVE

1. Describe the indications and important imaging features of neoplastic and nonneoplastic conditions of the spleen.

The spleen is located in the left upper quadrant, supported by gastrosplenic, splenorenal, and phrenicocolic ligaments. The spleen is mainly supplied by the splenic artery, which divides into approximately six branches at the splenic hilum. The blood flow through the spleen is approximately 50 mL/m, which represents approximately 5% of the cardiac output. Because of the high vascularity and fragility of splenic parenchyma, the spleen represents the most common and important organ affected involved in blunt trauma.

## CONGENITAL ANOMALIES

### Accessory Spleen

A splenule or accessory spleen is a small focus of normal splenic tissue which is noncontiguous from the spleen. This can be due to either failure of fusion of the components of the forming spleen during the embryologic phase or from prior trauma.[1] Usually, a clinically insignificant incidental finding, a persistent splenule after splenectomy for hypersplenism may result in persistent blood count abnormalities.[2] More commonly, a splenule may be misdiagnosed as a mass or enlarged lymph node, especially the rare intrapancreatic splenule.

A splenule will demonstrate imaging features similar to the spleen on US, CT, and MR studies. They are typically well-defined, round less than 2-cm focal lesion, most commonly located in the left upper quadrant, often posteromedial to the spleen (Fig. 11.1). On Doppler US, the vascular supply can be seen entering the accessory spleen. On arterial phase CT, the accessory spleen will show inhomogeneous striped enhancement pattern of the spleen. Intrapancreatic accessory spleen is hyperdense to pancreatic parenchyma on all phases of CT imaging and can be mistaken for neuroendocrine tumor, which are hyperdense to pancreatic parenchyma only on arterial phase imaging.

Tc-99m–labeled heat-damaged RBC scintigraphy is a specific imaging test to confirm the diagnosis.

### Splenosis

Splenosis refers to autotransplantation of splenic tissue secondary to disruption of splenic capsule in patients with a history of splenic trauma or splenectomy. They have imaging features, similar to the accessory spleen, but are often more numerous and more widespread than the accessory spleen (Fig. 11.2). As with the accessory spleen, Tc-99m–labeled heat-damaged RBC scintigraphy is the most accurate test to make the diagnosis (Fig. 11.3). Tc-99m sulfur colloid scan can also be used to make the diagnosis (Fig. 11.4).

### Heterotaxy Syndrome

The term situs is used to describe the positions of the heart and abdominal viscera relative to the midline.

*Situs solitus:* It represents the normal position of the viscera.

*Situs inversus:* Abdominal viscera is positioned in the mirror image of situs solitus.

*Heterotaxy syndrome:* They can be divided into two main subgroups: right-sided isomerism with asplenia and left-sided isomerism with polysplenia (Fig. 11.5).

1. In right-sided isomerism with asplenia, the patients generally have severe congenital heart diseases. Unlike the polysplenia group, the asplenic grouping usually has a normal IVC.[3] However, total anomalous pulmonary venous return is frequently seen with asplenia.
2. Polysplenia, or left-sided isomerism, reflects multiple noncontiguous segments of splenic tissue. The noncontiguous splenic tissue may be on the right or left but is always ipsilateral to the stomach. It can be associated with severe congenital cardiac anomalies, but these are generally less severe than patients with right-sided isomerism. Polysplenia may also be associated with vascular malformations (interrupted IVC with azygos or hemiazygos continuation), midline liver, and bilobed lungs.[4]

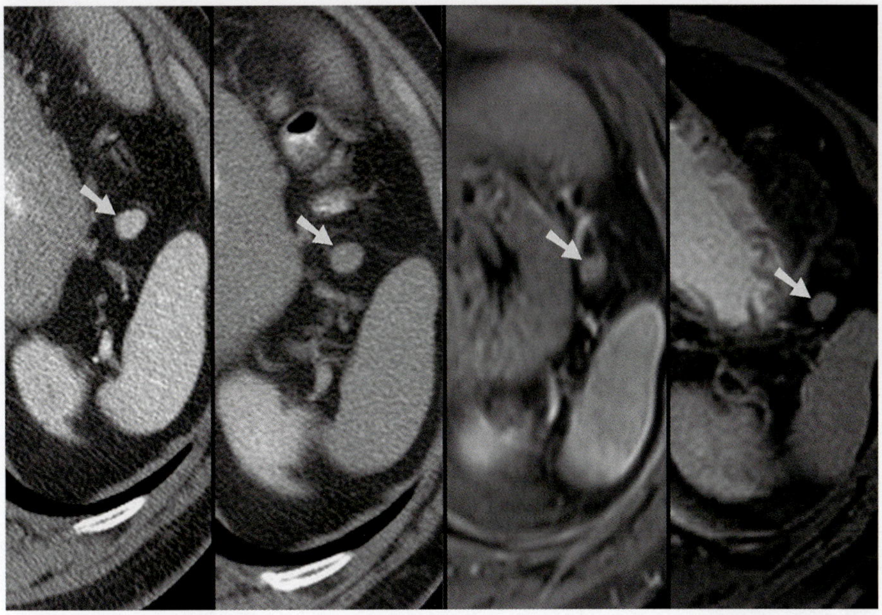

**FIG. 11.1 • Accessory spleen.** Arterial and portal venous phase contrast-enhanced CT and MR imaging demonstrates isointensity of the accessory spleen (*arrows*) with the splenic parenchyma.

## Wandering Spleen

Wandering spleen refers to abnormal position of the spleen due to laxity or absence of ligamentous attachments of the spleen. Less than 600 cases have been reported, and they tend to occur most commonly in young adult females. Wandering spleen may present a palpable mass or as acute abdominal pain related to torsion.

On CT, the left upper quadrant is empty, and the spleen is located more caudally in the abdomen. There may be torsion of the vessels, identified by their swirling appearance and splenic infarcts (Figs. 11.6 and 11.7). The treatment is surgical (splenectomy for infarction, splenopexy if no infarction).

## True Simple Cyst

A true simple cyst is uncommon compared to other solid visceral organs and has a surrounding epithelial lining. They are congenital in origin, accounting for 10% of splenic cysts. On imaging, they are seen as an ovoid fluid-filled structure without internal vascularity or enhancement (Fig. 11.8). They may cause elevation of tumor markers such as CEA, CA125, and CA19-9, despite a completely benign condition.[5] A true cyst may demonstrate thin septations, which may help to distinguish it from a posttraumatic pseudocyst.

## Pseudocyst

Pseudocysts can be posttraumatic or secondary to infection or infarct. They are seen on imaging as well-circumscribed, fluid-attenuating lesion without peripheral enhancement. Unlike a true splenic cyst, septations are uncommon with pseudocysts. Mural calcifications are more common, and wall thickness is greater in pseudocysts (Fig. 11.9).

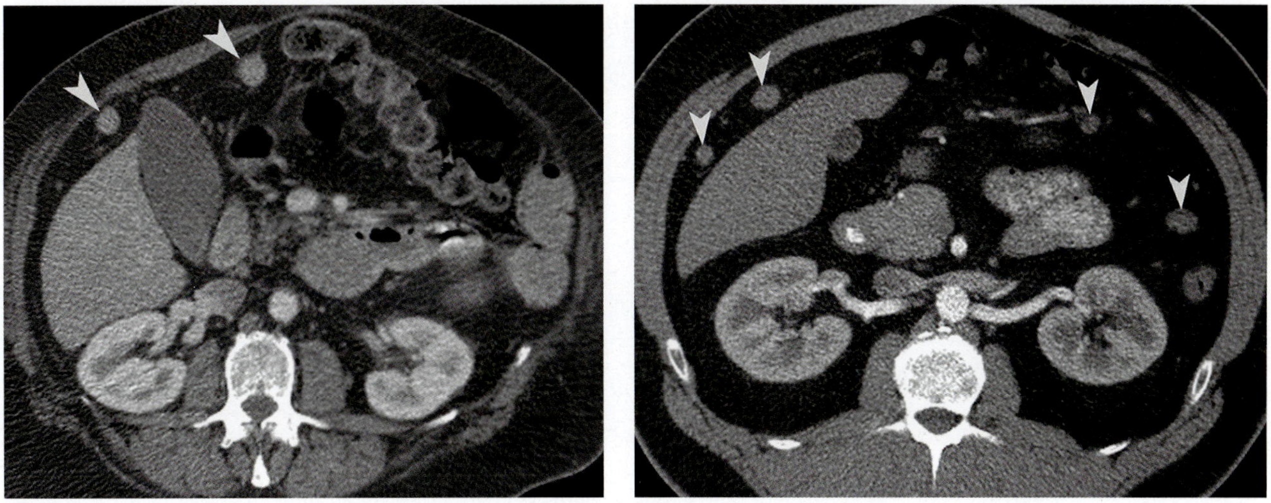

A B

**FIG. 11.2 • Splenosis.** Multiple enhancing soft tissue density nodules, representing splenosis (*arrows*), are seen in the greater omentum in a patient with prior history of splenectomy.

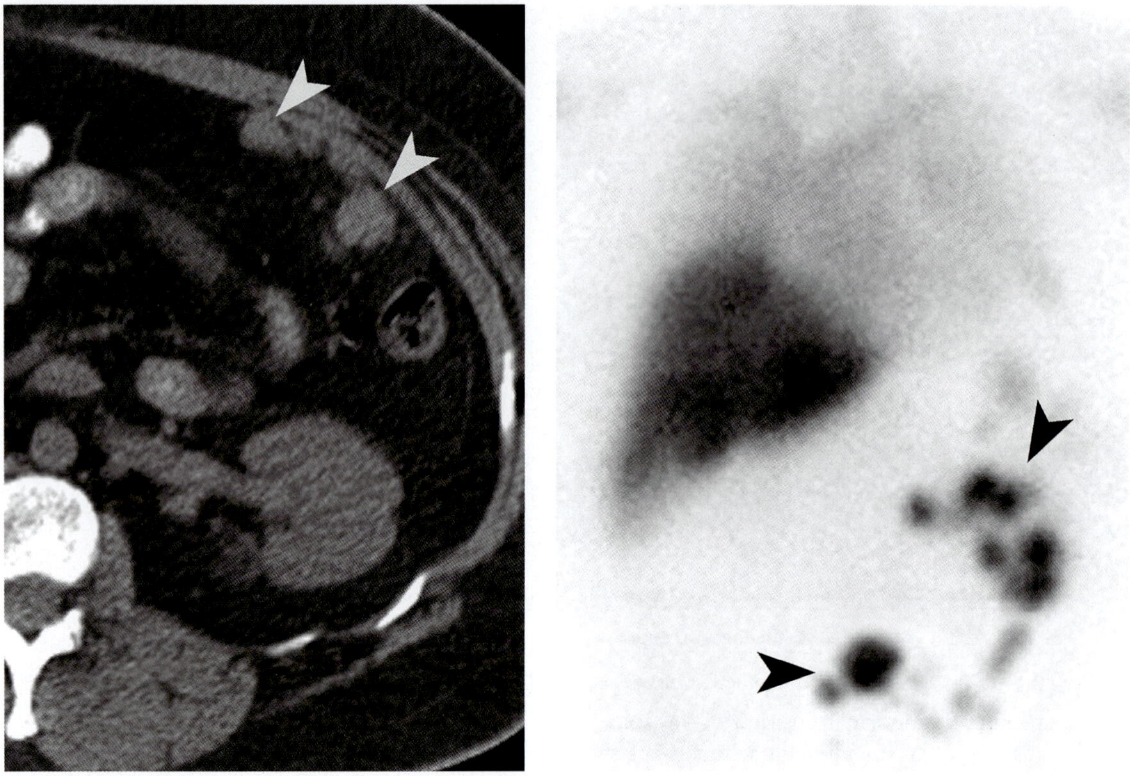

A B

**FIG. 11.3 • Splenosis.** Axial CT scan (**A**) and technetium-99m heat-damaged RBC scan (**B**) demonstrating multiple focal nodules in the left greater omentum, consistent with splenosis (*arrowheads*).

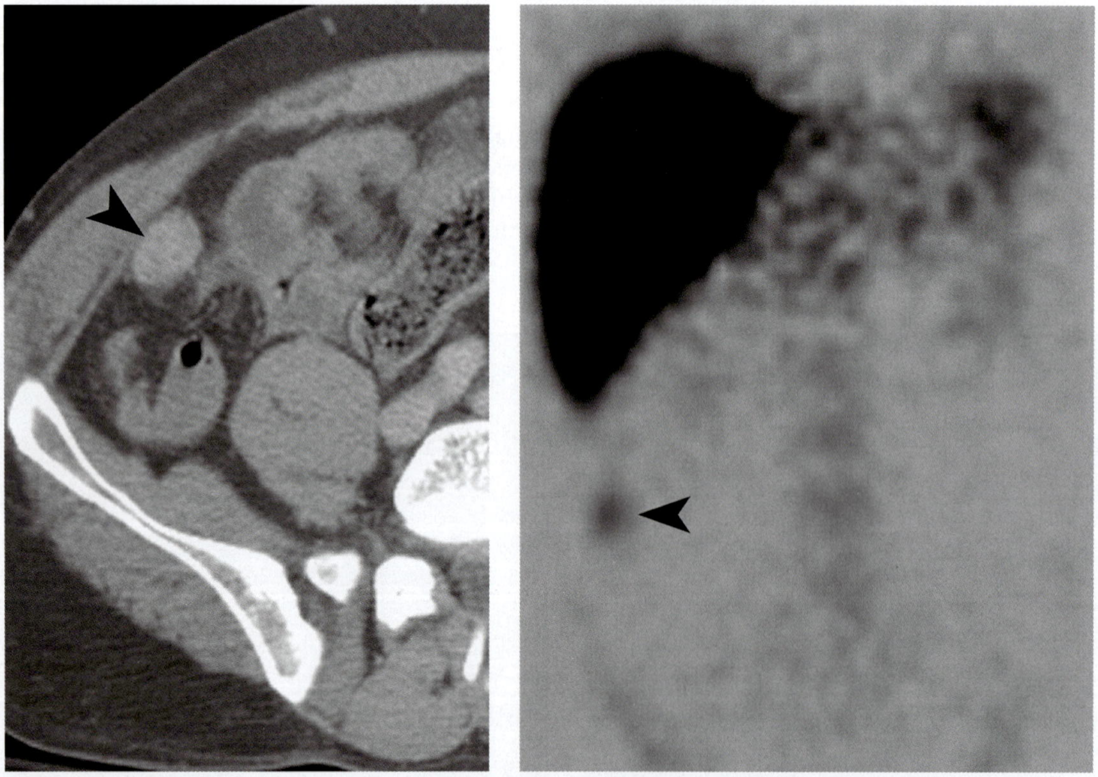

A B

**FIG. 11.4 • Splenosis. A:** Axial CT demonstrates a soft tissue density nodular lesion (*arrowhead*) in the right lower quadrant, centered within the greater omentum. **B:** Technetium-99m sulfur colloid scan of the same patient demonstrates focal area of radiotracer activity in the right lower quadrant (*arrowhead*), corresponding to the CT finding and consistent with splenic tissue.

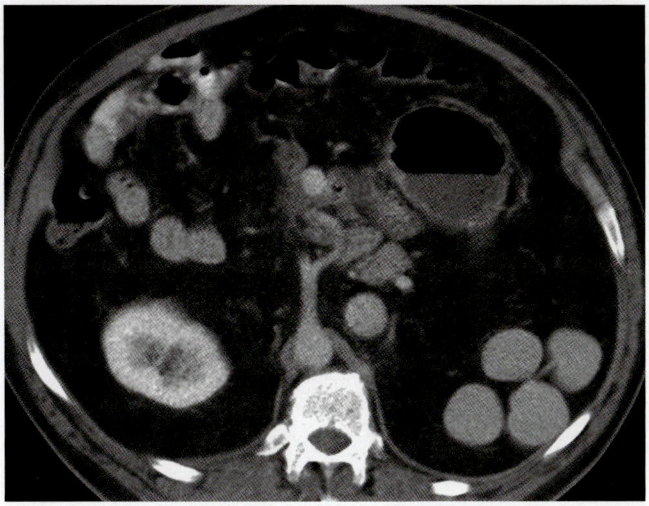

**FIG. 11.5 • Polysplenia in a patient with dextrocardia.** Axial contrast-enhanced CT demonstrates polysplenia in the left upper abdomen, in a patient with dextrocardia.

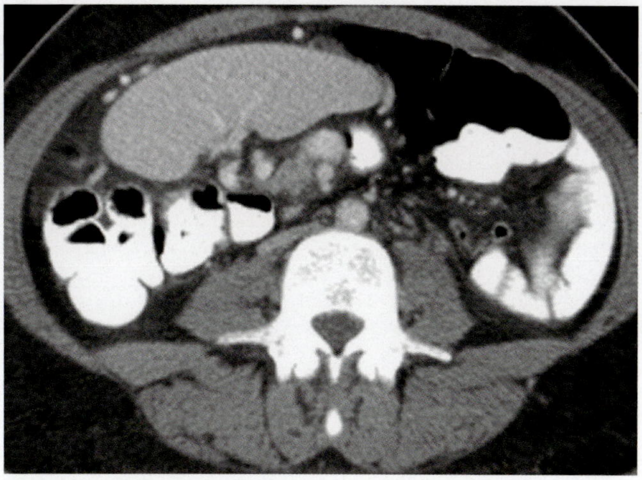

**FIG. 11.7 • Wandering spleen.** Axial contrast-enhanced CT demonstrates the spleen located in the right lower abdomen. There is no infarct seen in the spleen.

## Lymphangioma

Splenic lymphangiomas are a rare, benign neoplasm that may be solitary or multiple. Lymphangiomas appear as subcapsular, multilocular cystic lesions with thin septations. Postcontrast images may show septal enhancement.

## Fungal and Pyogenic Abscess

Fungal infections are seen most commonly in immunocompromised patients and are most often due to *Candida* species. The US findings include multiple sub cm hypoechoic foci and sometimes wheel-within-a-wheel appearance. The outer wheel is due to fibrosis, and inner echogenic wheel is caused by inflammatory cells. On CT, fungal abscesses are multiple, small hypodense (hypointense on T1 and hyperintense on T2) foci with enhancing rim (Fig. 11.10).

Pyogenic abscess is most often seen in patients with sepsis and is due to disseminated infection. On imaging, they are seen as fluid-density cystic collections, which are larger than the ones seen with fungal abscesses (Fig. 11.11). They have enhancing rims and may rarely contain air.

## Hydatid Disease

Hydatid disease is caused by *Echinococcus granulosus* larva forming cystic lesions, most commonly in the lungs and liver. The spleen is less commonly affected than the liver. On US, hydatid cyst appearance can vary from cysts with internal echoes or septations to calcified lesions. On CT, a hydatid cyst is seen as a cystic lesion with smooth well-defined wall (Fig. 11.12). Sometimes, the daughter cysts may be identified within the mother cyst. In late stage, the hydatid cyst may completely calcify.

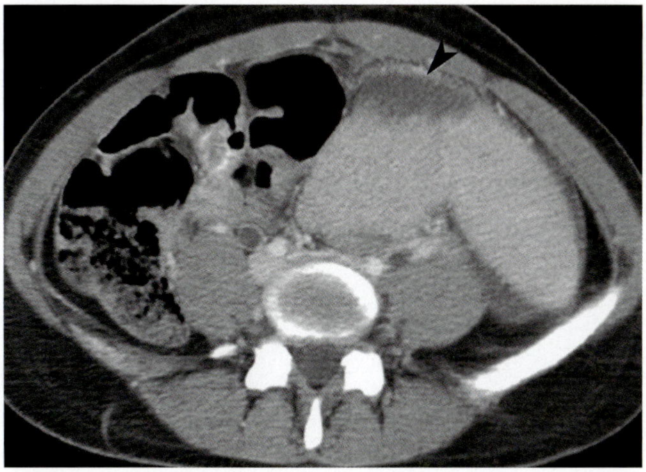

**FIG. 11.6 • Wandering spleen with splenic infarct.** Axial contrast-enhanced CT demonstrates the spleen located in the left lower quadrant. Low-density area present peripherally within the splenic parenchyma (*arrowhead*) represents an infarct.

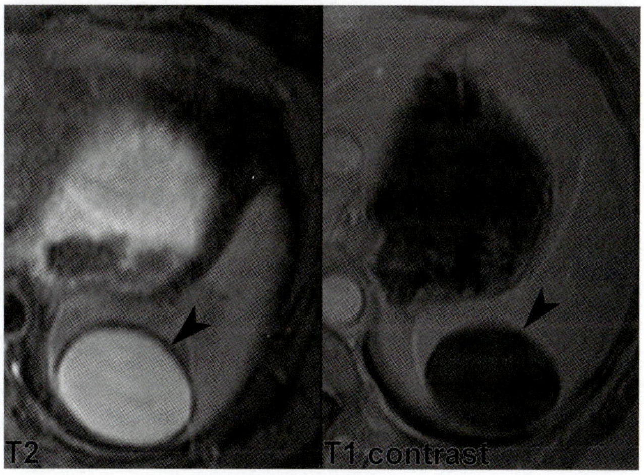


**FIG. 11.8 • Simple splenic cyst.** T2WI and postgadolinium T1WI demonstrates a simple cyst located in the splenic parenchyma (*arrowhead*). There is no wall nodularity or septation within the cyst.

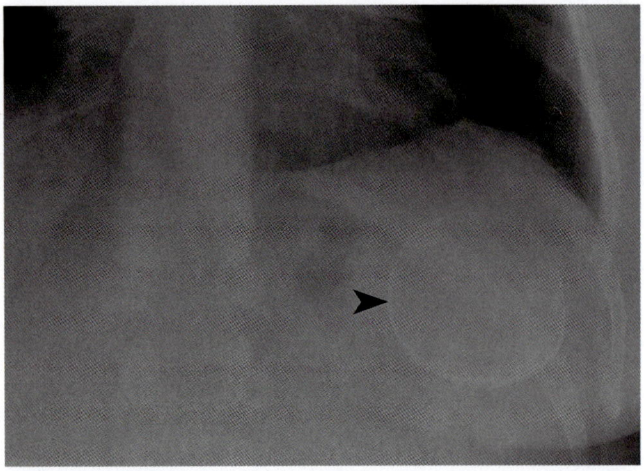

**FIG. 11.9 • Intrasplenic pseudocyst.** Plain x-ray of the upper abdomen demonstrates rim calcification in the left upper quadrant (*arrowhead*), which was located in the wall of an intrasplenic pseudocyst.

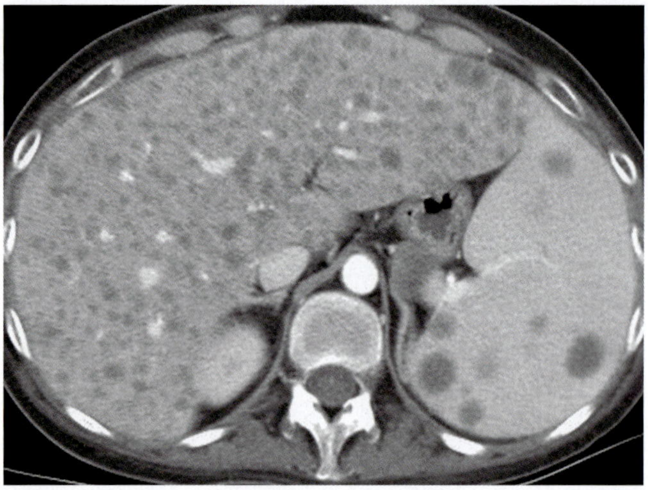

**FIG. 11.10 • Fungal abscesses in the liver and spleen.** Axial contrast-enhanced CT demonstrates innumerable less than 1.5-cm-diameter abscesses in the liver parenchyma. There are fewer abscesses located in the enlarged spleen.

## Splenic Infarct

Splenic infarcts may be seen in patients with hemolytic anemia, endocarditis, and sickle cell disease.[6] On CT, a splenic infarct is typically a wedge of devascularized hypodense splenic parenchyma with the apex facing the hilum and the base along the capsule (Fig. 11.13). As the vascular insult progresses, the wedge of devascularized tissue may resolve, fibrose, and retract the capsule or liquefy (Fig. 11.14).

## Sarcoidosis

Sarcoidosis is characterized by multiple nodular noncaseating granulomas. On imaging, the findings of sarcoidosis include splenomegaly and multiple less than 3-cm-diameter nodules (Fig. 11.15). These nodules are comprised of coalescent sarcoid granulomas and demonstrate low signal on all MR sequences. On postcontrast imaging, the nonenhancing nodules will be conspicuous against the strongly enhancing parenchyma.

## Inflammatory Pseudotumor

Splenic inflammatory pseudotumor is a nodular conglomeration of inflammatory exudate and cellular debris of uncertain etiology. It has a variable appearance and often seen as a well-circumscribed, heterogeneous enhancing mass, which may mimic the appearance of a more aggressive lesion such as an angiosarcoma.[8]

## Gamna-Gandy Bodies

Gamna-Gandy bodies, also referred to as splenic siderotic nodules, are tiny punctate foci of calcium and iron deposited in the spleen usually seen in the setting of chronic microhemorrhage

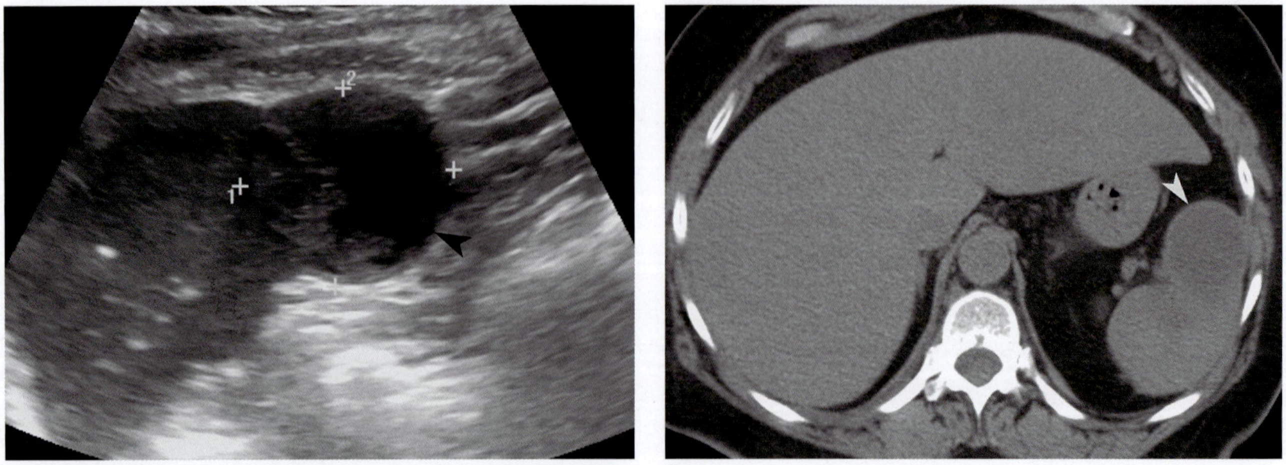

A B

**FIG. 11.11 • Pyogenic splenic abscess. A:** US demonstrates a complex cystic lesion (*arrowhead*) anteriorly in the splenic parenchyma. **B:** Noncontrast axial CT scan study demonstrates low-density abscess (*arrowhead*) in the anterior aspect of the spleen, bulging the splenic capsule.

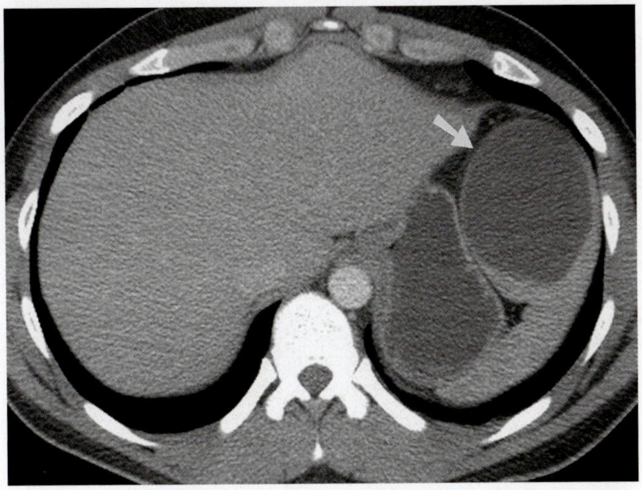

**FIG. 11.12 • Hydatid cyst of the spleen.** Axial contrast-enhanced CT scan study demonstrates a well-defined cyst (*arrow*) located anteriorly in the splenic parenchyma. There are no calcifications or septations within the cyst.

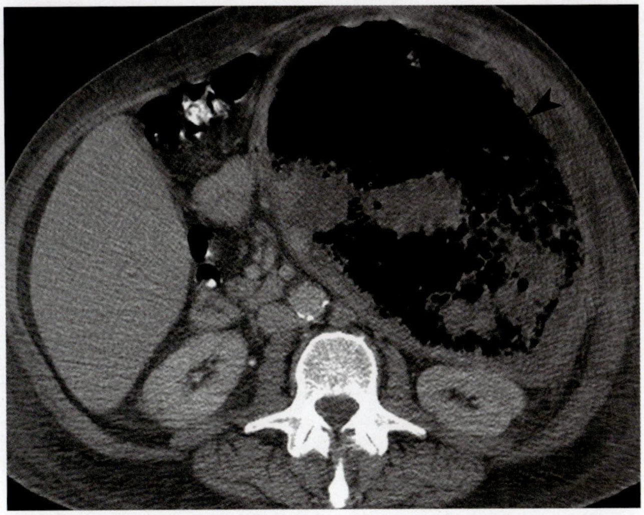

**FIG. 11.14 • Splenic infarction.** Contrast-enhanced CT of the abdomen demonstrates gross splenomegaly with central necrosis after embolization of the splenic artery. There is air as well as necrotic tissue present within the splenic outline (*arrowhead*).

secondary to portal hypertension.[9] They are seen as hypointense foci due to susceptibility on T1 and T2WI (Fig. 11.16). Gradient echo sequence is most sensitive for the detection of hemosiderin found in the nodules.

## Traumatic Injury

The spleen is the most frequently injured abdominal organ in blunt trauma. Although the majority of splenic injuries occur immediately after trauma, delayed sequelae including rupture can occur more than 48 hours after injury and is referred to as a delayed splenic rupture. The 48-hour period from splenic injury to rupture is known as the latent period of Baudet.[10] The American Association for the Surgery of Trauma classification of splenic injury grades splenic injury from grades I to V (Table 11.1). In general, the treatment of stable patients with grade I, II, and III injuries is conservative, while the treatment of grade IV and V injuries is surgical (Figs. 11.17 and 11.18).

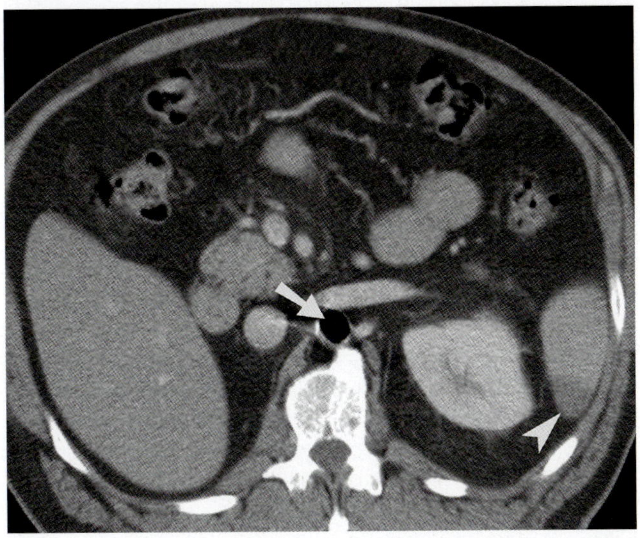

**FIG. 11.13 • Splenic infarct from intra-aortic balloon pump.** Axial contrast-enhanced CT scan study demonstrates low-density infarct (*arrowhead*) at the inferior margin of the spleen. Intra-aortic balloon pump (*arrow*) is located within the abdominal aorta.

Nontraumatic or spontaneous splenic rupture is a rare condition most often associated with underlying pathology such as infectious mononucleosis, malaria, lymphoma, and leukemia (Fig. 11.19). Malaria is the overall most common cause of spontaneous splenic rupture.

## Splenomegaly

The normal adult spleen normally measures around 12 cm in sagittal dimension with an upper limit of 15 cm.[11] The oblong orientation and shape of the spleen makes accurate volumetric analysis difficult. By US, a sagittal dimension of greater than 12 cm is generally considered to be enlarged. Causes of splenomegaly are numerous and include hematologic, hemodynamic, infectious, metabolic, and neoplastic etiologies.[11]

## Splenic Hemangiomas

Hemangiomas are the most common benign neoplasm of the spleen, seen most often in young and middle-aged adults. They are most commonly slow-flow cavernous malformation.

On CT, they are iso- to hypoattenuating on precontrast and hyperenhancing on postcontrast study with progressive centripetal enhancement. Some hemangiomas may show immediate enhancement on the postcontrast images. On MR, hemangiomas are iso- or hypointense on T1WI and hyperintense on T2WI (Fig. 11.20). They enhance peripherally; however, the characteristic nodular enhancement seen in hepatic hemangiomas is less common in the spleen. Some hemangiomas may have a complex cystic appearance and can show calcifications.

Nuclear medicine scintigraphy utilizing Tc-99m–labeled RBCs would show increased activity within the hemangioma on delayed images; however, Tc-99m sulfur colloid scanning may show ambiguous activity. Splenic hemangiomas are

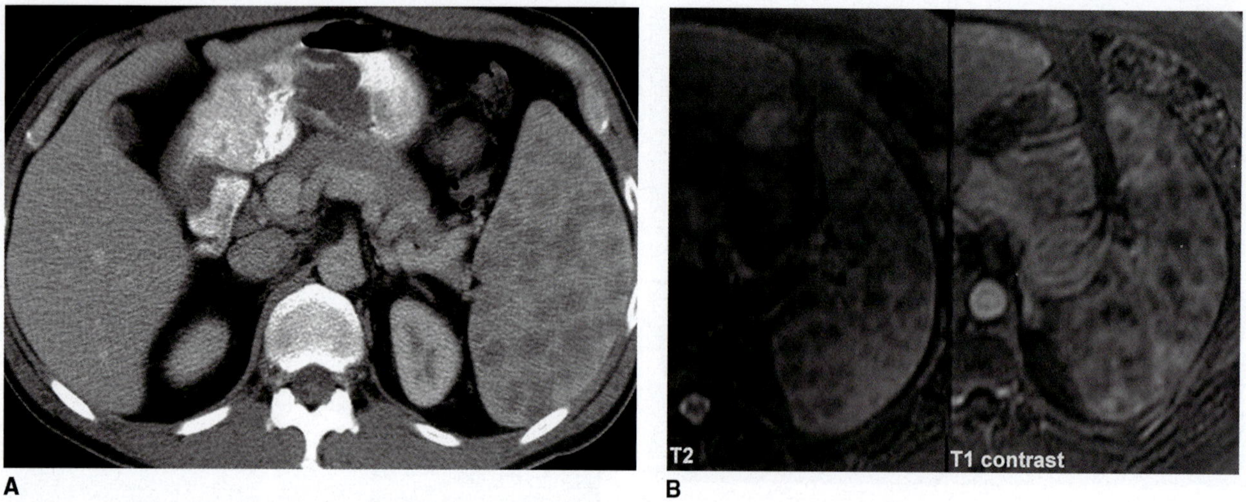


**FIG. 11.15 • Splenic sarcoidosis. A:** Axial contrast-enhanced CT demonstrates innumerable subcentimeter low-density foci in the enlarged spleen. **B:** T2WI and postgadolinium T1WI demonstrates innumerable subcentimeter hypointense foci.

commonly associated with Kasabach-Merritt syndrome and Klippel-Trenaunay-Weber syndrome.

## Splenic Hamartoma

Splenic hamartomas are solitary benign lesions comprised of irregular red pulp elements and reticuloendothelial cell proliferation in the splenic parenchyma. It is associated with tuberous sclerosis, anemia, pancytopenia, and thrombocytopenia.

Splenic hamartomas are generally well circumscribed, iso- or mildly hypodense compared to the spleen on pre- as well as postcontrast CT and is often recognized only by contour abnormality (Fig. 11.21). When large, they may show heterogeneous enhancement. On MR, a hamartoma is well-defined, iso- or slightly hyperintense mass on T1WI. They are heterogeneously hyperintense on T2WI. They show heterogeneous enhancement on early and more uniform enhancement on delayed phase MR. There are reports of Tc-99m sulfur colloid uptake by splenic hamartomas due to the presence of reticuloendothelial cells. Definitive diagnosis is usually not possible on imaging alone because of overlap of imaging features with other splenic neoplasm.

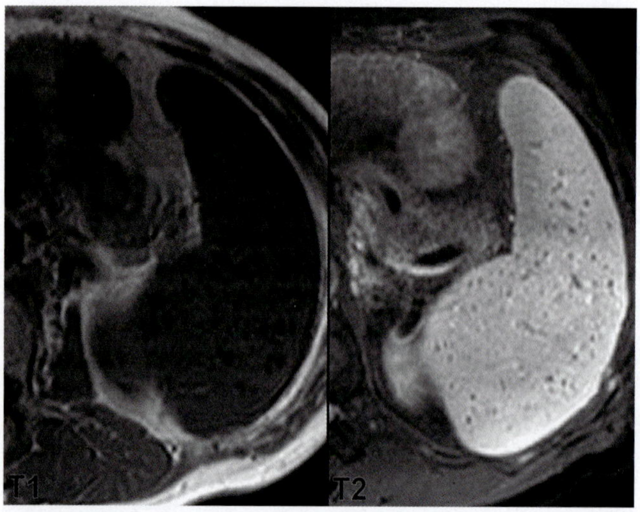


**FIG. 11.16 • Gamna-Gandy bodies.** T1WI and T2WI demonstrate multiple hypointense foci in the splenic parenchyma caused by iron as well as calcium deposition.

Table 11.1 **GRADING OF SPLENIC INJURY (1994 REVISION)**

| Grade | Injury Type | Description |
|---|---|---|
| I | Hematoma | Subcapsular, <10% surface area |
| | Laceration | Capsular tear, <1 cm parenchymal depth |
| II | Hematoma | Subcapsular, 10–50% surface area<br>Intraparenchymal, <5 cm diameter |
| | Laceration | 1–3 cm parenchymal depth not involving a parenchymal vessel |
| III | Hematoma | Subcapsular, >50% surface area or expanding; ruptured subcapsular or parenchymal hematoma; intraparenchymal hematoma >5 cm |
| | Laceration | >3 cm parenchymal depth or involving trabecular vessels |
| | Laceration | Laceration of segmental or hilar vessels producing major devascularization (>25% of the spleen) |
| IV | Laceration | Completely shattered spleen |
| V | Vascular | Hilar vascular injury that devascularized spleen |

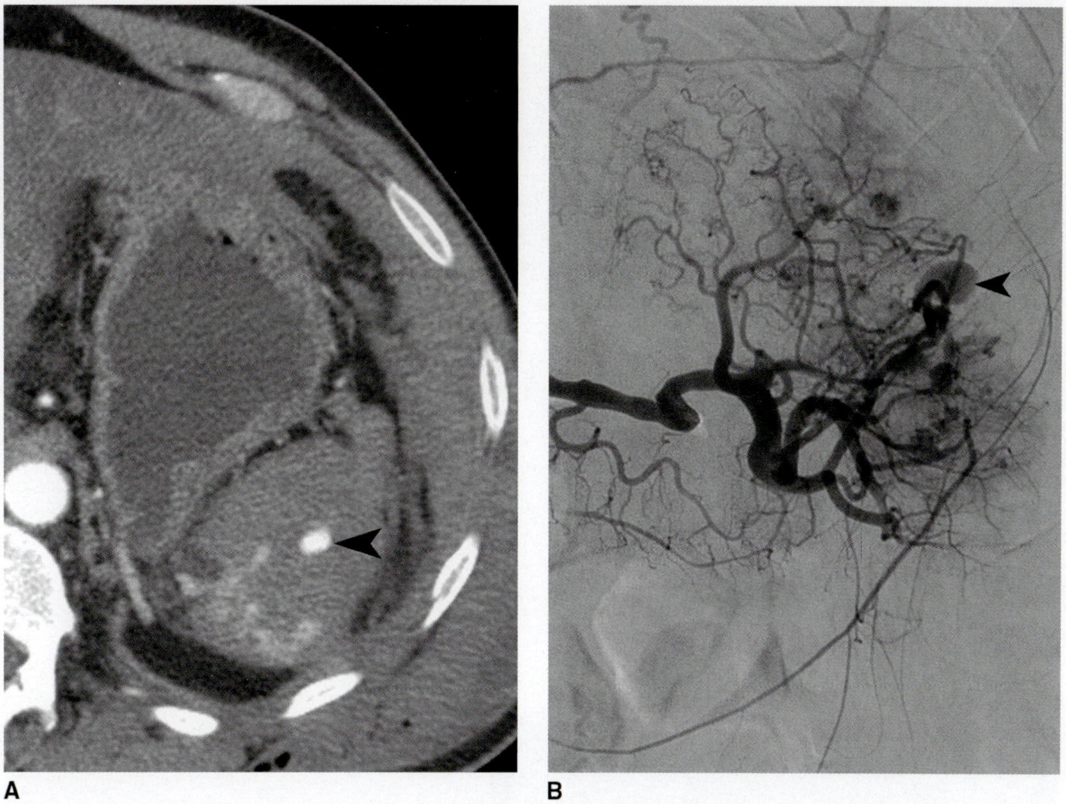

FIG. 11.17 • **Splenic laceration. A:** Contrast-enhanced CT of the upper abdomen demonstrates low-density splenic laceration, containing a focus of pseudoaneurysm (*arrowhead*). **B:** Splenic artery angiogram demonstrates pseudoaneurysm (*arrowhead*) located within the splenic parenchyma, which was subsequently embolized.

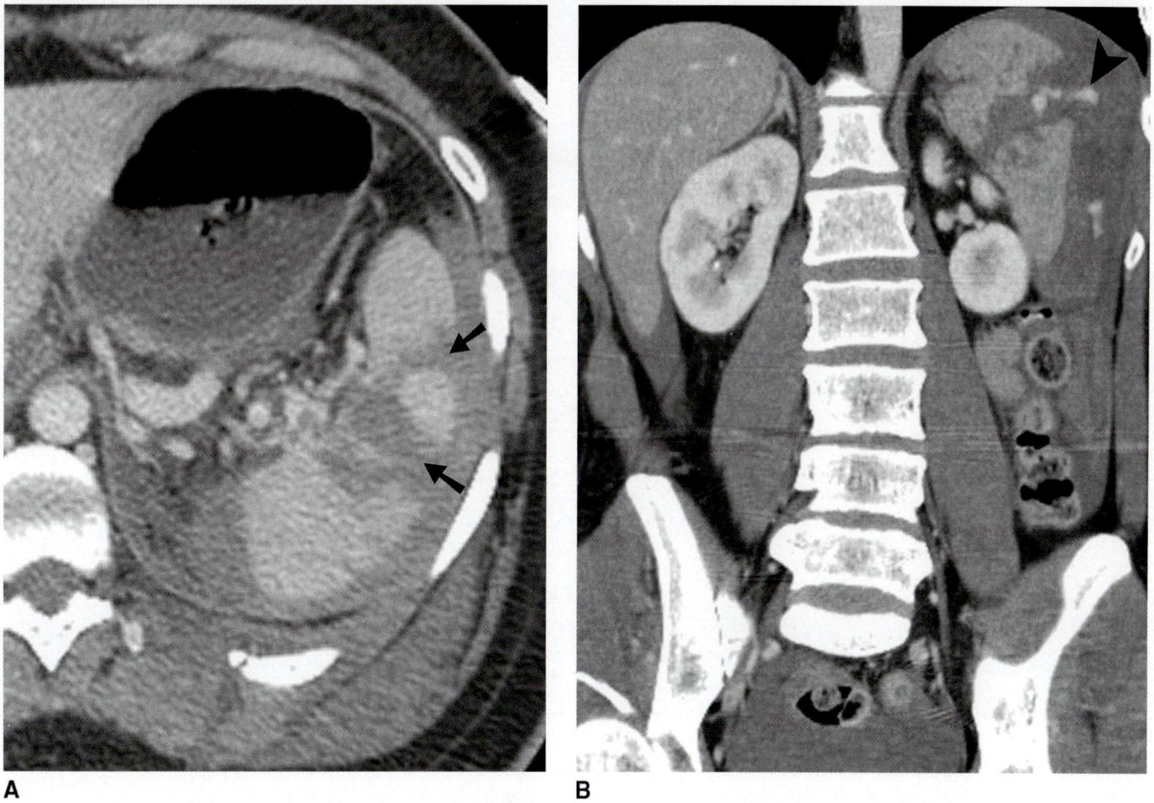

FIG. 11.18 • **Shattered spleen. A, B:** Axial and coronal CT of the abdomen demonstrates splenic lacerations (*arrows*) extending from the splenic capsule to the splenic hilum with active extravasation (*arrowhead*) of contrast and perisplenic hematoma.

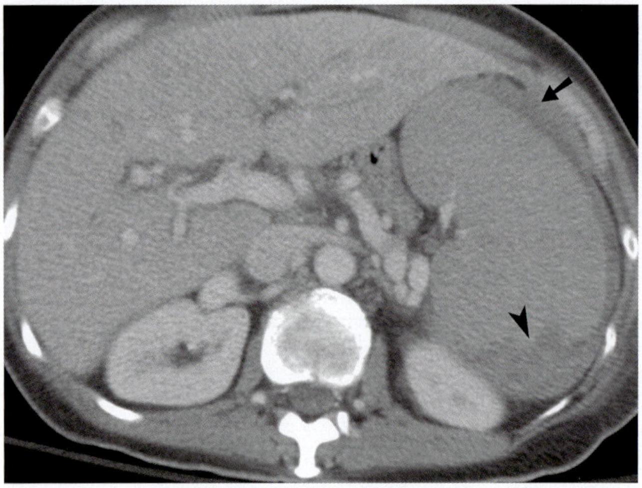

**FIG. 11.19 • Spontaneous splenic rupture.** Contrast-enhanced CT of the upper abdomen demonstrates splenomegaly and posteriorly located splenic laceration (*arrowhead*). There is small amount of perisplenic hematoma (*arrow*) identified in this patient with leukemia.

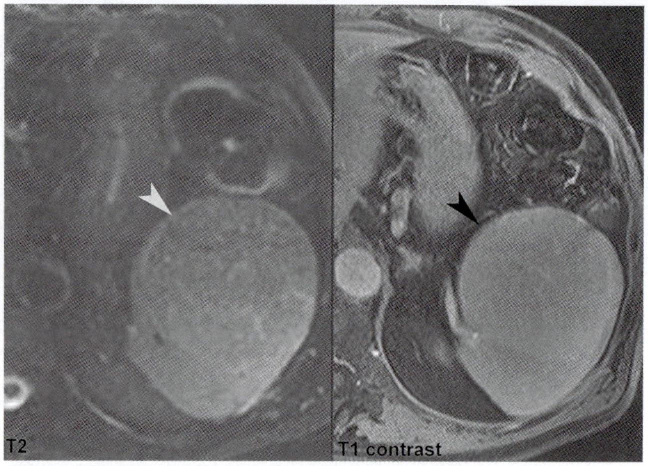


**FIG. 11.21 • Splenic hamartoma.** T2WI and postgadolinium T1WI demonstrate contour abnormality (*arrowheads*) of the spleen caused by an isointense splenic hamartoma.

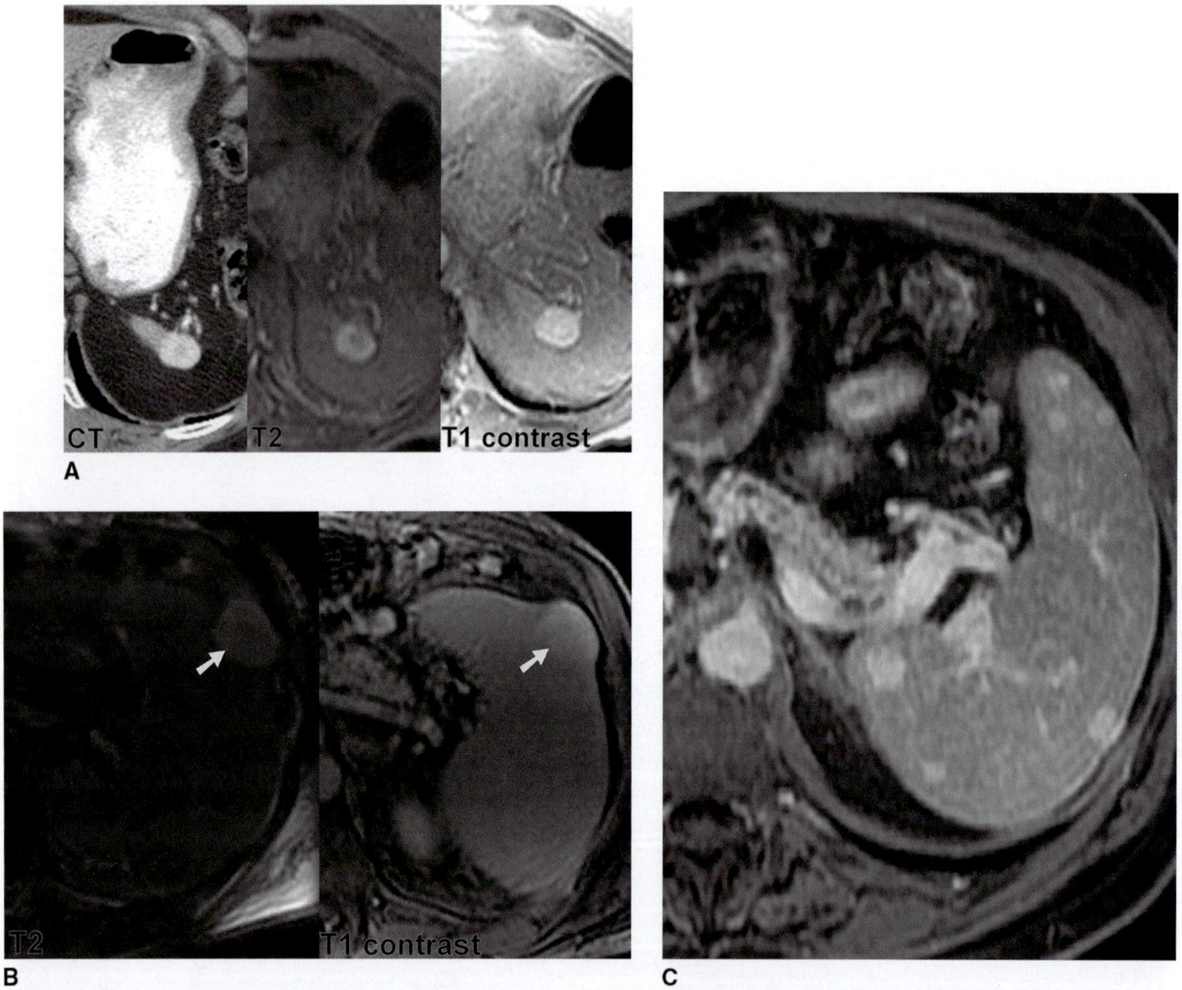


**FIG. 11.20 • Splenic hemangioma. A:** Axial contrast-enhanced CT, T2WI, and postgadolinium T1WI of the upper abdomen demonstrate the enhancing focal lesion in the splenic parenchyma, which is T2 hyperintense. **B:** T2W1 and postgadolinium T1WI demonstrates partially exophytic T2 hyperintense, intensely enhancing hemangioma (*arrows*) in the peripheral splenic parenchyma. **C:** Postgadolinium T1WI demonstrates multiple enhancing hemangiomas in the splenic parenchyma.

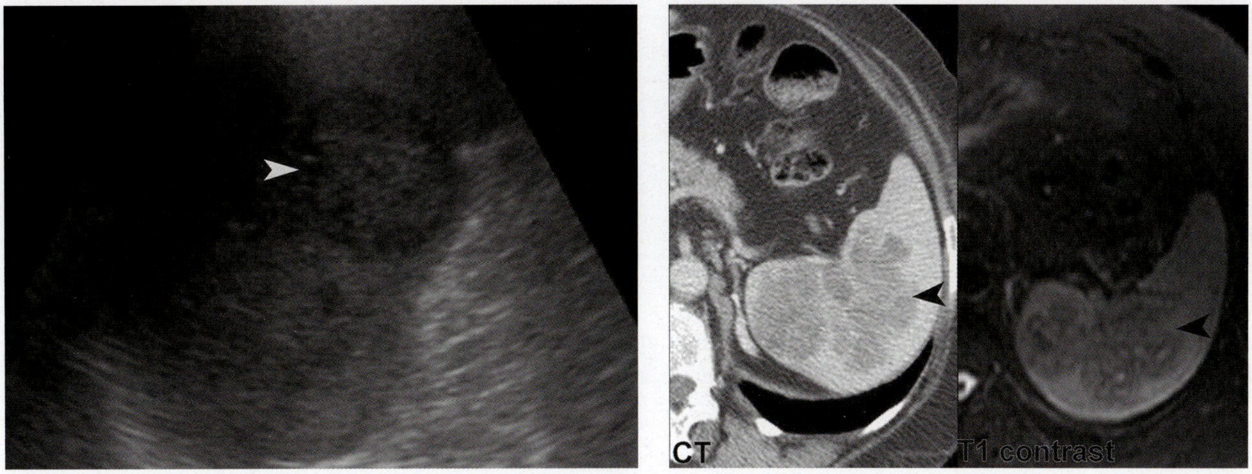


A B

**FIG. 11.22 • Splenic lymphoma. A:** US of the upper abdomen demonstrates a solid space-occupying lesion (*arrowhead*) in the spleen, which was biopsied and was found to represent B-cell lymphoma. **B:** Contrast-enhanced CT and postgadolinium T1WI demonstrate a lobulated space-occupying lesion (*arrowheads*) in the splenic parenchyma, consistent with lymphoma.

## Malignant Tumors

Although lymphoma is the most common malignancy of the spleen, angiosarcoma is the most common primary malignant tumor of the spleen (Fig. 11.22). These are highly malignant tumors that demonstrate early metastases and poor prognosis. They are seen most commonly after the age of 50 and have no association with Thorotrast exposure. CT findings consist of hypervascular masses with heterogeneous enhancement, areas of necrosis, and widespread metastases.

The most common neoplasm responsible for causing splenic metastases includes melanoma and ovarian cancer (Fig. 11.23).

## Thorotrast Retention

Thorotrast (thorium dioxide) was used as an intravenous contrast agent until the 1950s and suffers from the drawback of being retained by the reticuloendothelial system, most prominently in the liver, spleen, bone marrow, and lymph nodes. It has a biologic half-life of 22 years and is therefore retained in the body for the lifespan of the patient. Because of the release of alpha particles, there is increased risk of leukemia, angiosarcoma, and cholangiocarcinoma. On imaging, the common appearance is granular increased density of the small-sized spleen due to accumulation of thorium dioxide in the reticuloendothelial system (Fig. 11.24). The increase in the liver density is much less pronounced than the spleen.

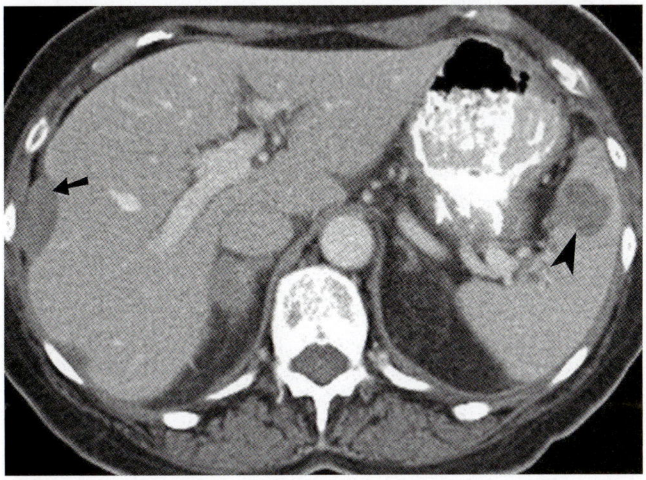

**FIG. 11.23 • Ovarian cancer metastasis to the spleen.** Axial contrast-enhanced CT demonstrates a hypodense focal lesion (*arrowhead*) in the splenic parenchyma. There is a peritoneal metastatic deposit (*arrow*) seen to the right of the liver, causing scalloping of the liver capsule.

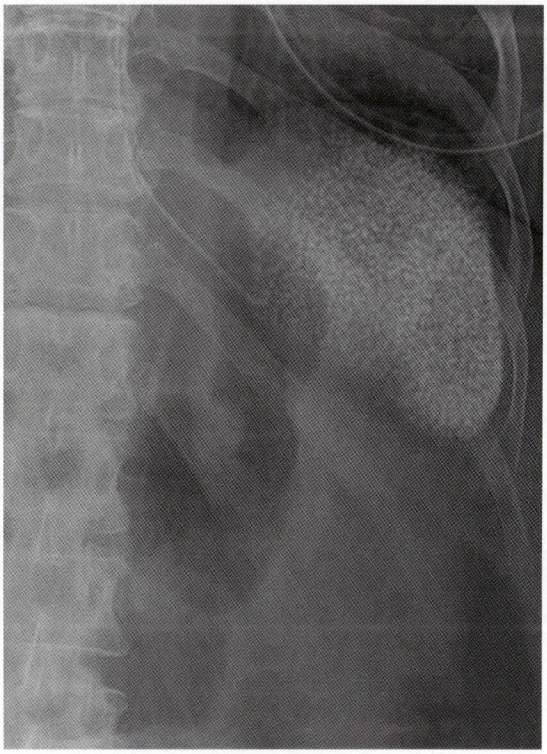

**FIG. 11.24 • Thorotrast exposure.** Plain radiograph demonstrates innumerable granular foci of increased density caused by thorium dioxide accumulation in the spleen.

## References


1. Gayer G, Zissin R, Apter S, et al. CT Findings in congenital anomalies of the spleen. *Br J Radiol.* 2001;74(884):767–772.
2. Thanarajasingam G, Vaidya R, Erie A, et al. Accessory splenectomy for refractory immune thrombocytopenic purpura. *Am J Hematol.* 2011;86:520–523. doi: 10.1002/ajh.22011.
3. Applegate KE, Goske MJ, Pierce G, et al. Situs revisited: imaging of the heterotaxy syndrome. *Radiographics.* 1999;19:837–852
4. Sutherland MJ, Ware SM. Disorders of left–right asymmetry: heterotaxy and situs inversus. *Am J Med Genet C: Semin Med Genet.* 2009;151(4):307–317.
5. Uludag M, Yetkin G, Citgez B, et al. Giant true cyst of the spleen with elevated serum markers, carbohydrate antigen 19-9 and cancer antigen 125. *BMJ Case Rep.* 2009;2009:bcr03.2009.1691.
6. Goerg C, Schwerk WB. Splenic infarction: sonographic patterns, diagnosis, follow-up, and complications. *Radiology.* 1990;174(3):803–807.
7. Warshauer DM, Lee JK. Imaging manifestations of abdominal sarcoidosis. *AJR Am J Roentgenol.* 2004;182(1):15–28.
8. Hsu C-W, Lin C-H, Yang T-L, et al. Splenic inflammatory pseudotumor mimicking angiosarcoma. *World J Gastroenterol.* 2008;14(41):6421–6424. doi: 10.3748/wjg.14.6421.
9. Chan YL, Yang WT, Sung JJ, et al. Diagnostic accuracy of abdominal ultrasonography compared to magnetic resonance imaging in siderosis of the spleen. *J Ultrasound Med.* 2000;19(8):543–547.
10. Resteghini N, Nielsen J, Hoimes ML, et al. Delayed splenic rupture presenting 70 days following blunt abdominal trauma. *Clin Imaging.* 2014;38(1):73–74.
11. Taylor AJ, Dodds WJ, Erickson SJ, et al. CT of acquired abnormalities of the spleen. *AJR Am J Roentgenol.* 1991;157(6):1213–1219.


## SELF-ASSESSMENT QUESTIONS

1. A patient has a T2 hyperintense lesion in the spleen with peripheral nodular enhancement. Which syndrome is commonly associated with this finding?
   A. Sturge-Weber syndrome
   B. Tuberous sclerosis
   C. Kasabach-Merritt syndrome
   D. Sickle cell

2. Gamna-Gandy bodies refer to which of the following?
   A. Small infarcts from sickle cell
   B. Siderotic nodules from microhemorrhages
   C. Noncaseating granulomas
   D. Paracytic cysts

3. What does the focal splenic lesion depicted on the CT represent?

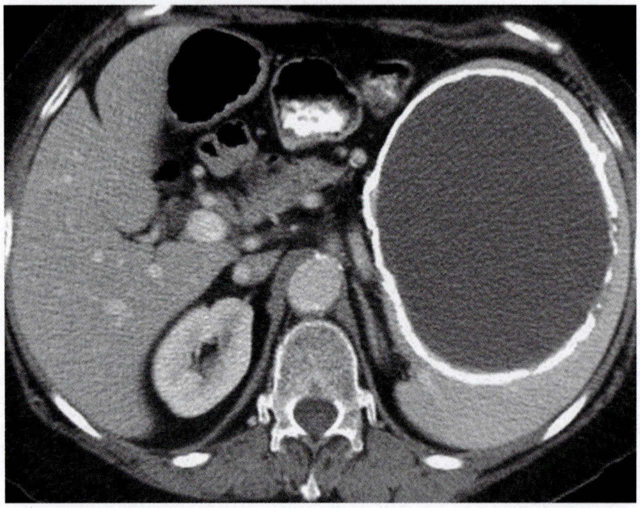

   A. Pseudocyst
   B. True epithelial cyst
   C. Hamartoma
   D. Hemangioma

4. What is the most likely cause of new CT imaging abnormality in the spleen in an immunocompromised patient?

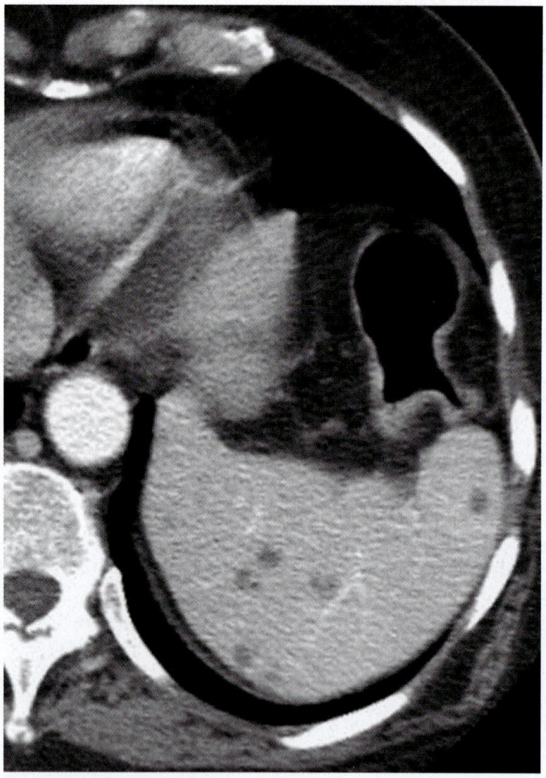

   A. Kaposi sarcoma
   B. Fungal abscesses
   C. Infarcts
   D. Hemangiomas

5. What is a likely cause of the numerous focal lesions seen on the CT?

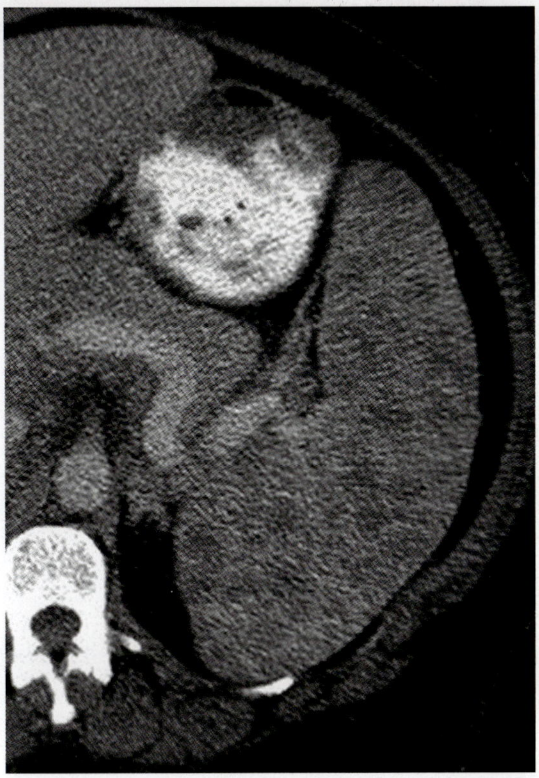

A. Cysts
B. Infarcts
C. Sarcoidosis
D. Angiosarcoma

## Answers to Self-Assessment Questions

**1. C.** Kasabach-Merritt syndrome. Splenic hemangiomas are commonly associated with Kasabach-Merritt syndrome and Klippel-Trenaunay-Weber syndrome.

**2. B.** Siderotic nodules from microhemorrhages. Gamna-Gandy bodies, also referred to as splenic siderotic nodules, are tiny punctate foci of calcium and iron deposited in the spleen usually seen in the setting of chronic microhemorrhage secondary to portal hypertension.

**3. A.** Pseudocyst. The CT depicts a cyst with rim calcification. Mural calcifications are more common, and wall thickness is greater in pseudocysts.

**4. B.** Fungal abscesses. Fungal abscesses are typically seen on CT as multiple, small hypodense foci with enhancing rim. The differential diagnosis include fungal abscesses, sarcoidosis, cysts, and hemangiomas. In this case, the splenic abnormalities are new and therefore exclude pathologies other than abscesses.

**5. C.** Sarcoidosis. In this patient, we see numerous noncystic hypodense splenic nodules and splenomegaly. This fits with CT imaging findings of sarcoidosis, which typically include splenomegaly and multiple less than 3-cm-diameter nodules.

# Self-Assessment Exam

## SELF-ASSESSMENT QUESTIONS

1. What is the gastric antral abnormality (arrowhead) detected on upper GI series of a man with epigastric pain for 8 weeks?

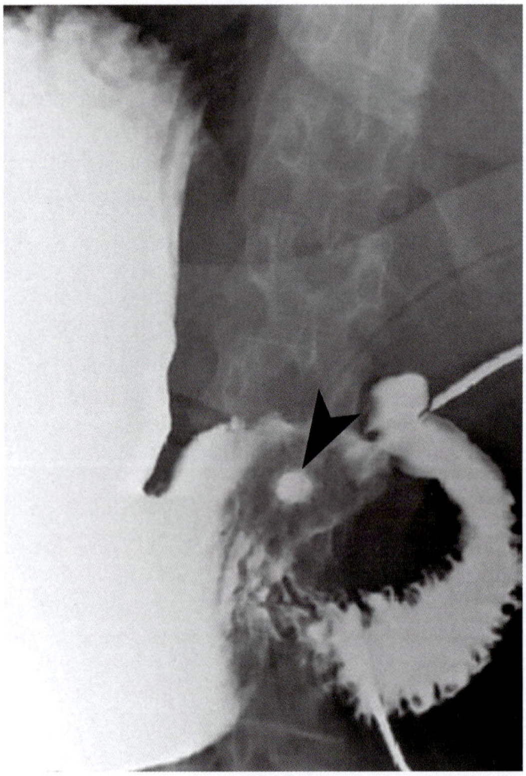

   A. Polyp
   B. Diverticulum
   C. Ulcer
   D. Perforation

2. Mexican hat sign is seen in which pathology on barium study?
   A. Diverticulum
   B. Ulcer
   C. Sessile polyp
   D. Pedunculated polyp

3. What type of diverticulum (arrowhead) is depicted on the upper GI series of a man with abdominal pain?

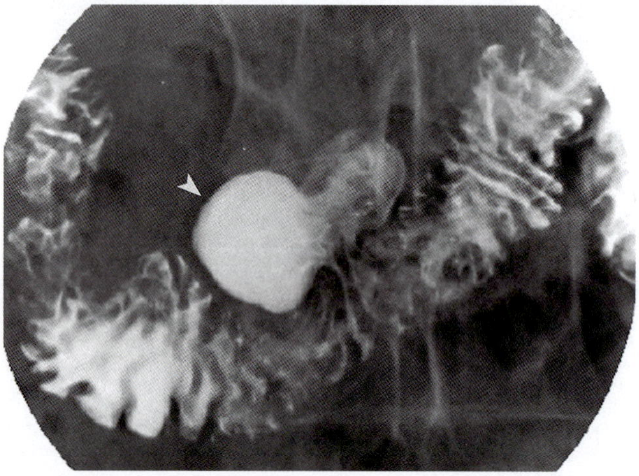

   A. True diverticulum
   B. Traction diverticulum
   C. False diverticulum
   D. Zenker diverticulum

4. What type of diverticulum (arrowhead) is depicted on the barium swallow?

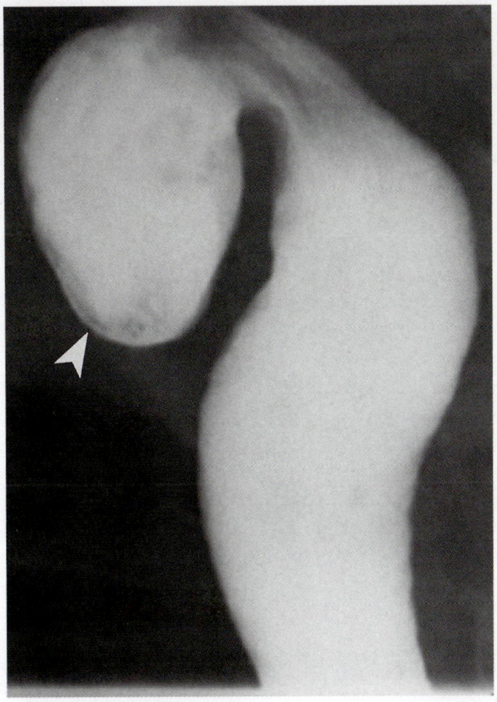

A. True diverticulum
B. Traction diverticulum
C. Pulsion diverticulum
D. Zenker diverticulum

5. What type of pathology is depicted on the upper GI series?

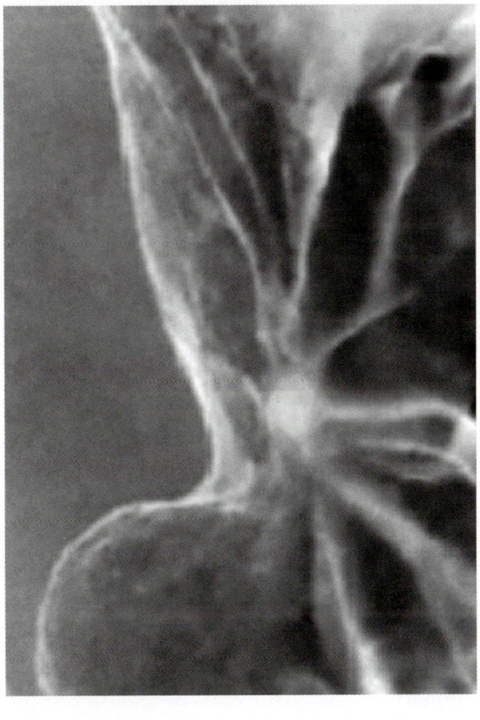

A. Carcinoid tumor
B. Malignant ulcer
C. Bull's-eye lesion
D. Benign ulcer

6. Based on the double-contrast esophagram study, what is the likely cause of esophagitis in an immunocompromised patient?

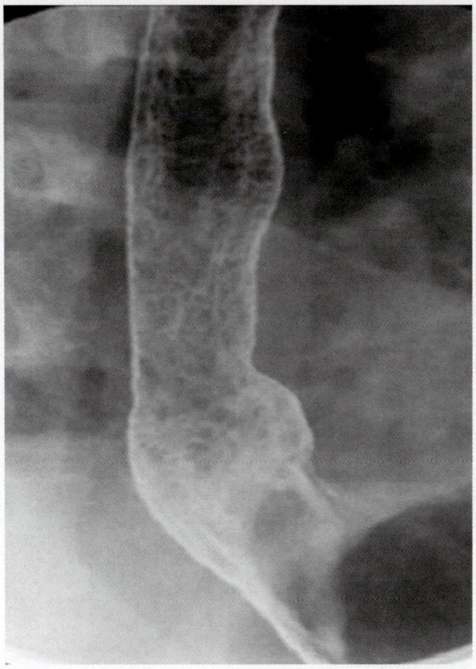

A. Candida
B. Herpes
C. CMV
D. HIV

7. Thin transient mucosal transverse folds were seen during fluoroscopy in an immunocompromised patient. What is the diagnosis?

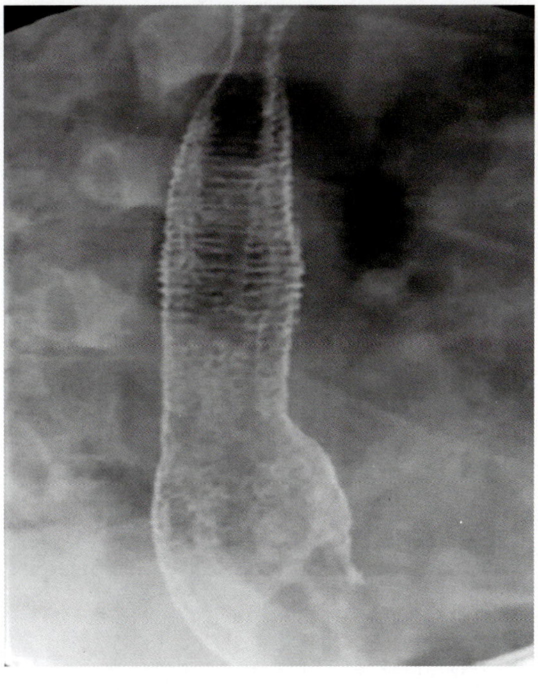

A. Candida esophagitis
B. Feline esophagus
C. Reflux esophagitis
D. Lacerated esophagus

8. What is the likely diagnosis on the given chest radiograph?

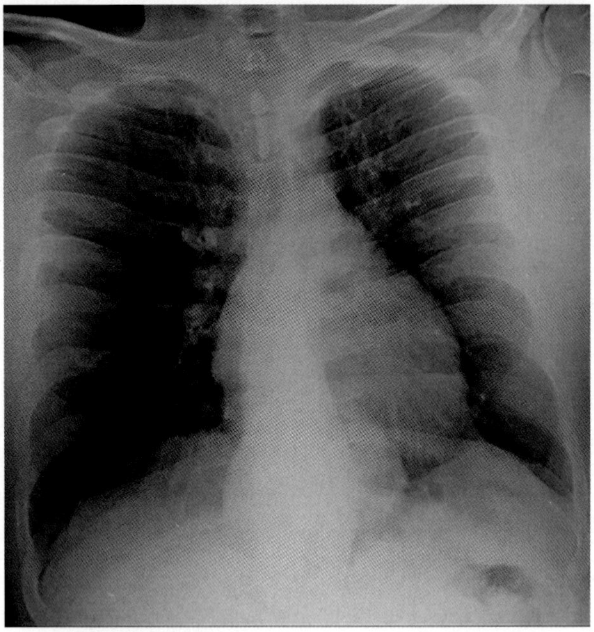

A. Aortic aneurysm
B. Hiatus hernia
C. Pneumomediastinum
D. Lung atelectasis

9. What is the cause of the dysphagia in the patient whose single-contrast barium swallow is shown?

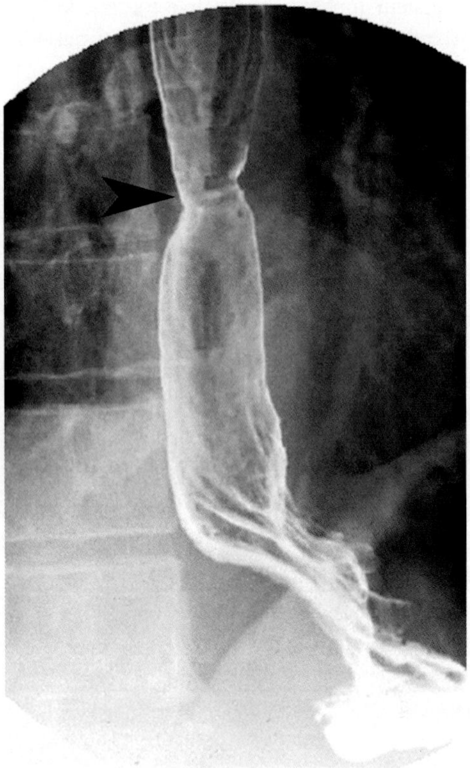

A. Malignant stricture
B. Benign stricture
C. Esophageal dysmotility
D. Extrinsic compression

10. What is the cause of small filling defects on the barium swallow?

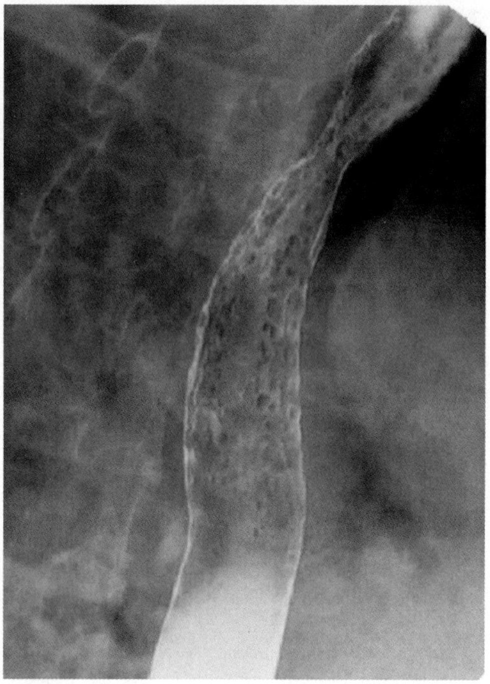

A. Normal variant
B. Kaposi sarcoma
C. Breast cancer
D. Candidiasis

11. What type of diverticulum (arrowhead) is seen on the barium swallow study?

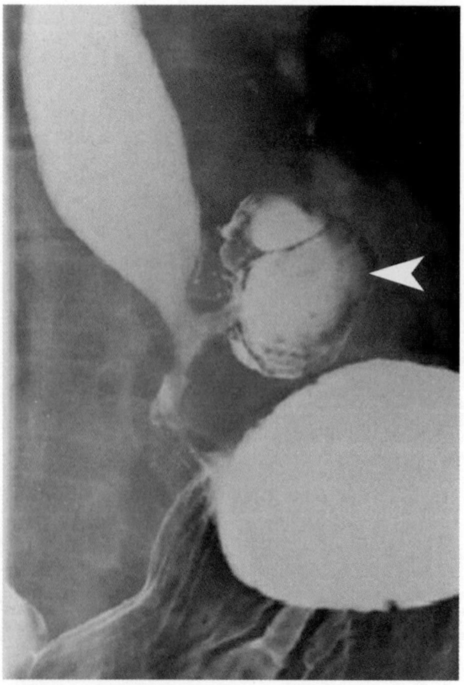

A. Zenker diverticulum
B. Traction diverticulum
C. Epiphrenic diverticulum
D. Killian-Jamieson diverticulum

12. What is the likely cause for the patient's abdominal symptoms on the CT scan study?

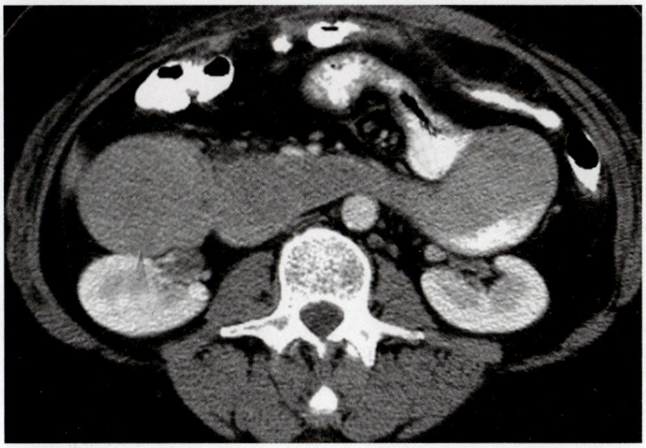

A. Intussusception
B. Bowel obstruction
C. Volvulus
D. Bowel ischemia

13. Where is heterotopic pancreas usually located?

A. Body
B. Fundus
C. Cardia
D. Antrum

14. What is the most common location of gastric diverticulum?

A. Body
B. Antrum
C. Pylorus
D. Cardia

15. Where is the morphologic abnormality seen on the double-contrast upper GI study?

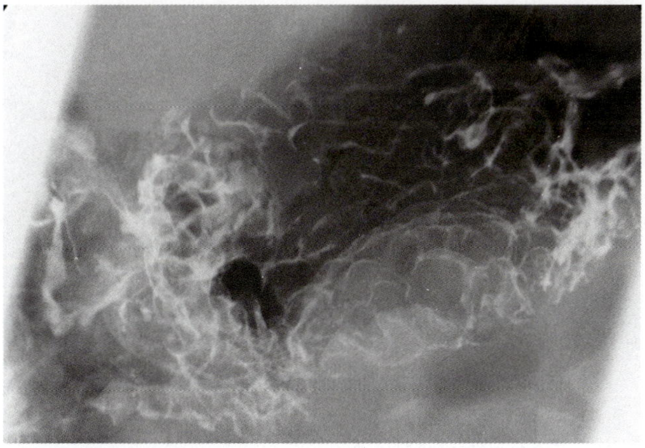

A. Area gastrica
B. Greater curvature
C. Lesser curvature
D. Rugal folds

16. Which of the following gastric malignancy is most likely to cause ovarian enlargement shown on the MR?

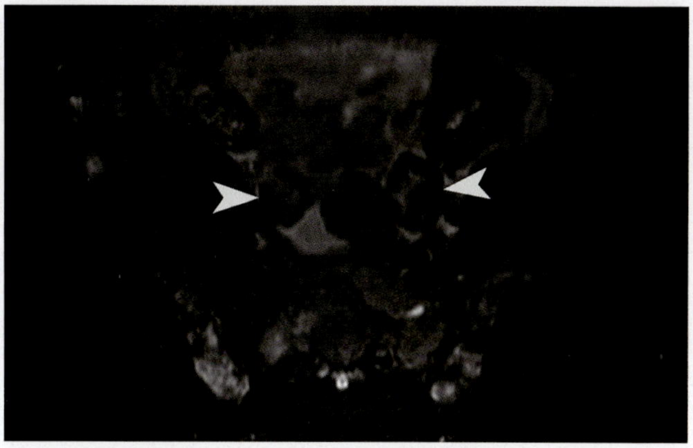

A. Adenocarcinoma
B. Lymphoma
C. GIST
D. Carcinoid

17. What is the most likely histologic diagnosis of the pathology shown on the upper GI study?

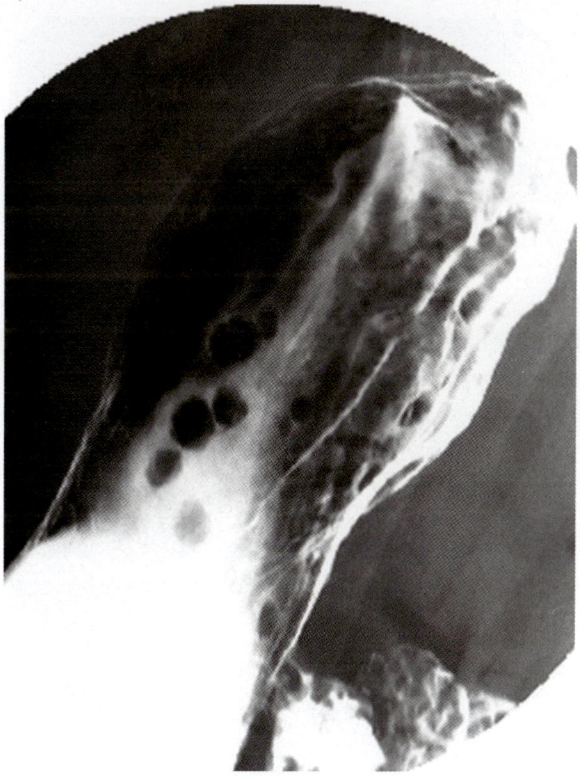

A. Hyperplastic polyp
B. Fundic gland polyp
C. Inflammatory polyp
D. Adenomatous polyp

18. What is the focal gastric antral pathology (arrow) depicted on the upper GI study?

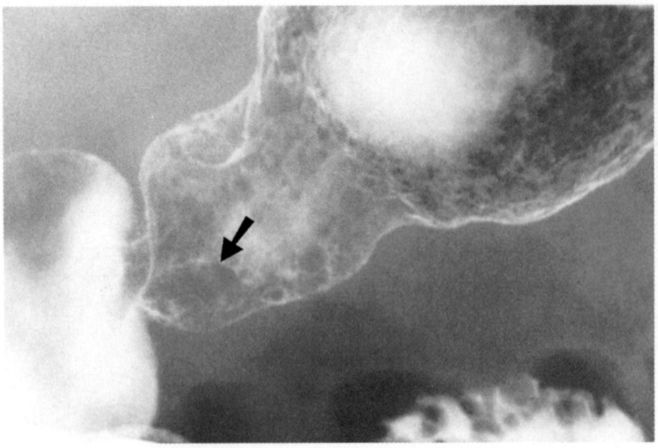

A. Mucosal polyp
B. Submucosal mass
C. Extrinsic mass
D. Malignant ulcer

19. Which of the following is the likely location of the pathology shown on the upper GI study?

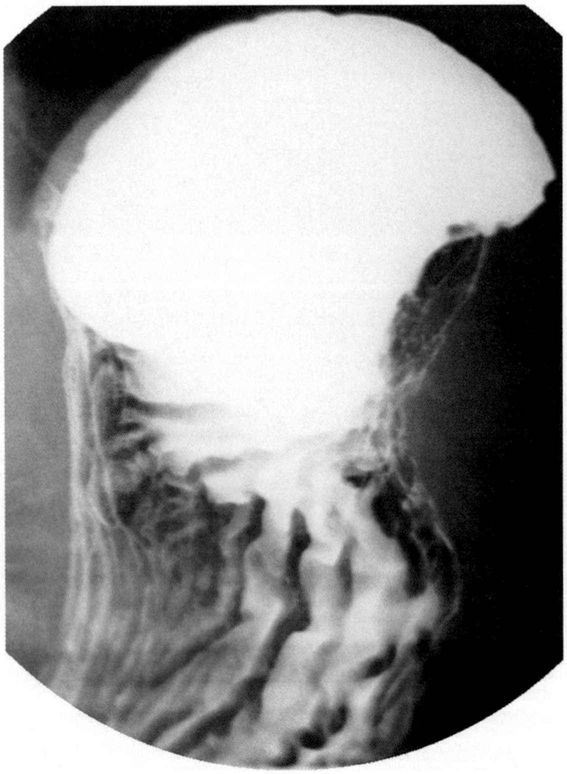

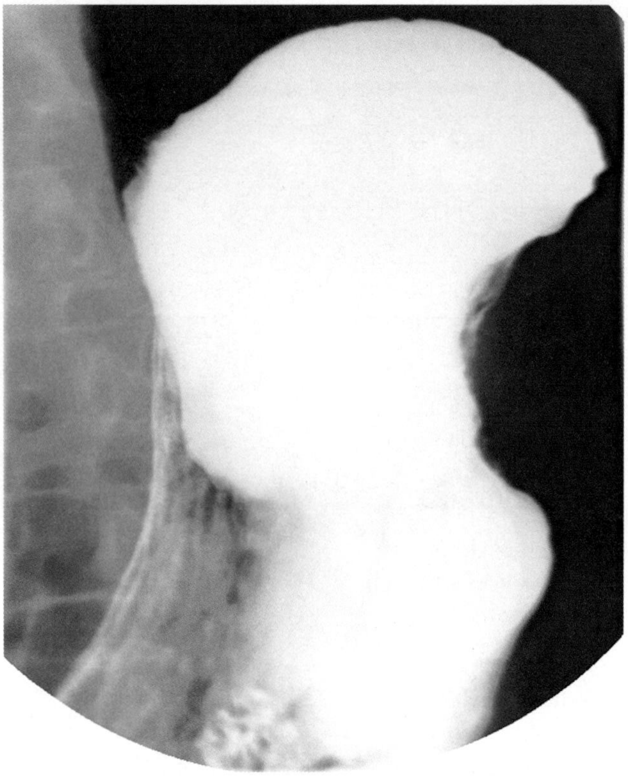

A. Mucosal
B. Submucosal
C. Extrinsic
D. Intraluminal

20. What is the abnormality seen on the single-contrast UGI study?

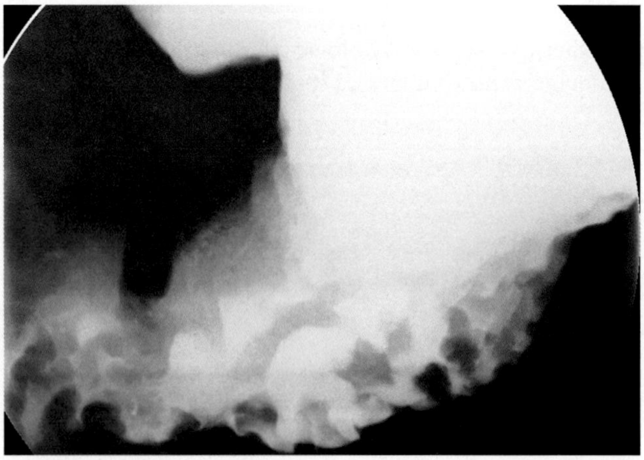

A. Mucosal fold thickening
B. Mucosal ulceration
C. Prominent area gastrica
D. Mucosal polyps

21. What is the likely cause of the CT finding (arrowhead) in a patient who has extensive systemic lymphadenopathy?

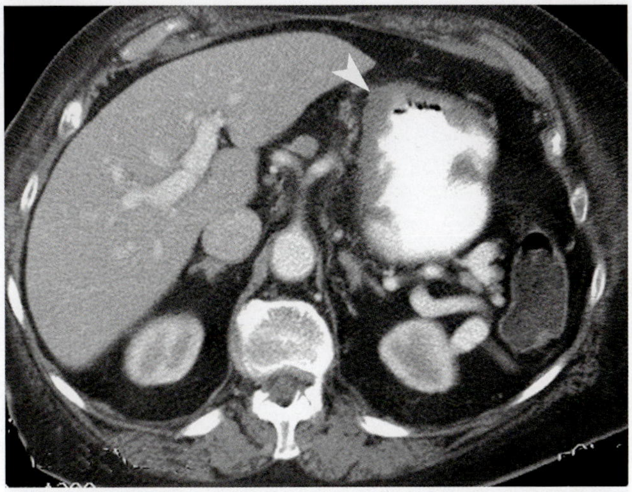

A. Adenocarcinoma
B. Lymphoma
C. GIST
D. Carcinoid

22. What is the likely cause of the CT findings in a young adult patient?

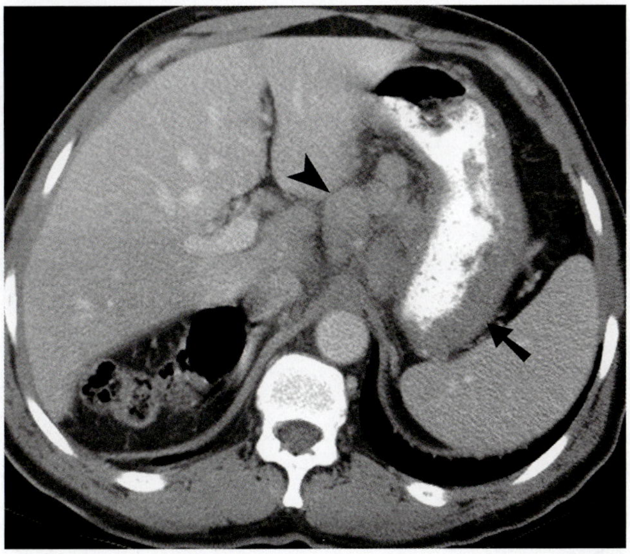

A. Gastric adenocarcinoma
B. Gastric lymphoma
C. Gastrointestinal stromal tumor
D. Gastric carcinoid

23. What is the likely histology of the abnormality depicted on the upper GI study?

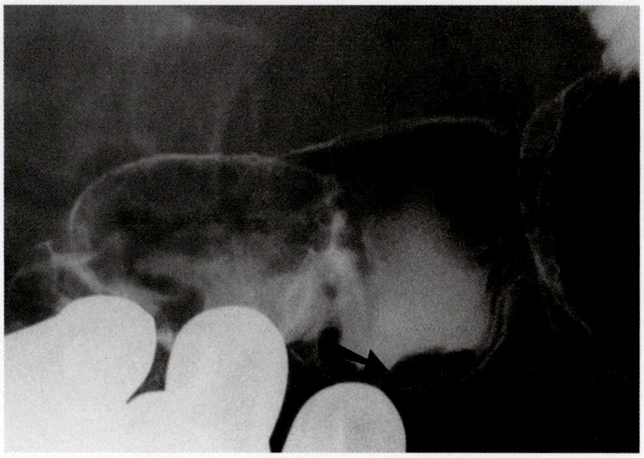

A. Hyperplastic polyp
B. Fundic gland polyp
C. Adenomatous polyp
D. Brunner gland hamartoma

24. What is the cause of the patient's vomiting shown on upper GI study in a young adult patient?

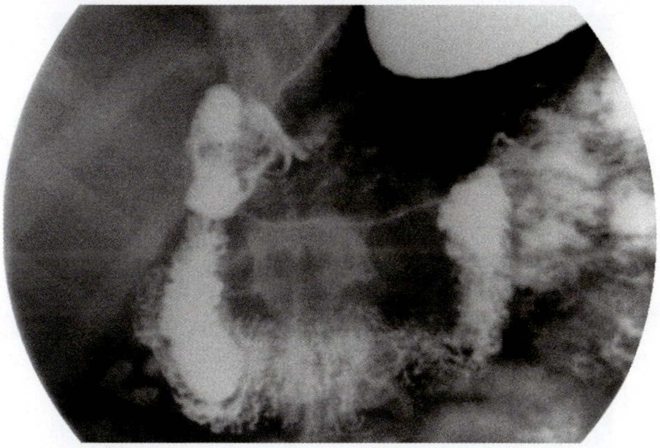

A. Duodenal ulcer
B. Duodenal web
C. Duodenal diverticulitis
D. Duodenal adenocarcinoma

25. What is the cause of duodenal obstruction in this patient who had recently suffered steering wheel injury to the abdomen 1 week ago?

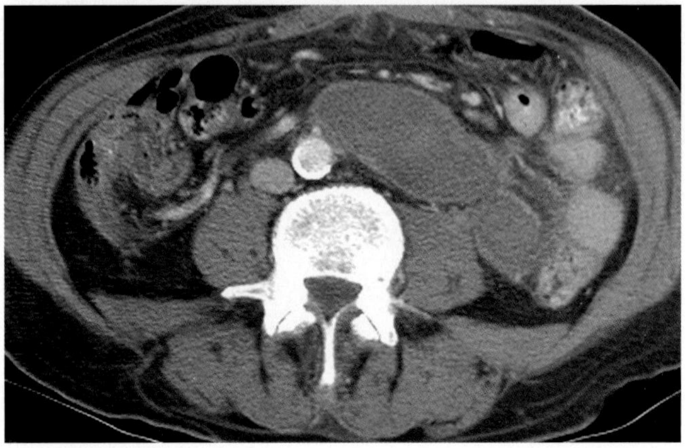

A. Lymphoma
B. Adenocarcinoma
C. Hematoma
D. Perforation

26. What is the incidental finding on the coronal CT reformation?

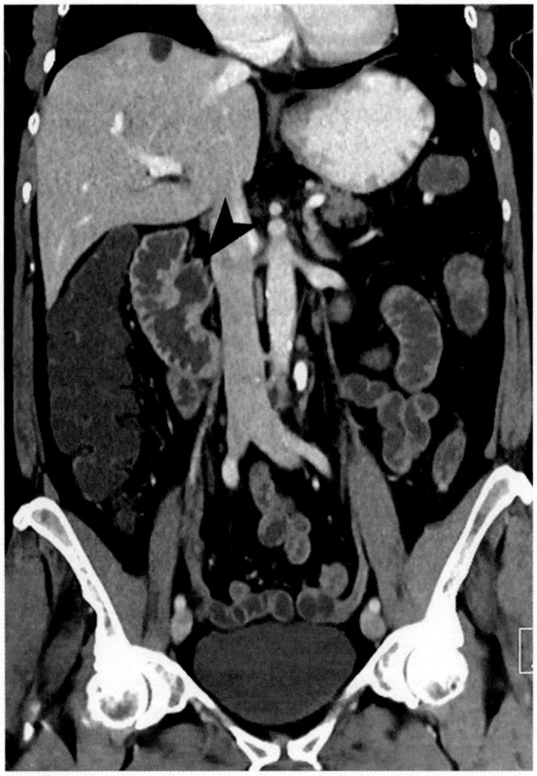

A. IPMN
B. Diverticulum
C. Intussusception
D. Cystic neoplasm

27. What is the cause (arrowheads) of the abdominal pain seen on CT of this patient?

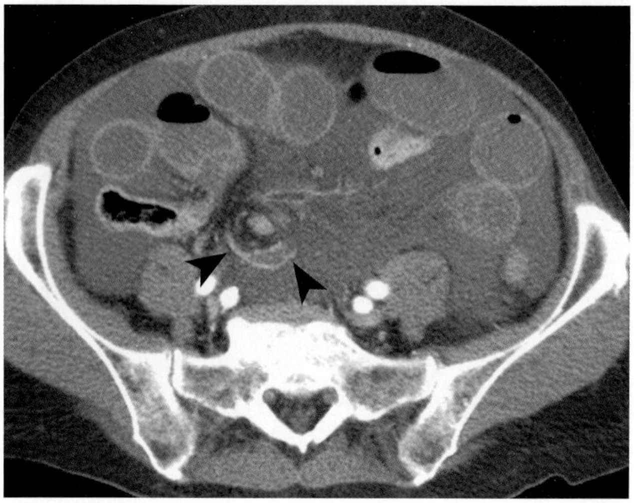

A. Adhesions
B. Gallstone
C. Ischemia
D. Volvulus

28. What is the underlying disease seen on the SBFT of a young adult patient with chronic diarrhea?

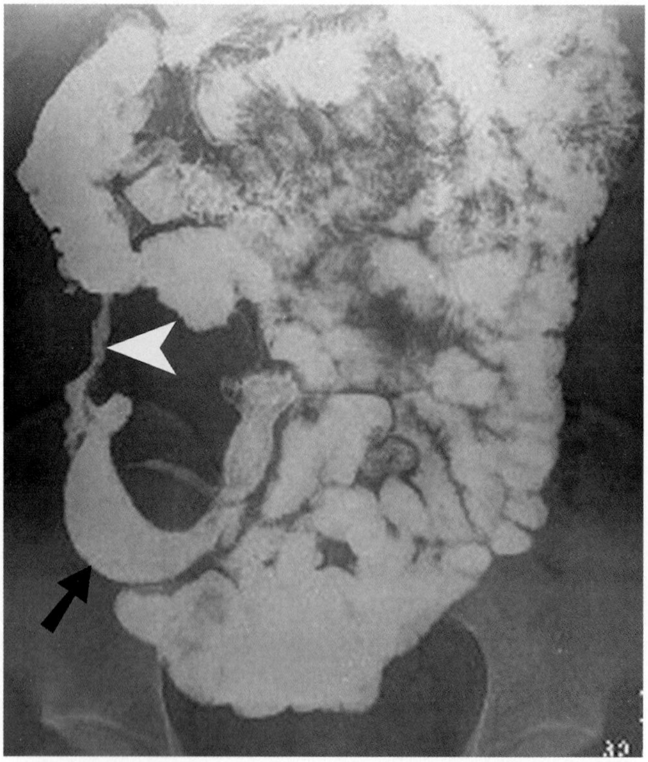

A. Cystic fibrosis
B. Typhlitis
C. Diverticulitis
D. Crohn disease

29. What is the small bowel pathology (arrowhead) seen on the CT of a patient with acute abdomen?

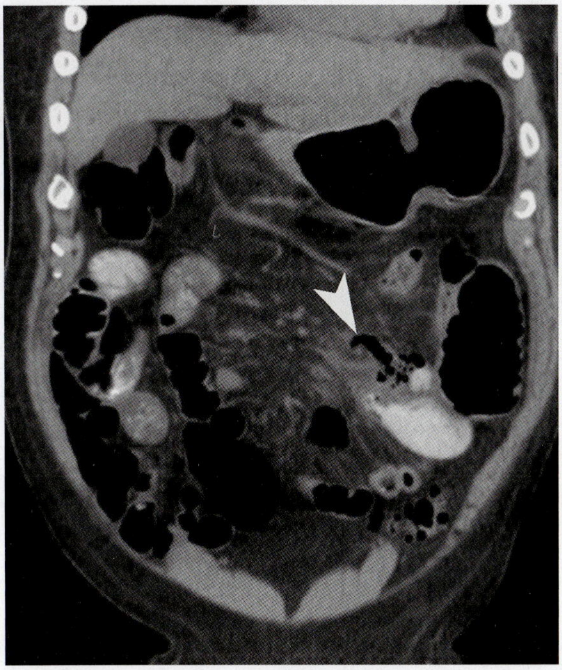

A. Diverticulitis
B. Crohn disease
C. Infarction
D. Malrotation

30. A patient has an SBFT study that demonstrated nodular thickening of bowel wall folds in the small bowel. What should be included in the differential?

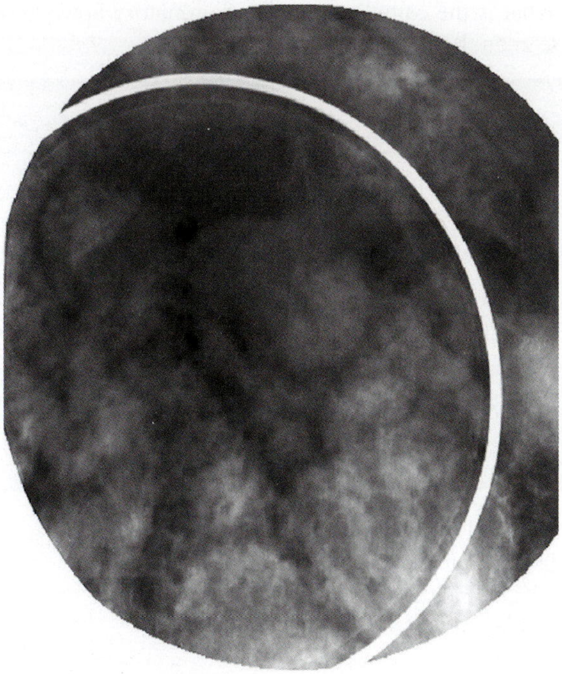

A. Hypoproteinemia
B. Lymphatic obstruction
C. Small bowel ischemia
D. Cystic fibrosis

31. Which is true regarding small bowel diverticula?
   A. Majority are true diverticula involving all three layers of the bowel wall.
   B. Most commonly arise along the antimesenteric border of the small bowel.
   C. There is higher prevalence than colonic diverticula.
   D. Bacterial overgrowth can occur leading to malabsorption.

32. What is the most common primary small bowel malignancy?
   A. Carcinoid tumor
   B. Adenocarcinoma
   C. Lymphoma
   D. GIST

33. Which is true regarding the small bowel neoplasm seen on CT?

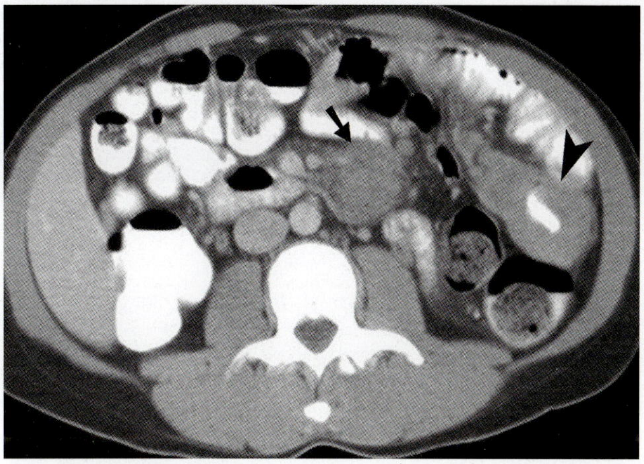

   A. It most commonly arises in the proximal jejunum.
   B. It rarely causes obstruction.
   C. Small bowel is the most common bowel location of this neoplasm.
   D. It is the most common bowel neoplasm.

34. What is the abnormality seen on the upper GI study of a patient with intermittent vomiting?

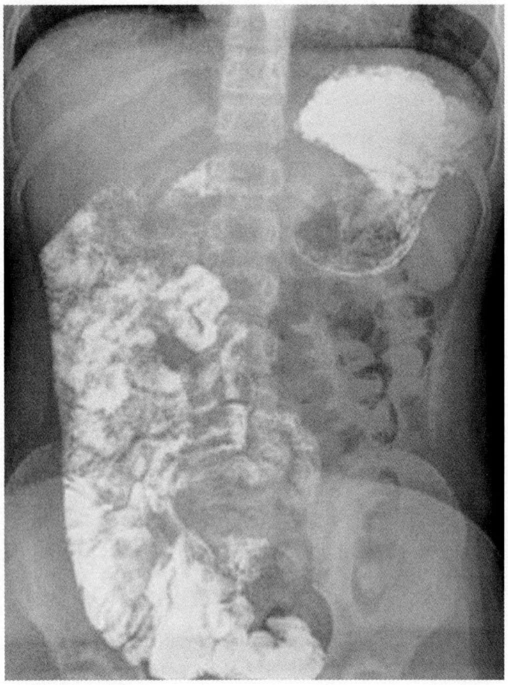

A. Paraduodenal hernia
B. Bowel malrotation
C. Annular pancreas
D. Intussusception

35. Thirty-four-year-old man presenting with recurrent pain in the abdomen. What is the finding on barium enema?

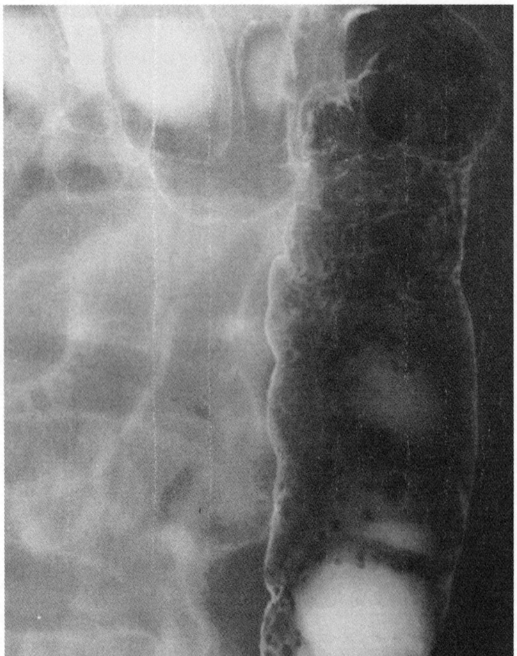

A. Pseudopolyps
B. Fistula
C. Malignancy
D. Deep ulcers

36. What is the diagnosis on the double-contrast barium enema?

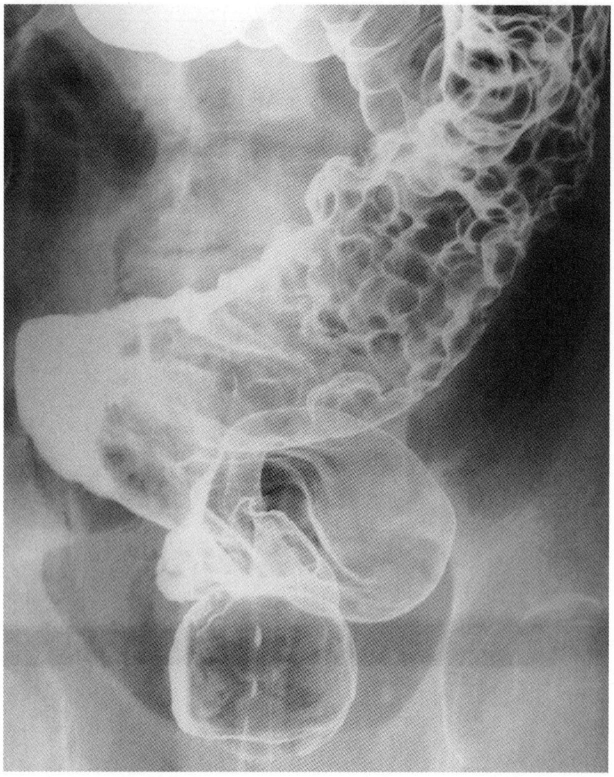

A. Diverticulosis
B. Pneumatosis cystoides intestinalis
C. Stool impaction
D. Ectopic pancreas

37. What is the complication of inflammatory bowel disease seen on the CT?

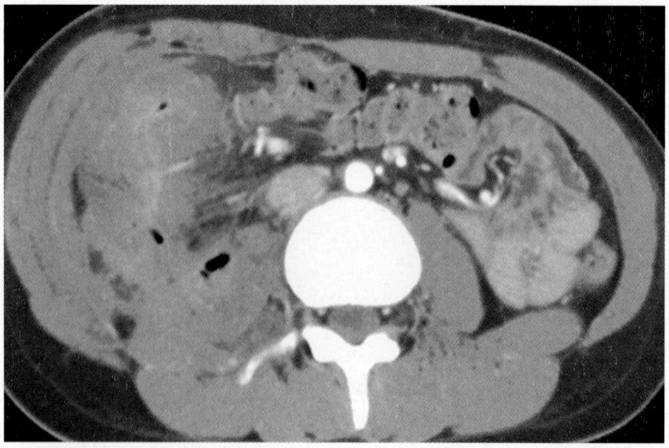

A. Cecal carcinoma
B. Psoas abscess
C. Colonic stricture
D. Colonic ischemia

38. What is the radiologic sign on the supine radiograph?

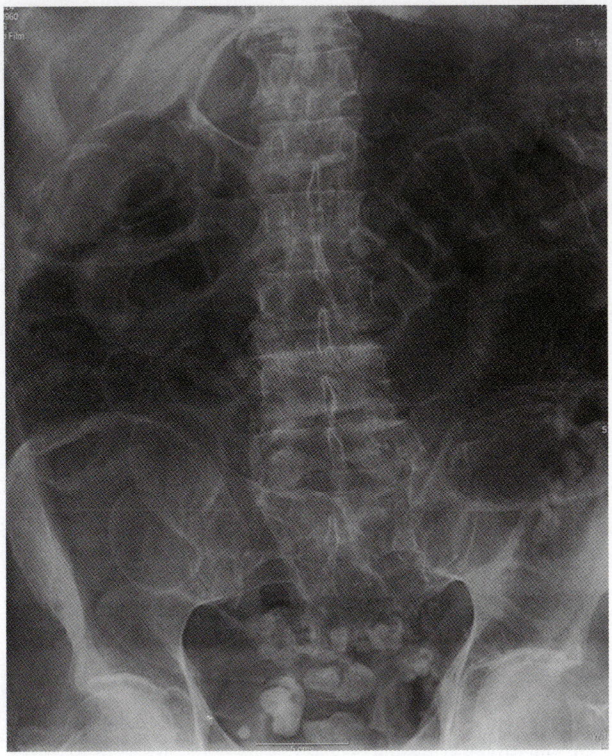

A. Rigler sign
B. Football sign
C. Doge cap sign
D. Cupola sign

39. Thirty-five-year-old man with recurrent pain in the abdomen. What is the radiologic sign seen on barium enema?

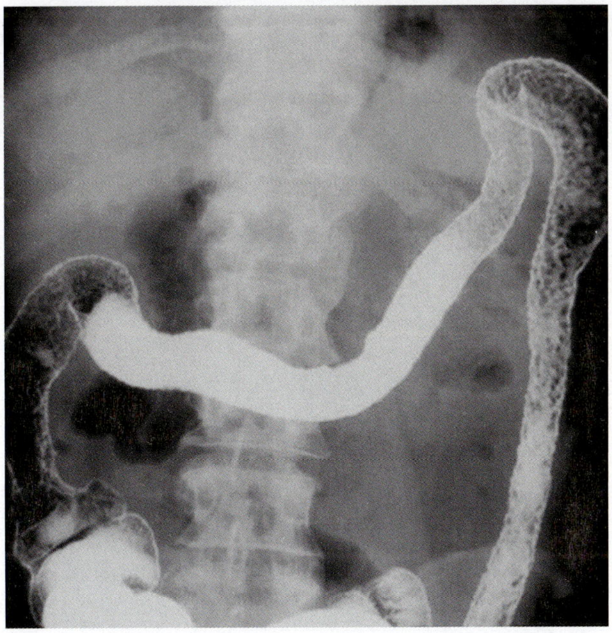

A. Lead pipe
B. Gooseneck
C. String sign
D. Accordion sign

40. What is the cause of the colonic obstruction (arrowhead) on the single-contrast barium enema?

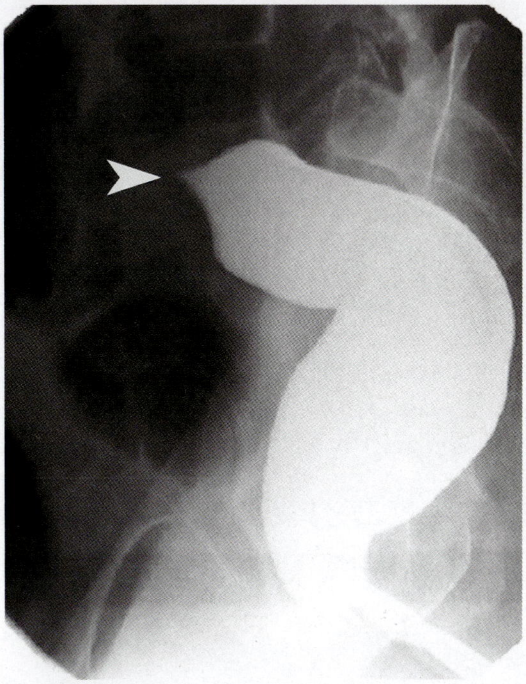

A. Adenocarcinoma
B. Diverticulitis
C. Volvulus
D. Hirschsprung disease

41. What is the imaging finding seen in the colonic lumen on barium enema?

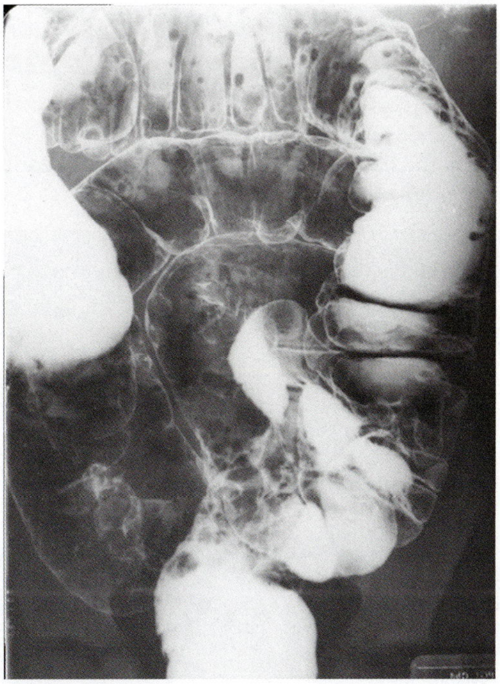

A. Diverticula
B. Polyps
C. Ulcers
D. Fecal matter

42. What is the most likely cause of mucocele appendix?
    A. Cecal carcinoma
    B. Mucinous neoplasm of appendix
    C. Carcinoid appendix
    D. Appendix mucosal hyperplasia

43. What is the cause of acute abdomen seen on the CT?

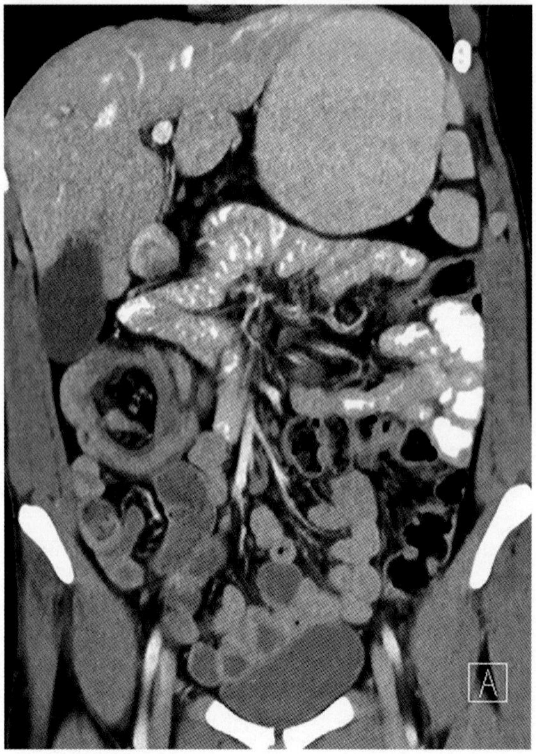


    A. Carcinoma
    B. Adenoma
    C. Intussusception
    D. Metastases

44. What is the likely lead point (arrow) for intussusception shown on the CT?

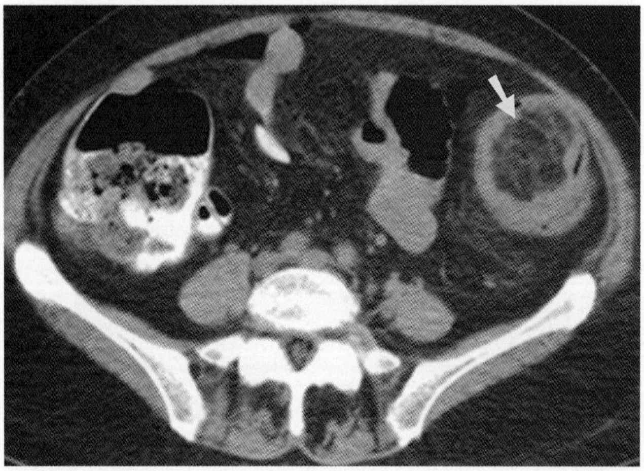

    A. Adenocarcinoma
    B. Lymphoma
    C. Carcinoid
    D. Lipoma

45. What is the plain radiographic finding in this patient with chronic diarrhea?

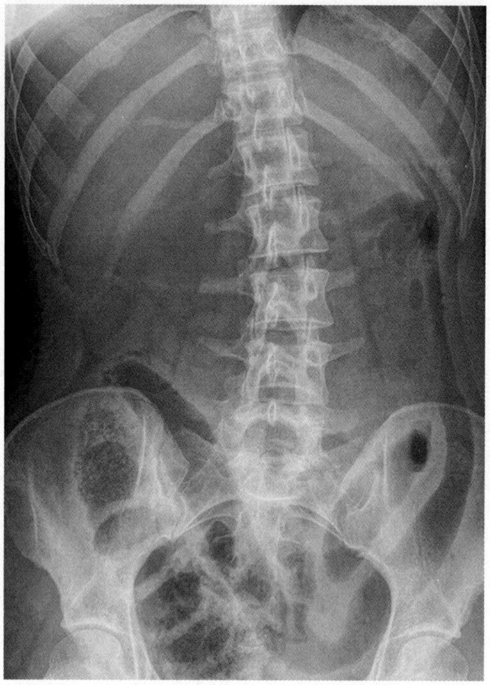

    A. Featureless bowel
    B. Dilated bowel
    C. Free air
    D. Volvulus

46. What is the likely cause of the pathology depicted on the barium enema?

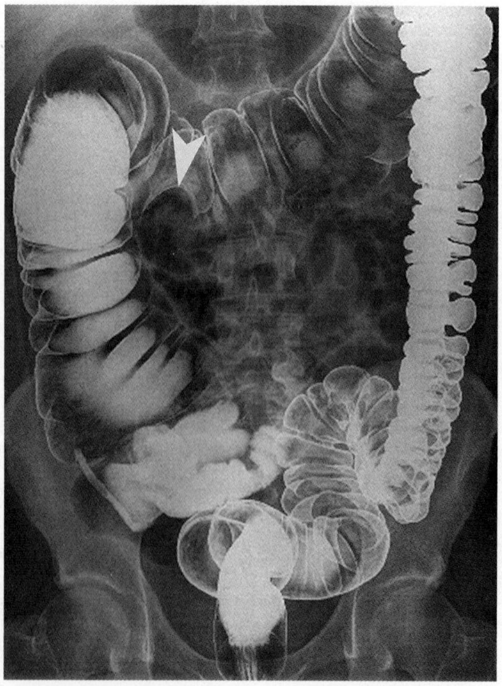

    A. Mucosal mass
    B. Submucosal mass
    C. Exophytic mass
    D. Infiltrating mass

47. A patient with history of appendiceal tumor presents with abdominal distention. Based on the CT scan study, what is the likely diagnosis?

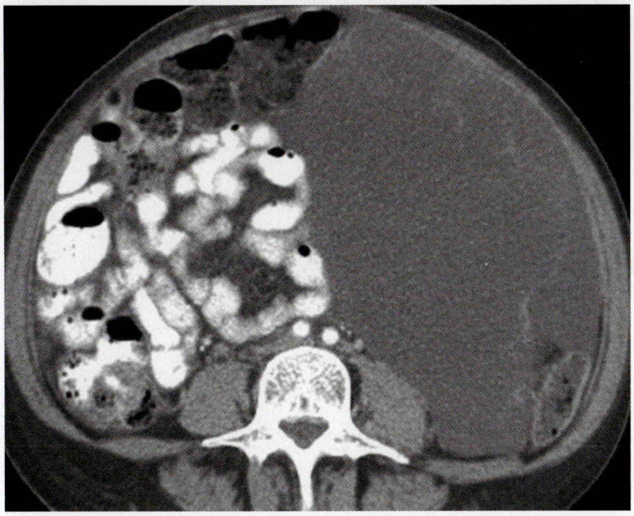

A. Volvulus
B. Pseudomyxoma peritonei
C. Appendiceal abscess
D. Mesenteric cyst

48. What is the most appropriate imaging modality in a 10-year-old male with clinical suspicion of acute appendicitis?
A. US
B. CT
C. MR
D. Plain radiograph

49. What is the most appropriate imaging modality for the evaluation of right lower quadrant pain in a pregnant patient?
A. US
B. CT
C. MR
D. Plain radiograph

50. What is the most common location of the appendix, in relation to cecum?
A. Anterior
B. Lateral
C. Posterolateral
D. Posteromedial

51. Which arrow points to the transverse mesocolon on the CT scan?

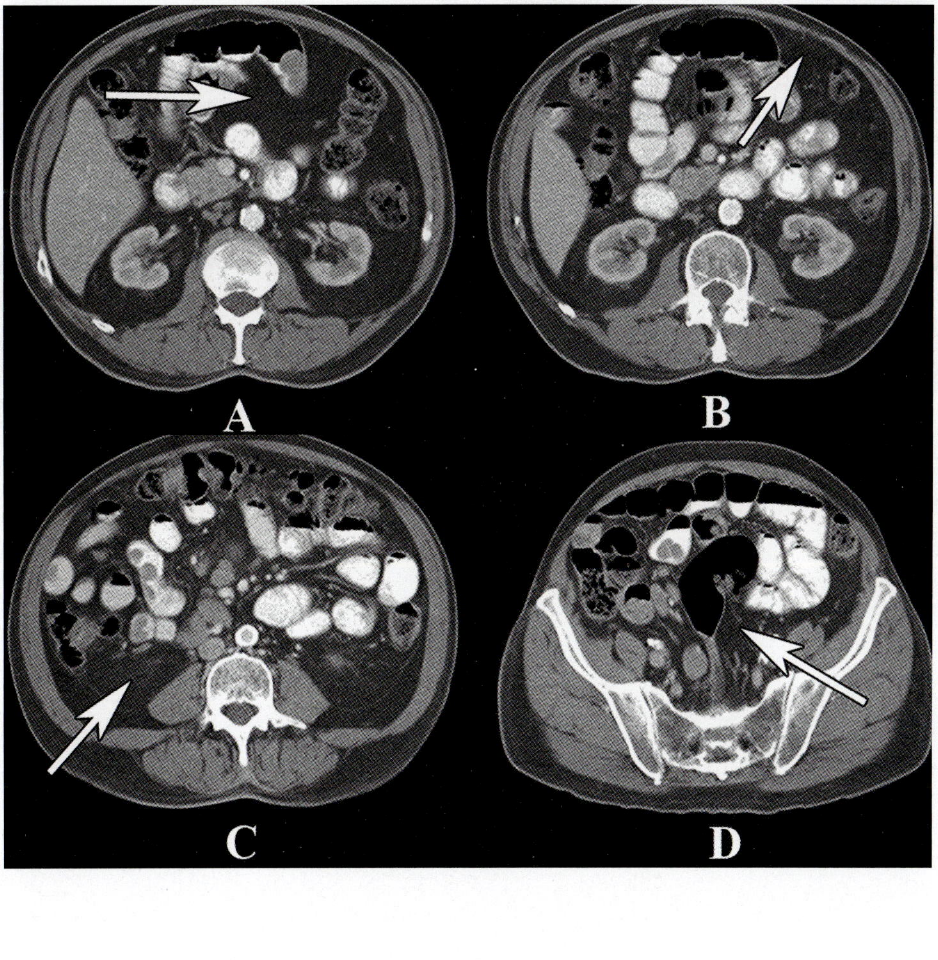

52. In this patient with a history of familial adenomatous polyposis, what is the most likely diagnosis?

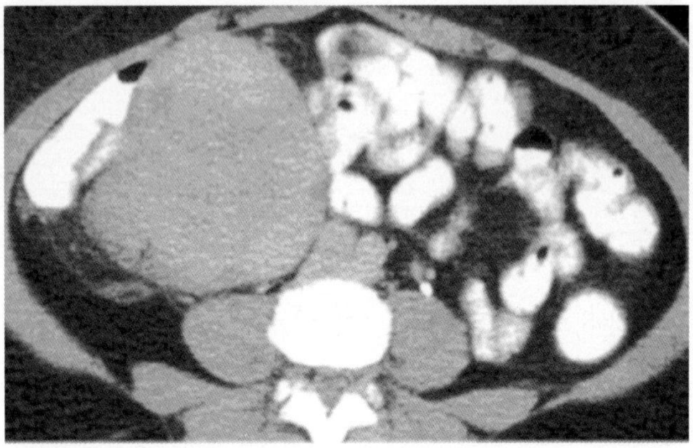

A. Sclerosing mesenteritis
B. Lymphoma
C. Desmoid tumor
D. Peritoneal carcinomatosis

53. What is the likely diagnosis (arrowhead) based on the CT in a patient with normal pentetreotide scan?

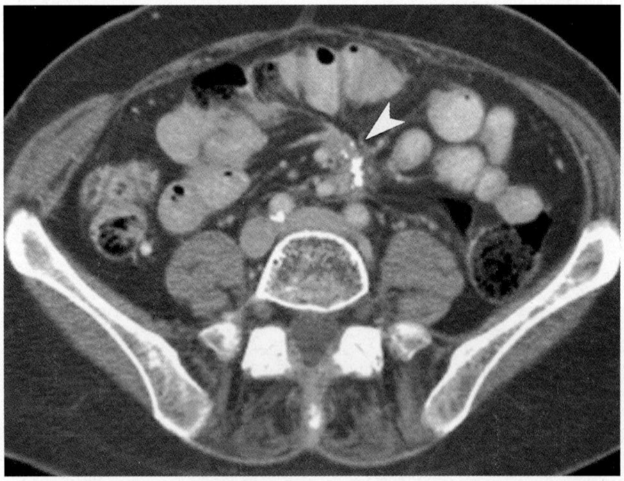

A. Peritoneal mesothelioma
B. Peritoneal carcinomatosis
C. Tuberculous peritonitis
D. Sclerosing mesenteritis

54. Elderly female presenting with abdominal distention. What is the likely diagnosis?

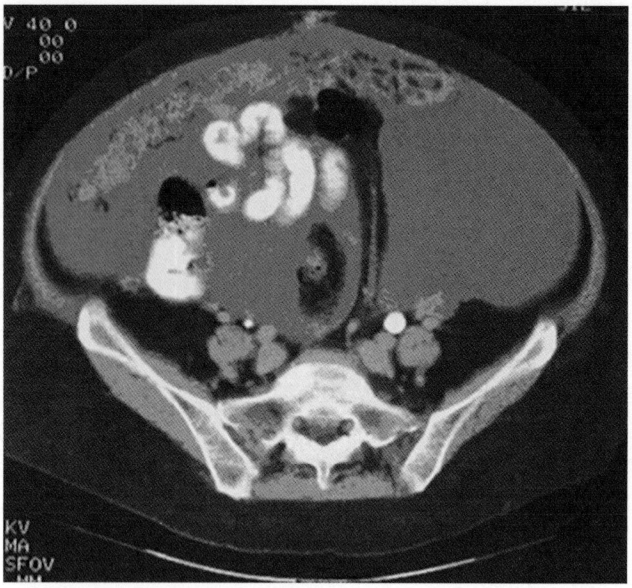

A. Peritoneal carcinomatosis
B. Tuberculous peritonitis
C. Mesenteric panniculitis
D. Pseudomyxoma peritonei

55. What is the likely etiology of the imaging findings in a patient with hypotension?

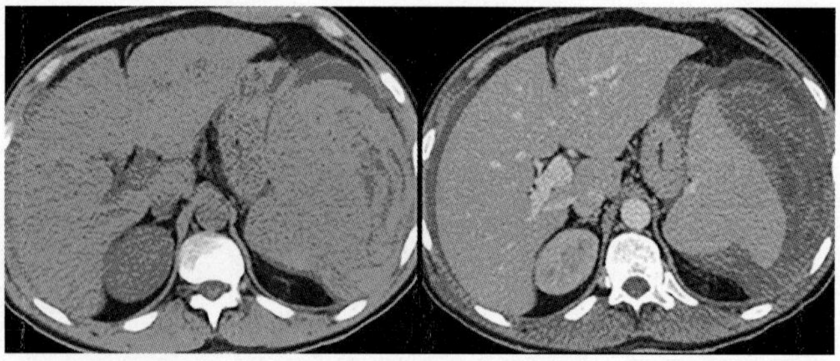

A. Ruptured appendiceal tumor
B. Bacterial peritonitis
C. Splenic rupture
D. Peritoneal mesothelioma

56. What is the cause of peritoneal signs in this patient with abdominal pain?

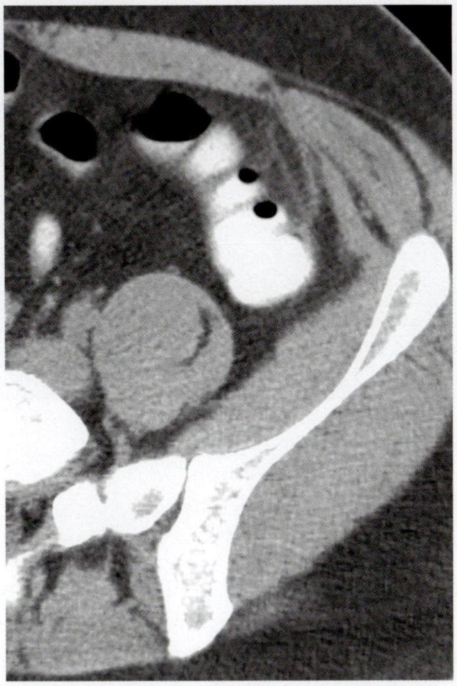

A. Acute epiploic appendagitis
B. Segmental omental infarction
C. Acute sigmoid colonic diverticulitis
D. Small bowel diverticulitis

57. What is the most likely diagnosis on the CT scan of a man with abdominal distension?

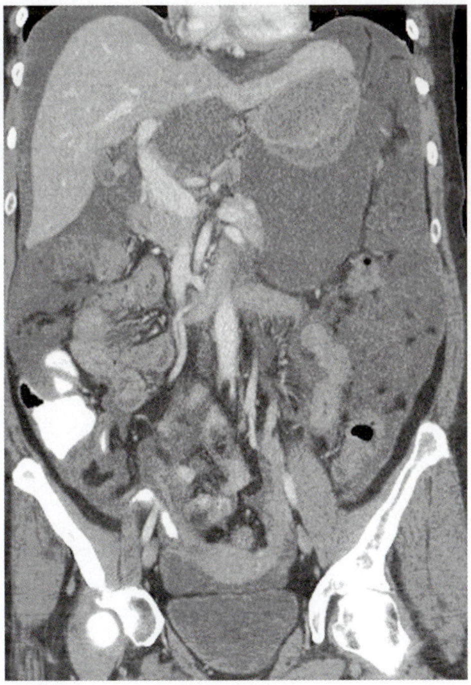

A. Ascites
B. Pseudomyxoma peritonei
C. Sclerosing mesenteritis
D. Peritoneal carcinomatosis

58. What is the most optimal treatment of the pathology depicted on the CT?

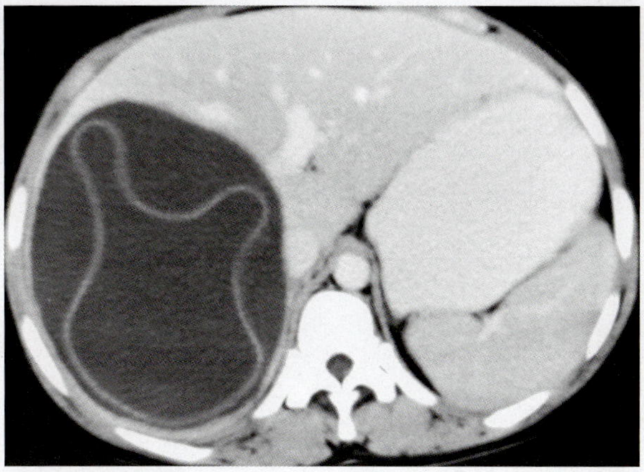

A. Ampicillin
B. Albendazole
C. Metronidazole
D. Adriamycin

59. A 75-year-old woman, with recent history of Whipple surgery and intra-aortic balloon pump placement. A CT was obtained for elevated LFT and abdominal pain. What is the most likely diagnosis in this patient?

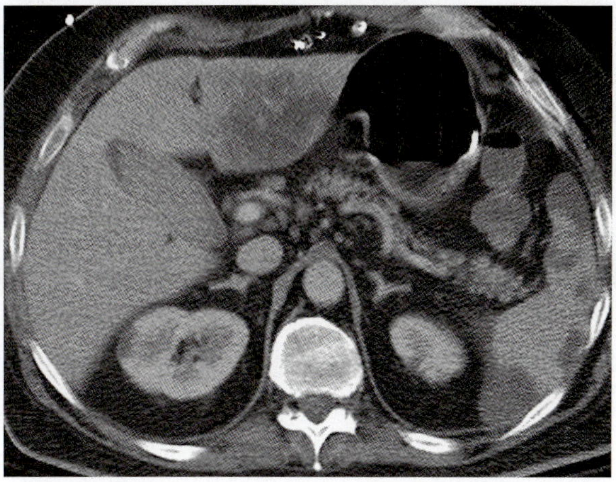

A. Tumor
B. Infection
C. Infarct
D. Cholangitis

60. Which of the followings is the most common vascular complication after liver transplantation?
A. Hepatic artery stenosis
B. Hepatic artery thrombosis
C. Hepatic artery pseudoaneurysm
D. IVC stenosis

61. Which of the following primary tumors is most likely to produce hypervascular hepatic metastasis?
A. Lung
B. Colon
C. Thyroid
D. Pancreas

62. Based on the CT and MR, which is the most likely diagnosis?

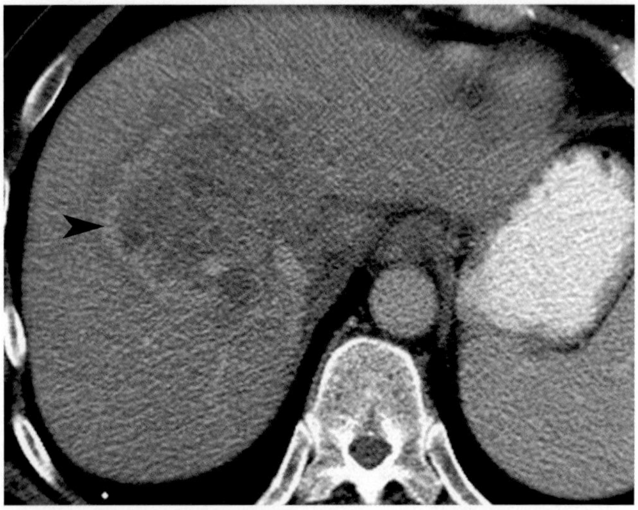

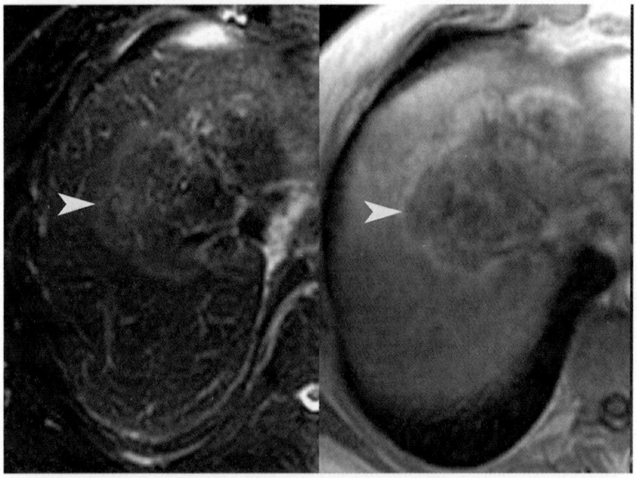

A. Hemangioma
B. FNH
C. Hepatocellular carcinoma
D. Abscess

63. Which of the following focal liver lesions shows imaging features depicted on the CT and MR studies?

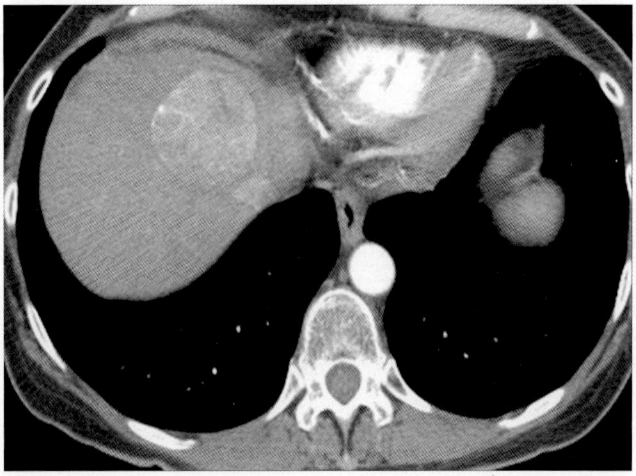

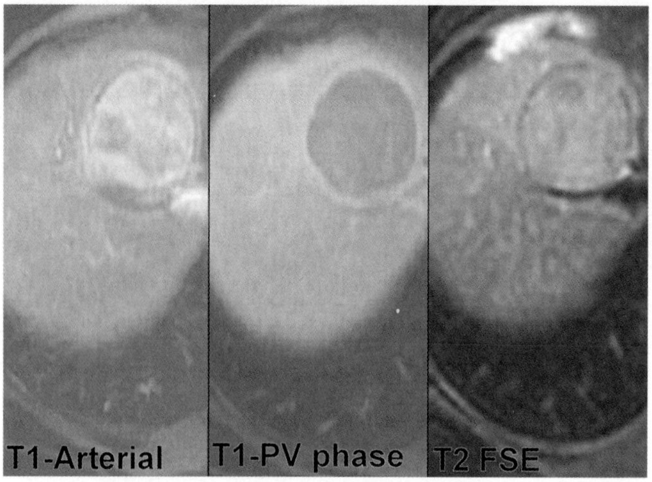


A. Hemangioma
B. Neuroendocrine metastasis
C. Hepatic cholangiocarcinoma
D. Hepatocellular carcinoma

64. What is the risk of metastases from the liver pathology depicted on the CT of a patient with no history of chronic liver disease?

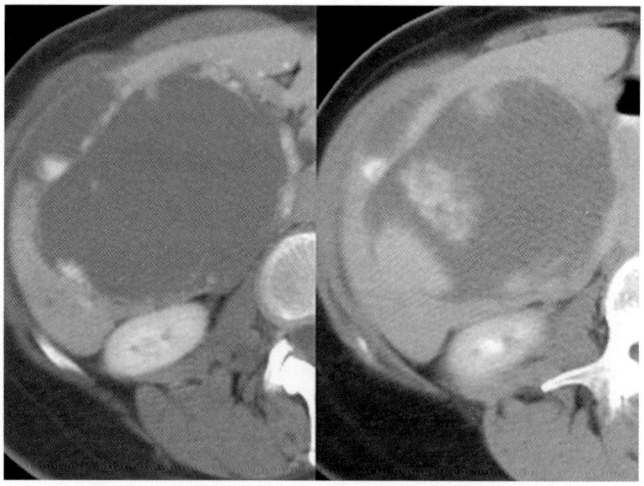

A. 0%
B. 10%
C. 50%
D. 80%

65. What is the pathology depicted on the portal venous phase CT?

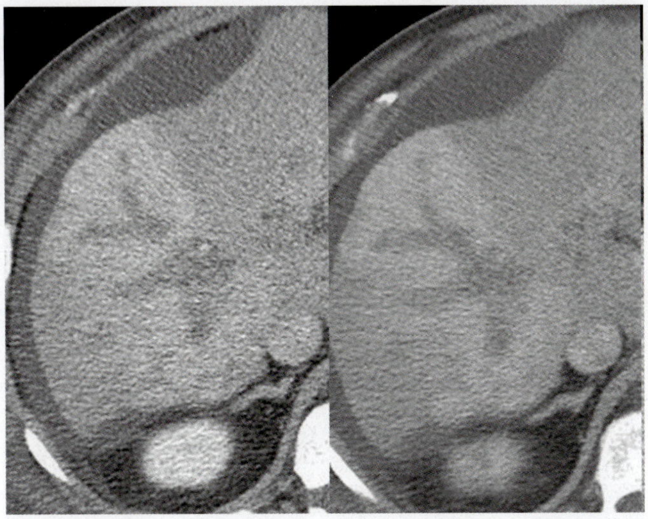

A. Fatty liver
B. Budd-Chiari syndrome
C. Portal vein thrombosis
D. Normal liver

66. Which of the following suggests that the gall bladder abnormality found incidentally on US imaging is more likely to be benign?

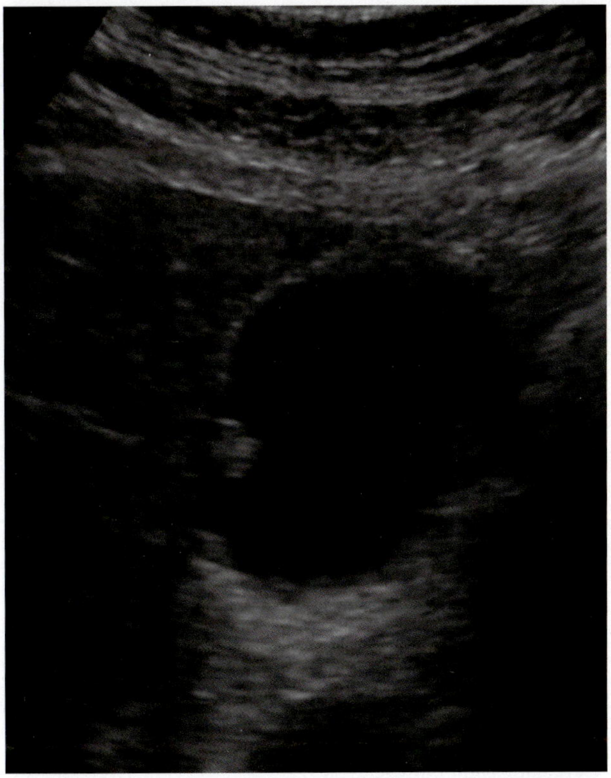

A. Size less than 10 mm
B. Thick wall
C. Doppler flow
D. Calcification

67. Which of the following provides the best likelihood for detection of choledocholithiasis on CT?

A. Axial images
B. Stone in the distal CBD
C. Stone size less than 5 mm
D. Presence of CBD dilatation

68. Which of the following describes the characteristic imaging feature of cholangiocarcinoma of the bile duct?

A. Discrete mass
B. Biliary stricture
C. Delayed enhancement
D. Bulging off the liver contour

69. Which of the following condition is depicted on the CT of a patient with chronic abdominal pain?

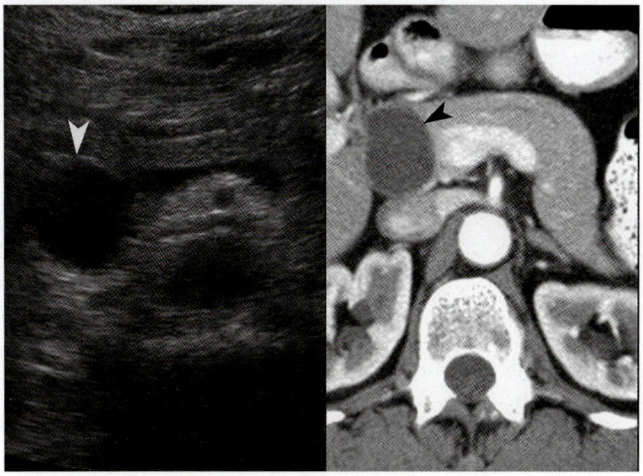

A. Aberrant pancreaticobiliary junction
B. CBD stone
C. Choledochocele
D. Parasitic infestation

70. What imaging finding is seen on the cholescintigraphy study of a patient with acute right upper quadrant pain?

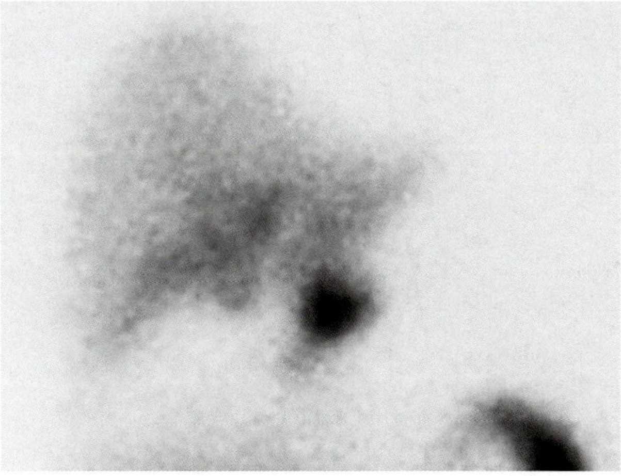

A. Rim sign
B. Dilated CBD
C. Dilated bowel
D. Delayed excretion

71. A peripheral hypoattenuating halo can be seen in what pancreatic condition?
   A. Annular pancreas
   B. Acute pancreatitis
   C. Autoimmune pancreatitis
   D. Pancreatic sarcoidosis

72. What is the cause of the pancreatic pathology depicted on the CT?

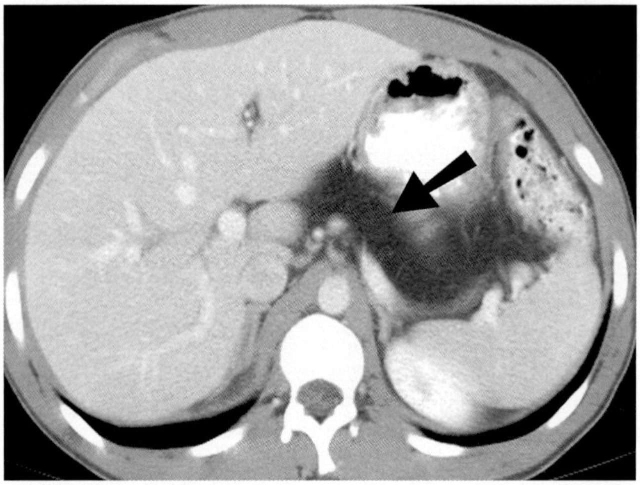

   A. Non-Hodgkin lymphoma
   B. Acute trauma
   C. Cystic fibrosis
   D. Acute pancreatitis

73. In a patient with pancreatic pseudocyst, what important finding is depicted on the CT scan study?

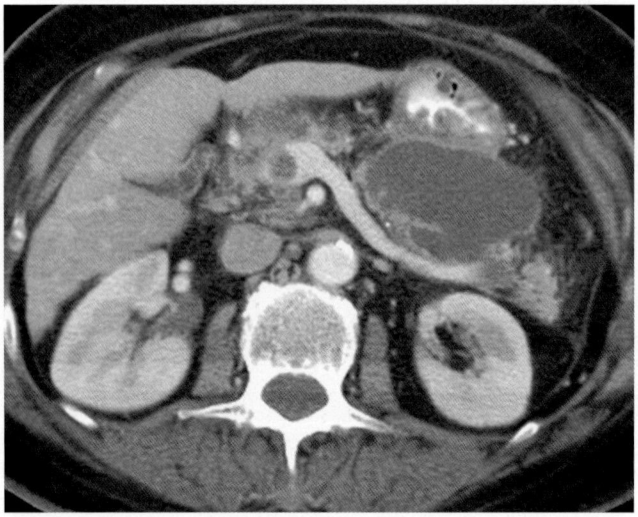

   A. Biliary obstruction
   B. Pancreatic necrosis
   C. Pancreatic duct disruption
   D. Portal vein thrombosis

74. Enhancing thrombus within the portal vein on CT is likely secondary to:
   A. Tumor thrombus
   B. Thrombus secondary to pancreatitis
   C. Thromboembolic disease
   D. Hypercoagulable state

75. What is the pathology (arrowheads) depicted on the CT of a patient with recent history of acute pancreatitis?

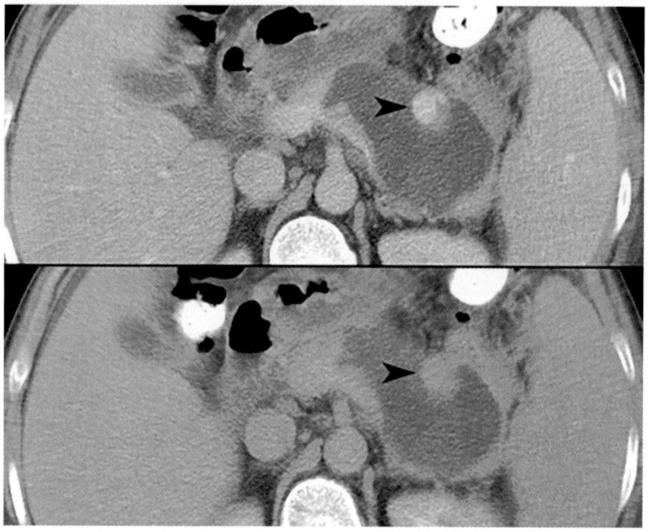

   A. Aneurysm
   B. Tumor
   C. Infection
   D. Sludge

76. What is the best diagnosis on the CT of a patient with history of acute abdomen?

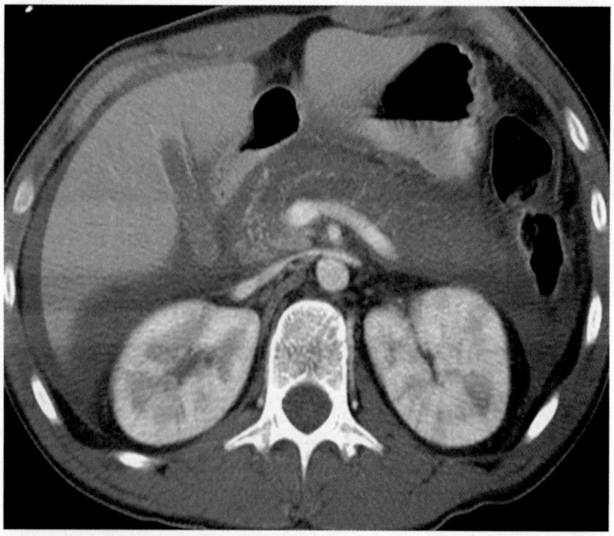

   A. Gallstone pancreatitis
   B. Autoimmune pancreatitis
   C. Necrotizing pancreatitis
   D. Pancreatic lipodystrophy

77. What is the cause of pancreatitis depicted on the ERCP study?

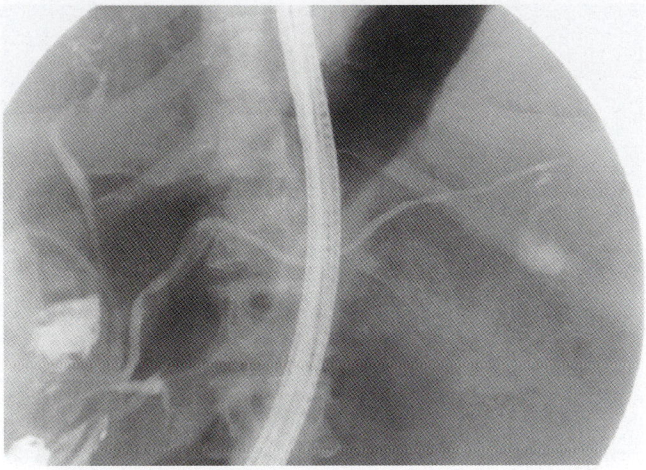

A. Pancreatic duct stone
B. Pancreatic duct disruption
C. Side-branch IPMN
D. Pancreatic neoplasm

78. What is the management of the focal pancreatic lesion seen on the CT study?

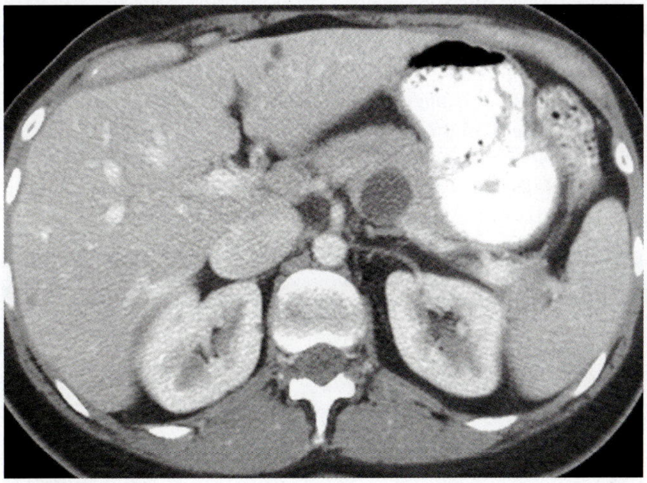

A. Surgery
B. Biopsy
C. No further workup
D. Follow-up CT

79. What is the most likely type of tumor depicted on the CT?

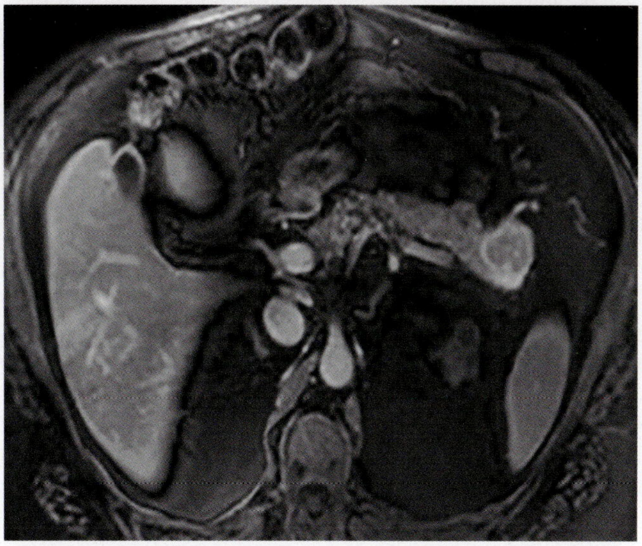

A. Adenocarcinoma
B. Metastases
C. Insulinoma
D. Lymphoma

80. What is the treatment of the pathology depicted on the CT?

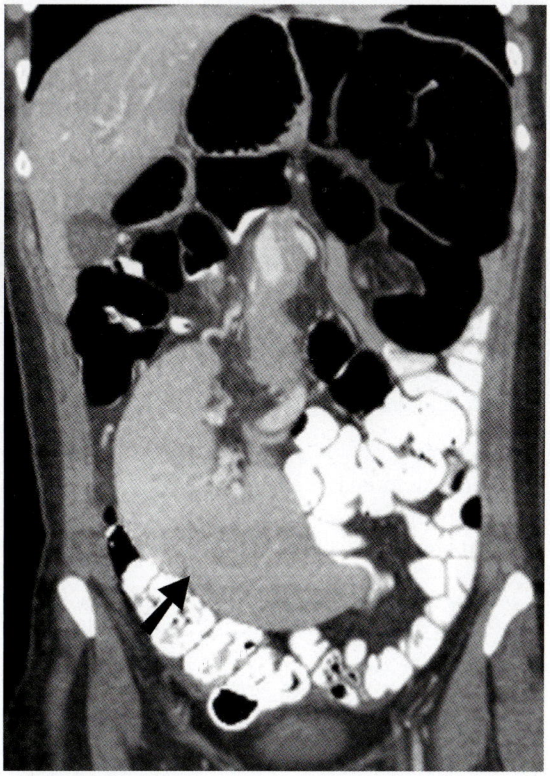

A. Splenectomy
B. Chemotherapy
C. Splenopexy
D. Radiotherapy

81. What is the upper GI series finding responsible for the patient's acute epigastric pain symptoms?

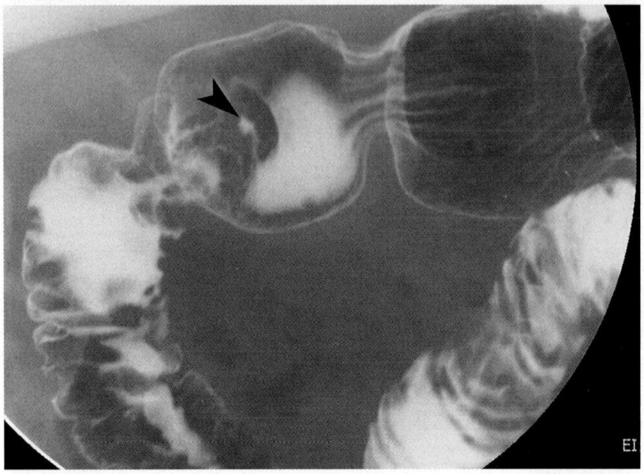


A. Ulcer
B. Polyp
C. Carcinoma
D. Erosions

82. Which is the most likely neoplastic condition causing abnormality (arrowheads) of the stomach?

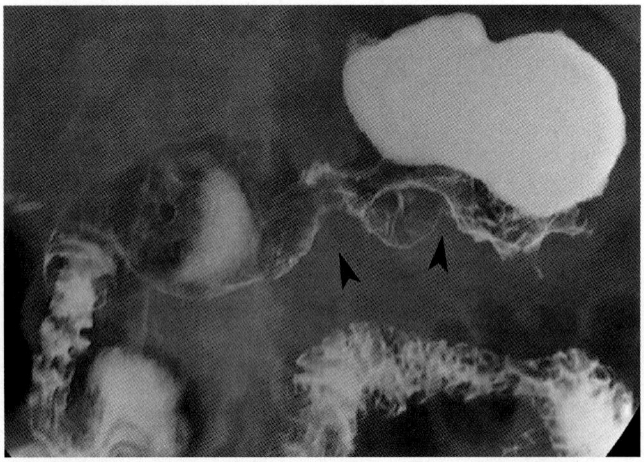

A. Carcinoid
B. Adenocarcinoma
C. Leiomyosarcoma
D. Lymphoma

83. What is the incidental gastric finding (arrowhead) seen on the contrast-enhanced CT scan study?

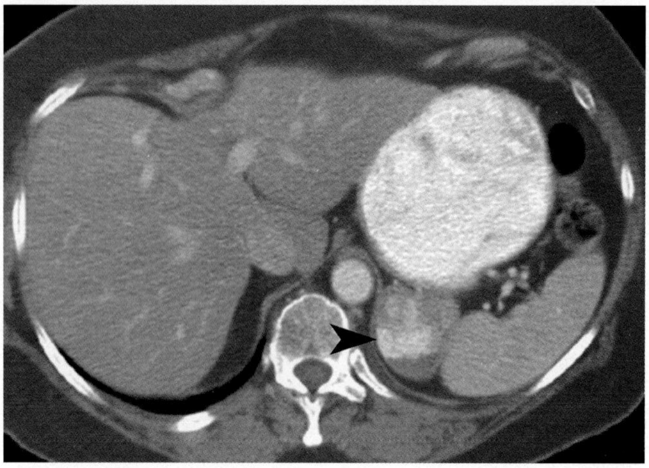

A. Gastric perforation
B. Gastric neoplasm
C. Gastric ulcer
D. Gastric diverticulum

84. What is early gastric cancer?
A. Cancer limited to the mucosa and submucosa regardless of nodal or distant colonization
B. Cancer limited to the mucosa and submucosa with no extragastric involvement
C. Mucosal cancer with or without distant metastasis
D. Stage 0 adenocarcinoma

85. What is the abnormality (arrowhead) seen on CT in a young adult male with chronic nausea and vomiting?

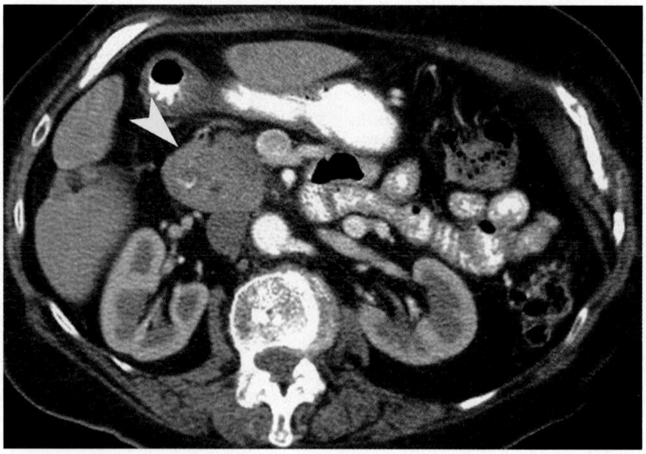

A. Annular pancreas
B. Pancreatitis
C. Duodenal web
D. Duodenal atresia

86. What is a morphologic abnormality seen on the upper GI study?

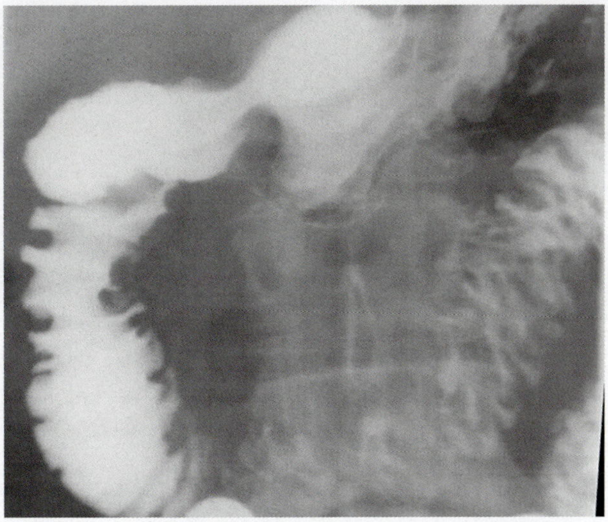

A. Duodenal diverticulitis
B. Duodenitis
C. Duodenal ulcer
D. Polyp

87. What is a likely cause of the CT finding (arrowhead) in a patient with acute abdomen?

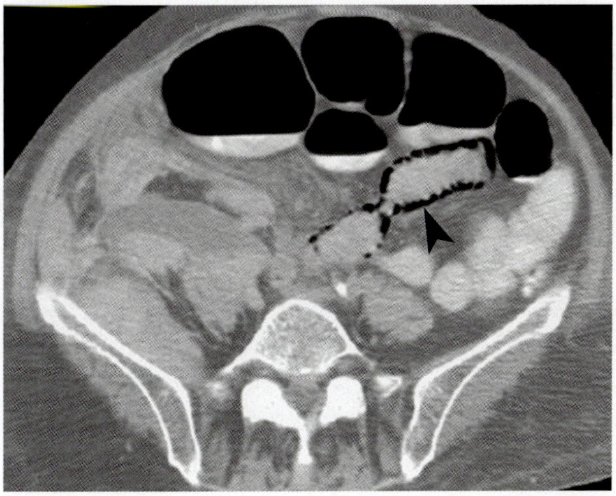

A. Tuberculosis
B. Ischemia
C. Typhlitis
D. Dysmotility

88. What is the classic imaging appearance of scleroderma in the small bowel?

A. Multiple contracted loops of bowel with uniformly thickened folds
B. Dilatation of small bowel loops with thin, crowded folds producing a hidebound appearance
C. Increased number of bowel wall folds of the ileum producing a jejunization appearance
D. Circumferential wall thickening with an abrupt transition from normal caliber lumen to narrowed lumen

89. What is the cause of small bowel obstruction seen on the CT of this 75-year-old female?

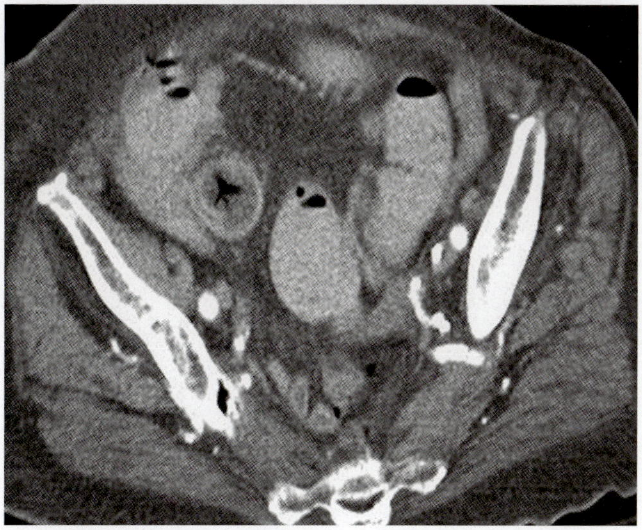

A. Adhesions
B. Gallstone
C. Volvulus
D. Neoplasm

90. What is the diagnosis?

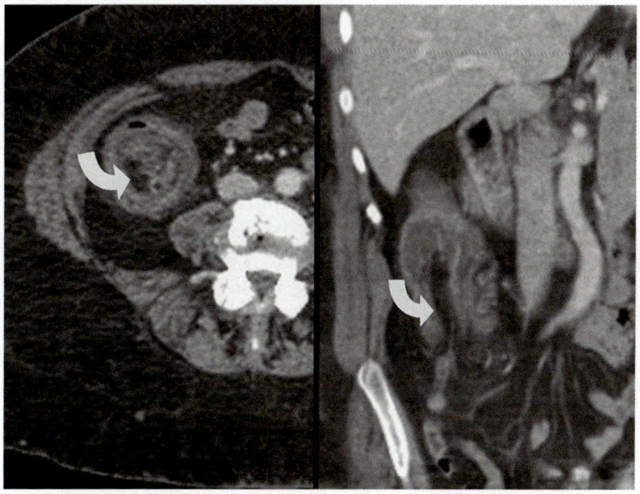

A. Volvulus
B. Abscess
C. Intussusception
D. Appendicitis

91. What is the pathology depicted on the barium enema?

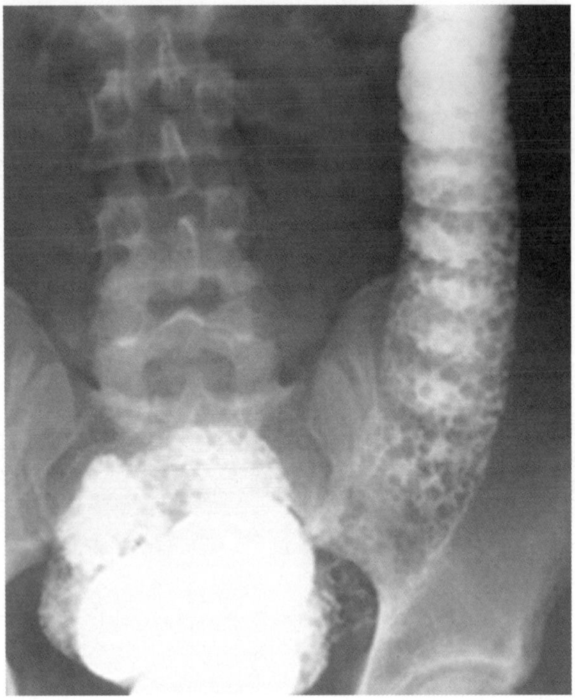

A. Familial adenomatous polyposis
B. Colonic diverticulosis
C. Fecal residues
D. Pseudomembranous colitis

92. What is the imaging abnormality seen on the double-contrast barium enema of a patient with ulcerative colitis?

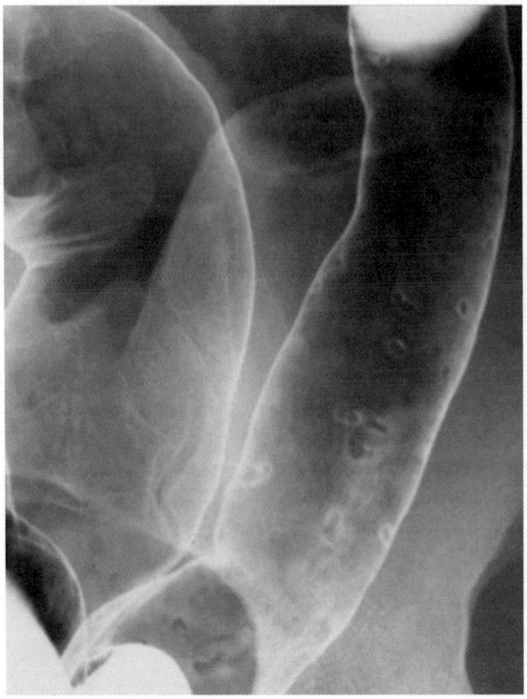

A. Polyps
B. Pseudopolyps
C. Diverticula
D. Mucosal ulcerations

93. What is the pathology seen coronal reformation of non-contrast CT of the abdomen?

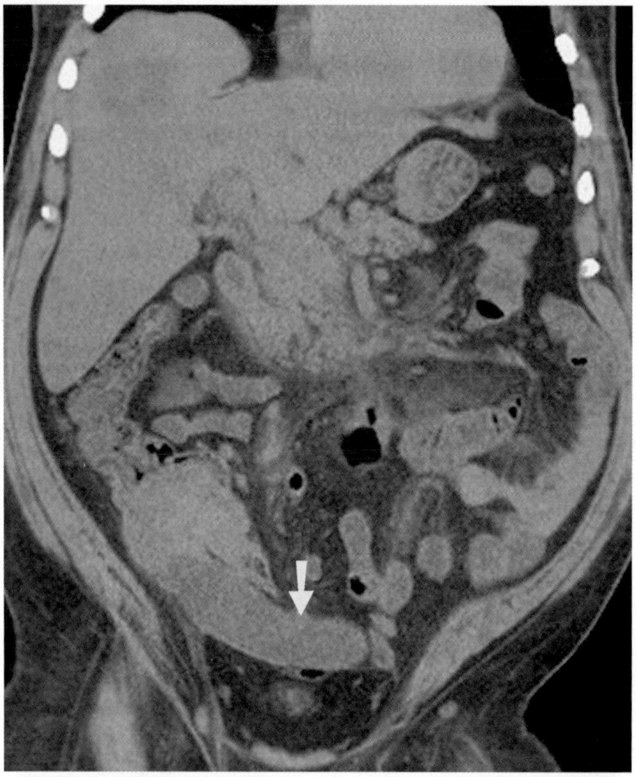

A. Diverticular abscess
B. Dilated distal ileum
C. Mucocele appendix
D. Cecal bascule

94. A 55-year-old man, known case of HBV, gets an MR to evaluate segment 4 abnormality (arrowheads) seen initially on CT. Which is the most likely diagnosis?

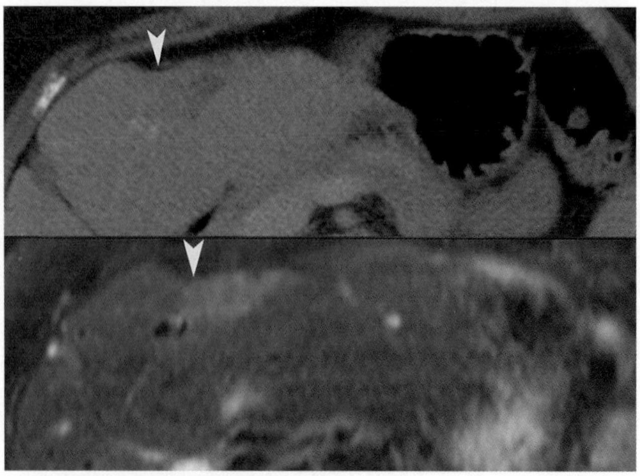

A. Confluent hepatic fibrosis
B. Focal fat infiltration
C. Hepatic infarction
D. Intrahepatic cholangiocarcinoma

95. A 30-year-old man, with underlying of thalassemia major, presents with abnormal liver function tests. His MRI reveals signal drop-off of the hepatic and splenic parenchyma on in-phase T1-gradient images when compared to opposed-phase images. The pancreatic parenchyma is relatively spared. What is the most likely condition in this patient?
   A. Wilson disease
   B. Hepatic steatosis
   C. Primary hemochromatosis
   D. Secondary hemochromatosis

96. Which of the following findings is considered atypical for focal nodular hyperplasia?
   A. Size 5 cm
   B. T2 hypointense scar
   C. T1 isointensity
   D. Isointensity

97. Which of the following factors is strongly associated with spontaneous rupture of hepatocellular carcinoma?
   A. Tumor diameter of greater than 5 cm
   B. Tumors with peripheral rim enhancement
   C. Tumors with fatty metamorphosis
   D. Centrally located tumors

98. Based on the arterial phase T1WI, what is the most likely diagnosis in young adult women on oral contraceptives?

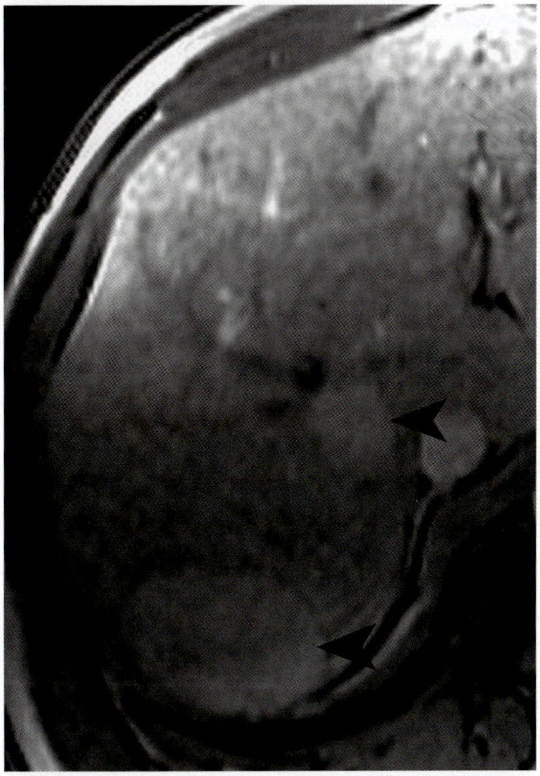

   A. HCC
   B. Hemangioma
   C. FNH
   D. Adenoma

99. A patient develops peripancreatic fluid 2 weeks after an episode of acute pancreatitis. What is the correct terminology for this finding?
   A. Acute peripancreatic fluid collection
   B. Pancreatic pseudocyst
   C. Abscess
   D. Necrotizing pancreatitis

100. What is the typical appearance on MRI for a pancreatic abscess?
   A. Increased T1 and T2 signal without restricted diffusion
   B. Decreased T1 and T2 signal without restricted diffusion
   C. Decreased T1 and increased T2 signal with restricted diffusion
   D. Increased T1 and decreased T2 signal with restricted diffusion

101. Acute complications of pancreatitis should be assessed at what point after initial onset?
   A. At presentation
   B. 24 hours after onset
   C. 48 hours after onset
   D. 72 hours after onset

102. Metastases to the pancreas is most frequently from which primary neoplasm?
   A. Lung cancer
   B. Breast cancer
   C. Oncocytoma
   D. Melanoma

103. In a patient with pancreatic head adenocarcinoma, what finding makes the tumor unresectable?
   A. Loss of fat planes around the superior mesenteric artery
   B. Ill-defined outline of the tumor
   C. Central necrosis
   D. Pancreatic ductal dilatation

104. What is the likely cause of jaundice in this patient?

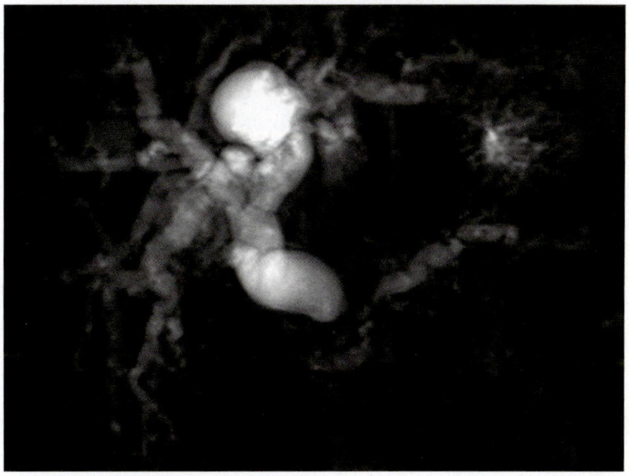

   A. Lymphoma
   B. Hepatocellular carcinoma
   C. Adenocarcinoma
   D. Islet cell tumor

105. Which of the following sequences constitutes the back bone of MRCP imaging of the pancreatic or biliary ductal system?
   A. SSFSE
   B. FIESTA
   C. T2-FSE
   D. STIR

106. A 27-year-old pregnant patient presented with acute abdominal pain and was investigated using noncontrast MRI study. What is the cause of the patient's abdominal pain?

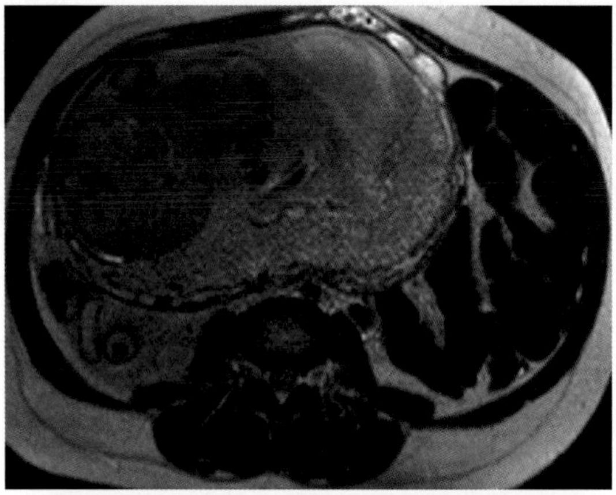

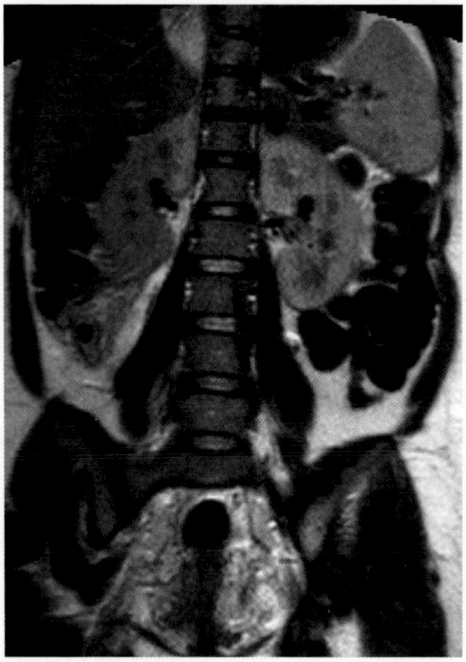

   A. Abruption placenta
   B. Small bowel obstruction
   C. Acute appendicitis
   D. Acute diverticulitis

107. What is the sensitivity of MRI study when compared with CT imaging for the evaluation of acute appendicitis?
   A. CT is more sensitive.
   B. MR is more sensitive.
   C. MR has sensitivity comparable to CT.
   D. MR sensitivity is variable.

108. A patient presented with gluteal pain. Based on the MR, what is the cause of the gluteal pain in this immunocompromised patient?

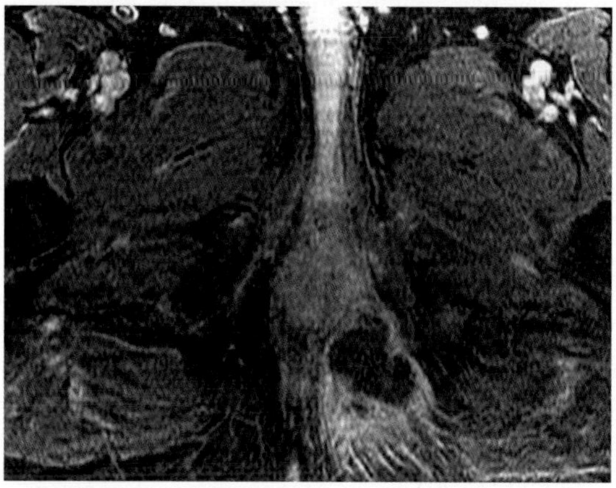

   A. Proctitis
   B. Abscess
   C. Fournier gangrene
   D. Myositis

109. A 62-year-old female patient had US-guided biopsy of the liver for the evaluation of liver mass. The patient started complaining of right upper quadrant pain and light-headedness after the procedure. Based on the noncontrast and postcontrast CT study, what is the likely cause of the patient's clinical complaints?

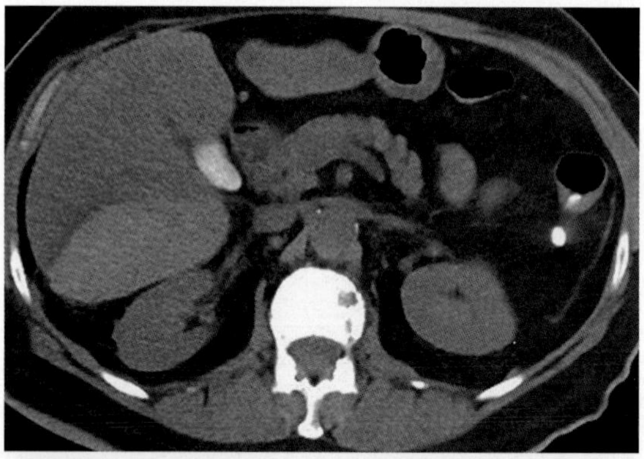

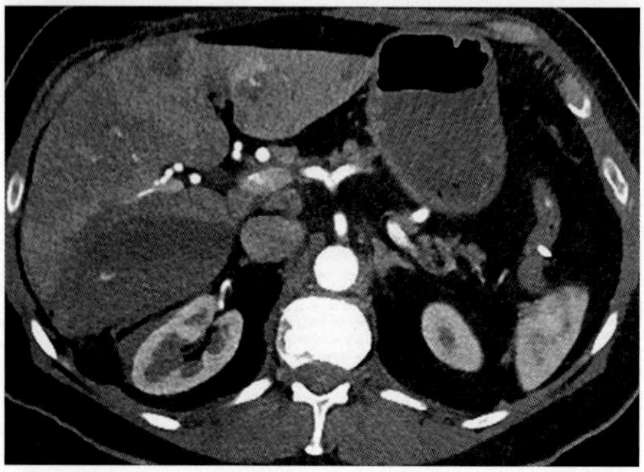

   A. Intrahepatic intraparenchymal hemorrhage
   B. Subcapsular hemorrhage
   C. Portal vein obstruction
   D. Hepatic rupture

110. What would be the next step in the management of this patient?
    A. Arterial embolization
    B. Watchful observation
    C. Manual compression
    D. Intravenous TPA

111. The CT scan study of a 25-year-old female patient demonstrated focal abnormality in the pancreas. What is the most likely cause of the abnormality?

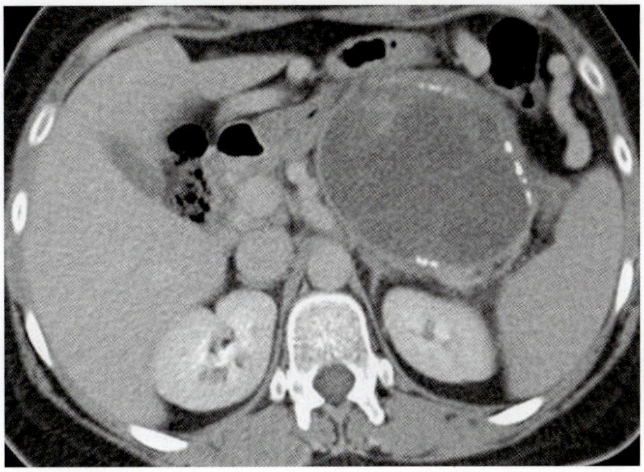

    A. Acute hemorrhage
    B. Abscess
    C. Neoplasm
    D. Pancreatic transection

112. Which is the most common type of islet cell tumor of the pancreas?
    A. VIPoma
    B. Gastrinomas
    C. Glucagonoma
    D. Insulinoma

113. A 35-year-old female presented with diarrhea and fever. What is the likely cause of the patient's symptoms, based on the MR study?

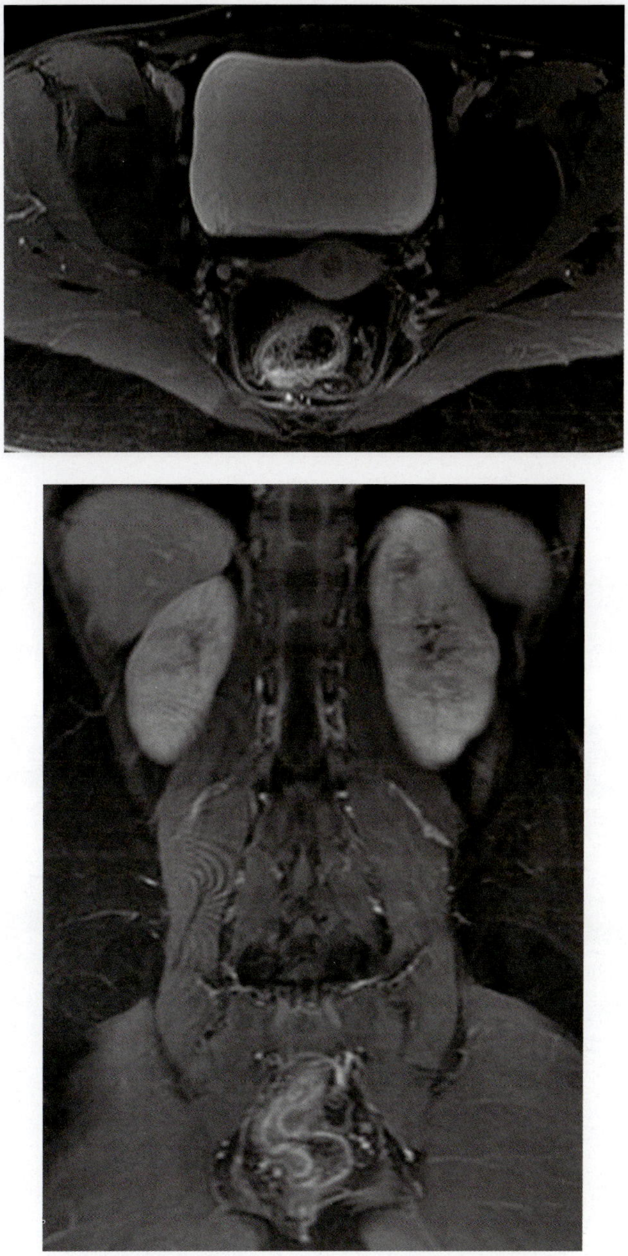

    A. Endometritis
    B. Inflammatory bowel disease
    C. Mesenteric lymphadenitis
    D. Rectal cancer

114. A 65-year-old male patient presents with weight loss, anorexia, and epigastric pain. What is the likely cause of the patient's presentation based on the MRI study?

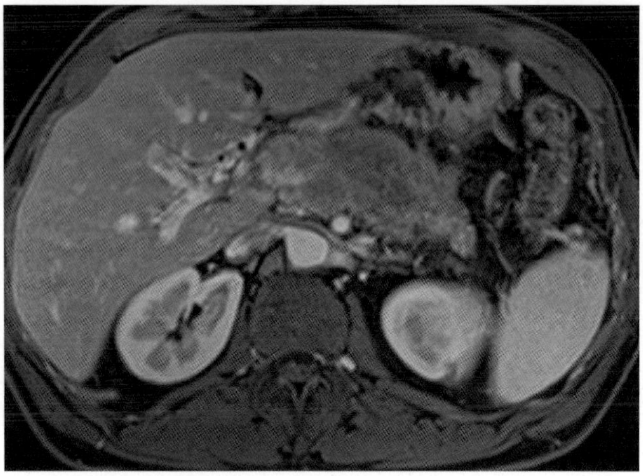

A. Cystic fibrosis
B. Pancreatic adenocarcinoma
C. Acute pancreatitis
D. Syndromic islet cell tumor

115. What underlying disease is likely to be associated with the pathology depicted on the MRI study?

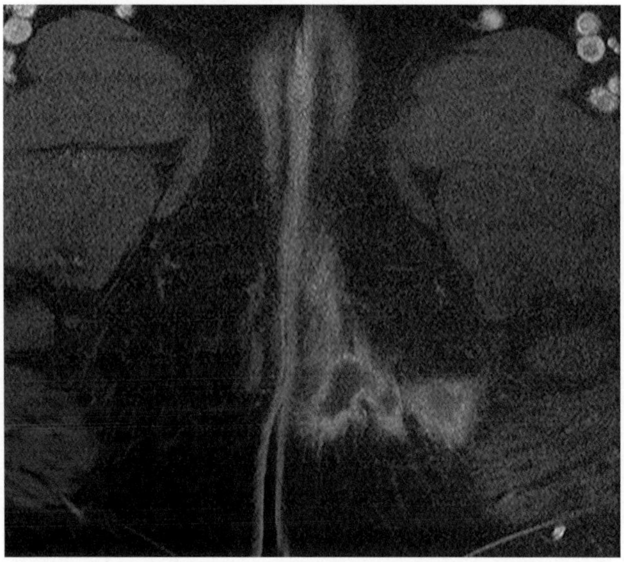

A. Tuberculosis
B. Crohn disease
C. Ulcerative colitis
D. Hepatitis

116. What is the second most common type of esophageal neoplasm?

A. Squamous cell carcinoma
B. Adenocarcinoma
C. Adenosquamous carcinoma
D. Carcinoid tumor

117. An elderly female presented with dysphagia for the last 3 months. What is the abnormality depicted on the barium swallow study?

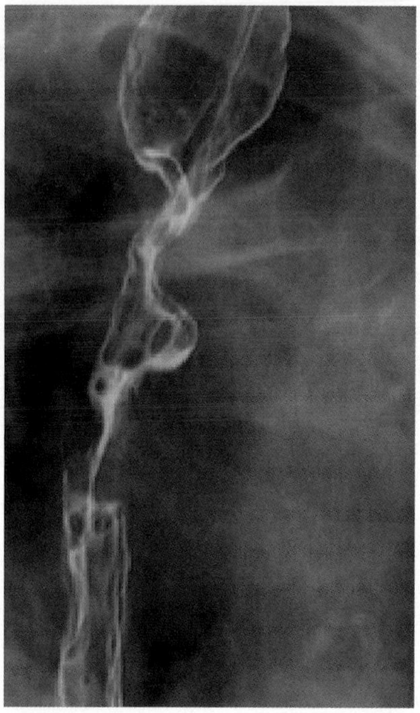

A. Lye stricture
B. Chemical esophagitis
C. Esophageal adenocarcinoma
D. Reflux esophagitis

118. What is the likely cause of the patient's multiple liver abscesses, depicted on the coronal CT reformation?

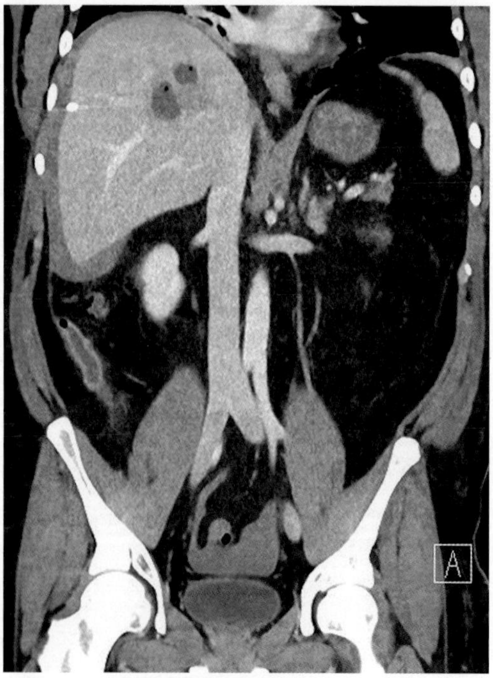


A. Acute diverticulitis
B. Acute gastritis
C. Acute appendicitis
D. Acute cholangitis

119. An 85-year-old female patient presented with episodes of flushing and palpitations. What abnormality seen on the CT scan study explains the patient's clinical presentation?

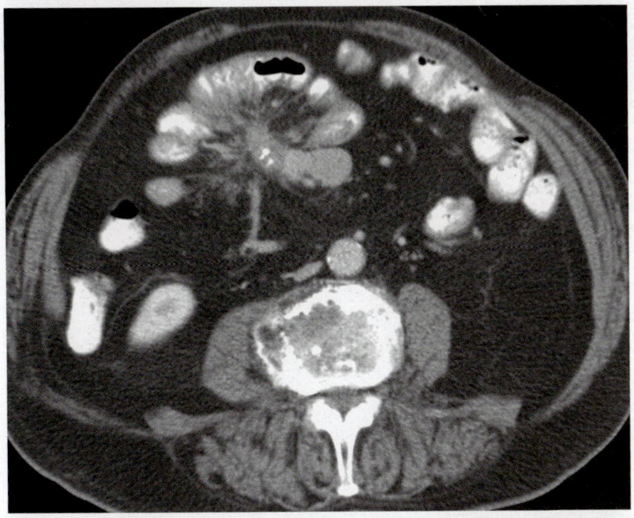

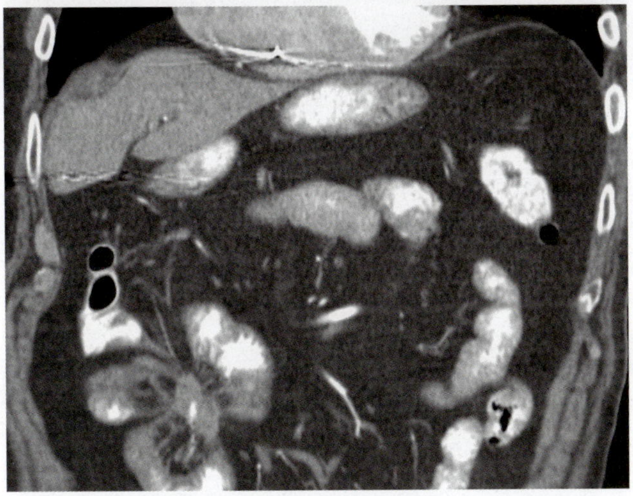

A. Carcinoid tumor
B. Desmoid
C. Retractile mesenteritis
D. Lymphoma

120. A 20-year-old patient presented to the hospital with right upper quadrant pain. What is the cause of the patient's clinical presentation based on the contrast-enhanced CT scan study?

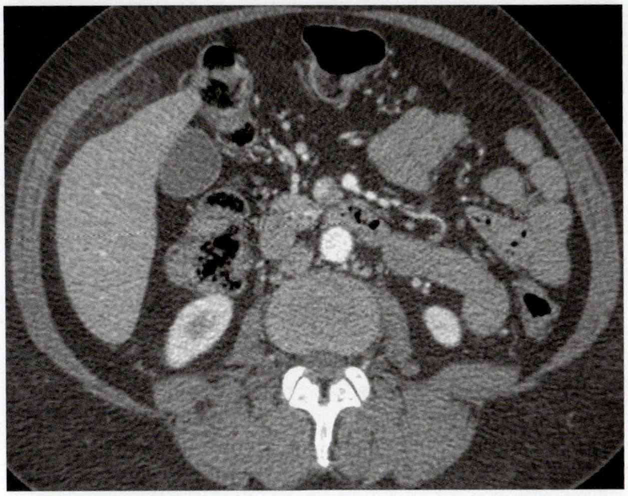

A. Acute epiploic appendagitis
B. Segmental omental infarction
C. Acute cholecystitis
D. Acute hepatitis

121. A 50-year-old male patient with a history of repeated small bowel obstruction presents with acute abdominal pain. What imaging finding is depicted by the arrows on the US study?

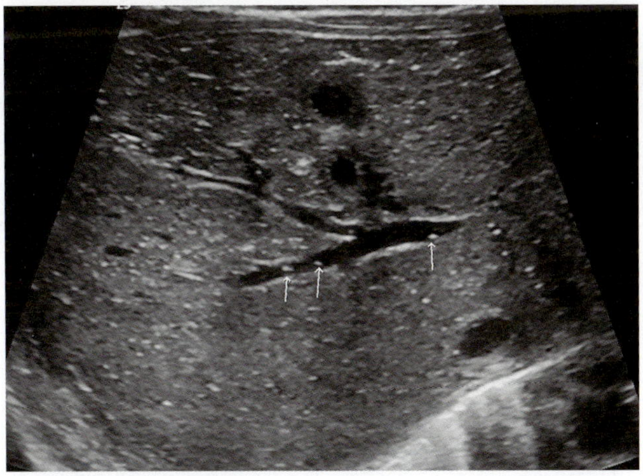

A. Choledocholithiasis
B. Pneumobilia
C. Portal vein gas
D. Calcifications

122. What is the most likely underlying cause of the abnormality depicted on the axial and coronal CT images of a patient with abdominal pain?

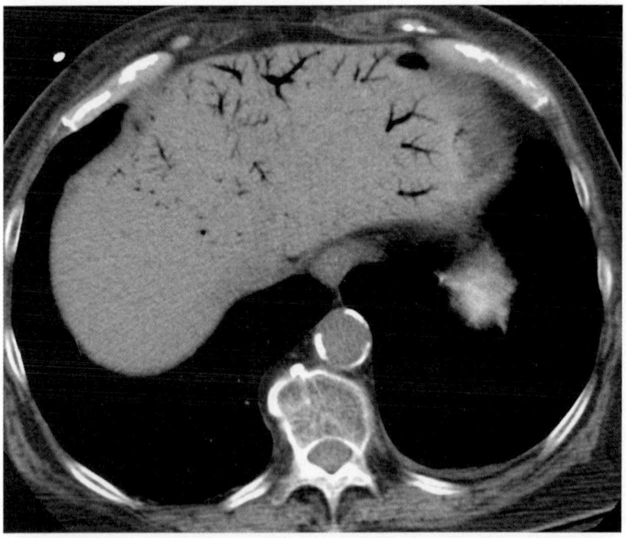

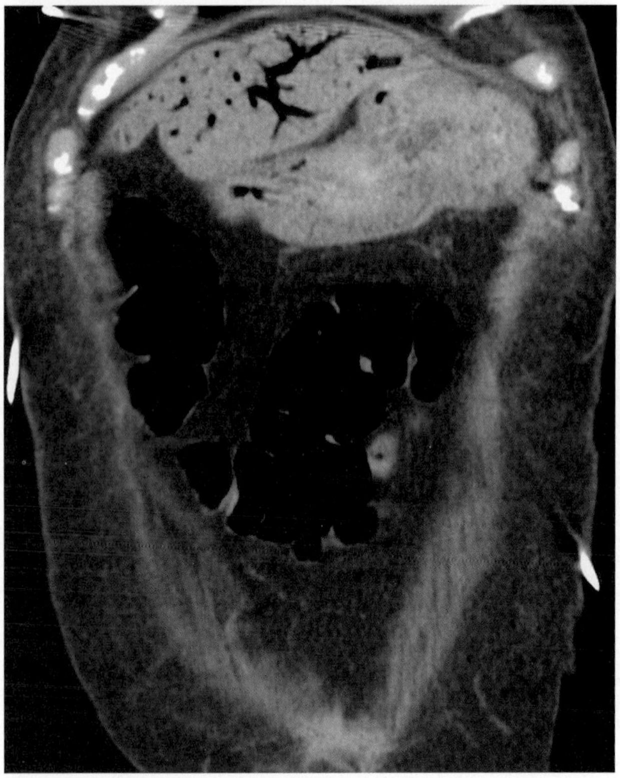

A. Asthma
B. Steroids
C. Infection
D. Ischemia

123. What is the cause of portal venous gas detected on the contrast-enhanced CT scan study of an elderly patient presenting with abdominal pain?

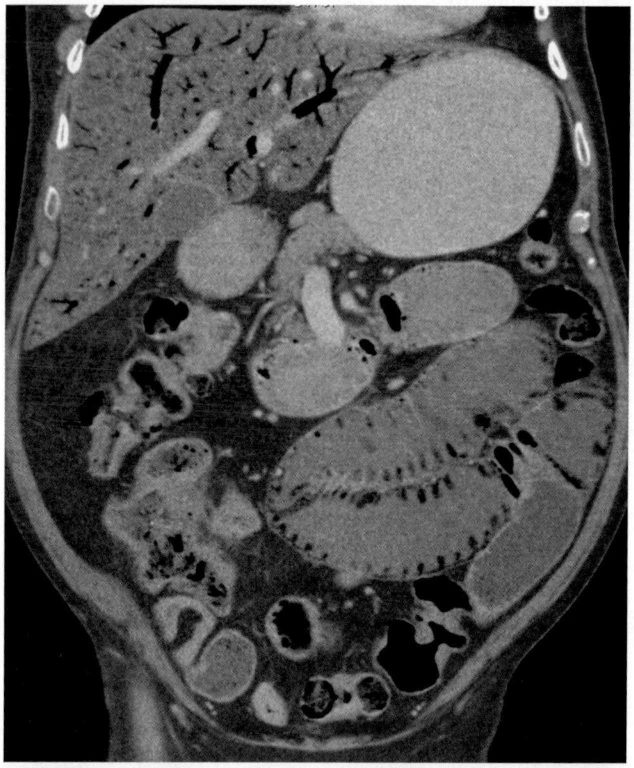

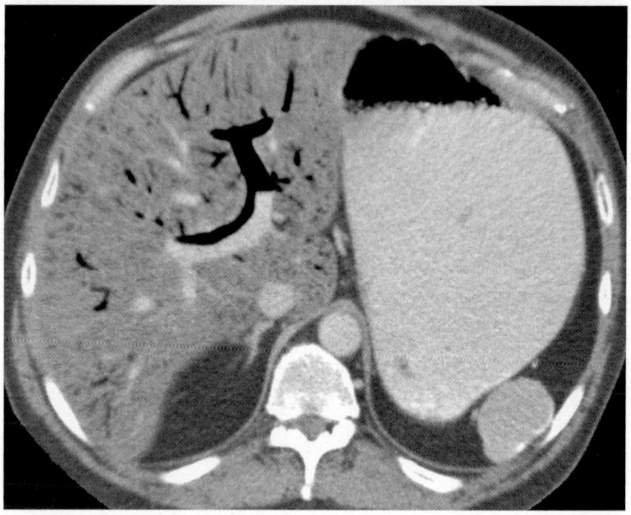

A. Graft versus host disease
B. Crohn disease
C. Ulcerative colitis
D. Small bowel ischemia

124. How does the sensitivity of the US study for the diagnosis depicted on the image compares with CT and MRI study?

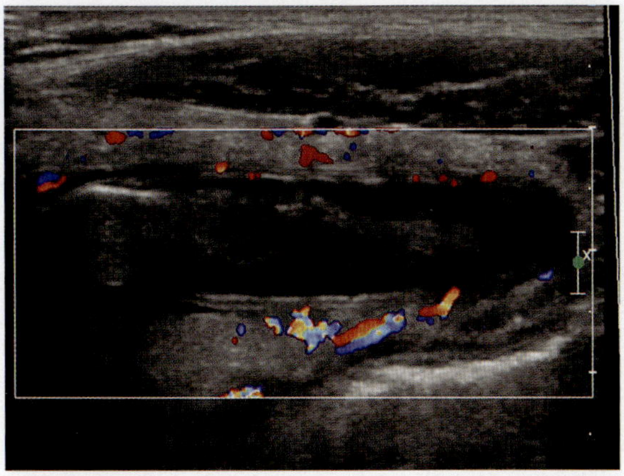

A. US is more sensitive than CT.
B. CT is more sensitive than US.
C. CT and US have similar sensitivity.
D. US is more sensitive than MR.

125. What is the likely cause of the right lower quadrant pain in a patient whose CT was performed using rectal and intravenous (100-second delay) contrast?

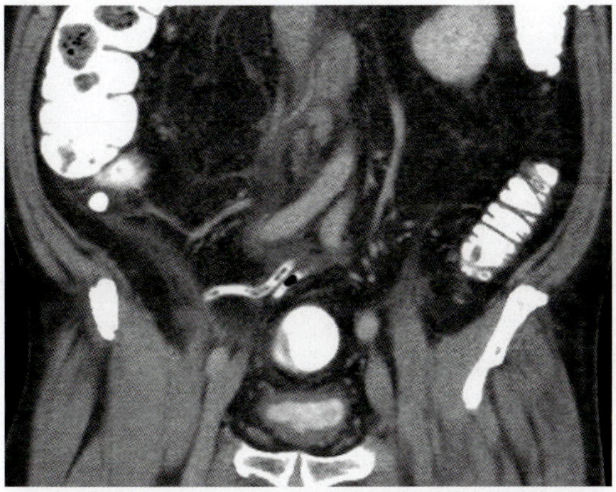

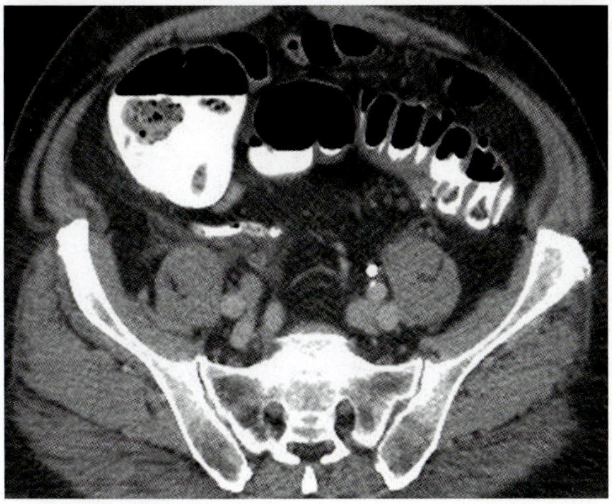

A. Acute appendicitis
B. Acute diverticulitis
C. Typhlitis
D. Ureteric obstruction

126. Based on the CT study, what is the likely diagnosis in a pediatric patient presenting with lower abdominal pain and fever?

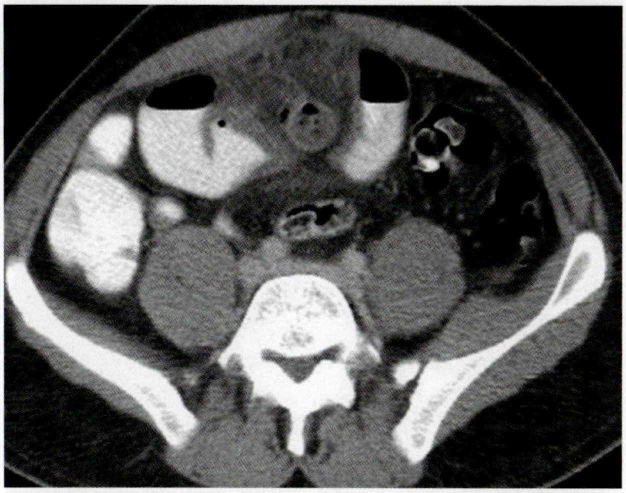

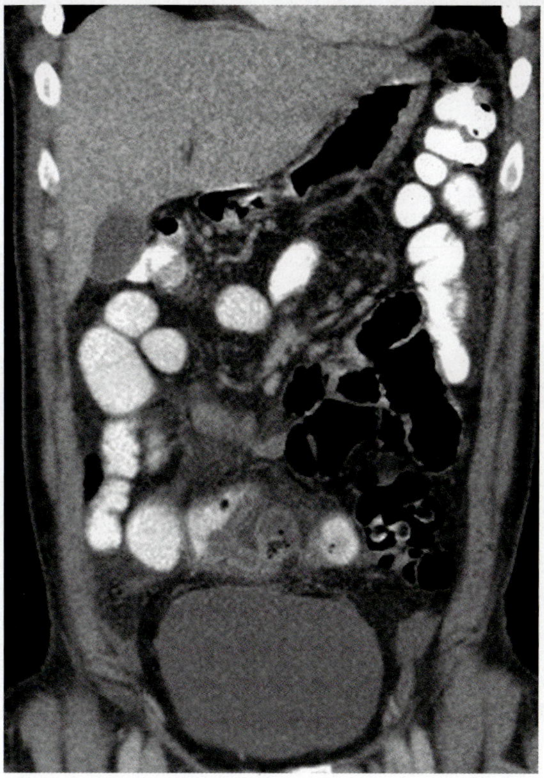

A. Intussusception
B. Cystitis
C. Meckel diverticulitis
D. Bowel obstruction

127. What is the abnormality detected on the CT scan study of a patient presenting with weight loss?

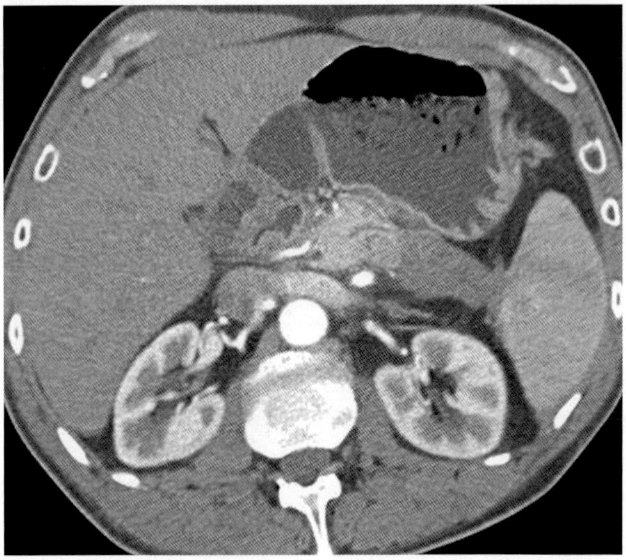

A. IVC thrombosis
B. Pancreatic neoplasm
C. Gastritis
D. Pyelonephritis

128. What is true about the rectal cancer depicted on the axial postcontrast T1WI and T2WI?

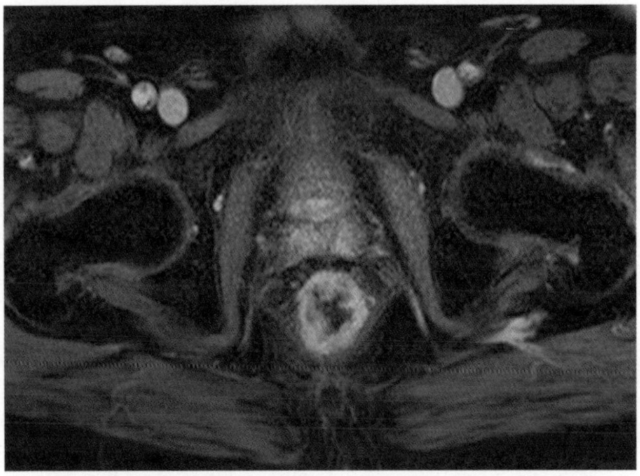

A. Extension into the pelvic floor muscles
B. Pelvic lymphadenopathy
C. Extension beyond the serosa
D. Bony metastasis

129. What are the hepatic abnormalities seen on the postgadolinium T1WI?

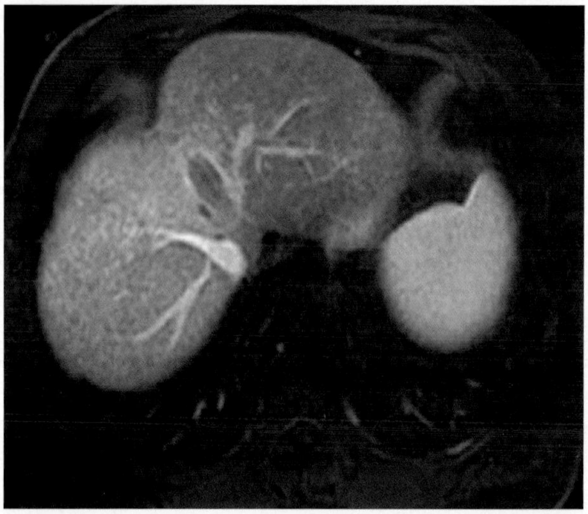

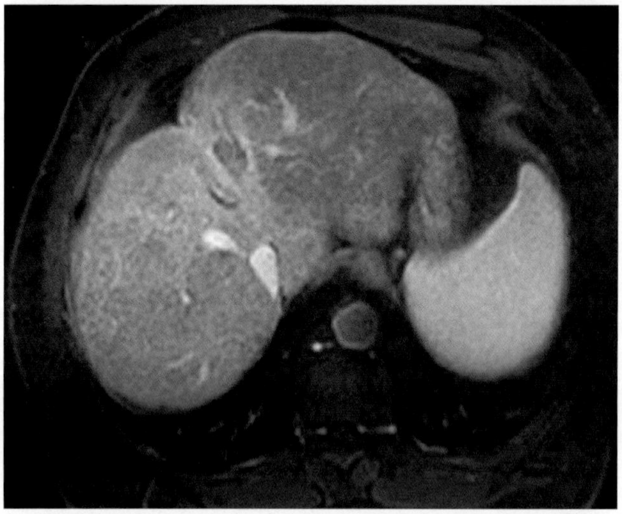

A. IVC thrombus
B. Portal vein thrombus
C. Hepatic vein thrombosis
D. Mattingly and stenosis

130. What is the most significant finding depicted on the abdominal radiograph of a patient presenting with abdominal pain?

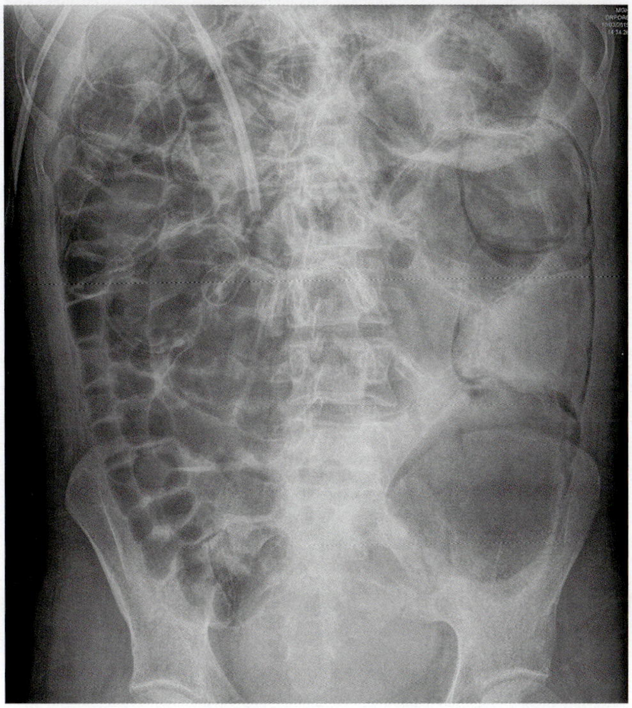

A. Bowel obstruction
B. Paralytic ileus
C. Pneumatosis
D. Portal venous gas

131. What radiologic sign is used to describe the most significant finding seen on the upright film of the abdomen?

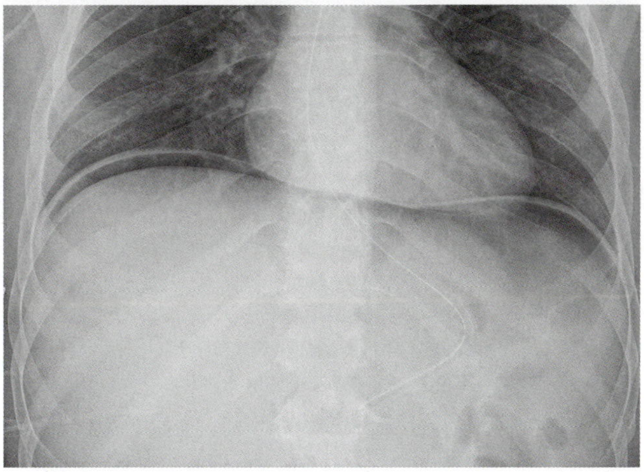

A. Doge cap sign
B. Continuous diaphragm sign
C. Football sign
D. Rigler sign

132. What is the imaging diagnosis based on the plain radiograph of abdomen in a premature baby with sepsis?

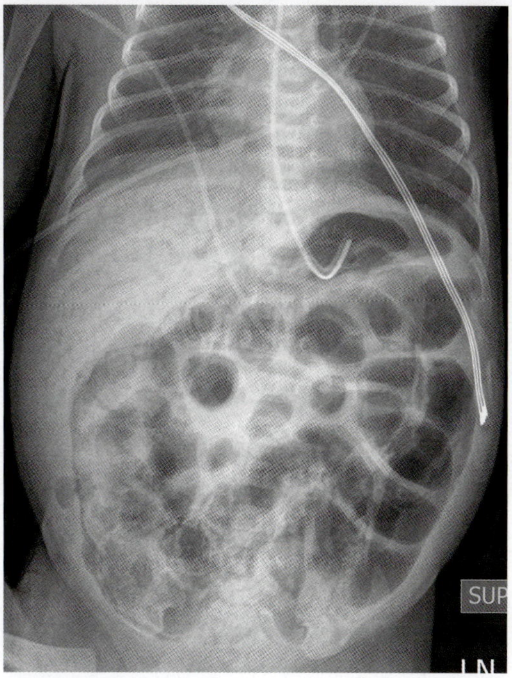


A. Intussusception
B. Volvulus
C. Bowel obstruction
D. Necrotizing enterocolitis

133. What is the likely underlying pathology in the patient whose plain radiograph is depicted?

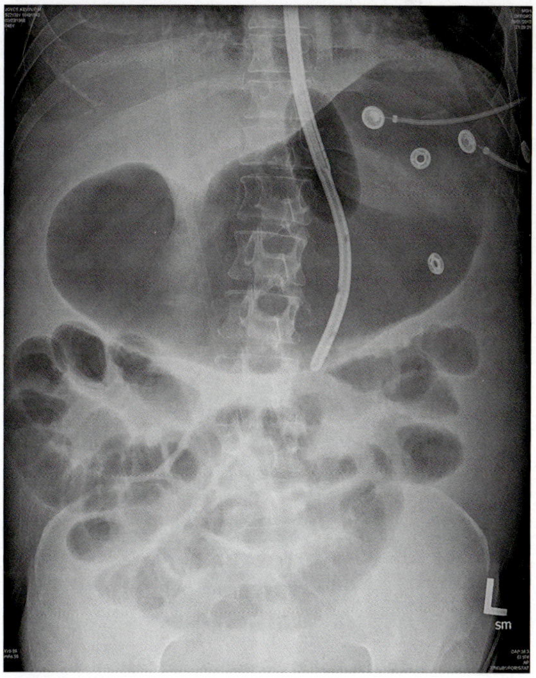


A. Thalassemia
B. Cirrhosis
C. Ulcerative colitis
D. Kartagener syndrome

134. Which of the following is the most ominous sign on the supine film of the abdomen in a patient with abdominal pain?

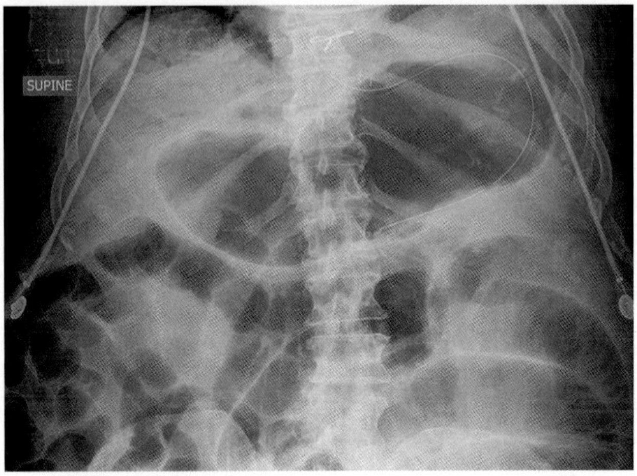


A. Bowel distention
B. Stomach distention
C. Free air
D. Portal vein gas

135. What is the likely location of the abnormality depicted on the upright film of the abdomen?

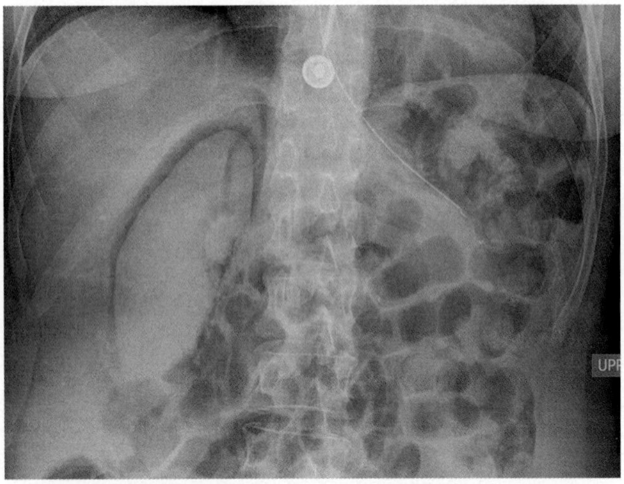

A. Intraperitoneal
B. Retroperitoneal
C. Properitoneal
D. Intraluminal

136. What pathology does the lateral view radiograph depict in a premature baby?

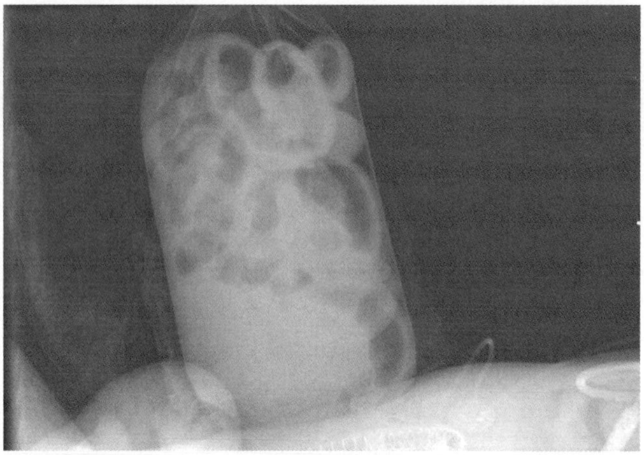

A. Gastroschisis
B. Omphalocele
C. Traumatic hernia
D. Prune belly syndrome

137. What pathology does the lateral view radiograph depicts a premature baby?

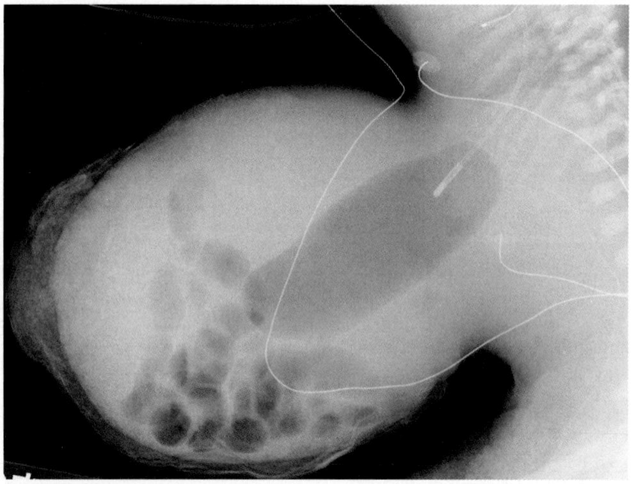

A. Gastroschisis
B. Omphalocele
C. Traumatic hernia
D. Prune belly syndrome

138. What is the likely histopathologic diagnosis of the focal abnormality detected on the postgadolinium T1WI image of the upper abdomen?

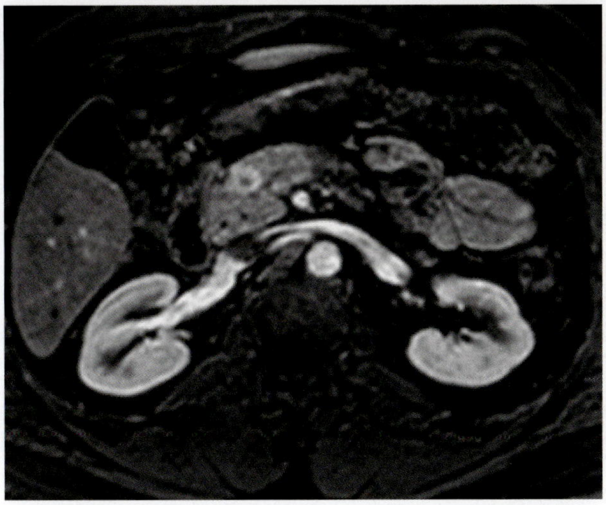

A. Neuroendocrine tumor
B. Adenocarcinoma
C. IPMN
D. Lymphoma

139. What is the pathology depicted on the plain x-ray of the abdomen in a patient with chronic abdominal pain?

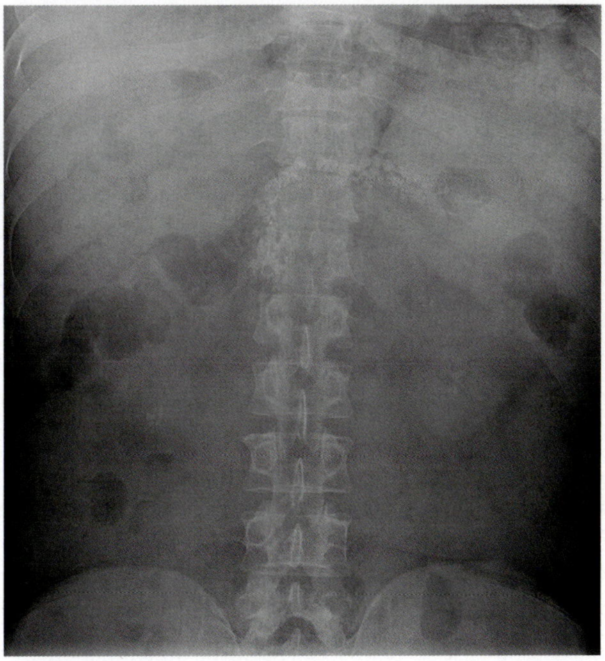

A. Chronic pancreatitis
B. Free air
C. Bowel obstruction
D. Acute cholecystitis

## Answers to Self-Assessment Questions

**1. C.** Ulcer. The upper GI series demonstrates a benign gastric antral ulcer crater (arrowhead) surrounded by smooth ulcer mound.

**2. D.** Pedunculated polyp. Mexican hat sign is seen with pedunculated polyp hanging down from the nondependent wall of the bowel and is as two concentric rings, with the outer ring representing the head and with the inner ring representing the stalk of the polyp.

**3. C.** False diverticulum. False diverticulum lacks all the layers of the bowel wall and is seen along the mesenteric border of a small bowel loop. True diverticulum has all layers of the bowel and arises from the antimesenteric border of the small bowel. The diverticulum arising along the medial border margin of the second portion of the duodenum has a smooth margin and represents a pulsion diverticulum (not true diverticulum).

**4. C.** Pulsion diverticulum. The diverticulum seen on the barium swallow has a smooth outline and represents a pulsion diverticulum. Majority of esophageal diverticula are false diverticula, which are associated with motility disorder and increased intraluminal pressure in the esophagus.

**5. D.** Benign ulcer. The gastric ulcer depicted demonstrates radiating mucosal folds extending to the edge of the ulcer crater, a feature of benignity.

**6. A.** Candida. On double-contrast esophagram, discrete longitudinally, irregular plaque-like lesions and some shaggy areas are consistent with candida esophagitis. Herpetic esophagitis is characterized by multiple small superficial ulcers against the background of normal mucosa usually in the mid-to-upper esophagus.

**7. B.** Feline esophagus. The esophagram study demonstrates fine, transverse mucosal folds measuring 1 to 2 mm in thickness, present circumferentially, and caused by contraction of muscularis mucosae. It is associated with gastroesophageal reflux.

**8. B.** Hiatus hernia. The plain chest radiograph demonstrates retrocardiac density extending on both sides of the midline and statistically most likely to represent a hiatus hernia. The differential diagnosis includes posterior mediastinal mass (e.g., neurogenic tumor), aortic aneurysm, and paraspinal abscess from tuberculosis.

**9. B.** Benign stricture. The double-contrast barium swallow shows multiple plaque-like filling defects and esophageal narrowing from candida esophagitis.

**10. D.** Candidiasis. The presence of multiple plaque-like filling defects is suggestive of candida esophagitis.

**11. C.** Epiphrenic diverticulum. The barium swallow study shows smooth epiphrenic diverticula, which usually arise just proximal to the lower esophageal sphincter and are caused by herniation of the esophageal mucosa and submucosa through weakness in the muscular layer, secondary to increased intraluminal pressure.

**12. B.** Bowel obstruction. The contrast-enhanced CT shows dilated duodenum and proximal jejunum, with bowel loops present more anteriorly in the upper abdomen.

This patient had small bowel obstruction with transition at Roux-en-Y anastomosis site.

**13. D.** Antrum. Ectopic pancreas is most often located along the greater curvature of the gastric antrum.

**14. D.** Cardia. Majority of the gastric diverticula were located in the posterior wall of the fundus of the stomach and 2 cm below the esophagogastric junction.

**15. D.** Rugal folds. The double-contrast study demonstrates prominent gastric rugal folds. In a normal stomach, the gastric rugal folds are most prominent in the proximal stomach fundus and body. Typically, the rugal fold is less than 5 mm in thickness in the distended stomach.

**16. A.** Adenocarcinoma. The MR shows mild bilateral ovarian enlargement, in addition to T2 hyperintense bone metastases and pelvic free fluid. Krukenberg tumor (metastases to the ovary) is classically due to gastrointestinal tract malignancy, most commonly from gastric adenocarcinoma.

**17. A.** Hyperplastic polyps. The upper GI series shows multiple polyps in the gastric body, outlined by barium. Majority of the gastric polyps are hyperplastic polyps.

**18. B.** Submucosal mass. The double-contrast upper GI series demonstrates a smoothly marginated submucosal mass (arrow) in the gastric antrum. There is a second submucosal mass also seen more cranially in the antrum.

**19. C.** Extrinsic. The upper GI series demonstrates extrinsic impression along the greater curvature of the stomach. Note the absence of mucosal irregularity or rugal fold thickening in the stomach.

**20. A.** Mucosal fold thickening. The upper GI series demonstrates rugal fold thickening along the greater curvature of the stomach. The normal gastric rugal fold thickness is less than 5 mm.

**21. B.** Lymphoma. The contrast-enhanced CT shows gastric wall thickening, which in presence of extensive systemic lymphadenopathy would favor the diagnosis of lymphoma over other neoplasms.

**22. B.** Gastric lymphoma. The contrast-enhanced CT shows gastric wall thickening with bulky gastrohepatic ligament lymphadenopathy. These findings favor the diagnosis of gastric lymphoma over adenocarcinoma.

**23. C.** Adenomatous polyp. Adenomatous polyps are more than 1 cm in diameter and may be sessile or pedunculated. Subcentimeter polyps in the stomach are most often hyperplastic polyps.

**24. B.** Duodenal web. The upper GI series depicts wind sock sign, which is seen with intraluminal duodenal diverticulum. The upper GI study shows a barium-filled sac in the second portion of the duodenum, outlined by radiolucent rim, which reflects the duodenal web.

**25. C.** Hematoma. The CT demonstrates an intramural hematoma in the fourth portion of the duodenum.

**26. B.** Diverticulum. The coronal CT reformation depicts fluid-filled diverticulum arising from the second portion of the duodenum.

**27. D.** Volvulus. The contrast-enhanced CT shows whorled appearance (arrowheads) of the mesentery surrounding the superior mesenteric vessels, indicating small bowel volvulus.

**28. D.** Crohn disease. The small bowel follow-through study shows stricture (arrowhead) of the terminal ileum with dilatation of the bowel segment (arrow) proximal to it. Tuberculosis and Crohn disease would be in the differential diagnosis.

**29. A.** Diverticulitis. The coronal CT reformation depicts a perforated small bowel diverticulum (arrowhead) with surrounding inflammation.

**30. D.** Cystic fibrosis. The differential diagnosis of nodular mucosal folds in the small bowel includes giardiases, Whipple disease, cystic fibrosis, Crohn disease, etc.

**31. D.** Bacterial overgrowth can occur leading to malabsorption. Majority of small bowel diverticula are false diverticula and are present along the mesenteric border of the small bowel. Colonic diverticula are more common than small bowel diverticula.

**32. A.** Carcinoid tumor is the most common, and adenocarcinoma is the second most common small bowel malignancy.

**33. B.** It rarely causes obstruction. The contrast-enhanced CT shows aneurysmal dilatation of a small bowel loop with wall thickening (arrowhead). There are multiple mesenteric lymph nodes (arrow) identified. These imaging features indicate the presence of small bowel lymphoma, which rarely causes bowel obstruction.

**34. B.** Bowel malrotation. The small bowel follow-through study shows the small bowel loops located to the right side of the midline. The duodenojejunal flexure is located on the right side. The colon is located to the left of the midline.

**35. A.** Pseudopolyps. The double-contrast barium enema in this patient with ulcerative colitis shows multiple round and worm-like filling defects, which represent residual mucosa.

**36. B.** Pneumatosis cystoides intestinalis. The barium enema demonstrates multiple polypoidal filling defects in the sigmoid colon, caused by cystic collection of air in the bowel wall. The patient did not have any colonic wall ischemia.

**37. B.** Psoas abscess. The contrast-enhanced CT of a patient with Crohn disease shows extension of inflammation from the right colon into the right psoas muscle. There is an air-containing cavity seen in the right psoas major muscle.

**38. A.** Rigler sign. Rigler sign or double wall sign is seen on plain radiograph of the abdomen and is characterized by the presence of air outlining the inside and outside of the bowel. Doge cap sign refers to triangular air lucency due to air in the Morrison pouch. Football sign refers to large air lucency in the shape of an American football seen on supine abdominal radiograph.

**39. A.** Lead pipe. Lead pipe appearance of the colon in chronic ulcerative colitis is characterized by loss of haustral markings in the diseased segment of the colon, producing a cylindrical appearance of the large bowel. Accordion sign is seen with pseudomembranous colitis due to trapping of barium between edematous haustral folds.

**40. C.** Volvulus. The single-contrast study in a patient with sigmoid volvulus demonstrates tapered narrowing at the rectosigmoid junction, described as the bird-beak sign.

**41. B.** Polyps. Barium enema exam demonstrates multiple polyps in the colon, in a patient with familial adenomatous polyposis.

**42. B.** Mucinous neoplasm of the appendix. Mucocele of the appendix is characterized by appendiceal distention due to retained mucus, often caused by mucinous cystoadenoma or cystadenocarcinoma.

**43. C.** Intussusception. The coronal CT reformation demonstrates ileocolonic intussusception in the ascending colon. The terminal ileum is the intussuscipiens and is surrounded by mesenteric fat.

**44. D.** Lipoma. The axial CT image shows a large fat density lipoma (arrowhead) as the lead point of the colocolonic intussusception in the sigmoid colon.

**45. A.** Featureless bowel. The plain radiograph of the abdomen of a patient with ulcerative colitis demonstrates lack of haustra and featureless appearance of the left colon.

**46. B.** Submucosal mass. The double-contrast barium enema shows a smooth hemispherical submucosal mass with obtuse angle between the mass and the colonic wall. Mucosal mass would make acute angle with the adjacent bowel wall.

**47. B.** Pseudomyxoma peritonei. The CT depicts loculated fluid density lesion with internal septation, displacing the bowel loops to the right side. Among the four choices, pseudomyxoma is the best choice.

**48. A.** US. US is considered the most appropriate imaging modality for the assessment of children and pregnant patients with suspected appendicitis.

**49. A.** US. US and MR are considered the first-line and second-line imaging modalities for the assessment of pregnant patients with suspected appendicitis.

**50. D.** Posteromedial. The appendix is most often located from 2 o'clock to 6 o'clock position, in relation to the cecum.

**51. A.** Transverse mesocolon. B and D represent greater omentum and sigmoid mesocolon, respectively. C represents retroperitoneal fat.

**52. C.** Desmoid tumor. The patients with familial adenomatous polyposis are at increased risk of developing colorectal cancer, hepatoblastoma, and desmoid tumor. The CT depicts a large soft tissue mass in the abdomen in a patient with prior colectomy.

**53. D.** Sclerosing mesenteritis. The contrast-enhanced CT demonstrates a spiculated mesenteric mass with calcifications. The differential diagnosis will include sclerosing mesenteritis, and carcinoid tumor. Since pentetreotide scan is normal, the likely nononcologic cause is sclerosing mesenteritis.

**54. A.** Peritoneal carcinomatosis. The CT findings of peritoneal carcinomatosis seen here include tumor studding of the peritoneum, malignant ascites, and omental caking.

**55. C.** Splenic rupture. The noncontrast and contrast-enhanced CT shows perisplenic sentinal clots, suggesting splenic origin of the hemoperitoneum.

**56. A.** Acute epiploic appendagitis. The CT depicts the classic findings of epiploic appendagitis, including fat density tubular lesion with surrounding inflamed visceral peritoneum, arising from the anterior aspect of the sigmoid colon.

**57. B.** Pseudomyxoma peritonei. The CT demonstrates large amount of fluid in the peritoneal cavity. The primary finding, which favors pseudomyxoma peritonei, is the presence of scalloping of the liver outline (on the cranial aspect of the left lobe of the liver).

**58. B.** Albendazole is the treatment of hydatid cyst. The contrast-enhanced CT depicts a hepatic hydatid cyst containing a daughter cyst.

**59. C.** Infarct. The CT demonstrates multiple infarcts in the spleen, kidneys, and left lobe of the liver.

**60. B.** Hepatic artery thrombosis is the most common vascular complication after liver transplant and can lead to hepatic infarction, biliary ischemia, and biloma formation.

**61. C.** Thyroid. Hypervascular liver metastases are from renal cell carcinoma, thyroid carcinoma, neuroendocrine tumors, choriocarcinoma, melanoma, and breast cancer.

**62. C.** Hepatocellular carcinoma. The solid mass depicted on the CT and MR (T2WI and postcontrast T1WI) has continuous rim enhancement, thereby making abscess and hemangioma unlikely. The mass enhances heterogeneously, thereby making FNH an unlikely possibility.

**63. D.** Hepatocellular carcinoma. The arterial phase CT demonstrates a hyperenhancing liver mass, which shows continuous pseudocapsule enhancement on portal venous phase T1WI. These features favor the diagnosis of hepatocellular carcinoma.

**64. A.** 0%. The portal venous and delayed phase CT show discontinuous, peripheral nodular enhancement with progressive centripetal filling. These features are consistent with liver hemangioma.

**65. C.** Portal vein thrombosis. The contrast-enhanced CT demonstrates lack of enhancement of portal vein branches due to the presence of thrombosis.

**66. A.** Size less than 10 mm. Generally, polyps of less than 5 mm are considered unlikely to be malignant, while those greater than 10 mm are suspicious for malignancy.

**67. D.** Presence of CBD dilatation. Imaging detection of choledocholithiasis is greater if stones are larger and located more proximally within the CBD and biliary ductal dilatation is present.

**68. C.** Delayed enhancement. Cholangiocarcinoma with significant fibrosis shows delayed enhancement.

**69. C.** Choledochocele. The US and CT demonstrate cystic lesion in the periampullary region, ruling out A, B, and D.

**70. A.** Rim sign. The rim sign refers to increased hepatic activity surrounding the gall bladder fossa on cholescintigraphy. It is due to the spread of inflammation from the gall bladder to the liver parenchyma.

**71. C.** Autoimmune pancreatitis. Imaging features of autoimmune pancreatitis include diffuse enlargement of the pancreas with a peripheral halo of hypoattenuation on CT or hypointense signal on T2WI.

**72. C.** Cystic fibrosis. The CT depicts pancreatic lipomatosis, which can be seen with Shwachman-Diamond syndrome, Cushing syndrome, cystic fibrosis, and Johanson-Blizzard syndrome.

**73. D.** Portal vein thrombosis. The contrast-enhanced CT demonstrates a round thrombus in the portal vein.

**74. A.** Tumor thrombus. Because of the presence of vascularity within tumor thrombus, they can enhance on postcontrast CT and MR.

**75. A.** Aneurysm. The CT demonstrates a pseudoaneurysm in the arterial and portal venous phase with surrounding fluid collection.

**76. C.** Necrotizing pancreatitis. The contrast-enhanced CT shows lack of enhancement of the pancreatic parenchyma, thereby suggesting necrotizing pancreatitis.

**77. B.** Pancreatic duct disruption. The ERCP demonstrates leakage of contrast from the pancreatic duct, into a collection located caudal to the pancreatic tail.

**78. D.** Follow-up CT. The contrast-enhanced CT depicts a well-defined cystic lesion measuring less than 2 cm in diameter. These are likely benign in etiology and can be followed on serial CT exams.

**79. C.** Insulinoma. Arterial phase T1WI shows a hypervascular neuroendocrine tumor arising from the pancreatic tail.

**80. C.** Splenopexy. The coronal CT reformation depicts wandering spleen located in the right lower quadrant. Since there are no splenic infarcts, these patients can be managed with splenopexy rather than splenectomy.

**81. A.** Ulcer. The upper GI series shows barium collection in an ulcer crater (arrowhead) with surrounding mucosal edema in the gastric antrum.

**82. B.** Adenocarcinoma. The upper GI series depicts a large polypoidal mass (arrowheads) along the greater curvature of the stomach, which is statistically most consistent with an adenocarcinoma.

**83. D.** Gastric diverticulum. The contrast-enhanced CT depicts a gastric diverticulum (arrowhead) in its most common location posterior to the gastric cardia. The diverticulum is filling with oral contrast, which is helpful in distinguishing it from an adrenal mass.

**84. A.** Early gastric cancer is cancer limited to the mucosa and submucosa regardless of nodal or distant colonization. It is minimally protruding (endoluminal), plaque-like, or shallow ulcerated lesion.

**85. A.** Annular pancreas. The CT depicts pancreatic tissue posterolateral and anterolateral (arrowhead) to the second part of the duodenum, consistent with annular pancreas.

**86. B.** Duodenitis. Upper GI series demonstrates diffuse thickening of the mucosal folds in the duodenum.

**87. B.** Ischemia. The CT demonstrates pneumatosis intestinalis (arrowhead) in the left lower quadrant, which is most often associated with small bowel wall ischemia.

**88. B.** Dilatation of small bowel loops with thin, crowded folds producing a hidebound appearance. Thinning and crowding of the valvulae conniventes producing a hidebound or stack of coins appearance is seen in greater than 60% of cases of scleroderma.

**89. B.** Gallstone. The contrast-enhanced CT demonstrates dilated small bowel loops caused by an obstructing gallstone in the right lower quadrant. The triradiate central lucency caused by nitrogen in the obstructing gallstone is called the Mercedes-Benz sign.

**90. C.** Intussusception. The CT study depicts intussusceptum located within the intussuscipiens, separated by mesenteric fat.

**91. A.** Familial adenomatous polyposis. The barium enema demonstrates innumerable polyps in the descending and sigmoid colon, a feature of familial adenomatous polyposis. Peutz-Jeghers syndrome polyps are most frequently located, in order of prevalence in the jejunum, ileum, duodenum, colon, and stomach.

**92. B.** Pseudopolyps. The double-contrast barium enema demonstrates polypoidal filling defects caused by islands of normal mucosa, surrounded by denuded colon in a patient with inflammatory bowel disease.

**93. C.** Mucocele appendix. The coronal CT reformation demonstrates a sausage-shaped cystic structure arising from the base of the cecum, consistent with mucocele of the appendix.

**94. A.** Confluent hepatic fibrosis. The contrast-enhanced CT and T2WI shows a solitary wedge-shaped abnormality with a wide base toward the hepatic capsule and capsular retraction from volume loss. The involvement of the segments IV and VIII is typical of confluent hepatic fibrosis.

**95. D.** Secondary hemochromatosis is characterized by excess iron deposition in the reticuloendothelial system, resulting in deposition in the liver, spleen, and bone marrow. The pancreas is spared in secondary hemochromatosis.

**96. B.** T2 hypointense scar. Focal nodular hyperplasia is isointense on both T1- and T2WI with a central scar, which is T1 hypointense and T2 hyperintense.

**97. A.** Tumor diameter of greater than 5 cm. Maximum tumor diameter greater than 5 cm and high Child-Pugh grade are associated with spontaneous rupture.

**98. D.** Adenoma. The history of oral contraceptive intake and the presence of multiple enhancing hepatic masses are suggestive of multiple hepatic adenomas.

**99. A.** Acute peripancreatic fluid collection. Fluid collections occurring in or around the pancreas within the first 4 weeks of the onset of necrotizing pancreatitis are termed acute necrotic collections.

**100. C.** Decreased T1 and increased T2 signal with restricted diffusion. A pancreatic abscess is typically low signal on T1 and high signal in T2WI. DWI will demonstrate restricted diffusion within the infected collection.

**101. D.** 72 hours after onset. The optimal time for assessing acute complications of acute pancreatitis is approximately 72 hours after symptom onset.

**102. A.** Lung cancer. Metastases to the pancreas are most frequently from renal cell carcinoma and lung cancer.

**103. A.** Loss of fat planes around the superior mesenteric artery. On CT, more than 180 degrees contact between superior mesenteric artery and tumor indicates arterial encasement.

**104. C.** Adenocarcinoma. The MRCP demonstrates dilatation of the biliary as well as pancreatic duct, suggesting the presence of pathology in the pancreatic head. Pancreatic head adenocarcinoma and periampullary carcinoma are the two most common causes of this appearance on MRCP, also described as double duct sign.

**105. A.** SSFSE. SSFSE sequence is the single most important MRCP sequence that allows the evaluation of the ducts with thick slab as well as thin-slice MRCP images. SSFSE has the advantage of absence of motion artifact and very short acquisition time.

**106. C.** Acute appendicitis. The axial and coronal SSFSE sequence demonstrates dilated tortuous tubular structure in the right lower quadrant, containing an appendicolith. The findings are consistent with acute appendicitis.

**107. C.** MR has sensitivity comparable to CT. The sensitivity of MR for the evaluation of acute appendicitis is more than 90% and is comparable to contrast-enhanced CT scan study. The drawback of MR imaging of acute appendicitis is the high cost, longer scan, and lack of availability.

**108. B.** Abscess. The contrast-enhanced T1WI demonstrates a left ischiorectal fossa abscess with enhancing margins.

**109. B.** Subcapsular hemorrhage. The CT scan study demonstrates a subcapsular hematoma posterior to the segment 6 of the liver, which on postcontrast CT demonstrates a focus of active extravasation of contrast.

**110. A.** Arterial embolization. Given the active extravasation of contrast seen into the subcapsular hematoma, catheter-guided arterial embolization procedure could be performed to stop the active bleeding.

**111. C.** Neoplasm. The focal hypodense lesion in the pancreatic body and tail region demonstrates peripheral rim of calcification, ruling out the acute pathologies listed above. This patient has a solid and cystic papillary tumor, which is most commonly seen in young adult females and often seen in the pancreatic body and tail region.

**112. D.** Insulinoma. Insulinoma is the most common islet cell tumor of the pancreas. Unlike glucagonoma, VIPoma, gastrinoma, and somatostatinoma, insulinomas are rarely cancerous.

**113. B.** Inflammatory bowel disease. The contrast-enhanced T1WI demonstrates thickening of the rectal wall with intense mucosal enhancement, consistent with proctitis. This patient has known Crohn proctocolitis with acute flare-up.

**114. B.** Pancreatic adenocarcinoma. The postcontrast T1WI demonstrates a large mass lesion involving the pancreatic body and tail region, consistent with a neoplastic process. Syndromic islet cell tumors are much less common than pancreatic adenocarcinoma and usually do not reach this size and are typically less than 4 cm in diameter.

**115. B.** Crohn disease. The postgadolinium T1WI demonstrates multiple ring-enhancing abscesses in the left ischiorectal fossa. Perianal manifestation of Crohn disease is seen in 15% of the patients with Crohn ileitis.

**116. B.** Adenocarcinoma. Adenocarcinoma has progressively increased over the last 30 years and currently constitutes a little over 50% of the esophageal cancers. Squamous cell cancers are most common esophageal malignancy in the upper third of the esophagus, while adenocarcinoma is the most common esophageal malignancy involving the lower third of the esophagus.

**117. C.** Esophageal adenocarcinoma. The double contrast barium swallow study demonstrates a neoplastic growth in the upper thoracic esophagus with multiple filling defects and distal shouldering. The features of a malignant growth in the esophagus typically include eccentric stricture with nodular filling defects and shouldering.

**118. C.** Acute appendicitis. The CT depicts dilated appendix with enhancing wall in the right lower quadrant. The origin of the liver abscess in this patient was believed to be secondary to liver seeding from the inflamed appendix.

**119. A.** Carcinoid tumor. The CT scan study demonstrates a mesenteric mass with calcifications and spiculated margins. These imaging features can be associated with carcinoid tumor and retractile mesenteritis. The clinical symptoms of carcinoid syndrome in this patient would favor the diagnosis of carcinoid tumor over retractile mesenteritis.

**120. B.** Segmental omental infarction. The CT scan study demonstrates inflammatory densities in the omental fat anterior to the liver, consistent to the diagnosis of acute segmental omental infarction. Unlike omental infarction, acute epiploic appendagitis is typically located in the left lower quadrant, abutting colonic wall and associated with the hyperdense ring of inflamed visceral peritoneum.

**121. C.** Portal vein gas. Portal venous gas can be recognized as small mobile echogenic foci of gas bubbles resembling a string of pearls traveling in the direction of the blood flow. The numerous foci of increased echogenicity within the liver represent gas foci lodged within the liver.

**122. D.** Ischemia. The contrast-enhanced CT images depict extensive portal venous gas in branching pattern located predominantly in the peripheral liver. The most common cause of portal venous gas is bowel ischemia.

**123. D.** Small bowel ischemia. The contrast-enhanced CT of the patient with extensive portal vein demonstrates pneumatosis intestinalis and dilatation of small bowel loops in the left abdomen, consistent with the diagnosis of small bowel ischemia.

**124. B.** CT is more sensitive than US. The sensitivity of the US for the diagnosis of acute appendicitis is approximately 78%, while the sensitivity of CT and MR for the diagnosis of acute appendicitis is generally reported to be in excess of 90%.

**125. D.** Ureteric obstruction. The contrast-enhanced CT demonstrates a normal appendix filling up with radiopaque contrast, ruling out the possibility of acute appendicitis. Inflammatory stranding seen in the right lower abdomen is related to obstructive uropathy caused by right distal ureteric stone (not seen on the image). Note that the left ureter opacifies with radiopaque contrast while the right ureter does not opacify with contrast on this 100-second delay CT study.

**126. C.** Meckel diverticulitis. The axial and coronal contrast-enhanced CT demonstrates a small bowel diverticulum arising from the antimesenteric border of the distal small bowel, consistent with a true ileal diverticulum. This diverticulum demonstrates wall thickening and surrounding inflammatory changes, consistent with the presence of Meckel diverticulitis.

**127. B.** Pancreatic carcinoma. Contrast-enhanced CT scan study demonstrates an infiltrating mass lesion in the distal pancreatic body and tail region consistent with the diagnosis of pancreatic adenocarcinoma.

**128. C.** Extension beyond the serosa. The axial contrast-enhanced CT and T2-weighted sequences demonstrate irregular thickening of the rectal wall with focal extension beyond the serosa on the right anterior aspect.

**129. C.** Hepatic vein thrombosis. The gadolinium-enhanced T1WI demonstrates thrombus distending the entire left hepatic vein. The hepatic veins and the right lobe of the liver show normal contrast enhancement.

**130. C.** Pneumatosis. The supine x-ray of the abdomen demonstrates extensive pneumatosis in the colonic wall, involving the hepatic flexure, transverse colon, splenic flexure, and descending colon. This patient had transmural infarction of the colon.

**131. B.** Continuous diaphragm sign. Upright film of the abdomen demonstrates subdiaphragmatic lucency, which is seen to extend across the midline, outlining the entire undersurface of the diaphragm, commonly described as continuous diaphragm sign.

**132. D.** Necrotizing enterocolitis. The radiograph of the abdomen demonstrates extensive pneumatosis intestinalis and portal venous gas, which in a premature baby is highly suggestive of necrotizing enterocolitis.

**133. B.** Cirrhosis. The plain radiograph depicts a Blakemore tube with inflated gastric and esophageal bulbs. This is used to control variceal bleeding in patients with portal hypertension.

**134. D.** Portal vein gas. The plain radiograph of the abdomen demonstrates extensive portal venous gas, which is typically seen with bowel ischemia and associated with up to 80% mortality rate.

**135. B.** Retroperitoneal. The upright film of the abdomen demonstrates air outlining the right kidney, indicating the right retroperitoneal location of the pathology.

**136. A.** Gastroschisis. The plain x-ray of the abdomen demonstrates multiple small bowel loops outside the abdomen in a silo without overlying skin covering.

**137. B.** Omphalocele. The plain x-ray of the abdomen demonstrates multiple small bowel loops covered with a membrane. Unlike gastroparesis, omphalocele has higher association with other congenital anomalies, including trisomy 18, trisomy 13, trisomy 21, congenital heart disease, CNS malformation, and genitourinary malformations.

**138. A.** Neuroendocrine tumor. The postgadolinium T1WI of the abdomen depicts an arterially enhancing 2-cm focal lesion in the pancreatic head, most consistent with a neuroendocrine tumor. Adenocarcinoma and lymphoma do not usually demonstrate arterial phase hyperenhancement compared to the pancreatic parenchyma.

**139. A.** Chronic pancreatitis. Supine film of the abdomen demonstrates extensive calcifications in the pancreatic head, body, and tail region, consistent with chronic calcific pancreatitis. These calcifications are intraductal and most often seen with alcohol abuse. The patient also has incidental multiple renal stones.

# INDEX

*Note*: Page numbers followed by "*f*" indicate figures, those followed by "*t*" indicate tables.

## M



## N